1995 CodeLink

Plastic Surgery

DISCLAIMER

This book is intended to offer guidance and information related to basic CPT, HCPCS, and ICD–9–CM coding principles as well as the logical associations between procedure and diagnosis codes. This book is not, nor should it be considered, a substitute for the Amercian Medical Association's CPT book or the HCPCS or ICD–9–CM coding systems. The interpretations herein are those of the author and do not necessarily represent the views of the American Medical Association, Health Care Financing Administration or other medical society or governmental agency. Neither the author nor the publisher may be held responsible for any misuse or misinterpretation of the guidelines in this text. Information provided is believed and intended to be reliable, but accuracy is not guaranteed by the author or the publisher.

1995 CodeLink

Plastic Surgery

Context Software Systems Inc.

McGraw-Hill Inc.

New York St. Louis San Francisco Auckland Bogotá Caracas Lisbon
London Madrid Mexico Milan Montreal New Delhi Paris
San Juan Singapore Sydney Tokyo Toronto

A product of McGraw–Hill, Inc.

CODELINK FOR PLASTIC SURGERY

1 2 3 4 5 6 7 8 9 0 BKM BKM 95

ISBN 0–07–600763–4

NOTICE:

CPT is a listing of descriptive terms and five–digit numeric identifying codes and modifiers for reporting medical services performed by physicians. This presentation includes only CPT descriptive terms, numeric identifying codes and modifiers for reporting medical services and procedures that were selected by McGraw–Hill, for inclusion in this publication.

The most current CPT is available from the American Medical Association.

No fee schedules, basic unit values, relative value guides, conversion factors or scales are included in CPT. The AMA is not recommending that any specific relative values, fees, fee schedules, or related listings, be attached to CPT. Any relative listings assigned to the CPT codes are not those of the AMA and such assignment should not be construed as a recommendation for use of these relative values by the AMA.

The AMA assumes no responsibility for the consequences attributable to or related to any use or interpretation of any information contained or not contained in this Publication.

NOTICE REGARDING COPYRIGHT DATES:

The AMA CPT for 1995 is published by the AMA in calendar year 1994 and carries a 1994 copyright. These are the valid CPT codes to be used for 1995.

This book was composed and set in Helvetica using Wordperfect®, Ventura Publisher® and an IBM LaserPrinter® by Context Software Systems, Inc.

TABLE OF CONTENTS

PREFACE

The opening paragraph of the original Preface for the *CodeLink* series began with a quote attributed to Alcott: "That is a good book which is opened with expectation and closed with profit." Much to our delight, judging by the widely growing popularity of the the *CodeLink* series, it seems we have met the challange of providing a "good" book. The series began with *CodeLink* manuals for Oral & Maxillofacial Surgery, Orthopaedics, and Ophthalmology. Due to popular demand, we will be adding titles on Otolaryngology and Plastic Surgery this year, with additional titles to follow as this series continues to grow.

CodeLink was designed to provide a unique tool that will help your practice submit more accurate claims, to lift from your shoulders a bit of the burden of dealing with third party payers, and, as a result, increase your income. This manual helps guide you in the selection of proper codes by providing frequently used ICD–9–CM linkages to CPT codes used within each specialty.

This text would not have been possible without the tireless efforts of many individuals. Bill Elliott, Senior Vice President at Context, worked his computer magic on tens of millions of claims — the starting point of this text. Suzanne McGuire spent endless hours checking and validating the links between CPT and ICD–9–CM codes, working directly with the Editorial Panel members. Leslie Garvey integrated the CPT and Medicare rules, and designed and typeset the manual. Suzanne and Leslie proofed and edited the text Maureen Cirnitski at McGraw–Hill spent numerous hours tying together all the loose ends to ensure the production quality of the series.

We again thank our Editorial Panel members, listed on pages ix through x of this book, for taking time away from their busy schedules to provide guidance on the contents of the text and the links between codes.

We welcome your constructive comments and suggestions on ways of making this text more usable to your practice. Please send them to my attention at the address below.

Gary M. Knaus
President
Context Software Systems, Inc.
241 South Frontage Road, Suites 38–39
Burr Ridge, Illinois 60521

EDITORIAL PANEL

The CPT to ICD–9–CM linkages found in this text are derived from claims actually submitted to third party payers. To help guarantee the quality and integrity of this information, a panel of expert plastic surgeons reviewed and validated the linkages. The following persons offered their time and expertise in this process. Their help is gratefully acknowledged.

Walter L. Erhardt, Jr., M.D.

Albany, Georgia

Dr. Erhardt is Chairman of the Department of Surgery and Chairman of the Division of Plastic Surgery at Phoebe Putney Memorial Hospital in Albany, Georgia. He is also the Director of the Crippled Children's Plastic Surgery Clinic, and maintains a solo private practice in Albany, Georgia. Dr. Erhardt's many publications and presentations include the American Society of Plastic and Reconstructive Surgeons (ASPRS) instructional course, "Entering Practice – the Real World" and articles in the *Journal of the Medical Association of Georgia* and *Annals of Plastic Surgery*. In addition to active membership in many professional societies, he serves on the following committees for the ASPRS: Finance (Chairman), Practice Development, Publications, Strategic Planning, and CPT coding. He has been a member of medical mission teams to India and El Salvador. Dr. Erhardt graduated *cum laude* from Roanoke College in Salem, Virginia, and received his M.D. from the University of Virginia School of Medicine in Charlottesville. He is a Diplomate of the American Board of Plastic Surgery and the National Board of Medical Examiners.

Kevin L. Smith, M.D.

Charlotte, North Carolina

In addition to maintaining a private practice in Charlotte, North Carolina, Dr. Smith is an Assistant Clinical Professor and Resident Program Director of the Department of Plastic Surgery, Charlotte Division, of the University of North Carolina – Chapel Hill. He has authored numerous articles and book chapters on hand rehabilitation. As Director of the Physicians for Peace/Carolinas Medical Center International Medical Scholars Program, he teaches plastic surgery techniques to visiting doctors. He has also been a Visiting Professor at many international universities and hospitals, including the Philippines, Jordan, Syria, and Egypt. Dr. Smith is Vice–Chairman of the Department of Plastic Surgery and of the Operating Room Committee for the Carolinas Medical Center, and he is Chairman of the Quality Assurance Sub–Committee for the Department of Plastic Surgery. He is a Certified member of the American Board of Surgery and the American Board of Plastic Surgery and a Diplomate of the National Board of Medical Examiners. He received his A.B. at Princeton University, his M.Sc. at George Washington University and his M.D. at Eastern Virginia Medical School in Norfolk, Virginia.

Paul C. Zweibal, M.D., D.M.D.

Littleton, Colorado

Dr. Zweibel is a Board Certified member of the American Board of Plastic Surgery, the National Board of Dental Examiners and the National Board of Medical Examiners, as well as a Fellow of the American College of Surgeons. A past President, Vice–President and Secretary/Treasurer of the Colorado State Society of Plastic and Reconstructive Surgeons, Dr. Zwiebel is active in numerous professional and civic organizations. He received his M.D. from the Mount Sinai School of Medicine in New York City, his D.M.D. from the Harvard School of Dental Medicine in Boston, and fellowships in Microvascular Surgery, Cranio–Maxillofacial Surgery and Craniofacial Surgery at Massachusetts General Hospital, UCLA and Paris. He is in private practice in Littleton, Colorado.

INTRODUCTION

To receive proper reimbursement from third party payers, plastic surgery practices are by now familiar with and using the CPT, HCPCS, and ICD–9–CM coding systems. They are also probably familiar with the guidelines regarding appropriate circumstances to use each system. However, what they may not be familiar with is the increasing scrutiny third party payers are applying to insurance claims.

Attempting to better control costs, payers are increasingly looking at the medical necessity of a procedure or service before deciding to pay for it. If it seems reasonable based on the patient's problem, it is paid. If it does not seem reasonable, it probably is not paid. This process of verifying the medical necessity is done by testing the relationships, or linkages, between the procedure and diagnosis codes submitted on the claim form. These linkages can set the stage for a paid or denied claim.

Therefore, the purpose of this text is to provide this linkage information, as well as the basic reimbursement and coding guidelines necessary to bill properly. Please be aware that this book is not to be considered a replacement for your CPT, HCPCS, or ICD–9–CM books. This manual should be used after location of the correct codes in the coding manuals to verify that your code selections make sense.

CODE LINKAGES

The code linkages in this text were derived from actual claims submitted by plastic surgeons. The linkages were statistically validated, meaning that if a linkage was infrequently reported, it was not included in this volume.

Please note that this text has limitations. While the linkages provided herein should cover the vast majority of codes reported by plastic surgery practices, they are not intended, nor does the author or publisher purport to provide a "complete" or "all–inclusive" list. While confident of the quality and integrity of the linkages, the author and publisher make no claim that those provided are "absolute." The linkages are based on actual claims submitted to third party payers which means they are representative of the actual linkages used by plastic surgery practices. The exclusion of a code from the linkage list does not indicate that the code may not be medically appropriate; it means only that it is infrequently reported by plastic surgery practices. For these less–than–common linkages, you may need to submit support documentation to the third party payer to justify and explain the reasons for the procedure/service.

CPT to ICD–9–CM Linkages

The CPT to ICD–9–CM linkages provide the logically–related diagnosis code (ICD–9–CM) relationships to an individual CPT code. This information can be used to validate the diagnosis code choice when the procedure code (CPT) is already known. An example from this section of the book is provided on the next page.

CODELINK for PLASTIC SURGERY 103

CPT CODE **SERVICE**

11700* Debridement of nails, manual; five or less

11701 Debridement of nails, manual; each additional five or less

CPT NOTES

- For drainage of paronychia or onychia, see 10060, 10061.

ICD–9–CM

110.1	Dermatophytosis of nail
112.3	Cutaneous candidiasis
117.x	Mycosis
681.0x	Cellulitis and abscess, finger
703.x	Diseases of nail
757.5	Nail anomalies NEC
923.3	Contusion of finger
927.3	Crushing injury, finger
959.5	Finger injury NOS

REIMBURSEMENT INFORMATION

General

- Starred procedure. (11700)

Medicare

- Follow–up Days
  11700 — 0
  11701 — none; falls with global period of another procedure
- Assistant Surgeon — not paid
- Supply Charges — not allowed
- Outpatient Limit — applies
- Minor Surgery Rules Apply
- Fragments —64450

Fourth– and Fifth–Digit Representation

You will note that in some cases, ICD–9–CM codes are listed as "123.4x," "123.x.," or "123.xx." The "x" indicates that fourth or fifth digits apply to this code. However, in the interest of conserving space, not all codes are fully expanded, but instead are listed in this way. Be sure to check your ICD–9–CM manual for the fourth– and fifth–digit code applicable to your coding situation.

HOW TO USE THIS MANUAL

This manual is arranged in sections as follows:

Coding Guidelines.	This section explains the basic coding conventions and guidelines which all users of the coding systems need to know. While it is not exhaustive, it does provide an overview of topics such as the global surgical package, billing starred procedures, the basics of ICD–9–CM and CPT coding, etc.
CPT to ICD–9–CM Linkages.	This section contains the "what's and why's"; that is, the logical relationships between procedures and diagnoses. A single CPT code number is listed in the left column with the logically related diagnosis (ICD–9–CM) code(s) listed in the right column. In addition, you will find general coding reminders, notes from CPT relevant to each code, and pertinent Medicare reimbursement information. Within this section, the linkages are grouped and divided according to the sections of CPT.

To make best use of this manual, it is recommended that you become familiar with the organization of and notations used in this text. An overview of the organization was provided above. The specific notations used are discussed below.

OVERVIEW AND EXPLANATION OF NOTATIONS

Additional coding and reimbursement information is provided in the CPT to ICD–9–CM Linkages section of this manual. A sample page is shown on the next page and an explanation of the notations is provided following the sample.

CPT CODE **SERVICE**

▲ **25240** Excision distal ulna partial or complete, (eg, Darrach type or matched resection)

CPT NOTES

- For implant replacement, distal ulna, see 25442.
- For obtaining fascia for interposition, see 20920, 20922.

ICD-9-CM Code Number(s)/Link(s)

CPT Code Number

CPT Description

New/Changed Code Marker

CPT Notes

General Reimbursement Information

Medicare Reimbursement Information

ICD-9-CM

170.5	M-Neoplasm, Wrist/Hand bones
213.5	B-Neoplasm, Wrist/Hand bones
238.0	UB-Neoplasm, Bone
239.2	Bone/Skin neoplasm NOS
714.0	Rheumatoid arthritis
714.30	Juvenile rheumatoid arthritis NOS
714.31	Juvenile acute rheumatoid arthritis
714.32	Pauciarticular juv rheum arthritis
714.33	Monoarticular juv rheum arthritis
715.13	Loc prim osteoarthritis, forearm
715.33	Loc osteoarthritis NOS, forearm
716.13	Traumatic arthropathy, forearm
716.14	Traumatic arthropathy, hand
718.03	Articular cartilage dis, forearm
719.43	Pain in joint, forearm
906.2	Late effect of superficial injury

ICD-9-CM Description(s)

REIMBURSEMENT INFORMATION

General

- See notes on page 286.
- Description changed in 1995 CPT.

Medicare

- Follow-up Days — 90
- Assistant Surgeon — paid
- Supply Charges — not allowed
- Outpatient Limit — does not apply
- Major Procedure Rules

CPT CODE–SERVICE

This is the code number and full description as it appears in CPT 1995.

CPT NOTES

Pertinent parenthetical or other notes found in CPT which apply specifically to the code listed are printed here for your reference. Where applicable, notes relative to an entire section of codes are reproduced as a single entry before that group of codes. For example, the notes from CPT 1995 from the Musculoskeletal section are included as a single entry on page 286. A note in the right column under "General Information" refers you to the appropriate page of this manual which you should reference should you wish to review these notes.

ICD–9–CM

These are the logically related ICD–9–CM 1995 code numbers and shortened descriptions. Please note again that this list is not intended to be all–inclusive nor should it be construed as any kind of recommendation of "correct" medical parameters. The linkages are provided for reference and guidance. If your situation dictates that you report a code not found on the list, you may wish to add the linkage. Conversely, you may wish to delete linkages not pertinent to your practice.

REIMBURSEMENT INFORMATION

General

This notation contains general reimbursement information, such as the references to section notes, whether the code is new or the description changed in 1995, and whether certain coding rules, such as separate procedure or starred procedure rules, apply.

For the notes found at the beginning of a section of codes in CPT which are reproduced in this book, the reference in this notation says "See notes on page xx." Refer to that page in this text to find these notes. For example, the note on page 424 of this text for CPT code number 24136 instructs you to "See notes on page 286." For the instructional notes related to these repairs, you would refer to page 286 of this text for those notes. You can refer also to the section guidelines of your CPT for more complete information.

Codes for which the description changed in 1995 are noted with both the triangle (CPT's symbol for change) as well as the notation "Description changed in 1995 CPT." New codes which were added to CPT 1995 are noted with both the circle (CPT's symbol for new) as well as the notation "New procedure, 1995 CPT."

Codes for which the starred procedure billing rules or the separate procedure billing rules apply have a note under this heading which states "Starred procedure" or "Separate procedure rules apply." These notes are provided to help the coder use the codes and bill properly. These coding rules are also discussed in this text in the Coding Guidelines section. Starred procedures are discussed beginning on page xxxiii and separate procedures are discussed beginning on page xxxvi.

Medicare

The notations under this heading provide information specific to Medicare. Each is explained below.

Follow–Up Days. This note indicates the number of surgical follow–up days applicable to the procedure. The numbers will be 0, 10 or 90, depending upon the procedure. If this note reads "none; included in global package of another procedure," you should interpret this to mean the procedure is actually a component of another procedure and so no follow–up days are assigned for performance of the procedure alone. A note which reads "global concept does not apply" indicates that this service is not considered surgical in nature so no follow–up days need to be assigned. A note which reads "determined by local carrier" indicates that the local carrier determines the follow–up days for this procedure on an individual basis. Typically, these are unlisted procedures.

Assistant Surgeon. This note tells you whether Medicare permits payment for an assistant surgeon for the procedure. "Paid" means Medicare may allow payment for an assistant for this procedure. "Not paid" means Medicare has determined that an assistant surgeon is not necessary for this procedure and so will not pay for one. (You are not permitted to attempt to charge the patient for the assistant.) A "by report" notation means that the individual carrier makes a determination as to whether an assistant is payable for this service.

Supply Charges. Medicare permits payment for supplies provided in the physician's office only for certain identified procedures (refer to the "Coding Guidelines" chapter of this manual for further information about this provision). This notation reminds you whether or not the supply of a surgical tray is payable separately. "Not allowed" means Medicare considers the tray to be part of the charge for the procedure; you cannot collect this charge from the patient. "Allowed" indicates you can charge Medicare an additional amount, using HCPCS National code A4550, for the provision of a surgical tray.

Outpatient Limit. Also called the site–of–service reduction, the outpatient limit refers to a 50 percent reduction in the practice expense component of the procedure's relative value units. The outpatient limit applies to certain identified procedures which, if provided in an outpatient department or hospital rather than the physician's office, will receive this reduction. A note which reads "applies" means that payment will be reduced if the place of service is other than the physician's office. A note which reads "does not apply" means Medicare will not adjust payment based on the place of service.

Minor or Major Procedure Rules. Medicare's global surgical package rules can be referenced with this note. "Minor Procedure Rules" means that the minor surgical package rules apply to this procedure. "Major Procedure Rules" means the major surgical package rules apply to this procedure. For more information about Medicare's surgical package definitions, refer to the Coding Guidelines chapter of this text.

Fragments The codes listed with this notation are considered by Medicare to be incidental or integral to the major procedure listed and should not be billed separately when the code listed is billed. This information is also available from your carrier under the heading of "Uniform Reporting of Physicians' Services" or "Correct Coding Initiative."

EVALUATION AND MANAGEMENT SERVICES

This section of code linkages deserves special mention. You will note an "Examples" notation following many of the evaluation and management (E&M) services codes. The information provided under this notation is a vignette, or illustration, of the level of care provided. These vignettes are found in the CPT code manual, either following the code or in Appendix D. They are included here for illustrative purposes.

Notes specific to a group of E&M codes are found prior to that group of codes in this manual and are referenced with the "See notes on page xx" notation. These are provided for your reference. For more complete information regarding the definitions of each component of an E&M code and other pertinent rules, refer to your CPT book.

Also, it is important to note that in some cases a limited set of ICD–9–CM linkages are provided for each level of E&M service. The author and publisher recognize that an almost unlimited set of diagnoses could be listed with each code. However, in the interest of space and to make the book easier to use, only a limited set are included. It is recommended that you add to or delete from this list as pertinent to your practice.

CODING GUIDELINES

OVERVIEW OF CODING SYSTEMS

The means by which plastic surgery practices communicate to third party payers is by the use of codes. That is, codes are reported to inform the insurance carrier what was done to the patient (procedures and services) and why (diagnoses). Plastic surgeons actually use three different coding systems. Procedures and services are reported using the American Medical Association's *Current Procedural Terminology* (CPT) and the *Health Care Financing Administration's (HCFA) Common Procedure Coding System* (HCPCS). The *International Classification of Diseases, Ninth Revision, Clinical Modification* (ICD–9–CM) coding system is used to report patient diagnoses. A brief discussion of each system is provided below because an understanding of how to use these coding systems is essential to proper reimbursement. For more information about coding and reimbursement issues, refer to McGraw–Hill's *Getting Paid For What You Do* and *ICD–9–CM Coding for Physicians' Offices.*

PHYSICIANS' CURRENT PROCEDURAL TERMINOLOGY (CPT)

Published by the American Medical Association and updated annually in December, CPT is the most widely used procedural coding system in the United States. CPT contains codes and descriptions for more than 7,000 procedures and services rendered by physicians. Codes listed in CPT consist of two parts: a five–digit code number and the associated description. The following is an example of a CPT code and its description:

13120 Repair, complex, scalp, arms, and/or legs; 1.1cm to 2.5 cm

All claims submitted by plastic surgery practices to their patients' medical insurance will contain CPT codes. Therefore, it is imperative that the reader have a grasp of the CPT system as a whole: the symbols and format utilized, modifiers, and the general rules guiding the choice and use of codes. Users of CPT need to be especially aware of the many notes contained in the coding system which provide information about how certain procedures and services are to be reported. These notes may appear before a group of codes, below a code, or at the end of a group of codes. In some cases, interpretation of these notes will vary from coder to coder, and from one third party payer to another. Experienced CPT coders have learned to accept that there is not always an absolute right way to code certain procedures and services.

Organization of the CPT Coding Manual

CPT is divided into six distinct sections of codes: Evaluation and Management (for visits and consultations); Anesthesia; Surgery (for procedures such as breast reconstructions and grafts); Radiology (for X–ray and magnetic resonance imaging (MRI) services); Pathology and Laboratory (for lab work such as urinalysis); and Medicine (for non-invasive services, such as injections and physical therapy). Each of the six sections are preceded by guidelines that contain rules and modifiers relevant to that section of codes.

In addition to codes, CPT also contains an introduction, four appendices, and an index. The CPT Introduction provides information about and rules related to use of the coding system and describes symbols and other important concepts. Appendix A lists all CPT modifiers and their definitions. Changes that have appeared since the previous year's volume are noted in Appendix B. (The use of symbols to indicate changes will be discussed later.) The third appendix (Appendix C) notes changes applying to those practices that use the CPT short procedure descriptions in their computer database. Appendix D contains clinical examples for E&M services. CPT's Index is located at the back of the book and is preceded by instructions related to helping the user locate codes.

Symbols

CPT utilizes three symbols that provide special information about the codes: the circle; the triangle; and the star. Each of these symbols is discussed below.

Circle (•)

A blackened circle, or bullet, is placed to the left of codes that are new to CPT. That is, these codes did not appear in the previous year's volume. Noting the circle serves two purposes. First, it allows users of CPT to quickly locate new procedures and services without having to refer back and forth between Appendix B and the code sections. Second, it reminds the coder that the procedure or service is new. This is important when billing because third party payers do not always implement new codes when they are released. Information related to patient conditions for which the procedure is appropriate, reasonable fees for the new procedures, etc., must be developed by the third party payers before the new procedure is routinely reimbursed. Therefore, when submitting new CPT codes to third party payers, it may be necessary to provide additional information that justifies both medical necessity and the charge being made. Once the third party payers begin paying for the new procedure or service on a routine basis, the supplementary support documentation may not be needed to ensure payment.

Triangle (▲)

The blackened triangle, or delta, to the left of a code signifies that the code's definition has been changed. Changes may be significant or minor, but in any case, for those codes used by the practice, a comparison of the current to the previous year's definition should be made. The comparison is important for reimbursement and audit liability reasons. To understand why, consider a procedure for which the definition has significantly changed, but the practice is unaware of the change and continues to bill as if the code describes something which it no longer does. In such a case the plastic surgeon is not reporting what was performed. Two unfortunate consequences may result. First, the plastic surgeon may be inappropriately reimbursed due to the fact that what was billed was not what was actually performed. Second, if audited, this could be interpreted as fraudulent billing and might create a host of problems for the practice.

Star (*)

In the Surgery section of CPT, stars appear to the right of several code numbers. The star notes that CPT's surgical package concept does not apply to the procedure. That is, preoperative and postoperative care are to be billed separately in addition to the starred procedure, subject to a set of rules found in the Surgery section guidelines. These rules are discussed on pages xxxii–xxxvii of this text.

HEALTH CARE FINANCING ADMINISTRATION'S COMMON PROCEDURE CODING SYSTEM (HCPCS)

Pronounced "hick-pix," this coding system was developed by Medicare (HCFA) and consists of the three levels of codes described below:

Level I — CPT

Level II — National Codes

Level III — Local Codes

Level I, CPT, was incorporated into HCPCS in 1984 with the permission of the American Medical Association. The Level II and III codes are created by HCFA and local Medicare carriers to supplement CPT. National Codes (Level II) contain listings of supplies and procedures not specified in CPT. These National codes may be differentiated from CPT codes in that they begin with a letter of the alphabet (A through V) followed by four numbers. An example of a National code is given below:

J7030 Infusion, normal saline solution, (1000 cc.)

Local codes (Level III) are created by each individual state's Medicare carrier and are for use only in that carrier's region. These codes can be distinguished from National codes in that they begin with the letter W, X, Y, or Z followed by four numbers. Local codes sometimes describe supplies, injections, and procedures that are very new, and therefore not yet listed in the CPT or National systems. In other cases, Local codes will describe variations on the services and supplies listed in the other levels. Furthermore, some states' Medicare carriers have Local codes that could be used by plastic surgery practices while, in other states, no codes would apply.

Use of HCPCS Codes

HCPCS codes are reported in the same manner on claim forms and superbills as CPT codes. Determining which codes to use — CPT, National, or Local — is a simple process if the following rules are kept in mind:

1. Use HCPCS codes when reporting services, procedures, and supplies to Medicare, and in some states, to Medicaid.

2. Use the HCPCS code which most completely describes the procedure, service, or supply.

Although in most cases the plastic surgeon will report CPT codes to Medicare and Medicaid, there are two groups of codes in the National system of interest. These are the medical and surgical supply codes (A4190–A5507) and the injection/chemotherapy codes (J0110–J9999). An example of using a HCPCS National code follows.

> The plastic surgeon treats a Medicare patient. During the visit, he/she injects 500 mg of Ampicillin intramuscularly. CPT provides an all–purpose intramuscular antibiotic injection code, 90788:
>
> 90788 Intramuscular injection of antibiotic (specify).
>
> For non–Medicare/Medicaid patients, this CPT code could be appropriate for reporting the injection and supply. The type of antibiotic and amount injected would be listed with the description. However, for Medicare and Medicaid patients the reporting rules differ. To report the supply of the antibiotic substance, the most specific code should be listed. The HCPCS National system contains more than 400 codes for different injectables, many of which are antibiotics. There is a code for ampicillin:
>
> J0290 Injection, Ampicillin, up to 500 mg.

Using the second rule above, since the J0290 code more exactly describes the service it should be reported to Medicare instead of the more general CPT antibiotic injection code, 90788. As a rule, never use the CPT therapeutic injection codes (90782–90799) when reporting the supply of injectables to Medicare (or possibly Medicaid). The appropriate "J" code for the supply should be listed instead.

Note that Medicare considers the administration of the injection to be included in the service provided. Separate billing is allowed, using the appropriate HCPCS National code, for the supply of the injected material only.

Local codes can also be important to plastic surgery practices. Their importance depends upon the specific codes used by the practice's local Medicare carrier. If the Medicare carrier has created codes for injections, supplies, procedures, and/or services, they should be reviewed for potential use by the practice. Optimal reimbursement from Medicare and Medicaid depends upon understanding the rules associated with these HCPCS National and Local codes. As such, plastic surgery practices need to obtain copies of both the HCPCS National and Local codes.

INTERNATIONAL CLASSIFICATION OF DISEASES, NINTH REVISION, CLINICAL MODIFICATION (ICD–9–CM)

The ICD–9–CM coding system was developed in the late 1970s by the National Center for Health Statistics as a statistical classification system. It was created to replace the older ICD–A system, and to allow for better reporting of both inpatient and outpatient conditions. Today, ICD–9–CM is used by virtually all third party payers as the coding system for describing patient conditions. ICD–9–CM is updated annually in October. It is expected that the next revision of ICD, ICD–10, will not be released until sometime after the year 2000.

Although the complete ICD–9–CM coding system consists of three volumes, plastic surgery practices need only concern themselves with Volumes 1 and 2, the Tabular List and Index, respectively. Volume 3, which contains procedures and an index to procedures, is used almost exclusively by hospitals. Volume 1, the Tabular Listing, contains diagnosis codes and their descriptions. Volume 2 is the index to the codes found in the Tabular Listing. The example below was taken from Volume 1 and demonstrates an ICD–9 code:

945.34 Burn of lower limb(s); full thickness skin loss (third degree NOS); lower leg

Organization and Use of ICD–9–CM

On April 1, 1989, a law requiring that all physicians use ICD–9–CM codes when reporting patient diagnoses to Medicare took effect. Serious penalties can result from lack of compliance on claims submitted to Medicare after June 1, 1989. Penalties range from possible non-payment of assigned claims to potential fines of $2,000 per occurrence on unassigned claims.

Although this law applies only to claims submitted to Medicare, the use of ICD–9–CM codes for reporting diagnoses to all third party payers is advisable for several reasons. First, if diagnosis codes are not used, payment may be denied or delayed. Second, when not used, the carrier's staff will locate an ICD–9–CM code based on the doctor's description of the patient's problem. This coding is usually performed by individuals with either no or very limited medical background. As a result, the codes selected by the carrier may not logically match with the procedure or service being reported, and the claim could be denied.

Finally, many third party payers have purchased or developed software programs that compare the CPT code to the ICD–9–CM code. These programs test for logical relationships. Should, for example, the procedure listed be the reduction of a fracture and the diagnosis is tonsillitis, the claim will be automatically denied for lack of medical necessity or reasonableness.

Therefore, it is becoming increasingly important that plastic surgery practices familiarize themselves with the ICD–9–CM coding system and its rules. To that end, discussed below is the organization of the ICD–9–CM coding manual, and the abbreviations, symbols, and notes, used throughout the system. The discussion is not intended to be exhaustive.

Organization

The complete ICD–9–CM consists of three volumes. Plastic surgery practices do not need the third volume, as it contains procedure codes for hospital use. Volume 1 of ICD–9–CM, the Tabular List, contains codes and descriptions for diseases, illnesses, injuries, complaints, symptoms, etc. It is organized into 17 chapters plus two supplementary sections. These later sections are for coding patients who are not being seen for a current illness ("V" codes) or where the patient's problem is due to an external cause related to injury or poisoning ("E" codes). Volume 2 of ICD–9–CM is the index to the first volume.

Codes can be either three–digits (called categories), four–digits (called classifications), or five–digits (called sub–classifications). Many category codes are further defined by the classification and subclassification codes. The additional fourth and fifth digits typically provide additional information to the category pertinent to the body area, site, or whether the patient did or did not present complications. An example of each level of code is shown below.

881. Open wound of elbow, forearm, and wrist

881.1 Complicated

881.12 Wrist

Symbols

Two symbols are used throughout the first volume of ICD–9–CM. The first symbol, the lozenge "□," is not relevant to plastic surgery practices. The second symbol, the section mark, "§," is important as it alerts the coder to the presence of fifth digits that need to be added to the code. In many instances, definitions for the fifth digits are found on pages preceding the code.

Abbreviations

Users of ICD–9–CM will be familiar with the two abbreviations, NEC and NOS. Each has a specific meaning and importance to coding and reimbursement.

Not Elsewhere Classifiable (NEC)

In some situations the coder will not have enough information available to determine a more specific code. This may occur in cases where highly specific codes exist. The ICD–9–CM Index provides references to specific codes when such cases arise, and uses the NEC abbreviation to help guide the coder. For example, the plastic surgeon determines that a patient has a neck anomaly but does not provide any further information about the condition. The ICD–9–CM Index lists anomaly as follows:

Anomaly, anomalous (congenital) (unspecified type) 759.9
neck (any part) 744.9
specified type NEC 744.89

The NEC abbreviation informs the coder that code 744.89 might be appropriate in the example cited above. A review of code 744.89 shows that it is indeed proper for this coding situation.

In other cases there may not be a code which completely describes the patient's condition. Not elsewhere classifiables will also be used in these situations. For example, suppose the plastic surgeon specified the type of a lower limb anomaly, but that particular diagnosis is not listed in ICD–9–CM. That is, it is not one of the types mentioned (e.g., coxa valga, coxa vara, macrodactylia, etc.). In this case, the Index reference to specified type NEC would apply to this coding situation. So, code 755.69 would be appropriate to use in this coding example where the anomaly is known, but the specific type is not listed in the ICD–9–CM book.

From a reimbursement standpoint, in such cases as cited above, it may be necessary to inform the third party payer of the specific diagnosis. That is, a brief description of the patient's illness may need to be submitted to help ensure proper payment.

Not Otherwise Specified (NOS)

This abbreviation appears throughout the Tabular List and is frequently associated with the "unspecified" codes. In fact, "not otherwise specified" means the same as "unspecified." Use of codes with NOS as part of their definition will often result when the coder does not have enough information to select a more definitive diagnosis. For example, suppose a patient is seen by the plastic surgeon for a deformity of the forearm, but the type has not been determined. ICD–9–CM provides a code for this situation, "736.00, Unspecified deformity of forearm."

When codes for unspecified conditions are reported to third party payers, special attention may need to be given to the claim if reimbursement is expected. Many carriers will often suspend for review claims that list an unspecified diagnosis code. Therefore, it may be necessary to attach a brief note to the claim explaining the patient's problem in more detail.

Notes

Users of ICD–9–CM have undoubtedly noticed the Includes and Excludes notes that appear with groups of codes as well as specific codes. These terms have specific meanings in ICD–9–CM. Includes notes further define or give an example of the contents of a group of codes. Consider the following code from ICD–9–CM:

891. Open wound of knee, leg (except thigh), and ankle

Includes: leg NOS
multiple sites of leg, except thigh

Patients suffering from an open wound of the leg could be coded using listings from the 891 series.

Excludes notes mean just the opposite of Includes notes. In ICD–9–CM, the term "Excludes:" is always surrounded by a printed box so that it is easily noticed. Coders need to be aware of conditions that are excluded from groups of codes, and therefore, should take notice of the Excludes notes. An example of an Excludes note appears on the next page:

876 Open wound of back

Excludes: *open wound into thoracic cavity (860.0–862.9)*
traumtic pneumothorax and hemothorax (860.1–860.5)

Thus, if a patient is suffering from an open wound into the thoracic cavity, codes from the 876 group would not be reported.

Fourth– and Fifth–Digit Codes

In many cases there will be fourth– and fifth–digit codes from which to select. If there is a fifth–digit code, it should always be used. If there are no fifth–digit codes, but there are fourth–digit codes, use a fourth–digit code. Only if there are no fourth– and fifth–digit codes may a third–digit code be used.

Fifth digits are presented in different ways in ICD–9–CM. Each fifth–digit code may be listed as is found under the series 872.0, "Open wound of external ear, without mention of complication." All possible fifth–digit codes are listed. Another method involves printing the fifth–digits themselves, with their definitions, prior to the fourth–digit codes to which they apply. An example of this is found for the three–digit category 942, "Burn of trunk" codes. The fifth–digit subclassifications for use with this category are found under the "Burn of trunk" heading before subcategory code 942.0. Seven fifth–digits apply to category 942, as shown below:

0 trunk, unspecified site

1 breast

2 chest wall, excluding breast and nipple

3 abdominal wall

4 back [any part]

5 genitalia

9 other and multiple sites of trunk

These would be applied to the fourth–digit codes in the 942 series as appropriate. As an example, for a patient suffering from a burn of unspecified degree of the intrascapular region, the fifth–digit "4" is required to indicate the location of the burn for a final code of 942.04. If the burn was classified as second degree, the final code would be 942.24. Claims not listing fifth– or fourth–digit diagnoses when required may be denied.

Symptoms, Signs, and Ill–Defined Conditions

Some patients may present symptoms or signs that defy immediate diagnosis. Nonetheless, if a claim is filed, a diagnosis must be listed, and special codes can be used in such cases. Chapter 16 in ICD–9–CM serves this purpose as it provides codes for these types of conditions. For example, an plastic surgeon is treating a patient with exanthem. Until a more definitive diagnosis is established, code 782.1 "Rash and other nonspecific skin eruption; exantham" can be listed.

"V" Codes

These codes appear toward the end of Volume One under the title "Supplementary Classification of Factors Influencing Health Status and Contact with Health Services." They are typically used when the patient is being seen for something other than a current illness or injury. A follow–up visit related to cancer that has not been present in a patient for several years would be an example.

Many plastic surgeons and staff are afraid to report "V" codes because they are aware that in most cases the patient's insurance policy will not cover services associated with "V" codes. But the problem is really not the physicians', as well meaning as they may be. Patients purchase specific coverages when they buy health insurance and few carriers today sell coverage for cosmetic services. Thus, it is the patient's responsibility to pay for non-covered services, and the plastic surgeon should not feel shy about reporting "V" codes when it is appropriate to do so.

"E" Codes

The "E" codes are supplementary and are used to describe external causes of injuries and poisonings. They are never reported by themselves, and are rarely used by plastic surgeons.

REPAIRS AND RECONSTRUCTION DIAGNOSES

Plastic surgeons should be aware of the following diagnosis coding issues related to repairs and reconstructive procedures:

1. In most case the surgeon should list the primary reason for the repair or reconstructive surgery, such as an open wound or the late effect of an original procedure (such as cancer surgery), rather than the original diagnosis (cancer). Failure to do so may result in a claim denial or lower reimbursement.

2. One of the most widely used diagnoses in plastic surgery is 611.8 for "surgical amastia" or "absence of breast, acquired." Note that although these conditions are not directly listed with code 611.8, by looking up "amastia" and "absence of breast, acquired" in the ICD–9–CM Index, you will find they are referenced to code 611.8.

3. In 1995, the diagnosis code for "seborrheic keratosis" (702.1) was split into two codes. Code 702.11 is for "inflamed seborrheic keratosis" and code 702.19 is for "other seborrheic keratosis." Medicare will pay only for 702.11.

EVALUATION AND MANAGEMENT (E&M) SERVICES

The 1992 CPT completely redefined both the code numbers and descriptions of all visit and consultation codes. The changes were intended to reduce the potential for differing interpretations of the codes and to increase the consistency of reporting by doctors in differing specialties. Medicare began requiring use of these codes effective for services rendered on or after January 1, 1992. Other payers phased the codes in over time.

Unlike with the old "visit" codes, it is no longer possible to make direct comparison between levels of service provided to new and established patients, or to services rendered in different locations. For example, a Level II new patient office visit is not defined in the same way as a Level II established patient office visit. General E&M coding rules and important factors associated with different types of E&M codes are covered below.

New and Established Patients

The definitions for new and established patients were changed in the 1992 CPT. New patients are those for whom the doctor has not provided professional services within the past three years. Obviously, patients provided professional services within the past three years are considered to be established. There are two key exceptions to this rule:

1. If you are on call or covering for another doctor (including locum tenens doctors, according to Medicare) and bill your services, you would report using the same code that would have been used by the physician for whom you are covering.

2. If you have never before provided professional services to a patient, but are a member of a group practice that bills under a group ID, and the patient received services within the last three years from a doctor of the same specialty in that group, then Medicare will consider the patient established. If the patient was seen by a practitioner of a different specialty, you may consider the patient new.

Definitions of E&M Services

Evaluation and management services (visits) are defined based upon three key components. Selection of a code requires the performance of each of the three components. Certain key words and phrases are used to define these components. The components, and their definitions, are described below.

History

The levels of E&M services recognize four types of history that are defined as follows:

- **Problem Focused.** History of the chief complaint; brief history of present illness or problem.

- **Expanded Problem Focused.** History of the chief complaint; brief history of present illness; problem pertinent system review.

- **Detailed.** History of the chief complaint; extended history of present illness; extended system review; pertinent past, family and/or social history.
- **Comprehensive.** History of the chief complaint; extended history of present illness; complete system review; complete past, family and social history.

Examination

The levels of E&M services recognize four types of examination that are defined as follows:

- **Problem Focused.** An examination that is limited to the affected body area or organ system.
- **Expanded Problem Focused.** An examination of the affected body area or organ system and other symptomatic or related organ systems.
- **Detailed.** An extended examination of the affected body area(s) and other symptomatic or related organ system(s).
- **Comprehensive.** A complete single system specialty examination or a complete multi–system examination.

Medical Decision Making

This refers to the complexity of establishing a diagnosis and/or selecting a management option as measured by:

- the number of possible diagnoses and/or the number of management options that must be considered.
- the amount and/or complexity of information (e.g., medical records, diagnostic tests, etc.) that must be obtained, reviewed and analyzed.
- the risk of significant complications, morbidity and/or mortality, as well as co-morbidities, associated with the patient's presenting problem(s), the diagnostic procedure(s), and/or the possible management options.

Four types of medical decision making are recognized: straightforward; low complexity; moderate complexity; and high complexity. For a service to qualify as involving a certain type of medical decision making, two of the three descriptions listed after each type of decision making in the following table must be met or exceeded.

Type of Decision Making	Number of Diagnoses or Management Options	Amount and/or Complexity of Data to be Reviewed	Risk of Complications and/or Morbidity or Mortality
Straightforward	Minimal	Minimal or None	Minimal
Low Complexity	Limited	Limited	Low
Moderate Complexity	Multiple	Moderate	Moderate
High Complexity	Extensive	Extensive	High

Comorbidities/underlying diseases, in and of themselves, are not considered in selecting a level of E&M service unless their presence significantly increases the complexity of the medical decision making.

Contributing Components

There are four contributory components which can affect code selection. Each of these contributory components is described below.

Nature of Presenting Problem

A presenting problem is a disease, condition, illness, injury, symptom, sign, finding, complaint, or other reason for an encounter, whether or not a diagnosis is established at the time of the encounter. Definitions for the five types of problems are found in the E&M Guidelines in your CPT.

Counseling/Coordination of Care

Counseling is a discussion with the patient and/or the family concerning one or more of the following areas:

- Diagnostic results, impressions and/or recommended diagnostic studies.
- Prognosis.
- Risks and benefits of management (treatment) options.
- Instructions for management (treatment) and/or follow–up.
- Importance of compliance with chosen management (treatment) options.
- Risk factor reduction.
- Patient and family education.

Coordination of care is not formally defined in CPT. However, it is self–explanatory.

Time

Time as an explicit factor is included to assist doctors in selecting the most appropriate level of service. It should be recognized that the specific times expressed in the visit code descriptors are averages, and therefore represent a range of times which may be higher or lower depending on actual clinical circumstances. Time is to be considered as a deciding factor in code selection only when counseling and/or coordination of care comprise more than 50 percent of the encounter.

Intra–service times are defined as face–to–face time for office and other outpatient visits and as unit/floor time for hospital and other inpatient visits. This distinction is necessary because most of the work of typical office visits takes place during the face–to–face time with the patient, while most of the work of typical hospital visits takes place during the time spent on the patient's floor or unit.

Consultations

A consultation is service provided by an plastic surgeon whose opinion or advice regarding evaluation and/or management of a specific problem is requested by another physician or other appropriate source. The request for a consultation from the attending doctor or other appropriate source and the need for the consultation must be documented in the patient's medical record. The consultant's opinion and any services that were ordered or performed must also be documented in the patient's medical record and communicated to the requesting doctor or other appropriate source. "Communicated" in this sense means that a written report must be provided to the requesting physician.

CPT provides four criteria for determining whether or not the service provided constitutes a consultation. These criteria are:

1. The opinion or advice is requested by another doctor or appropriate source.
2. During the consultation, the consultant–physician may initiate diagnostic and/or therapeutic services. (However, should the consultant continue to care for the patient, he or she should use the appropriate subsequent hospital visit or office visit codes.)
3. The request for the consultation must be documented in the patient's record.
4. The opinion and/or recommendations of the consultant must also be documented in the patient's record and communicated to the requesting physician or other source. This means that a written report containing the consultant's opinion and/or advice should be sent to the requesting physician.

Any specifically identifiable procedure performed on or subsequent to the date of the initial consultation should be reported separately. Additionally, any lab or other types of procedures/tests which are performed as part of the consultation should be reported separately.

CPT defines four types of consultation services:

- Office or other outpatient (office, ambulatory care facility, emergency department, etc.).
- Initial inpatient (hospital or nursing home).
- Follow-up inpatient (hospital or nursing home).
- Confirmatory (additional opinion).

A "consultation" initiated by a patient and/or the patient's family, and not requested by a physician, is not reported using the initial consultation codes but may be reported using the codes for confirmatory consultation or office visits, as appropriate.

Office or Other Outpatient Consultations

These codes are used to report consultations provided in the office or in an outpatient or other ambulatory facility, including an emergency department.

Follow–up visits in the consultant's office or other outpatient facility that are initiated by the physician–consultant are reported using office visit codes for established patients. If an additional request for an opinion or advice regarding the same or a new problem is received from the attending physician and is documented in the patient's record, the office consultation codes may be used again.

Initial Inpatient Consultations

These codes are used to report consultations provided to hospital inpatients or residents of nursing facilities. Only one initial consultation should be reported by a consultant per admission. Any additional visits to the patient during the same admission, providing you have not assumed care, should be coded as follow–up consultations. In cases where the plastic surgeon has assumed care of the patient's problem, use the subsequent hospital care codes. (Be aware of the possibility of concurrent care in a situation such as this.)

There are also codes for follow–up inpatient consultations and confirmatory consultations. Refer to your CPT book for further information regarding these services.

SURGICAL PROCEDURES

Billing for surgical services is complicated for plastic surgery practices because the CPT definition for what is considered to be included in the surgery charge is different from the definition used by Medicare. Both the AMA's and Medicare's definitions of the global surgical package are discussed below, as are reporting starred procedures and separate procedures. Refer also to your CPT and your Medicare carrier's bulletins for more information.

Surgical Package Rules

CPT's Global Surgical Package

The CPT system provides a definition of what is called the global surgical package. Discussed in the Surgery section guidelines, it specifies those components assumed to be included in the charge for a surgery. The components are:

- The operation itself;
- Local or topical anesthetics or digital blocks (if provided); and,
- The normal, uncomplicated follow–up care related to the procedure.

The above three items comprise the surgical package. Since anesthetics and digital blocks are itemized, the plastic surgeon should not bill separately for them; if provided, they are included in the charge for the surgery. However, questions may arise regarding follow–up care, such as what is considered normal and what is a complication. Traditionally, follow–up care is defined as the period of time after surgery during which the patient is not billed for visits, whether in the hospital or office. The amount of normal follow–up time varies by procedure. Estimates of normal follow–up days can be found in the major relative value guides, such as McGraw–Hill's *Relative Values for Physicians*. If the plastic surgeon is still seeing the patient after the "normal" period of time for the procedure (perhaps due to a secondary illness affecting his recovery such as diabetes), consider billing for the services. The treatment of all but the most minor complications following surgery may be also billed.

Conspicuously missing from this definition is reference to preoperative care, such as consultations, office visits, and initial hospital care. This was apparently omitted because practices have historically varied with respect to charging for preoperative services; some practices always billed them separately while others did not. Due to the omission in CPT, many third party payers created their own definitions of allowable preoperative billing. These range from allowing all reasonable charges to restricting claims submitted up to two weeks prior to surgery.

It should be noted that Medicare defines the surgical package differently than CPT. The Medicare definition delineates the number of pre– and postoperative days which are included in the package as well as the types of services which are included. Medicare's definition is provided later in this section under the heading, "Medicare's Global Surgical Package."

Starred Procedures

Starred procedures are those procedures in CPT for which a star (or asterisk) appears to the right of the code number, such as the example shown below:

> 11305* Shaving of epidermal or dermal lesion, single lesion, scalp, neck, hands, feet, genitalia; lesion diameter 0.5 cm or less

The star indicates that the surgical package as defined above <u>does not apply</u> to the starred procedure. A separate set of rules applies to billing these starred surgical procedures. Stars are usually given to minor procedures that typically don't have any significant associated postoperative care or where the care is so variable that the package concept won't work.

The logic of the global surgical package concept is based on the predictability of an operation and its follow–up. Major differences between patients aside, the preoperative services, the operation itself, and the follow–up for any particular surgical procedure involves approximately the same level of effort from one patient to the next. Thus, each surgical procedure can have a standard charge. However, for relatively minor surgeries, this logic does not hold. One patient who is treated for a soft tissue abscess by incision may not require a follow-up visit where another might. Thus, there are separate rules for billing preoperative and postoperative services for these minor procedures:

1. If the patient is new to the practice and the major service rendered is a starred procedure, the plastic surgeon can bill for both the procedure and a new patient visit. Usually the visit is billed with a special code, 99025, or with one of the patient office visit codes.
2. If the patient is established and the major service rendered is a starred procedure, bill only for the procedure.
3. If in addition to the starred procedure the patient is seen and treated or evaluated for other problems, additional service charges may be made as appropriate.
4. If to perform the starred procedure the patient must be hospitalized, the plastic surgeon may bill for hospital visits in addition to the starred procedure.

Note that Medicare uses a different definition of the surgical package for starred procedures. The Medicare definition is discussed below as part of Medicare's minor surgical package.

Medicare's Global Surgical Package

Medicare's definition of the global surgical package differs substantially from that found in CPT. First, according to Medicare, procedures are considered to be either major or minor. Second, Medicare defines more specifically than CPT which pre– and postoperative services are included in, and excluded from, the surgical package. Medicare's global surgical package for major surgeries includes:

- Preoperative visits. These include all preoperative visits, in or out of the hospital, by the surgeon beginning with the day before the day of surgery.
- Intra–operative services. This includes all intra–operative services that are normally a usual and necessary part of a surgical procedure.
- Complications following surgery. All additional medical or surgical services required of the surgeon providing the postoperative care within 90 days of the surgery to treat complications which do not require additional trips to the operating room are included.
- Postoperative visits. Follow–up visits within 90 days after surgery that are related to recovery from the surgery are included. These services may be provided in any setting, e.g., hospital, ambulatory surgery center, surgeon's office. Visits to a patient in an intensive care or critical care unit are also included if made by the surgeon.

- Post–surgical pain management. Pain management provided by the surgeon providing the postoperative care are included in the package.
- Supplies. Except for a surgical tray for certain procedures, all supplies are included in the package.
- Miscellaneous services. Included are items such as dressing changes; local incisional care; removal of operative pack, removal of cutaneous sutures and staples, lines, wires, tubes, drains, casts, and splints; insertion, irrigation and removal of urinary catheters, routine peripheral intravenous lines, nasogastric and rectal tubes; and changes and removal of tracheotomy tubes.

The package does not include:

- The initial evaluation or consultation of the problem by the surgeon to determine the need for surgery (even if performed the day of or the day before surgery).
- Services of other doctors except when the services included in a global package are furnished by more than one doctor.
- Visits unrelated to the diagnosis for which the surgery is performed.
- Treatment for the underlying condition or an added course of treatment which is not part of the normal recovery from surgery.
- Diagnostic tests and procedures, including radiological procedures.
- Clearly distinct surgical procedures during the postoperative period which are not re–operations or treatment for complications. (A new postoperative period begins with the subsequent procedure.) These services should be reported with modifier "–79."
- Treatment for postoperative complications which require a return trip to the operating room, including ambulatory surgery centers and hospital outpatient departments. (A reduced payment rate applies.) These services should be reported using modifier "–78." No new postoperative period begins in this case.
- The surgical tray for certain procedures performed in a doctor's office.

Medicare's package for minor surgery and nonincisional procedures, which include starred procedures and diagnostic/therapeutic nonincisional endoscopic procedures, is defined the same as that for the major surgeries with two exceptions:

- The postoperative period is 10 days for some procedures. Those procedures which do not have a 90 or 10 day postoperative period have 0 days, or no postoperative period. A complete list of codes and their associated postoperative period can be obtained from your Medicare carrier. For your reference, this text provides the postoperative follow–up days for Medicare for each procedure listed.

- Visits provided on the same day as a minor surgery or endoscopy are included in the package unless a documented, separately identifiable service is furnished (generally, for a problem different from that requiring surgery). These services should be reported using modifier "–24" or "–25."

Separate Procedure Concept

About 5 percent of surgeons account for 80 percent of surgical overbillings. How do these doctors overcharge? Most do so by "fragmenting" or "unbundling" their surgical charges, for example, billing for a biopsy in addition to an excision of a neoplasm of the upper lip instead of only for the excision (which would include the biopsy). Such "a la carte" billing results in higher charges.

Because fragmented and unbundled charging may result from ignorance, it is important to be familiar with the rule related to CPT's separate procedures. Refer to CPT code 11100.

11100 Biopsy of skin, subcutaneous tissue and/or mucous membrane (including simple closure), unless otherwise listed (separate procedure); single lesion

The definition for this code contains the parenthetical note "(separate procedure)." The separate procedure notation informs the plastic surgery practice not to bill for the procedure if it is performed as part of a larger, more global service.

Think of it this way: If a surgical procedure has the words "(separate procedure)" listed as part of the definition, and it is either the only procedure performed through the incision or is not related to other procedures being performed through the incision, then the plastic surgeon can charge for the separate procedure code.

Rules Associated With Billing For Assistant Surgeons

A normal surgical assist is billed by reporting the appropriate CPT surgery code (i.e., the code(s) used by the primary surgeon) plus the "–80" modifier. Many payers will pay the assistant a predetermined percentage of the amount paid to the primary surgeon. Medicare will make payment to the assistant surgeon at 16 percent of the fee schedule amount allowed for the primary surgeon.

If two surgeons with different skills perform surgery for a patient at the same time, they would be considered co–surgeons rather than primary/assistant surgeons. Note that Medicare and many other payers will not make payment for a surgical assist in addition to payment for co–surgeons. In other words, it has to be one or the other (assist or co–surgeons), not both.

For those services where, on a national level, assistants are used in less than 5 percent of the cases, Medicare will not allow payment for a surgical assistant. As you may have noted in the "Overview and Explanation of Notations" section in the "Introduction" to this text, a notation is provided in the Reimbursement notes in this manual to help alert you to those instances where Medicare restricts payment for an assistant surgeon. Recall that "paid" means Medicare may allow payment for an assistant for this procedure. "Not paid" means Medicare has determined that an assistant surgeon is not necessary for this procedure and so will not pay for one. (You are not permitted to attempt to charge the patient for the assistant.) A "by report" notation means that the individual carrier makes a determination as to whether an assistant is payable for this service.

BILLING SUPPLIES

The code you will use for items supplied to the patient will be CPT code 99070. Think of it as the all–purpose, generic code for supplies. When billing a patient for supplies you need to keep the following factors in mind.

1. If you are billing for the first time for supplies that were previously included in the charge for the service, you are "unbundling" and thus might not be reimbursed by the carrier for the supply. Consider the plastic surgeon who in the past always provided a surgical tray as needed when performing minor surgeries in his office. Upon discovering the supply code for a surgical tray, he decides to list a separate charge for the tray in addition to his usual charge for the minor surgery. Summed together, the two charges (tray and procedure) are greater than what he had been charging when the tray was included. This is unbundling and might be interpreted by payers as an increase in charges.

2. When billing a patient for more than one supply on the same claim, list code 99070 more than once. Next to each use of 99070, describe the supply and list the charge for each.

3. When determining whether or not to bill for supplies, consider factors related to patient satisfaction. If you feel that your patients will complain that you are "padding" your bills with charges for supplies, the patient may seek care from a different plastic surgeon in the future. Use common sense when billing for supplies.

Most Medicare and Medicaid carriers reject charges for supplies when CPT code 99070 is used. Recall from the discussion of HCPCS that Medicare's HCPCS codes provide hundreds of specific codes for billing supplies. These codes should be used instead of 99070 when billing Medicare and Medicaid for supplies.

Note, however, that Medicare reimburses separately for supplies, such as surgical trays, for only a certain number of identified "facility–based" procedures which are performed in a doctor's office instead of the facility. For your reference, this text provides reference to whether Medicare will reimburse for a supply under the "Reimbursement Information" column. Be sure that the procedure for which you wish to bill the tray is identified as one for which Medicare will pay for the supply of a surgical tray. If it is not, the charge for the tray should be considered to be included as part of your charge for the procedure. You may not bill the patient for the tray, either.

CPT MODIFIERS

CPT provides two–digit modifiers which can be attached to codes. Modifiers communicate additional information to the carrier, usually that circumstances that affected the performance of a procedure or service occurred. A discussion of those modifiers relevant to plastic surgery practices is provided below.

"–20" Microsurgery

Surgical procedures for which charges are increased due to the use of microsurgical techniques require the addition of the "–20" modifier. There are three exceptions to this rule. First, if the procedure is always performed microsurgically, use of the modifier may be considered inappropriate. Second, some procedures are described as involving microsurgical techniques. In such cases, use of the modifier would be redundant. As an example of this latter point, refer to code 64727, which is for internal neurolysis requiring use of an operating microscope. When billing code 64727 you do not need to also list the "–20" modifier because the description includes it. Finally, when reporting nerve repair by suture procedures (range 64831–64876), instead of the "–20" modifier you add an additional code, 64830, to report the use of microsurgical technique.

"–21" Prolonged Evaluation and Management Services

This modifier is for use exclusively with E&M codes. In situations where the E&M service(s) provided is prolonged or otherwise greater than that usually required for the highest level of E&M service within a given category, this modifier should be used with the highest level code to report that circumstance. A special report explaining the situation may be necessary to ensure proper payment.

"–22" Unusual Service

The unusual service modifier is primarily used to denote circumstances for which a procedure or service was significantly more difficult than usual to perform or when it required significantly more time than usual to perform. Typically, the plastic surgeon also adds an additional charge for the extra time or work. This modifier is used in these circumstances. Note, however, that addition of the modifier does not guarantee increased payment. Most carriers will require support documentation for this modifier.

"–24" Unrelated Evaluation and Management Service by the Same Physician During a Postoperative Period

There are times during the follow–up period of a surgery when the plastic surgeon provides E&M services for a problem unrelated to that for which the surgery was performed. To indicate that the E&M service is not part of the global surgical package, this modifier is listed next to the E&M code. Medicare requires that support documentation be submitted when this modifier is used.

"–25" Significant, Separately Identifiable Evaluation and Management Service by the Same Physician on the Day of a Procedure

Medicare and other payers do not allow separate payment for non–surgical services provided to a patient on the day of a surgery. However, for situations where the patient's condition requires that the surgeon provide E&M services above and beyond the usual pre– and post-operative care associated with the procedure, this modifier should be used. Such services may be warranted if the patient has a condition that requires E&M services for a condition unrelated to that for which surgery is being performed, for example.

"–26" Professional Component

Many procedures include both technical and professional aspects. When billing for the professional aspects, use this modifier on the appropriate CPT code.

"–32" Mandated Services

Mandated services are those requested by an insurance carrier, peer review organization, utilization review panel, HMO, PPO or other entity. Typically, the request is for a second or third opinion regarding a patient illness or treatment. When mandated services are requested, the doctor performing the service is usually required to accept assignment from the payer, and in turn, the payer reimburses the doctor 100 percent of the payer's allowable for the service. An example of a mandated service would be a Level 2 additional opinion consultation. This would be reported as:

99272–32

The "–32" modifier is used to alert the payer's claim processors to the fact that the service was mandated and should receive special handling.

"–50" Bilateral Procedures

In 1990, all specifically listed bilateral procedure codes were deleted from CPT. Procedures are assumed to be unilateral unless they are either always performed bilaterally or are otherwise noted.

Plastic surgery practices are sometimes confused by the definition of bilateral. Bilateral procedures are identical procedures (i.e., use of the same CPT code) performed on the same anatomic site but on opposite sides of the body. Furthermore, each procedure should be performed through its own separate incision to qualify for bilateral.

The most commonly accepted method of reporting bilateral procedures is to list the procedure twice and add the "–50" modifier to the second procedure as shown below for reduction mammoplasty:

19318	Reduction mammoplasty, LEFT
19318–50	Reduction mammoplasty, RIGHT

Note that the words "right" and "left" have been added to clarify that the procedures were indeed performed bilaterally. Also, it is common to report your full charge for each procedure and let the payer reduce the amount on the second, or bilateral, procedure.

Some payers will accept an alternative method of billing bilateral procedures. This method involves listing the procedure once and adding the "–50" modifier as shown below:

19318–50 Reduction mammoplasty, bilateral

If this method is used, place a "2" in the UNITS column of the claim form so that the payer is aware that two procedures are being listed on one line. The charge reported on the claim for the procedures is typically twice that of what the doctor charges for performing one of the procedures.

"–51" Multiple Procedures

This modifier has traditionally been used to identify multiple surgical procedures performed on a patient during the same operative session. For example, debridement of skin and removal of 10 skin tags would be coded as:

11044 Debridement; skin, subcutaneous tissue, muscle, and bone
11200*–51 Removal of skin tags, multiple fibrocutaneous tags, any area; up to and including 15 lesions

Note that the higher charge procedure (for the debridement, in this case) is listed first and the multiple procedure modifier is added to the lesser or secondary service. If three procedures had been performed, the services would be ranked from highest to lowest charge on the claim form and the "–51" modifier would be added to all but the first (highest charge) procedure.

The definition of multiple procedures was expanded in the 1990 CPT to include not only multiple procedures performed during the same operative session, but to extend to multiple medical and/or surgical services performed for a patient on the same day.

Although it is acceptable to use the "–51" modifier when reporting multiple services and procedures, it is not known how many, if any, payers which require the "–51" modifier under these circumstances. Use of the "–51" modifier is usually limited to reporting multiple surgeries performed in the same operative session. However, payer policies can change overnight and OMS practices should keep abreast of the requirements of their major payers with regard to use of this modifier.

"–52" Reduced Services

When the plastic surgeon performs only a portion of, rather than the complete or total service, this modifier can be used to denote the situation. Fees for these reduced services are invariably lowered due to the fact that only part of the service was provided.

"–54" Surgical Care Only
"–55" Postoperative Management Only
"–56" Preoperative Management Only

These three modifiers may be used, as appropriate, to report that portion(s) of surgery provided by a surgeon in situations where the surgeon does not perform all the services as defined by the surgical package. For example, if the surgeon performs preoperative and intra–operative services and a different doctor handles the patient's postoperative care, then the surgeon would list modifiers "–56" and "–54" on his claim next to the appropriate surgery code. The doctor taking responsibility for the postoperative care would list the "–55" modifier.

"–57" Decision For Surgery

Many payers, including Medicare, now bundle some or all of the surgical preoperative services as part of the global surgical package. An exception is typically allowed for the evaluation and management visit during which the decision for surgery was made. If the decision for surgery was made during the period of time normally included in the global surgical package, the evaluation and management visit may be billed by adding the "–57" modifier to the reported code. For example, with one exception, Medicare does not allow for billing of preoperative services related to a surgery that are performed the day of or day before the surgery. Medicare will, however, pay for the E&M service during which the decision for surgery was made even if it was provided the day of or the day before. If the decision was made during a Level IV established patient office visit, it would be reported as 99214–57.

"–58" Staged or Related Procedure or Service by the Same Physician During the Postoperative Period.

This new modifier has been created to allow for billing of staged or related procedures that are performed by the doctor during the postoperative (follow–up) period for a procedure. It is intended for use under the following circumstances:

1. If at the time of the original procedure it was known that an additional procedure(s) would be performed, add the "–58" modifier to the additional procedure(s) when reporting it (them).
2. If a surgery during the postoperative period was more extensive or difficult than the initial procedure, add the "–58" modifier to the postop surgical procedure code.
3. When therapeutic services are provided following diagnostic surgical procedures, add the "–58" modifier to the therapy service codes.

"–62" Two Surgeons

This modifier is reported when two surgeons are acting as co–surgeons. That is, each surgeon is acting as a "primary" surgeon performing a different aspect of a complex procedure. As an example of two surgeons acting as co–surgeons, consider procedures such as a cranioplasty performed jointly by a neurosurgeon and a plastic surgeon. Each doctor might list the following on his/her claim:

62147–62 Cranioplasty with autograft (includes obtaining bone grafts); larger than 5 cm diameter

Third party payers often allow 60 percent of the prevailing to each surgeon in such cases. Medicare allows 125 percent of its global fee for the service, dividing the payment equally between the two surgeons.

"–76" Repeat Procedure By Same Physician
"–77" Repeat Procedure By Different Physician

These two modifiers are reported to note that a procedure which was previously performed was repeated. You may find it helpful to submit an explanation with the claim to justify the need to repeat the procedure and to clarify that you are not double billing for the procedure.

"–78" Return Trip to the Operating Room for a Related Procedure During the Postoperative Period

This modifier is reported for a return trip to the operating room for a related procedure during a postoperative period. This modifier is used, for instance, for complications from surgery, to indicate that another procedure was performed during the postoperative period of a related procedure.

"–79" Unrelated Procedure By the Same Physician During the Postoperative Period

During the follow–up period for a surgery, use this modifier to indicate that the performance of a service or procedure was unrelated to the original surgery. This modifier is used only on surgical services; the "–24" modifier is used for unrelated E&M services.

"–80" Assistant Surgeon
"–81" Minimum Assistant Surgeon
"–82" Assistant Surgeon (Where Qualified Resident Not Available)

These modifiers are used to identify surgical services provided by assistants. A normal surgical assist is billed by reporting the appropriate CPT surgery code (that is, the code(s) used by the primary surgeon) plus the addition of the "–80" modifier. In cases where a second assistant surgeon is warranted, his/her surgery code(s) would also list the "–81" minimum assistant surgeon modifier. It is important to note that assistant surgeons submit their charges on claims separate from those of the primary surgeon, even if both are from the same group practice or clinic. The reason is straightforward: each doctor must submit under his/her unique identification number, and by doing so, accept responsibility for the services he/she provided.

Many hospitals have surgical residency programs that provide qualified resident assistants. In hospitals where qualified residents are available, most payers will not reimburse for the services of a non–resident assistant surgeon, arguing that the fees they pay for the patient's hospitalization, use of the surgical suite, etc., include the services of the resident assistant. With one exception, the non–resident assistant's services in such situations will usually not be covered. The exception exists when (for whatever reason) a qualified resident assistant was not available at the time of the patient's surgery. In these cases the non–resident assistant surgeon may bill for the assist by adding the "–82" modifier to the surgery code(s). However, the assistant needs to obtain a note or letter from the hospital's administration stating that a qualified resident was not available, thus necessitating the services of the non–resident assistant surgeon. A copy of the note or letter should be submitted with the claim for the assistant surgeon's services. Of course, if a hospital does not have a surgical residency program, the assistant surgeon will use the "–80" modifier.

MAJOR HCPCS NATIONAL MODIFIERS

"–LT" Left Side

This modifier is used to identify procedures performed on the left side of the body.

"–RT" Right Side

This modifier is used to identify procedures performed on the right side of the body.

EVALUATION AND MANAGEMENT

OFFICE OR OTHER OUTPATIENT SERVICES
99201—99215

These codes are used to report evaluation and management services provided in the physician's office or in an outpatient or other ambulatory facility. A patient is considered an outpatient until inpatient admission to a health care facility occurs.

To report services provided to a patient who is admitted to a hospital or nursing facility in the course of an encounter in the office or other ambulatory facility, see the notes for initial hospital inpatient care (page 16) or comprehensive nursing facility assessments (see your CPT).

For services provided by physicians in the Emergency Department, see 99281–99285.

For observation care, see 99217–99220 in your CPT.

For definitions of key components, see Evaluation and Management Services Guidelines in your CPT.

New Patient
99201–99205

Established Patient
99211–99215

For definitions of new and established patients, refer to page 1 in the Coding Guidelines section of this text.

CPT CODE	SERVICE
99201	Office or other outpatient visit for the evaluation and management of a NEW patient, which requires these three key components: • a problem focused history • a problem focused examination; and • straightforward medical decision making. Counseling and/or coordination of care with other providers or agencies are provided consistent with the nature of the problem(s) and the patient's and/or family's needs. Usually, the presenting problem(s) are self limited or minor. Physicians typically spend 10 minutes face-to-face with the patient and/or family.

EXAMPLES

- ♦ Initial office visit with 65–year–old male for reassurance about an isolated seborrheic keratosis on the upper back.
- ♦ Initial office visit with 5-year old female to remove sutures from simple wound, placed by another physician.

ICD–9–CM

173.x	Malignant neoplasm, Skin
214.0	Lipoma, Skin of face
214.1	Lipoma, Skin NEC
216.x	Benign neoplasm, Skin
229.8	Benign neoplasm NEC
232.3	CA in situ, Skin of face NEC
238.2	UB-Neoplasm, Skin
701.x	Hypertrophic/atrophic skin
702.x	Other dermatosis
707.1	Chronic ulcer of the leg
709.9	Skin disorder NOS
727.03	Trigger finger
728.6	Contracture of palmar fascia
782.2	Localized superficial swelling
883.x	Open wound of finger(s)

REIMBURSEMENT INFORMATION

General

- ♦ See notes on page 3.

Medicare

- ♦ Outpatient Limit — applies

CPT CODE	SERVICE
99202	Office or other outpatient visit for the evaluation and management of a NEW patient, which requires these three key components: • an expanded problem focused history • an expanded problem focused examination; and • straightforward medical decision making. Counseling and/or coordination of care with other providers or agencies are provided consistent with the nature of the problem(s) and the patient's and/or family's needs. Usually the presenting problem(s) are of low to moderate severity. Physicians typically spend 20 minutes face-to-face with the patient and/or family.

EXAMPLE

♦ Initial office visit for a patient presenting with itching and discussion of treatment of rhinophyma.

ICD–9–CM

173.x	Malignant neoplasm, Skin
195.0	M-Neoplasm, Head/face/neck
214.1	Lipoma, Skin NEC
216.x	Benign neoplasm, Skin
229.8	Benign neoplasm NEC
232.3	CA in situ, Skin of face NEC
238.2	UB-Neoplasm, Skin
354.0	Carpal tunnel syndrome
374.3x	Ptosis of eyelid
611.x	Disorders of breast
701.x	Hypertrophic/atrophic skin
702.x	Other dermatosis
706.2	Sebaceous cyst
707.x	Chronic ulcer of skin
709.0	Dyschromia
709.2	Scar/fibrosis of skin
714.0	Rheumatoid arthritis
882.x	Open wound of hand
883.x	Open wound of finger(s)
891.x	Open wound of knee, leg, ankle

REIMBURSEMENT INFORMATION

General

♦ See notes on page 3.

Medicare

♦ Outpatient Limit — applies

CPT CODE	SERVICE
99203	Office or other outpatient visit for the evaluation and management of a NEW patient, which requires these three key components: • a detailed history • a detailed examination; and • medical decision making of low complexity. Counseling and/or coordination of care with other providers or agencies are provided consistent with the nature of the problem(s) and the patient's and/or family's needs. Usually, the presenting problems are of moderate severity. Physicians typically spend 30 minutes face-to-face with the patient and/or family.

EXAMPLE

- Initial office visit of 49-year-old male with nasal obstruction. Detailed exam with topical anesthesia.

ICD–9–CM

173.x	Malignant neoplasm, Skin
195.0	M-Neoplasm, Head/face/neck
216.1	B-Neoplasm, Skin of eyelid/canthus
216.2	B-Neoplasm, Skin of ear
216.3	B-Neoplasm, Skin of face NEC
232.3	CA in situ, Skin of face NEC
238.2	UB-Neoplasm, Skin
239.2	Bone/Skin neoplasm NOS
470.	Deviated nasal septum
611.1	Hypertrophy of breast
611.8	Breast disorders NEC
701.1	Keratoderma, acquired
702.0	Actinic keratosis
707.x	Chronic ulcer of skin
709.2	Scar/fibrosis of skin
709.9	Skin disorder NOS
727.0x	Synovitis and tenosynovitis
728.6	Contracture of palmar fascia
882.x	Open wound of hand
883.x	Open wound of finger(s)
891.x	Open wound of knee, leg, ankle

REIMBURSEMENT INFORMATION

General

- See notes on page 3.

Medicare

- Outpatient Limit — applies

CPT CODE	SERVICE
99204	Office or other outpatient visit for the evaluation and management of a NEW patient, which requires these three components:

- a comprehensive history
- a comprehensive examination; and
- medical decision making of moderate complexity.

Counseling and/or coordination of care with other providers or agencies are provided consistent with the nature of the problem(s) and the patient's and/or family's needs.

Usually, the presenting problem(s) are of moderate to high severity. Physicians typically spend 45 minutes face-to-face with the patient and/or family.

EXAMPLE

♦ Initial office visit for evaluation of 70–year–old female with polyarthralgia.

ICD–9–CM

173.x	Malignant neoplasm, Skin
216.1	B-Neoplasm, Skin of eyelid/canthus
216.5	B-Neoplasm, Skin of trunk
216.6	B-Neoplasm, Skin of arm
232.3	CA in situ, Skin of face NEC
238.2	UB-Neoplasm, Skin
239.2	Bone/Skin neoplasm NOS
374.3x	Ptosis of eyelid
611.1	Hypertrophy of breast
611.7x	Signs and symptoms in breast
611.8	Breast disorders NEC
707.x	Chronic ulcer of skin
709.x	Skin & subcutaneous tissue disorder
727.0x	Synovitis and tenosynovitis
728.6	Contracture of palmar fascia
785.4	Gangrene
800.00	Closed skull vault Fx
801.00	Closed skull base fracture
802.4	Fx malar/maxillary, closed
996.54	Breast prosthesis malfunction

REIMBURSEMENT INFORMATION

General

♦ See notes on page 3.

Medicare

♦ Outpatient Limit — applies

CPT CODE	SERVICE
99205	Office or other outpatient visit for the evaluation and management of a NEW patient, which requires these three key components: • a comprehensive history • a comprehensive examination; and • medical decision making of high complexity. Counseling and/or coordination of care with other providers or agencies are provided consistent with the nature of the problem(s) and the patient's and/or family's needs. Usually, the presenting problem(s) are of moderate to high severity. Physicians typically spend 60 minutes face-to-face with the patient and/or family.

EXAMPLE

- ♦ Initial office visit for a severely diabetic patient with multiple leg ulcers.

ICD–9–CM

173.1	M-Neoplasm, Skin of eyelid/canthus
173.3	M-Neoplasm, Skin of face NEC
174.x	Malignant neoplasm, Female breast
216.3	B-Neoplasm, Skin of face NEC
238.2	UB-Neoplasm, Skin
374.3x	Ptosis of eyelid
611.8	Breast disorders NEC
707.0	Decubitus ulcer
707.1	Chronic ulcer of the leg
709.9	Skin disorder NOS
728.6	Contracture of palmar fascia

REIMBURSEMENT INFORMATION

General

- ♦ See notes on page 3.

Medicare

- ♦ Outpatient Limit — applies

CPT CODE	SERVICE
99211	Office or other outpatient visit for the evaluation and management of an ESTABLISHED patient, that may not require the presence of a physician. Usually, the presenting problem(s) are minimal. Typically, 5 minutes are spent performing or supervising these services.

EXAMPLES

- Office visit for a 50-year-old male, established patient, for removal of uncomplicated sutures.
- Office visit for a 19-year-old established patient, for removal of sutures from a two cm. laceration of forehead, which you placed four days ago in ER.
- Office visit for a 69-year-old female, established patient, for partial removal of antibiotic gauze from an infected wound site.

ICD–9–CM

173.x	Malignant neoplasm, Skin
174.x	Malignant neoplasm, Female breast
195.0	M-Neoplasm, Head/face/neck
216.x	Benign neoplasm, Skin
232.3	CA in situ, Skin of face NEC
238.2	UB-Neoplasm, Skin
454.x	Varicose veins of lower extremity
611.1	Hypertrophy of breast
682.6	Cellulitis of leg
701.x	Hypertrophic/atrophic skin
702.x	Other dermatosis
706.0	Acne varioliformis
706.1	Acne NEC
706.3	Seborrhea
707.x	Chronic ulcer of skin
709.00	Dyschromia, unspecified
709.9	Skin disorder NOS
V10.83	Hx of skin malignancy NEC
V51.	Aftercare w/plastic surgery
V58.3	Attention to surg dressing/suture
V67.0	Surgery follow-up
V71.1	Observation, suspect malignant neop

REIMBURSEMENT INFORMATION

General

- See notes on page 3.

Medicare

- Outpatient Limit — applies

CPT CODE	SERVICE
99212	Office or other outpatient visit for the evaluation and management of an ESTABLISHED patient, which requires at least TWO of these three key components:

- a problem focused history
- a problem focused examination
- straightforward medical decision making.

Counseling and/or coordination of care with other providers or agencies are provided consistent with the nature of the problem(s) and the patient's and/or family's needs.

Usually, the presenting problem(s) are self limited or minor. Physicians typically spend 10 minutes face-to-face with the patient and/or family.

EXAMPLE

- ♦ Office visit for 22-year-old male, established patient, one month after I & D of "wrestler's ear."
- ♦ Office visit for an established patient with an irritated skin tag for reassurance.

ICD–9–CM

173.x	Malignant neoplasm, Skin
195.0	M-Neoplasm, Head/face/neck
216.x	Benign neoplasm, Skin
232.3	CA in situ, Skin of face NEC
611.1	Hypertrophy of breast
611.8	Breast disorders NEC
701.1	Keratoderma, acquired
702.0	Actinic keratosis
702.1	Seborrheic keratosis
707.x	Chronic ulcer of skin
785.4	Gangrene
883.x	Open wound of finger(s)
891.x	Open wound of knee, leg, ankle
892.x	Open wound of foot
998.3	Postop wound disruption
V10.82	Hx of malignant skin melanoma
V10.83	Hx of skin malignancy NEC
V67.0	Surgery follow-up

REIMBURSEMENT INFORMATION

General

- ♦ See notes on page 3.

Medicare

- ♦ Outpatient Limit — applies

CPT CODE	SERVICE
99213	Office or other outpatient visit for the evaluation and management of an ESTABLISHED patient, which requires at least TWO of these three key components: • an expanded problem focused history • an expanded problem focused examination • medical decision making of low complexity. Counseling and coordination of care are provided consistent with the nature of the problem(s) and the patient's and/or family's needs. Usually, the presenting problem(s) are of low to moderate severity. Physicians typically spend 15 minutes face-to-face with the patient and/or family.

EXAMPLE

◆ Office visit for a 70-year-old female, established patient, one year post excision of basal cell carcinoma of nose with nasolabial flap. Now presents with new suspicious recurrent lesion and suspicious lesion of the back.

ICD–9–CM

173.x	Malignant neoplasm, Skin
216.x	Benign neoplasm, Skin
354.0	Carpal tunnel syndrome
454.2	Varicose leg w/ulcer+inflammation
611.1	Hypertrophy of breast
611.8	Breast disorders NEC
682.x	Cellulitis and abscess
701.1	Keratoderma, acquired
701.4	Keloid scar
706.2	Sebaceous cyst
707.x	Chronic ulcer of skin
709.2	Scar/fibrosis of skin
727.03	Trigger finger
728.6	Contracture of palmar fascia
883.x	Open wound of finger(s)
892.x	Open wound of foot
V10.83	Hx of skin malignancy NEC
V67.0	Surgery follow-up

REIMBURSEMENT INFORMATION

General

◆ See notes on page 3.

Medicare

◆ Outpatient Limit — applies

CPT CODE	SERVICE	ICD–9–CM

99214 Office or other outpatient visit for the evaluation and management of an ESTABLISHED patient, which requires at least TWO of these three key components:

- a detailed history
- a detailed examination
- medical decision making of moderate complexity.

Counseling and/or coordination of care with other providers or agencies are provided consistent with the nature of the problem(s) and the patient's and/or family's needs.

Usually, the presenting problem(s) are of moderate to high severity. Physicians typically spend 25 minutes face-to-face with the patient and/or family.

EXAMPLE

◆ Office visit for a 25-year-old female, established patient, for evaluation of progressive saddle nose deformity of unknown etiology.

ICD–9–CM	
173.x	Malignant neoplasm, Skin
216.x	Benign neoplasm, Skin
238.2	UB-Neoplasm, Skin
250.00	Diabetes, uncomplicated, type II
454.0	Leg varicosity w/ulcer
611.1	Hypertrophy of breast
611.72	Lump or mass in breast
611.8	Breast disorders NEC
696.1	Other psoriasis
707.x	Chronic ulcer of skin
882.x	Open wound of hand
883.x	Open wound of finger(s)
891.x	Open wound of knee, leg, ankle
V10.3	Hx of breast malignancy
V10.83	Hx of skin malignancy NEC

REIMBURSEMENT INFORMATION

General

◆ See notes on page 3.

Medicare

◆ Outpatient Limit — applies

99215 Office or other outpatient visit for the evaluation and management of an ESTABLISHED patient, which requires at least TWO of these three key components:

- a comprehensive history
- a comprehensive examination
- medical decision making of high complexity.

Counseling and/or coordination of care with other providers or agencies are provided consistent with the nature of the problem(s) and the patient's and/or family's needs.

Usually, the presenting problem(s) are of moderate to high severity. Physicians typically spend 40 minutes face-to-face with the patient and/or family.

EXAMPLE

◆ Office visit for an established patient, two years post–burn with bilateral ectropion, hypertrophic facial burn scars, near absence of left breast, and burn syndactyly of both hands. Discussion of treatment options following examination.

ICD–9–CM	
173.x	Malignant neoplasm, Skin
238.2	UB-Neoplasm, Skin
707.x	Chronic ulcer of skin
714.0	Rheumatoid arthritis
729.6	Old foreign body in soft tissue
882.x	Open wound of hand
883.x	Open wound of finger(s)
891.x	Open wound of knee, leg, ankle
892.x	Open wound of foot

REIMBURSEMENT INFORMATION

General

◆ See notes on page 3.

Medicare

◆ Outpatient Limit — applies

HOSPITAL OBSERVATION SERVICES 99217–99220

These codes are used to report evaluation and management services provided to patients designated/admitted as "observation status" in a hospital. It is not necessary that the patient be located in an observation area designated by the hospital. If such an area does exist in a hospital (as a separate unit in the hospital, in the emergency department, etc.), these codes are to be utilized if the patient is placed in such an area.

For definitions of key components and commonly used terms, please see Evaluation and Management Services Guidelines in your CPT.

Typical times have not yet been established for this category of services.

Observation Care Discharge Services 99217

Observation care discharge of a patient from "observation status" includes final examination of the patient, discussion of the hospital stay, instructions for continuing care, and preparation of discharge records.

Initial Observation Care 99218–99220

These codes are used to report the encounter(s) by the supervising physician with the patient when designated as "observation status." This refers to the initiation of observation status, supervision of the care plan for observation and performance of periodic reassessments. For observation encounters by other physicians, see Office or Other Outpatient Consultation codes (pages 22–23).

To report services provided to a patient who is admitted to the hospital after receiving hospital observation care services on the same date, see the notes for initial hospital inpatient care (page 16). For a patient admitted to the hospital on a date subsequent to the date of observation status, the hospital admission would be reported with the appropriate Initial Hospital Care Codes (page 16). Do not report observation discharge in conjunction with the hospital admission.

When "observation status" is initiated in the course of an encounter in another site of service (e.g., hospital emergency department, physician's office, nursing facility) all evaluation and management services provided by the supervising physician in conjunction with initiating "observation status" are considered part of the initial observation care when performed on the same date. The observation care level of service reported by the supervising physician should include the services related to initiating "observation status" provided in the other sites of service as well as in the observation setting.

Evaluation and management services on the same date provided in sites that are not related to initiating "observation status" should NOT be reported separately.

These codes may not be utilized for post–operative recovery if the procedure is considered part of the surgical "package." This code applies to all Evaluation and Management services that are provided on the same date of initiating "observation status."

CPT CODE	SERVICE	ICD–9–CM
99217	Observation care discharge day management	

CPT NOTES

- This code is to be utilized by the physician to report all services provided to a patient on discharge from "observation status" if the discharge is on other than the initial date of "observation status." To report services to a patient designated as "observation status" who is discharged on the same date, use only the codes for Initial Observation Services (99218-99220).

REIMBURSEMENT INFORMATION

General

- See notes on page 13.

Medicare

- Outpatient Limit — does not apply

99218 Initial observation care, per day, for the evaluation and management of a patient which requires these three key components:

- a detailed or comprehensive history
- a detailed or comprehensive examination; and
- straightforward or low complexity medical decision making.

Counseling and/or coordination of care with other providers or agencies are provided consistent with the nature of the problem(s) and the patient's and/or family's needs.

Usually, the problem(s) requiring admission to "observation status" are of low severity.

354.0	Carpal tunnel syndrome
454.0	Leg varicosity w/ulcer
707.x	Chronic ulcer of skin
749.1x	Cleft lip
749.2x	Cleft palate w/cleft lip
813.21	Fx radius shaft, closed
813.23	Fx shaft radius w/ulna, closed

REIMBURSEMENT INFORMATION

General

- See notes on page 13.

Medicare

- Outpatient Limit — does not apply

CPT CODE	SERVICE	ICD-9-CM
99219	Initial observation care, per day, for the evaluation and management of a patient, which requires these three key components: • a comprehensive history • a comprehensive examination; and • medical decision making of moderate complexity. Counseling and/or coordination of care with other providers or agencies are provided consistent with the nature of the problem(s) and the patient's and/or family's needs. Usually, the problem(s) requiring admission to "observation status" are of moderate severity.	802.4 Fx malar/maxillary, closed 813.41 Colles' fracture, closed 892.1 Open wound of foot, complicated **REIMBURSEMENT INFORMATION** General ◆ See notes on page 13. Medicare ◆ Outpatient Limit — does not apply
99220	Initial observation care, per day, for the evaluation and management of a patient, which requires these three key components: • a comprehensive history • a comprehensive examination; and • medical decision making of high complexity. Counseling and/or coordination of care with other providers or agencies are provided consistent with the nature of the problem(s) and the patient's and/or family's needs. Usually, the problem(s) requiring admission to "observation status" are of high severity.	173.3 M-Neoplasm, Skin of face NEC 802.x Fracture of face bones 948.00 Burn, 0-10% surface, 0-9% 3rd deg **REIMBURSEMENT INFORMATION** General ◆ See notes on page 13. Medicare ◆ Outpatient Limit — does not apply

HOSPITAL INPATIENT SERVICES
99221–99238

These codes are used to report evaluation and management services provided to hospital inpatients. Hospital inpatient services include those services provided to patients in a "partial hospital" setting. These codes are to be used to report these partial hospitalization services. See also psychiatry notes in the full text of CPT.

For definitions of key components and commonly used terms, please see Evaluation and Management Services Guidelines in your CPT. For hospital observation services, see 99218–99220.

Initlal Hospital Care
New Or Established Patient
99221–99223

These codes are used to report the first hospital inpatient encounter with the patient by the admitting physician. For initial inpatient encounters by physicians other than the admitting physician, see initial inpatient consultation codes (99251–99255) or subsequent hospital care codes (99231–99233) as appropriate.

When the patient is admitted to the hospital as an inpatient in the course of an encounter in another site of service (e.g., hospital emergency department, observation status in a hospital, physician's office, nursing facility) all evaluation and management services provided by that physician in conjunction with that admission are considered part of the initial hospital care when performed on the same date as the admission. The inpatient care level of service reported by the admitting physician should include the services related to the admission he/she provided in the other sites of service as well as the inpatient setting.

Evaluation and management services on the same date provided in sites other than the hospital that are related to the admission should NOT be reported separately.

Subsequent Hospital Care
99231–99233

All levels of subsequent hospital care include reviewing the medical record and reviewing the results of diagnostic studies and changes in the patient's status (i.e., changes in history, physical condition and response to management) since the last assessment by the physician.

Hospital Discharge Services
99238

Final hospital discharge of a patient includes final examination of the patient, discussion of the hospital stay, instructions for continuing care, and preparation of discharge records.

CPT CODE	SERVICE	ICD–9–CM	
99221	Initial hospital care, per day, for the evaluation and management of a patient which requires these three key components: • a detailed or comprehensive history • a detailed or comprehensive examination; and • straightforward or low complexity medical decision making. Counseling and/or coordination of care with other providers or agencies are provided consistent with the nature of the problem(s) and the patient's and/or family's needs. Usually, the problem(s) requiring admission are of low severity. Physicians typically spend 30 minutes at the bedside and on the patient's hospital floor or unit.	173.3 250.x 681.x 682.x 707.x 785.4 802.x 882.x 891.x 941.20 942.20 943.x 944.x 945.x	M-Neoplasm, Skin of face NEC Diabetes mellitus Cellulitis/abscess of finger/toe Cellulitis and abscess Chronic ulcer of skin Gangrene Fracture of face bones Open wound of hand Open wound of knee, leg, ankle 2nd deg burn, face/head/unspec 2nd deg burn trunk NOS Burn of upper limb Burn of wrist and hand Burn of lower limb

EXAMPLE

- ♦ Initial hospital visit for a 12-year-old patient with a laceration of the upper eyelid, involving the lid margin and superior canaliculus, admitted prior to surgery for IV antibiotic therapy.

REIMBURSEMENT INFORMATION

General

- ♦ See notes on page 16.

Medicare

- ♦ Outpatient Limit — does not apply

CPT CODE	SERVICE	ICD–9–CM	
99222	Initial hospital care, per day, for the evaluation and management of a patient, which requires these three key components: • a comprehensive history • a comprehensive examination; and • medical decision making of moderate complexity. Counseling and/or coordination of care with other providers or agencies are provided consistent with the nature of the problem(s) and the patient's and/or family's needs. Usually, the problem(s) requiring admission are of moderate severity. Physicians typically spend 50 minutes at the bedside and on the patient's hospital floor or unit.	173.3 681.x 682.x 707.x 802.x 941.20 942.20 943.x 944.x 945.x	M-Neoplasm, Skin of face NEC Cellulitis/abscess of finger/toe Cellulitis and abscess Chronic ulcer of skin Fracture of face bones 2nd deg burn, face/head/unspec 2nd deg burn trunk NOS Burn of upper limb Burn of wrist and hand Burn of lower limb

EXAMPLE

- ♦ Initial hospital visit for a 5–year–old patient with 2nd degree durns over face and neck.

REIMBURSEMENT INFORMATION

General

- ♦ See notes on page 16.

Medicare

- ♦ Outpatient Limit — does not apply

CPT CODE	SERVICE
99223	Initial hospital care, per day, for the evaluation and management of a patient, which requires these three key components: • a comprehensive history • a comprehensive examination; and • medical decision making of high complexity. Counseling and/or coordination of care with other providers or agencies are provided consistent with the nature of the problem(s) and the patient's and/or family's needs. Usually, the problem(s) requiring admission are of high severity. Physicians typically spend 70 minutes at the bedside and on the patient's hospital floor or unit.

EXAMPLES

- ♦ Initial hospital visit for a 26-year-old female for evaluation of severe facial fractures (LeFort's II/III).
- ♦ Initial hospital visit for a 55-year-old female for bilateral mandibular fractures resulting in flail mandible and airway obstruction.

ICD–9–CM

173.x	Malignant neoplasm, Skin
682.x	Cellulitis and abscess
707.x	Chronic ulcer of skin
728.6	Contracture of palmar fascia
883.1	Open wound of finger, complicated
891.1	Open wound of knee/leg/ankle, compl
941.20	2nd deg burn, face/head/unspec
942.20	2nd deg burn trunk NOS
943.x	Burn of upper limb
944.x	Burn of wrist and hand
945.x	Burn of lower limb

REIMBURSEMENT INFORMATION

General

- ♦ See notes on page 16.

Medicare

- ♦ Outpatient Limit — does not apply

CPT CODE	SERVICE
99231	Subsequent hospital care, per day, for the evaluation and management of a patient, which requires at least TWO of these three key components:

- a problem focused interval history
- a problem focused examination
- straightforward or low complexity medical decision making.

Counseling and/or coordination of care with other providers or agencies are provided consistent with the nature of the problem(s) and the patient's and/or family's needs.

Usually, the patient is stable, recovering or improving. Physicians typically spend 15 minutes at the bedside and on the patient's hospital floor or unit.

EXAMPLES

- ♦ Subsequent hospital visit for a 27-year-old male two days after open reduction and internal fixation for malar complex fracture.
- ♦ Subsequent hospital visit for a 36-year-old female with stable post-rhinoplasty epistaxis.

ICD–9–CM

250.x	Diabetes mellitus
443.x	Peripheral vascular disease
454.0	Leg varicosity w/ulcer
599.0	Urinary tract infection NOS
682.x	Cellulitis and abscess
686.9	Local skin infection NOS
707.x	Chronic ulcer of skin
728.9	Muscle/ligament disorder NOS
802.4	Fx malar/maxillary, closed
802.6	Fx orbital floor, closed
873.x	Open wound of head
876.x	Open wound of back
877.x	Open wound of buttock
879.0	Open wound of breast
891.x	Open wound of knee, leg, ankle
892.x	Open wound of foot
906.x	Late effect of skin/tissue injury
941.20	2nd deg burn, face/head/unspec
945.32	3rd deg burn, foot

REIMBURSEMENT INFORMATION

General

- ♦ See notes on page 16.

Medicare

- ♦ Outpatient Limit — does not apply

CPT CODE	SERVICE
99233	Subsequent hospital care, per day, for the evaluation and management of a patient, which requires at least TWO of these three key components:

- a detailed interval history
- a detailed examination
- medical decision making of high complexity.

Counseling and/or coordination of care with other providers or agencies are provided consistent with the nature of the problem(s) and the patient's and/or family's needs.

Usually, the patient is unstable or has developed a significant complication or a significant new problem. Physicians typically spend 35 minutes at the bedside and on the patient's hospital floor or unit.

EXAMPLE

◆ Subsequent hospital visit for a 44–year–old patient with electrical burns to the left arm with ascending infection.

ICD–9–CM

454.0	Leg varicosity w/ulcer
682.7	Cellulitis of foot
707.x	Chronic ulcer of skin
730.x	Infections involving bone
785.4	Gangrene
879.0	Open wound of breast
879.1	Open wound of breast, complicated
945.32	3rd deg burn, foot
949.3	3rd degree burn, NOS

REIMBURSEMENT INFORMATION

General

◆ See notes on page 16.

Medicare

◆ Outpatient Limit — does not apply

CPT CODE	SERVICE
99238	Hospital discharge day management (final day of a multiple day stay)

CPT NOTES

- This code is to be utilized by the physician to report all services provided to a patient on the date of discharge, if other than the initial date of inpatient status. To report services to a patient who is admitted as an inpatient, and discharged on the same date, use only the codes for Initial Hospital Inpatient Services, 99221-99223. To report concurrent care services provided by a physician(s) other than the attending physician, use subsequent hospital care codes (99231-99233) on the day of discharge.
- For Observation Care Discharge, use 99217.

ICD–9–CM

038.1	Staphylococcal septicemia
216.6	B-Neoplasm, Skin of arm
250.x	Diabetes mellitus
354.0	Carpal tunnel syndrome
459.9	Circulatory disease NOS
681.x	Cellulitis/abscess of finger/toe
682.x	Cellulitis and abscess
707.x	Chronic ulcer of skin
784.7	Epistaxis
785.4	Gangrene
958.3	Posttraumatic wound infection NEC
998.1	Hemorrhage complicating a procedure

REIMBURSEMENT INFORMATION

General

- See notes on page 16.

Medicare

- Outpatient Limit — does not apply

CONSULTATIONS
99241–99275

A consultation is a type of service provided by a physician whose opinion or advice regarding evaluation and/or management of a specific problem is requested by another physician or other appropriate source.

A physician consultant may initiate diagnostic and/or therapeutic services.

The request for a consultation from the attending physician or other appropriate source and the need for consultation must be documented in the patient's medical record. The consultant's opinion and any services that were ordered or performed must also be documented in the patient's medical record and communicated to the requesting physician or other appropriate source.

A "consultation" initiated by a patient and/or family, and not requested by a physician, is not reported using the initial consultation codes but may be reported using the codes for confimatory consultation or office visits, as appropriate. If a confirmatory consultation is required, e.g., by a third party payor, the modifier "–32" or 09932, mandated services, should also be reported.

Any specifically identifiable procedure (i.e., identified with a specific CPT code) performed on or subsequent to the date of the initial consultation should be reported separately.

If subsequent to the completion of a consultation, the consultant assumes responsibility for management of a portion or all of the patient's condition(s), the follow–up consultation codes should not be used. In the hospital setting, the physician receiving the patient for partial or complete transfer of care should use the appropriate inpatient hospital consultation code for the initial encounter and then subsequent hospital care codes (not follow–up consultation codes). In the office setting, the appropriate established patient code should be used.

There are four subcategories of consultations: office, initial inpatient, follow–up inpatient, and confirmatory. See each subcategory for specific reporting instructions.

For definitions of key components and commonly used terms, please see Evaluation and Management Services Guidelines in your CPT.

Office or Other Outpatient Consultations
New or Established Patient
99241–99245

These codes are used to report consultations provided in the physician's office or in an outpatient or other ambulatory facility, including hospital observation services, home services, domiciliary, rest home, custodial care, or emergency department (see consultation definition above).

Follow–up visits in the consultant's office or other outpatient facility that are initiated by the physician consultant are reported using office visit codes for established patients (99211–99215). If an additional request for an opinion or advice regarding the same or a new problem is received from the attending physician and documented in the medical record, the office consultation codes may be used again.

CONSULTATIONS, cont'd.

Initial Inpatient Consultations
New or Established Patient
99251–99255

These codes are used to report physician consultations provided to hospital inpatients, residents of nursing facilities, or patients in a partial hospital setting. Only one initial consultation should be reported by a consultant per admission.

Follow–Up Inpatient Consultations
Established Patient
99261–99263

Follow–up consultations are visits to complete the initial consultation OR subsequent consultative visits requested by the attending physician. A follow–up consultation includes monitoring progress, recommending management modifications or advising on a new plan of care in response to changes in the patient's status.

If the physician consultant has initiated treatment at the initial consultation, and participates thereafter in the patient's management, the codes for subsequent hospital care should be used (99231–99233).

These codes are used to report follow–up consultations provided to hospital inpatients or nursing facility residents only. For consultative services provided in other settings, the codes for office or other outpatient consultations should be reported (99241–99245).

Confirmatory Consultations
New or Established Patient
99271–99275

These codes are used to report the evaluation and management services provided to patients when the consulting physician is aware of the confirmatory nature of the opinion sought (e.g., when a second/third opinion is requested or required on the necessity or appropriateness of a previously recommended medical treatment or surgical procedure). Confirmatory consultations may be provided in any setting.

A physician consultant providing a confirmatory consultation is expected to provide an opinion and/or advice only. Any services subsequent to the opinion are coded at the appropriate level of office visit, established patient, or subsequent hospital care. If a confirmatory consultation is required, e.g., by a third party payor, the modifier "–32" or 09932, mandated services, should also be reported. (See also Consultation Notes, above.)

Typical times have not yet been established for this subcategory of services.

CPT CODE	SERVICE
99241	Office consultation for a new or established patient, which requires these three key components: • a problem focused history • a problem focused examination; and • straightforward medical decision making. Counseling and/or coordination of care with other providers or agencies are provided consistent with the nature of the problem(s) and the patient's and/or family's needs. Usually, the presenting problem(s) are self limited or minor. Physicians typically spend 15 minutes face-to-face with the patient and/or family.

ICD–9–CM

173.x	Malignant neoplasm, Skin
214.0	Lipoma, Skin of face
214.1	Lipoma, Skin NEC
216.x	Benign neoplasm, Skin
238.2	UB-Neoplasm, Skin
239.2	Bone/Skin neoplasm NOS
354.0	Carpal tunnel syndrome
701.1	Keratoderma, acquired
701.4	Keloid scar
702.x	Other dermatosis
707.x	Chronic ulcer of skin
709.2	Scar/fibrosis of skin
709.9	Skin disorder NOS
782.2	Localized superficial swelling
V50.1	Plastic surgery NEC

REIMBURSEMENT INFORMATION

General

- ◆ See notes on pages 22–23.

Medicare

- ◆ Outpatient Limit — applies

CPT CODE	SERVICE
99242	Office consultation for a new or established patient, which requires these three key components: • an expanded problem focused history • an expanded problem focused examination; and • straightforward medical decision making. Counseling and/or coordination of care with other providers or agencies are provided consistent with the nature of the problem(s) and the patient's and/or family's needs. Usually, the presenting problem(s) are of low severity. Physicians typically spend 30 minutes face-to-face with the patient and/or family.

EXAMPLE

- ♦ Initial office consultation for a 66-year-old female with wrist and hand pain, numbness of finger tips, suspected median nerve compression by carpal tunnel syndrome.

ICD–9–CM

173.x	Malignant neoplasm, Skin
195.0	M-Neoplasm, Head/face/neck
216.x	Benign neoplasm, Skin
238.2	UB-Neoplasm, Skin
239.2	Bone/Skin neoplasm NOS
354.0	Carpal tunnel syndrome
374.34	Blepharochalasis
454.0	Leg varicosity w/ulcer
611.1	Hypertrophy of breast
611.8	Breast disorders NEC
659.3	Generalized infection during labor
690.	Erythematosquamous dermatosis
692.9	Dermatitis NOS
701.4	Keloid scar
707.x	Chronic ulcer of skin
727.x	Disorders of synovium/tendon/bursa
802.x	Fracture of face bones
883.x	Open wound of finger(s)
891.x	Open wound of knee, leg, ankle
892.x	Open wound of foot

REIMBURSEMENT INFORMATION

General

- ♦ See notes on pages 22–23.

Medicare

- ♦ Outpatient Limit — applies

CPT CODE	SERVICE	ICD-9-CM
99243	Office consultation for a new or established patient, which requires these three key components: • a detailed history • a detailed examination; and • medical decision making of low complexity. Counseling and/or coordination of care with other providers or agencies are provided consistent with the nature of the problem(s) and the patient's and/or family's needs. Usually, the presenting problem(s) are of moderate severity. Physicians typically spend 40 minutes face-to-face with the patient and/or family.	173.x Malignant neoplasm, Skin 216.x Benign neoplasm, Skin 238.2 UB-Neoplasm, Skin 239.2 Bone/Skin neoplasm NOS 354.0 Carpal tunnel syndrome 374.34 Blepharochalasis 611.1 Hypertrophy of breast 611.8 Breast disorders NEC 701.4 Keloid scar 706.2 Sebaceous cyst 707.x Chronic ulcer of skin 714.0 Rheumatoid arthritis 728.6 Contracture of palmar fascia 891.x Open wound of knee, leg, ankle 892.x Open wound of foot **REIMBURSEMENT INFORMATION** General ♦ See notes on pages 22–23. Medicare ♦ Outpatient Limit — applies
99244	Office consultation for a new or established patient, which requires these three key components: • a comprehensive history • a comprehensive examination; and • medical decision making of moderate complexity. Counseling and/or coordination of care with other providers or agencies are provided consistent with the nature of the problem(s) and the patient's and/or family's needs. Usually, the presenting problem(s) are of moderate to high severity. Physicians typically spend 60 minutes face-to-face with the patient and/or family.	172.3 Malignant melanoma, Face NEC/NOS 173.x Malignant neoplasm, Skin 174.x Malignant neoplasm, Female breast 195.0 M-Neoplasm, Head/face/neck 238.2 UB-Neoplasm, Skin 374.3x Ptosis of eyelid 470. Deviated nasal septum 611.1 Hypertrophy of breast 611.8 Breast disorders NEC 686.9 Local skin infection NOS 701.4 Keloid scar 707.x Chronic ulcer of skin 709.2 Scar/fibrosis of skin 802.4 Fx malar/maxillary, closed 996.54 Breast prosthesis malfunction **REIMBURSEMENT INFORMATION** General ♦ See notes on pages 22–23. Medicare ♦ Outpatient Limit — applies

CPT CODE	SERVICE	ICD-9-CM
99245	Office consultation for a new or established patient which requires these three key components: • a comprehensive history • a comprehensive examination; and • medical decision making of high complexity. Counseling and/or coordination of care with other providers or agencies are provided consistent with the nature of the problem(s) and the patient's and/or family's needs. Usually, the presenting problem(s) are of moderate to high severity. Physicians typically spend 80 minutes face-to-face with the patient and/or family.	172.9 Malignant melanoma, Skin NOS 173.x Malignant neoplasm, Skin 174.x Malignant neoplasm, Female breast 216.x Benign neoplasm, Skin 354.0 Carpal tunnel syndrome 374.3x Ptosis of eyelid 611.1 Hypertrophy of breast 611.71 Mastodynia 611.8 Breast disorders NEC 701.9 Hypertrophic/atrophic skin NOS 707.x Chronic ulcer of skin 709.2 Scar/fibrosis of skin 730.0x Acute osteomyelitis 730.1 Chronic osteomyelitis 736.x Acquired deformity of limbs 754.0 Congen skull/face/jaw deformity 886.x Traumatic finger amputation 996.54 Breast prosthesis malfunction **REIMBURSEMENT INFORMATION** General ♦ See notes on pages 22–23. Medicare ♦ Outpatient Limit — applies
99251	Initial inpatient consultation for a new or established patient, which requires these three key components: • a problem focused history • a problem focused examination; and • straightforward medical decision making. Counseling and/or coordination of care with other providers or agencies are provided consistent with the nature of the problem(s) and the patient's and/or family's needs. Usually, the presenting problem(s) are self limiting or minor. Physicians typically spend 20 minutes at the bedside and on the patient's hospital floor or unit.	173.x Malignant neoplasm, Skin 216.x Benign neoplasm, Skin 238.2 UB-Neoplasm, Skin 239.2 Bone/Skin neoplasm NOS 454.0 Leg varicosity w/ulcer 682.x Cellulitis and abscess 707.x Chronic ulcer of skin 873.x Open wound of head 875.x Open wound of chest (wall) 877.x Open wound of buttock 884.x Open wound of upper limb 890.x Open wound of hip and thigh 891.x Open wound of knee, leg, ankle 892.x Open wound of foot 920. Contusion face/scalp/neck 998.3 Postop wound disruption 998.5 Postoperative infection **REIMBURSEMENT INFORMATION** General ♦ See notes on pages 22–23. Medicare ♦ Outpatient Limit — does not apply

CPT CODE	SERVICE
99252	Initial inpatient consultation for a new or established patient, which requires these three key components:

- an expanded problem focused history
- an expanded problem focused examination; and
- straightforward medical decision making.

Counseling and/or coordination of care with other providers or agencies are provided consistent with the nature of the problem(s) and the patient's and/or family's needs.

Usually, the presenting problem(s) are of low severity. Physicians typically spend 40 minutes at the bedside and on the patient's hospital floor or unit.

ICD–9–CM

173.x	Malignant neoplasm, Skin
216.x	Benign neoplasm, Skin
354.0	Carpal tunnel syndrome
454.x	Varicose veins of lower extremity
681.x	Cellulitis/abscess of finger/toe
682.x	Cellulitis and abscess
686.9	Local skin infection NOS
707.x	Chronic ulcer of skin
730.0x	Acute osteomyelitis
730.1x	Chronic osteomyelitis
802.x	Fracture of face bones
875.x	Open wound of chest (wall)
877.x	Open wound of buttock
879.x	Open wound NOS, except limbs
881.x	Elbow/forearm/wrist open wound
882.x	Open wound of hand
883.x	Open wound of finger(s)
884.x	Open wound of upper limb
890.x	Open wound of hip and thigh
891.x	Open wound of knee, leg, ankle
892.x	Open wound of foot
998.5	Postoperative infection

REIMBURSEMENT INFORMATION

General

- ◆ See notes on pages 22–23.

Medicare

- ◆ Outpatient Limit — does not apply

CPT CODE **SERVICE**

99253 Initial inpatient consultation for a new or established patient, which requires these three key components:

- a detailed history
- a detailed examination; and
- medical decision making of low complexity.

Counseling and/or coordination of care with other providers or agencies are provided consistent with the nature of the problem(s) and the patient's and/or family's needs.

Usually, the presenting problem(s) are of moderate severity. Physicians typically spend 55 minutes at the bedside and on the patient's hospital floor or unit.

EXAMPLE

♦ Initial hospital consultation for a 60–year–old diabetic male with gangrene of the foot.

ICD–9–CM

173.x	Malignant neoplasm, Skin
216.x	Benign neoplasm, Skin
238.2	UB-Neoplasm, Skin
682.x	Cellulitis and abscess
707.x	Chronic ulcer of skin
730.0x	Acute osteomyelitis
785.4	Gangrene
802.x	Fracture of face bones
873.x	Open wound of head
875.x	Open wound of chest (wall)
877.x	Open wound of buttock
886.x	Traumatic finger amputation
890.x	Open wound of hip and thigh
891.x	Open wound of knee, leg, ankle
892.x	Open wound of foot
894.x	Open wound of lower limb
946.3	3rd deg burn, multiple sites
998.1	Hemorrhage complicating a procedure
998.3	Postop wound disruption
998.5	Postoperative infection
998.9	Surgical complication NOS

REIMBURSEMENT INFORMATION

General

♦ See notes on pages 22–23.

Medicare

♦ Outpatient Limit — does not apply

CPT CODE	SERVICE	ICD-9-CM
99254	Initial inpatient consultation for a new or established patient, which requires these three key components: • a comprehensive history • a comprehensive examination; and • medical decision making of moderate complexity. Counseling and/or coordination of care with other providers or agencies are provided consistent with the nature of the problem(s) and the patient's and/or family's needs. Usually, the presenting problem(s) are of moderate to high severity. Physicians typically spend 80 minutes at the bedside and on the patient's hospital floor or unit. **EXAMPLE** ◆ Initial hospital consultation for 35-year-old multiple trauma male patient with complex facial fractures, to evaluate and formulate management plan.	173.x Malignant neoplasm, Skin 174.x Malignant neoplasm, Female breast 238.2 UB-Neoplasm, Skin 440.2x Atherosclerosis, extremity artery 457.1 Other lymphedema 682.x Cellulitis and abscess 707.x Chronic ulcer of skin 730.2x Osteomyelitis 784.2 Swelling in head/neck 785.4 Gangrene 802.6 Fx orbital floor, closed 802.8 Fx facial bone NEC, closed 873.1 Open wound of scalp, complicated 875.x Open wound of chest (wall) 890.x Open wound of hip and thigh 891.x Open wound of knee, leg, ankle 892.x Open wound of foot 893.x Open wound of toe(s) 998.3 Postop wound disruption 998.5 Postoperative infection **REIMBURSEMENT INFORMATION** General ◆ See notes on pages 22–23. Medicare ◆ Outpatient Limit — does not apply
99255	Initial inpatient consultation for a new or established patient, which requires these three key components: • a comprehensive history • a comprehensive examination; and • medical decision making of high complexity. Counseling and/or coordination of care with other providers or agencies are provided consistent with the nature of the problem(s) and the patient's and/or family's needs. Usually, the presenting problem(s) are of moderate to high severity. Physicians typically spend 110 minutes at the bedside and on the patient's floor or unit.	730.2x Osteomyelitis 875.1 Open wound of chest, complicated 891.1 Open wound of knee/leg/ankle, compl 946.x Burns of multiple sites 998.5 Postoperative infection **REIMBURSEMENT INFORMATION** General ◆ See notes on pages 22–23. Medicare ◆ Outpatient Limit — does not apply

CPT CODE	SERVICE	ICD-9-CM
99261	Follow-up inpatient consultation for an established patient, which requires at least TWO of these three key components: • a problem focused interval history • a problem focused examination • straightforward or low complexity medical decision making. Counseling and/or coordination of care with other providers or agencies are provided consistent with the nature of the problem(s) and the patient's and/or family's needs. Usually, the patient is stable, recovering or improving. Physicians typically spend 10 minutes at the bedside and on the patient's hospital floor or unit.	173.x Malignant neoplasm, Skin 681.x Cellulitis/abscess of finger/toe 682.x Cellulitis and abscess 707.x Chronic ulcer of skin 730.2x Osteomyelitis 785.4 Gangrene 877.x Open wound of buttock 879.x Open wound NOS, except limbs 881.x Elbow/forearm/wrist open wound 884.x Open wound of upper limb 890.x Open wound of hip and thigh 891.x Open wound of knee, leg, ankle 892.x Open wound of foot 893.x Open wound of toe(s) 906.0 Late effect, open wound head/trunk 945.26 2nd deg burn, thigh **REIMBURSEMENT INFORMATION** General ♦ See notes on pages 22–23. Medicare ♦ Outpatient Limit — does not apply
99262	Follow-up inpatient consultation for an established patient, which requires at least TWO of these three key components: • an expanded problem focused interval history • an expanded problem focused examination • medical decision making of moderate complexity Counseling and/or coordination of care with other providers or agencies are provided consistent with the nature of the problem(s) and the patient's and/or family's needs. Usually, the patient is responding inadequately to therapy or has developed a minor complication. Physicians typically spend 20 minutes at the bedside and on the patient's hospital floor or unit.	457.1 Other lymphedema 682.x Cellulitis and abscess 686.9 Local skin infection NOS 692.9 Dermatitis NOS 707.x Chronic ulcer of skin 802.x Fracture of face bones 875.x Open wound of chest (wall) 890.x Open wound of hip and thigh 891.x Open wound of knee, leg, ankle 892.x Open wound of foot 894.x Open wound of lower limb 945.26 2nd deg burn, thigh 998.5 Postoperative infection **REIMBURSEMENT INFORMATION** General ♦ See notes on pages 22–23. Medicare ♦ Outpatient Limit — does not apply

CPT CODE	SERVICE	ICD-9-CM

99263 Follow-up inpatient consultation for an established patient, which requires at least TWO of these three key components:

- a detailed interval history
- a detailed examination
- medical decision making of high complexity.

Counseling and/or coordination of care with other providers or agencies are provided consistent with the nature of the problem(s) and the patient's and/or family's needs.

Usually, the patient is unstable or has developed a significant complication or a significant new problem. Physicians typically spend 30 minutes at the bedside and on the patient's hospital floor or unit.

707.x	Chronic ulcer of skin
891.x	Open wound of knee, leg, ankle
894.x	Open wound of lower limb
998.3	Postop wound disruption
998.5	Postoperative infection
999.2	Vascular complications med care NEC

REIMBURSEMENT INFORMATION

General

- ◆ See notes on pages 22–23.

Medicare

- ◆ Outpatient Limit — does not apply

99271 Confirmatory consultation for a new or established patient, which requires these three key components:

- a problem focused history
- a problem focused examination; and
- straightforward medical decision making.

Counseling and/or coordination of care with other providers or agencies are provided consistent with the nature of the problem(s) and the patient's and/or family's needs.

Usually, the presenting problem(s) are self limited or minor.

173.x	Malignant neoplasm, Skin
238.2	UB-Neoplasm, Skin
374.34	Blepharochalasis
754.4	Congenital genu recurvatum
891.0	Open wound of knee/leg/ankle
V10.83	Hx of skin malignancy NEC

REIMBURSEMENT INFORMATION

General

- ◆ See notes on pages 22–23.

Medicare

- ◆ Outpatient Limit — applies

CPT CODE	SERVICE	ICD–9–CM

99272 Confirmatory consultation for a new or established patient, which requires these three key components:

- an expanded problem focused history
- an expanded problem focused examination; and
- straightforward medical decision making.

Counseling and/or coordination of care with other providers or agencies are provided consistent with the nature of the problem(s) and the patient's and/or family's needs.

Usually the presenting problem(s) are of low severity.

173.x	Malignant neoplasm, Skin
333.6	Idiopathic torsion dystonia
611.1	Hypertrophy of breast
681.x	Cellulitis/abscess of finger/toe
686.9	Local skin infection NOS
743.61	Congenital ptosis
784.49	Voice disturbance NEC
873.52	Open wound of forehead, complicated
883.1	Open wound of finger, complicated
V10.83	Hx of skin malignancy NEC

REIMBURSEMENT INFORMATION

General

- ♦ See notes on pages 22–23.

Medicare

- ♦ Outpatient Limit — applies

99273 Confirmatory consultation for a new or established patient, which requires these three key components:

- a detailed history
- a detailed examination; and
- medical decision making of low complexity

Counseling and/or coordination of care with other providers or agencies are provided consistent with the nature of the problem(s) and the patient's and/or family's needs.

Usually, the presenting problem(s) are of moderate severity.

172.4	Malignant melanoma, Scalp/neck
173.3	M-Neoplasm, Skin of face NEC
216.3	B-Neoplasm, Skin of face NEC
374.34	Blepharochalasis
707.x	Chronic ulcer of skin
892.x	Open wound of foot
909.3	Late effect of surg/med complic
V67.0	Surgery follow-up

REIMBURSEMENT INFORMATION

General

- ♦ See notes on pages 22–23.

Medicare

- ♦ Outpatient Limit — applies

CPT CODE	SERVICE	ICD-9-CM
99274	Confirmatory consultation for a patient, which requires these three key components: • a comprehensive history • a comprehensive examination; and • medical decision making of moderate complexity. Counseling and/or coordination of care with other providers or agencies are provided consistent with the nature of the problem(s) and the patient's and/or family's needs. Usually, the presenting problem(s) are of moderate to high severity.	173.x Malignant neoplasm, Skin 216.x Benign neoplasm, Skin 354.0 Carpal tunnel syndrome 682.x Cellulitis and abscess 754.0 Congen skull/face/jaw deformity 873.x Open wound of head **REIMBURSEMENT INFORMATION** General ♦ See notes on pages 22–23. Medicare ♦ Outpatient Limit — applies
99275	Confirmatory consultation for a patient, which requires these three key components: • a comprehensive history • a comprehensive examination; and • medical decision making of high complexity. Counseling and/or coordination of care with other providers or agencies are provided consistent with the nature of the problem(s) and the patient's and/or family's needs. Usually, the presenting problem(s) are of moderate to high severity.	801.0x Fracture of base of skull 891.x Open wound of knee, leg, ankle **REIMBURSEMENT INFORMATION** General ♦ See notes on pages 22–23. Medicare ♦ Outpatient Limit — does not apply

EMERGENCY DEPARTMENT SERVICES

New or Established Patient
99281–99285

These codes are used to report evaluation and management services provided in the emergency department. No distinction is made between new and established patients in the emergency department.

An emergency department is defined as an organized hospital–based facility for the provision of unscheduled episodic services to patients who present for immediate medical attention. The facility must be available 24 hours a day.

For critical care services provided in the emergency department, see Critical Care notes and 99291, 99292 in your CPT.

For evaluation and management services provided to a patient in an observation area of a hospital, see 99217–99220 in your CPT.

For definitions of key components and commonly used terms, see Evaluation and Management Services Guidelines in your CPT.

CPT CODE	SERVICE	ICD–9–CM
99281	Emergency department visit for the evaluation and management of a patient, which requires these three key components: • a problem focused history • a problem focused examination; and • straightforward medical decision making. Counseling and/or coordination of care with other providers or agencies are provided consistent with the nature of the problem(s) and the patient's and/or family's needs. Usually, the presenting problem(s) are self limited or minor.	173.x Malignant neoplasm, Skin 216.x Benign neoplasm, Skin 611.0 Inflammatory disease of breast 701.9 Hypertrophic/atrophic skin NOS 707.x Chronic ulcer of skin 729.6 Old foreign body in soft tissue 816.x Fracture of phalanges of hand 872.x Open wound of ear 873.x Open wound of head 881.x Elbow/forearm/wrist open wound 882.x Open wound of hand 883.x Open wound of finger(s) 884.x Open wound of upper limb 886.x Traumatic finger amputation 891.x Open wound of knee, leg, ankle 927.3 Crushing injury, finger 945.x Burn of lower limb 998.1 Hemorrhage complicating a procedure **REIMBURSEMENT INFORMATION** General ♦ See notes on page 35. Medicare ♦ Outpatient Limit — does not apply
99282	Emergency department visit for the evaluation and management of a patient, which requires these three key components: • an expanded problem focused history • an expanded problem focused examination; and • medical decision making of low complexity. Counseling and/or coordination of care with other providers or agencies are provided consistent with the nature of the problem(s) and the patient's and/or family's needs. Usually, the presenting problem(s) are of low to moderate severity.	707.x Chronic ulcer of skin 802.6 Fx orbital floor, closed 816.11 Fx mid/prox phalanx, hand, open 816.12 Fx distal phalanx, hand, open 873.x Open wound of head 882.x Open wound of hand 883.x Open wound of finger(s) 886.x Traumatic finger amputation 891.x Open wound of knee, leg, ankle 959.4 Hand injury NOS **REIMBURSEMENT INFORMATION** General ♦ See notes on page 35. Medicare ♦ Outpatient Limit — does not apply

CPT CODE	SERVICE	ICD–9–CM	
99283	Emergency department visit for the evaluation and management of a patient, which requires these three key components: • an expanded problem focused history • an expanded problem focused examination; and • medical decision making of moderate complexity. Counseling and/or coordination of care with other providers or agencies are provided consistent with the nature of the problem(s) and the patient's and/or family's needs. Usually, the presenting problem(s) are of moderate severity.	707.x 784.0 801.00 802.4 802.6 870.0 873.x 881.x 882.x 883.x 927.3 943.2x 998.3	Chronic ulcer of skin Headache Closed skull base fracture Fx malar/maxillary, closed Fx orbital floor, closed Laceration eyelid skin/periocular Open wound of head Elbow/forearm/wrist open wound Open wound of hand Open wound of finger(s) Crushing injury, finger Blisters, upper limb Postop wound disruption

REIMBURSEMENT INFORMATION

General

- ♦ See notes on page 35.

Medicare

- ♦ Outpatient Limit — does not apply

CPT CODE	SERVICE	ICD–9–CM	
99284	Emergency department visit for the evaluation and management of a patient, which requires these three key components: • a detailed history • a detailed examination; and • medical decision making of moderate complexity. Counseling and/or coordination of care with other providers or agencies are provided consistent with the nature of the problem(s) and the patient's and/or family's needs. Usually, the presenting problem(s) are of high severity, and require urgent evaluation by the physician but do not pose an immediate significant threat to life or physiologic function.	729.5 786.5x 816.12 870.0 873.x 881.x 882.x 883.x	Pain in limb Chest pain Fx distal phalanx, hand, open Laceration eyelid skin/periocular Open wound of head Elbow/forearm/wrist open wound Open wound of hand Open wound of finger(s)

REIMBURSEMENT INFORMATION

General

- ♦ See notes on page 35.

Medicare

- ♦ Outpatient Limit — does not apply

CPT CODE	SERVICE
99285	Emergency department visit for the evaluation and management of a patient, which requires these three key components within the constraints imposed by the urgency of the patient's clinical condition and mental status:

- a comprehensive history
- a comprehensive examination; and
- medical decision making of high complexity.

Counseling and/or coordination of care with other providers or agencies are provided consistent with the nature of the problem(s) and the patient's and/or family's needs.

Usually, the presenting problem(s) are of high severity and pose an immediate significant threat to life of physiologic function.

ICD–9–CM

374.2x	Lagophthalmos
682.x	Cellulitis and abscess
686.9	Local skin infection NOS
709.4	Foreign body granuloma, skin
873.x	Open wound of head
882.x	Open wound of hand
883.x	Open wound of finger(s)
884.x	Open wound of upper limb

REIMBURSEMENT INFORMATION

General

- ◆ See notes on page 35.

Medicare

- ◆ Outpatient Limit — does not apply

CRITICAL CARE SERVICES
99291–99292

Critical care includes the care of critically ill or injured patients in a variety of medical emergencies that requires the constant attendance of the physician (e.g., cardiac arrest, shock, bleeding, respiratory failure, postoperative complications). Critical care is usually, but not always, given in a critical care area, such as the coronary care unit, intensive care unit, respiratory care unit, or the emergency care facility.

Services for a patient who is not critically ill but happens to be in a critical care unit are reported using subsequent hospital care codes (see 99231–99233) or hospital consultation codes (see 99251–99263) as appropriate.

The following services are included in reporting critical care when performed during the critical period by the physician providing critical care: the interpretation of cardiac output measurements (93561, 93562), chest X–rays (71010, 71020), blood gases, and information data stored in computers (e.g., ECGs, blood pressures, hematologic data (99090)); gastric intubation (91105); temporary transcutaneous pacing (92953); ventilator management (94656, 94657, 94660, 94662); and, vascular access procedures (36000, 36410, 36415, 36600). Any services performed which are not listed above should be reported separately.

The critical care codes are used to report the total duration of time spent by a physician providing constant attention to a critically ill or injured patient, even if the time spent by the physician providing critical care services on that date is not continuous. Code 99291 is used to report the first hour of critical care on a given date. It should be used only once per date even if the time spent by the physician is not continuous on that date. Critical care of less than 30 minutes total duration on a given date should be reported with the appropriate E/M code. Code 99292 is used to report each additional 30 minutes beyond the first hour. It also may be used to report the final 15-30 minutes of critical care on a given date. Critical care of less than 15 minutes beyond the first hour or less than 15 minutes beyond the final 30 minutes is not reported separately.

The following examples illustrate the correct reporting of critical care services:

Total Duration of Critical Care	Codes
a. less than 30 minutes (less than 1/2 hour)	99232 or 99233
b. 30–74 minutes (1/2 hr. – 1 hr. 14 min.)	99291 x 1
c. 75–104 minutes (1 hr. 15 min. – 1 hr. 44 min.)	99291 x 1 AND 99292 x 1
d. 105–134 minutes (1 hr. 45 min. – 2 hr. 14 min.)	99291 x 1 AND 99292 x 2
e. 135–164 minutes (2 hr. 15 min. – 2 hr. 44 min.)	99291 x 1 AND 99292 x 3
f. 165–194 minutes (2 hr. 45 min. – 3 hr. 14 min.)	99291 x 1 AND 99292 x 4

CPT CODE	SERVICE	ICD–9–CM
99291	Critical care, evaluation and management of the critically ill or critically injured patient, requiring the constant attendance of the physician; first hour	681.x Cellulitis/abscess of finger/toe 941.3x 3rd degree burn NOS, face/head/neck 942.34 3rd deg burn trunk, back 942.44 Deep 3rd deg burn trunk, back 948.x Burns according to surface extent 998.1 Hemorrhage complicating a procedure **REIMBURSEMENT INFORMATION** General ◆ See notes on page 39. Medicare ◆ Outpatient Limit — does not apply
99292	Critical care, evaluation and management of the critically ill or critically injured patient, requiring the constant attendance of the physician; each additional 30 minutes	681.x Cellulitis/abscess of finger/toe 941.3x 3rd degree burn NOS, face/head/neck 942.34 3rd deg burn trunk, back 942.44 Deep 3rd deg burn trunk, back 948.x Burns according to surface extent 998.1 Hemorrhage complicating a procedure **REIMBURSEMENT INFORMATION** General ◆ See notes on page 39. Medicare ◆ Outpatient Limit — does not apply

NURSING FACILITY SERVICES
99301–99313

The following codes are used to report evaluation and management services to patients in Nursing Facilities (formerly called Skilled Nursing Facilities (SNFs), Intermediate Care Facilities (ICFs) or Long Term Care Facilities (LTCFs)).

These codes should also be used to report evaluation and management services provided to a patient in a psychiatric residential treatment center (a facility or a distinct part of a facility for psychiatric care, which provides a 24 hour therapeutically planned and professionally staffed group living and learning environment). If procedures such as medical psychotherapy are provided in addition to evaluation and management services, these should be reported in addition to the evaluation and management services provided.

Nursing facilities that provide convalescent, rehabilitative, or long term care are required to conduct comprehensive, accurate, standardized, and reproducible assessments of each resident's functional capacity using a Resident Assessment Instrument (RAI). All RAIs include the Minimum Data Set (MDS), Resident Assessment Protocols (RAPs) and utilization guidelines. The MDS is the primary screening and assessment tool; the RAPs trigger the identification of potential problems and provide guidelines for follow–up assessments.

Physicians have a central role in assuring that all residents receive thorough assessments and that medical plans of care are instituted or revised to enhance or maintain the residents' physical and psychosocial functioning.

Two subcategories of nursing facility services are recognized: Comprehensive Nursing Facility Assessments and Subsequent Nursing Facility Care. Both subcategories apply to new or established patients. Comprehensive Assessments may be performed at one or more sites in the assessment process: the hospital, office, nursing facility, domiciliary/non–nursing facility or patient's home.

For definitions of key components and commonly used terms, please see Evaulation and Management Services Guidelines in your CPT.

Comprehensive Nursing Facility Assessments
New or Established Patient
99301–99303

When the patient is admitted to the nursing facility in the course of an encounter in another site of service (e.g., hospital emergency department, physician's office), all evaluation and management services provided by that physician in conjunction with that admission are considered part of the initial nursing facility care when performed as part of the admission. The nursing facility care level of service reported by the admitting physician should include the services related to the admission he/she provided in the other sites of service as well as in the nursing facility setting. With the exception of hospital discharge services, evaluation and management services on the same date provided in sites other than the nursing facility that are related to the admission should NOT be reported separately. Hospital discharge services may be reported separately.

More than one comprehensive assessment may be necessary during an inpatient confinement.

NURSING FACILITY SERVICES (Cont'd.)

Subsequent Nursing Facility Care
New or Established Patient
99311–99312

These codes are used to report the services provided to residents of nursing facilities who do not require a comprehensive assessment, and/or who have not had a major, permanent change of status.

All levels include reviewing the medical record, noting changes in the resident's status since the last visit, and reviewing and signing orders.

CPT CODE	SERVICE	ICD–9–CM

99301 Evaluation and management of a new or established patient involving an annual nursing facility assessment which requires these three key components:

- a detailed interval history
- a comprehensive examination; and
- straightforward or low complexity medical decision making.

Counseling and/or coordination of care with other providers or agencies are provided consistent with the nature of the problem(s) and the patient's and/or family's needs.

Usually, the patient is stable, recovering or improving. The review and affirmation of the medical plan of care is required. Physicians typically spend 30 minutes at the bedside and on the patient's facility floor or unit.

344.0x	Quadriplegia NOS
344.1	Paraplegia NOS
454.2	Varicose leg w/ulcer+inflammation
707.x	Chronic ulcer of skin
709.8	Skin disorders NEC
876.x	Open wound of back
877.x	Open wound of buttock
891.x	Open wound of knee, leg, ankle
892.x	Open wound of foot

REIMBURSEMENT INFORMATION

General

- ♦ See notes on pages 41–42.

Medicare

- ♦ Outpatient Limit — does not apply

99302 Evaluation and management of a new or established patient involving a nursing facility assessment which requires these three key components:

- a detailed interval history
- a comprehensive examination; and
- medical decision making of moderate to high complexity.

Counseling and/or coordination of care with other providers or agencies are provided consistent with the nature of the problem(s) and the patient's and/or family's needs.

Usually, the patient has developed a significant complication or a significant new problem and has had a major permanent change in status. The creation of a new medical plan of care is required. Physicians typically spend 40 minutes at the bedside and on the patient's facility floor or unit.

173.x	Malignant neoplasm, Skin
198.89	M2-Neoplasm NEC
216.x	Benign neoplasm, Skin
344.0x	Quadriplegia NOS
344.1	Paraplegia NOS
454.2	Varicose leg w/ulcer+inflammation
707.x	Chronic ulcer of skin

REIMBURSEMENT INFORMATION

General

- ♦ See notes on pages 41–42.

Medicare

- ♦ Outpatient Limit — does not apply

CPT CODE	SERVICE	ICD-9-CM
99303	Evaluation and management of a new or established patient involving a nursing facility assessment at the time of initial admission to the facility, which requires these three key components: • a comprehensive history • a comprehensive examination; and • medical decision making of moderate to high complexity. Counseling and/or coordination of care with other providers or agencies are provided consistent with the nature of the problem(s) and the patient's and/or family's needs. The creation of a medical plan of care is required. Physicians typically spend 50 minutes at the bedside and on the patient's facility floor or unit.	707.x Chronic ulcer of skin 892.1 Open wound of foot, complicated **REIMBURSEMENT INFORMATION** General ♦ See notes on pages 41–42. Medicare ♦ Outpatient Limit — does not apply
99311	Subsequent nursing facility care, per day, for the evaluation and management of a new or established patient, which requires at least TWO of these three key components: • a problem focused interval history • a problem focused examination • straightforward or low complexity medical decision making. Counseling and/or coordination of care with other providers or agencies are provided consistent with the nature of the problem(s) and the patient's and/or family's needs. Usually, the patient is stable, recovering or improving. Physicians typically spend 15 minutes at the bedside and on the patient's facility floor or unit.	173.x Malignant neoplasm, Skin 216.x Benign neoplasm, Skin 238.2 UB-Neoplasm, Skin 454.2 Varicose leg w/ulcer+inflammation 686.8 Local skin infection NEC 701.1 Keratoderma, acquired 702.0 Actinic keratosis 707.x Chronic ulcer of skin 782.3 Edema 785.4 Gangrene 873.x Open wound of head 876.x Open wound of back 877.x Open wound of buttock 890.x Open wound of hip and thigh 891.x Open wound of knee, leg, ankle 892.x Open wound of foot 893.x Open wound of toe(s) 945.32 3rd deg burn, foot **REIMBURSEMENT INFORMATION** General ♦ See notes on pages 41–42. Medicare ♦ Outpatient Limit — does not apply

CPT CODE	SERVICE	ICD–9–CM

99312 Subsequent nursing facility care, per day, for the evaluation and management of a new or established patient, which requires at least TWO of these three key components:

- an expanded problem focused interval history
- an expanded problem focused examination
- medical decision making of moderate complexity.

Counseling and/or coordination of care with other providers or agencies are provided consistent with the nature of the problem(s) and the patient's and/or family's needs.

Usually, the patient is responding inadequately to therapy or has developed a minor complication. Physicians typically spend 25 minutes at the bedside and on the patient's facility floor or unit.

173.x	Malignant neoplasm, Skin
682.7	Cellulitis of foot
707.x	Chronic ulcer of skin
785.4	Gangrene
890.x	Open wound of hip and thigh

REIMBURSEMENT INFORMATION

General

- ♦ See notes on pages 41–42.

Medicare

- ♦ Outpatient Limit — does not apply

99313 Subsequent nursing facility care, per day, for the evaluation and management of a new or established patient, which requires at least TWO of these three components:

- a detailed interval history
- a detailed examination
- medical decision making of moderate to high complexity.

Counseling and/or coordination of care with other providers or agencies are provided consistent with the nature of the problem(s) and the patient's and/or family's needs.

Usually, the patient has developed a significant complication or a significant new problem. Physicians typically spend 35 minutes at the bedside and on the patient's facility floor or unit.

173.x	Malignant neoplasm, Skin
682.6	Cellulitis of leg
707.x	Chronic ulcer of skin
785.4	Gangrene
891.x	Open wound of knee, leg, ankle
892.x	Open wound of foot

REIMBURSEMENT INFORMATION

General

- ♦ See notes on pages 41–42.

Medicare

- ♦ Outpatient Limit — does not apply

DOMICILIARY, REST HOME (e.g., BOARDING HOME), or CUSTODIAL CARE SERVICES

New Patient
99321–99323

Established Patient
99331–99333

These codes are used to report evaluation and management services in a facility which provides room, board and other personal assistance services, generally on a long–term basis. The facility's services do not include a medical component.

For definitions of key components and commonly used terms, please see Evaluation and Management Services Guidelines in your CPT.

Typical times have not yet been established for this category of services.

CPT CODE	SERVICE

ICD–9–CM

99321 Domiciliary or rest home visit for the evaluation and management of a new patient, which requires these three key components:

- a problem focused history
- a problem focused examination; and
- straightforward or low complexity medical decision making.

Counseling and/or coordination of care with other providers or agencies are provided consistent with the nature of the problem(s) and the patient's and/or family's needs.

Usually, the presenting problem(s) are of low severity.

173.x	Malignant neoplasm, Skin
682.7	Cellulitis of foot
707.x	Chronic ulcer of skin
785.4	Gangrene
890.x	Open wound of hip and thigh

REIMBURSEMENT INFORMATION

General

- ♦ See notes on page 46.

Medicare

- ♦ Outpatient Limit — does not apply

99322 Domiciliary or rest home visit for the evaluation and management of a new patient, which requires these three key components:

- an expanded problem focused history
- an expanded problem focused examination; and
- medical decision making of moderate complexity.

Counseling and/or coordination of care with other providers or agencies are provided consistent with the nature of the problem(s) and the patient's and/or family's needs.

Usually, the presenting problem(s) are of moderate severity.

173.x	Malignant neoplasm, Skin
344.0x	Quadriplegia NOS
344.1	Paraplegia NOS
707.x	Chronic ulcer of skin

REIMBURSEMENT INFORMATION

General

- ♦ See notes on page 46.

Medicare

- ♦ Outpatient Limit — does not apply

CPT CODE	SERVICE
99323	Domiciliary or rest home visit for the evaluation and management of a new patient, which requires these three key components: • a detailed history • a detailed examination; and • medical decision making of high complexity. Counseling and/or coordination of care with other providers or agencies are provided consistent with the nature of the problem(s) and the patient's and/or family's needs. Usually, the presenting problem(s) are of high complexity.

ICD–9–CM

173.x	Malignant neoplasm, Skin
707.x	Chronic ulcer of skin
891.x	Open wound of knee, leg, ankle

REIMBURSEMENT INFORMATION

General

- ◆ See notes on page 46.

Medicare

- ◆ Outpatient Limit — does not apply

HOME SERVICES

New Patient
99341–99343

Established Patient
99351–99353

These codes are used to report evaluation and management services provided in a private residence.

For definitions of key components and commonly used terms, please see Evaluation and Management Services Guidelines in your CPT.

Typical times have not yet been established for this category of services.

CPT CODE	SERVICE	ICD–9–CM

99341 Home visit for the evaluation and management of a new patient, which requires these three key components:

- a problem focused history
- a problem focused examination; and
- straightforward or low complexity medical decision making.

Counseling and/or coordination of care with other providers or agencies are provided consistent with the nature of the problem(s) and the patient's and/or family's needs.

Usually, the presenting problem(s) are of low severity.

173.x	Malignant neoplasm, Skin
944.0x	Burn, wrist/hand, degree unspec
948.0x	Burn, less than 10% of body surface

REIMBURSEMENT INFORMATION

General

- ♦ See notes on page 49.

Medicare

- ♦ Outpatient Limit — does not apply

99342 Home visit for the evaluation and management of a new patient, which requires these three key components:

- an expanded problem focused history
- an expanded problem focused examination; and
- medical decision making of moderate complexity.

Counseling and/or coordination of care with other providers or agencies are provided consistent with the nature of the problem(s) and the patient's and/or family's needs.

Usually, the presenting problem(s) are of moderate severity.

344.0x	Quadriplegia NOS
344.1	Paraplegia NOS
354.0	Carpal tunnel syndrome
707.x	Chronic ulcer of skin
891.x	Open wound of knee, leg, ankle

REIMBURSEMENT INFORMATION

General

- ♦ See notes on page 49.

Medicare

- ♦ Outpatient Limit — does not apply

CPT CODE	SERVICE	ICD-9-CM
99351	Home visit for the evaluation and management of an established patient, which requires at least TWO of these three key components: • a problem focused interval history • a problem focused examination • straightforward or low complexity medical decision making. Counseling and/or coordination of care with other providers or agencies are provided consistent with the nature of the problem(s) and the patient's and/or family's needs. Usually, the patient is stable, recovering or improving.	454.0 Leg varicosity w/ulcer 701.4 Keloid scar 707.x Chronic ulcer of skin **REIMBURSEMENT INFORMATION** General ♦ See notes on page 49. Medicare ♦ Outpatient Limit — does not apply
99352	Home visit for the evaluation and management of an established patient, which requires at least TWO of these three key components: • an expanded problem focused interval history • an expanded problem focused examination • medical decision making of moderate complexity. Counseling and/or coordination of care with other providers or agencies are provided consistent with the nature of the problem(s) and the patient's and/or family's needs. Usually, the patient is responding inadequately to therapy or has developed a minor complication.	682.6 Cellulitis of leg 707.x Chronic ulcer of skin **REIMBURSEMENT INFORMATION** General ♦ See notes on page 49. Medicare ♦ Outpatient Limit — does not apply

CPT CODE	SERVICE
99353	Home visit for the evaluation and management of an established patient, which requires at least TWO of these three key components: • a detailed interval history • a detailed examination • medical decision making of high complexity. Counseling and/or coordination of care with other providers or agencies are provided consistent with the nature of the problem(s) and the patient's and/or family's needs. Usually, the patient is unstable or has developed a significant complication or a significant new problem.

ICD–9–CM

682.6	Cellulitis of leg
707.x	Chronic ulcer of skin

REIMBURSEMENT INFORMATION

General

- ◆ See notes on page 49.

Medicare

- ◆ Outpatient Limit — does not apply

CASE MANAGEMENT SERVICES

Team Conferences
99361—99362

Telephone Calls
99371–99373

Physician case management is a process in which a physician is responsible for direct care of a patient, and for coordinating and controlling access to or initiating and/or supervising other health care services needed by the patient.

CPT CODE	SERVICE
99373	Telephone call by a physician to patient or for consultation or medical management or for coordinating medical management with other health care professionals (eg, nurses, therapists, social workers, nutritionists, physicians, pharmacists); complex or lengthy (eg, lengthy counseling session with anxious or distraught patient, detailed or prolonged discussion with family members regarding seriously ill patient, lengthy communication necessary to coordinate complex services of several different health professionals working on different aspects of the total patient care plan)

ICD–9–CM

344.0x	Quadriplegia NOS
344.1	Paraplegia NOS
611.8	Breast disorders NEC
707.x	Chronic ulcer of skin
V58.3	Attention to surg dressing/suture

REIMBURSEMENT INFORMATION

General

- ♦ See notes on page 53.

Medicare

- ♦ Outpatient Limit — does not apply

SURGERY

CPT CODE	SERVICE
10040*	Acne surgery (eg, marsupialization, opening or removal of multiple milia, comedones, cysts, pustules)

CPT NOTES

- For excision, see 11400, et seq.

ICD–9–CM

680.2	Carbuncle of trunk
682.2	Cellulitis of trunk
695.3	Rosacea
704.09	Alopecia NEC
704.8	Hair diseases NEC
706.x	Diseases of sebaceous glands

REIMBURSEMENT INFORMATION

General

- Starred procedure.

Medicare

- Follow–up Days — 10
- Assistant Surgeon — not paid
- Supply Charges — not allowed
- Outpatient Limit — applies
- Minor Surgery Rules Apply

CPT CODE	SERVICE
10060*	Incision and drainage of abscess (eg, carbuncle, suppurative hidradenitis, and other cutaneous or subcutaneous abscess, cyst, furuncle, or paronychia); simple or single

CPT NOTES

- For excision, see 11400, et seq.

ICD-9-CM

372.75	Conjunctival cysts
373.1x	Deep inflammation of eyelid
373.2	Chalazion
374.84	Cysts of eyelids
375.32	Acute dacryocystitis
526.4	Inflammation of jaw
527.3	Salivary gland abscess
528.3	Cellulitis/abscess of mouth
528.5	Diseases of lips
529.0	Glossitis
680.x	Carbuncle and furuncle
681.x	Cellulitis/abscess of finger/toe
682.x	Cellulitis and abscess
683.	Acute lymphadenitis
705.83	Hidradenitis
706.2	Sebaceous cyst
910.5	Insect bite, head, infected
911.5	Insect bite, trunk, infected
912.5	Insect bite, shoulder/arm, infected
913.5	Insect bite, forearm, infected
914.5	Insect bite, hand, infected
915.5	Insect bite, finger, infected
916.5	Insect bite, hip/leg, infected
917.5	Insect bite, foot/toe, infected

REIMBURSEMENT INFORMATION

General

- Starred procedure.

Medicare

- Follow–up Days — 10
- Assistant Surgeon — not paid
- Supply Charges — not allowed
- Outpatient Limit — applies
- Minor Surgery Rules Apply
- Fragments — 64450

CPT CODE **SERVICE**

10061 Incision and drainage of abscess (eg, carbuncle, suppurative hidradenitis, and other cutaneous or subcutaneous abscess, cyst, furuncle, or paronychia); complicated or multiple

CPT NOTES

- For excision, see 11400, et seq.

ICD–9–CM

372.75	Conjunctival cysts
373.1x	Deep inflammation of eyelid
374.84	Cysts of eyelids
527.3	Salivary gland abscess
528.3	Cellulitis/abscess of mouth
528.5	Diseases of lips
529.0	Glossitis
680.x	Carbuncle and furuncle
681.x	Cellulitis/abscess of finger/toe
682.x	Cellulitis and abscess
683.	Acute lymphadenitis
705.83	Hidradenitis
706.2	Sebaceous cyst
910.5	Insect bite, head, infected
911.5	Insect bite, trunk, infected
912.5	Insect bite, shoulder/arm, infected
913.5	Insect bite, forearm, infected
914.5	Insect bite, hand, infected
915.5	Insect bite, finger, infected
916.5	Insect bite, hip/leg, infected
917.5	Insect bite, foot/toe, infected

REIMBURSEMENT INFORMATION.

Medicare

- Follow–up Days — 10
- Assistant Surgeon — not paid
- Supply Charges — not allowed
- Outpatient Limit — applies
- Minor Surgery Rules Apply
- Fragments — 64450

CPT CODE	SERVICE
10080*	Incision and drainage of pilonidal cyst; simple
10081	Incision and drainage of pilonidal cyst; complicated

CPT NOTES

- ◆ For excision, see 11400, et seq.
- ◆ For excision of pilonidal cyst, see 11770-11772.

ICD-9-CM

685.0	Pilonidal cyst w/abscess
685.1	Pilonidal cyst w/o abscess

REIMBURSEMENT INFORMATION

General

- ◆ Starred procedure. (10080)

Medicare

- ◆ Follow–up Days — 10
- ◆ Assistant Surgeon — not paid
- ◆ Supply Charges — not allowed
- ◆ Outpatient Limit — applies
- ◆ Minor Surgery Rules Apply

CPT CODE **SERVICE**

10120* Incision and removal of foreign body, subcutaneous tissues; simple

CPT NOTES

- For excision, see 11400, et seq.

ICD-9-CM

709.4	Foreign body granuloma, skin
729.6	Old foreign body in soft tissue
910.6	Foreign body, head
911.6	Foreign body, trunk
912.6	Foreign body, shoulder/arm
913.6	Foreign body, forearm
914.6	Foreign body, hand
915.6	Foreign body, finger
916.6	Foreign body, hip/leg
917.6	Foreign body, foot/toe
918.0	Superficial injury periocular
919.6	Superficial foreign body NEC
919.7	Superf foreign body NEC, infected
930.1	Foreign body in conjunctival sac
930.2	Foreign body in lacrimal punctum
998.4	Foreign body left during procedure

REIMBURSEMENT INFORMATION

General

- Starred procedure.

Medicare

- Follow-up Days — 10
- Assistant Surgeon — not paid
- Supply Charges — not allowed
- Outpatient Limit — applies
- Minor Surgery Rules Apply

CPT CODE	SERVICE
10121	Incision and removal of foreign body, subcutaneous tissues; complicated

CPT NOTES

- For excision, see 11400, et seq.

ICD–9–CM

709.4	Foreign body granuloma, skin
729.6	Old foreign body in soft tissue
910.7	Foreign body, head, infected
911.7	Foreign body, trunk, infected
912.7	Foreign body, should/arm, infected
913.7	Foreign body, forearm, infected
914.7	Foreign body, hand, infected
915.7	Foreign body, finger, infected
916.7	Foreign body, hip/leg, infected
917.7	Foreign body, foot/toe, infected
918.0	Superficial injury periocular
919.7	Superf foreign body NEC, infected
958.3	Posttraumatic wound infection NEC
998.5	Postoperative infection

REIMBURSEMENT INFORMATION

Medicare

- Follow–up Days — 10
- Assistant Surgeon — not paid
- Supply Charges — not allowed
- Outpatient Limit — applies
- Minor Surgery Rules Apply

CPT CODE **SERVICE**

10140* Incision and drainage of hematoma, seroma or fluid collection

CPT NOTES

- For excision, see 11400, et seq.

ICD–9–CM

380.31	Hematoma of auricle/pinna
527.6	Salivary gland mucocele
624.5	Hematoma of vulva
802.0	Nasal bone Fx, closed
802.1	Nasal bone Fx, open
802.37	Fx alveolar border mandible, open
802.38	Fx mandible body NEC, open
802.39	Multiple Fx mandible, open
802.4	Fx malar/maxillary, closed
802.5	Fx malar/maxillary, open
802.6	Fx orbital floor, closed
802.7	Fx orbital floor, open
802.8	Fx facial bone NEC, closed
802.9	Fx facial bone NEC, open
830.0	Dislocation jaw, closed
830.1	Dislocation jaw, open
848.1	Sprain of jaw
873.41	Open wound of cheek
905.0	Late effect, skull/face fracture
909.3	Late effect of surg/med complic
920.	Contusion face/scalp/neck
921.0	Black eye NOS
921.2	Contusion of orbital tissue
922.0	Contusion of breast
922.1	Contusion of chest wall
922.2	Contusion of abdominal wall
922.3	Contusion of back
923.1x	Contusion, elbow and forearm
923.20	Contusion of hand(s)
923.3	Contusion of finger
924.0x	Contusion, hip and thigh
924.1x	Contusion, knee and lower leg
924.20	Contusion of foot
924.3	Contusion of toe
924.5	Contusion of leg NOS
927.x	Crushing injury of upper limb
928.x	Crushing injury of lower limb
959.0	Face and neck injury NOS
998.1	Hemorrhage complicating a procedure

REIMBURSEMENT INFORMATION

General

- Starred procedure.

Medicare

- Follow–up Days — 10
- Assistant Surgeon — not paid
- Supply Charges — not allowed
- Outpatient Limit — applies
- Minor Surgery Rules Apply

CPT CODE	SERVICE	ICD-9-CM	
10160*	Puncture aspiration of abscess, hematoma, bulla, or cyst	373.13	Abscess of eyelid
		374.84	Cysts of eyelids
		380.11	Acute infection of pinna
		380.31	Hematoma of auricle/pinna
		473.0	Chronic maxillary sinusitis
		522.0	Pulpitis
		522.5	Periapical abscess w/o sinus
		522.8	Radicular cyst
		523.3	Acute periodontitis
		524.3	Tooth position anomaly
		526.0	Developmental odontogenic cysts
		526.1	Fissural cysts of jaw
		526.2	Jaw cysts NEC
		526.3	Jaw, central giant cell granuloma
		526.4	Inflammation of jaw
		527.3	Salivary gland abscess
		527.6	Salivary gland mucocele
		528.3	Cellulitis/abscess of mouth
		528.4	Oral soft tissue cyst
		528.5	Diseases of lips
		528.9	Oral soft tissue disease NEC
		529.0	Glossitis
		610.0	Solitary cyst of breast
		681.x	Cellulitis/abscess of finger/toe
		682.x	Cellulitis and abscess
		711.0x	Pyogenic arthritis
		744.42	Branchial cleft cyst
		750.26	Mouth anomaly NEC
		910.2	Blister, head
		910.3	Blister, head, infected
		911.2	Blister, trunk
		911.3	Blister, trunk, infected
		912.2	Blister, shoulder/arm
		912.3	Blister, shoulder/arm, infected
		913.2	Blister, forearm
		913.3	Blister, forearm, infected
		914.2	Blister, hand
		914.3	Blister, hand, infected
		915.2	Blister, finger
		915.3	Blister, finger, infected
		916.2	Blister, hip/leg
		916.3	Blister, hip/leg, infected
		917.2	Blister, foot/toe
		917.3	Blister, foot/toe, infected
		919.2	Blister NEC
		919.3	Blister NEC, infected
		920.	Contusion face/scalp/neck
		921.0	Black eye NOS
		921.2	Contusion of orbital tissue
		922.0	Contusion of breast
		922.1	Contusion of chest wall
		922.2	Contusion of abdominal wall
		922.3	Contusion of back
		923.1x	Contusion, elbow and forearm
		923.20	Contusion of hand(s)
		923.3	Contusion of finger
		924.0x	Contusion, hip and thigh

CPT NOTES

- ♦ For excision, see 11400, et seq.

CPT CODE	SERVICE
10160 (Cont'd.)	

ICD–9–CM

924.1x	Contusion, knee and lower leg
924.20	Contusion of foot
998.5	Postoperative infection

REIMBURSEMENT INFORMATION

General

- Starred procedure.

Medicare

- Follow–up Days — 10
- Assistant Surgeon — not paid
- Supply Charges — not allowed
- Outpatient Limit — applies
- Minor Surgery Rules Apply

CPT CODE	SERVICE
10180	Incision and drainage, complex, postoperative wound infection

CPT NOTES

- For excision, see 11400, et seq.
- For secondary closure of surgical wound, see 12020, 12021, 13160.

ICD–9–CM

681.10	Cellulitis, toe NOS
682.x	Cellulitis and abscess
998.5	Postoperative infection

REIMBURSEMENT INFORMATION

Medicare

- Follow–up Days — 10
- Assistant Surgeon — not paid
- Supply Charges — not allowed
- Outpatient Limit — does not apply
- Minor Surgery Rules Apply

CPT CODE	SERVICE
11000*	Debridement of extensive eczematous or infected skin; up to 10% of body surface

CPT NOTES

- For dermabrasions, see 15780-15791.
- For nail debridement, see 11700-11711.
- For burn(s), see 16000-16042.

ICD–9–CM

528.7	Oral epithelium disturbance NEC
528.9	Oral soft tissue disease NEC
684.	Impetigo
686.x	Skin/Subcutaneous tissue infection
692.x	Contact dermatitis and eczema
693.x	Dermatitis due to intern. substance
694.0	Dermatitis herpetiformis
694.2	Juvenile dermatitis herpetiformis
694.3	Impetigo herpetiformis
694.4	Pemphigus
694.8	Bullous dermatosis NEC
694.9	Bullous dermatosis NOS
696.1	Other psoriasis
701.5	Abnormal granulation tissue NEC
703.0	Ingrowing nail
707.x	Chronic ulcer of skin
709.3	Degenerative skin disorders
785.4	Gangrene
873.30	Open wound of nose NOS, complicated
873.31	Open wound nasal septum, complic
873.32	Open wound nasal cavity, complic
873.39	Multiple open nose wounds, complic
873.42	Open wound of forehead
873.5x	Face, complicated open wound
873.9	Open wound of head NEC, complicated
875.1	Open wound of chest, complicated
876.1	Open wound of back, complicated
877.1	Open wound of buttock, complicated
880.01	Open wound of scapula
880.11	Open wound of scapula, complicated
880.12	Open wound of axilla, complicated
880.13	Open wound of upper arm, complic
881.11	Open wound of elbow, complicated
881.12	Open wound of wrist, complicated
882.1	Open wound of hand, complicated
883.1	Open wound of finger, complicated
884.1	Open wound of arm mult/NOS, compl
890.1	Open wound of hip/thigh, complic
891.1	Open wound of knee/leg/ankle, compl
892.1	Open wound of foot, complicated
893.1	Open wound of toe, complicated
906.1	Late effect, open wound extremity
910.1	Abrasion, head, infected
911.1	Abrasion, trunk, infected
912.1	Abrasion, shoulder/arm, infected
913.1	Abrasion, forearm, infected
914.1	Abrasion, hand, infected
915.1	Abrasion, finger, infected
916.1	Abrasion, hip/leg, infected
917.1	Abrasion, foot/toe, infected
941.03	Burn NOS, lip
941.07	Burn NOS, face NEC

CPT CODE	SERVICE	ICD–9–CM
11000 (Cont'd.)		958.3 Posttraumatic wound infection NEC 998.3 Postop wound disruption 998.5 Postoperative infection

REIMBURSEMENT INFORMATION

General

- Starred procedure.

Medicare

- Follow–up Days — 10
- Assistant Surgeon — not paid
- Supply Charges — not allowed
- Outpatient Limit — applies
- Minor Surgery Rules Apply
- Fragments — 64450

CPT CODE **SERVICE**

11001 Debridement of extensive eczematous or infected skin; each additional 10% of the body surface

CPT NOTES

- For dermabrasions, see 15780-15791.
- For nail debridement, see 11700-11711.
- For burn(s), see 16000-16042.

ICD–9–CM

250.7	Diabetes w/circulatory disorders
454.0	Leg varicosity w/ulcer
454.1	Leg varicosity w/inflammation
454.2	Varicose leg w/ulcer+inflammation
528.7	Oral epithelium disturbance NEC
528.9	Oral soft tissue disease NEC
684.	Impetigo
686.x	Skin/Subcutaneous tissue infection
692.x	Contact dermatitis and eczema
693.x	Dermatitis due to intern. substance
694.0	Dermatitis herpetiformis
694.2	Juvenile dermatitis herpetiformis
694.3	Impetigo herpetiformis
694.4	Pemphigus
694.8	Bullous dermatosis NEC
694.9	Bullous dermatosis NOS
696.1	Other psoriasis
701.5	Abnormal granulation tissue NEC
703.0	Ingrowing nail
707.x	Chronic ulcer of skin
709.3	Degenerative skin disorders
785.4	Gangrene
873.42	Open wound of forehead
875.1	Open wound of chest, complicated
876.1	Open wound of back, complicated
877.1	Open wound of buttock, complicated
880.01	Open wound of scapula
880.1x	Open wound of shoulder/upper arm, complicated
881.11	Open wound of elbow, complicated
881.12	Open wound of wrist, complicated
882.1	Open wound of hand, complicated
883.1	Open wound of finger, complicated
884.1	Open wound of arm mult/NOS, compl
890.1	Open wound of hip/thigh, complic
891.1	Open wound of knee/leg/ankle, compl
892.1	Open wound of foot, complicated
893.1	Open wound of toe, complicated
906.1	Late effect, open wound extremity
910.1	Abrasion, head, infected
911.1	Abrasion, trunk, infected
912.1	Abrasion, shoulder/arm, infected
913.1	Abrasion, forearm, infected
914.1	Abrasion, hand, infected
915.1	Abrasion, finger, infected
916.1	Abrasion, hip/leg, infected
917.1	Abrasion, foot/toe, infected
958.3	Posttraumatic wound infection NEC
998.5	Postoperative infection

REIMBURSEMENT INFORMATION

Medicare

- Follow–up Days — none; falls within global period of another procedure
- Assistant Surgeon — not paid
- Supply Charges — not allowed
- Outpatient Limit — applies

CPT CODE	SERVICE
11040	Debridement; skin, partial thickness

CPT NOTES

- For dermabrasions, see 15780-15791.
- For nail debridement, see 11700-11711.
- For burn(s), see 16000-16042.

ICD-9-CM	
250.0	Diabetes mellitus w/o complication
250.7	Diabetes w/circulatory disorders
250.8	Diabetes w/manifestations
454.0	Leg varicosity w/ulcer
454.2	Varicose leg w/ulcer+inflammation
684.	Impetigo
686.x	Skin/Subcutaneous tissue infection
694.5	Pemphigoid
696.1	Other psoriasis
700.	Corns and callosities
701.1	Keratoderma, acquired
701.5	Abnormal granulation tissue NEC
701.8	Hypertrophic/atrophic skin NEC
707.x	Chronic ulcer of skin
709.3	Degenerative skin disorders
709.4	Foreign body granuloma, skin
709.8	Skin disorders NEC
785.4	Gangrene
870.1	Full-thickness laceration eyelid
873.30	Open wound of nose NOS, complicated
873.31	Open wound nasal septum, complic
873.32	Open wound nasal cavity, complic
873.39	Multiple open nose wounds, complic
873.5x	Face, complicated open wound
873.9	Open wound of head NEC, complicated
875.0	Open wound of chest
875.1	Open wound of chest, complicated
876.0	Open wound of back
876.1	Open wound of back, complicated
877.0	Open wound of buttock
877.1	Open wound of buttock, complicated
879.6	Open wound of trunk NEC
880.0x	Shoulder/upper arm, open wound
880.1x	Shoulder/upper arm, cplx open wound
881.00	Open wound of forearm
881.01	Open wound of elbow
881.10	Open wound of forearm, complicated
881.11	Open wound of elbow, complicated
882.0	Open wound of hand
882.1	Open wound of hand, complicated
883.0	Open wound of finger
883.1	Open wound of finger, complicated
886.x	Traumatic finger amputation
887.0	Amputation below elbow, unilateral
887.2	Amputation above elbow, unilateral
890.0	Open wound of hip/thigh
890.1	Open wound of hip/thigh, complic
891.0	Open wound of knee/leg/ankle
891.1	Open wound of knee/leg/ankle, compl
892.0	Open wound of foot
892.1	Open wound of foot, complicated
893.0	Open wound of toe
893.1	Open wound of toe, complicated
895.x	Traumatic amputation of toe(s)
896.0	Amputation of foot, unilateral
896.1	Amputation of foot, unilat, compl
897.0	Amputation below knee, unilateral

CPT CODE	SERVICE	ICD–9–CM	
11040 (Cont'd.)		897.1	Amputate below knee, unilat, compl
		897.2	Amputation above knee, unilateral
		910.0	Abrasion, head
		910.1	Abrasion, head, infected
		911.0	Abrasion, trunk
		911.1	Abrasion, trunk, infected
		912.0	Abrasion, shoulder/arm
		912.1	Abrasion, shoulder/arm, infected
		913.0	Abrasion, forearm
		913.1	Abrasion, forearm, infected
		914.0	Abrasion, hand
		914.1	Abrasion, hand, infected
		916.0	Abrasion, hip/leg
		916.1	Abrasion, hip/leg, infected
		917.0	Abrasion, foot/toe
		917.1	Abrasion, foot/toe, infected
		919.0	Abrasion NEC
		919.1	Abrasion NEC, infected
		927.3	Crushing injury, finger
		941.03	Burn NOS, lip
		941.07	Burn NOS, face NEC
		958.3	Posttraumatic wound infection NEC
		958.8	Early complications of trauma NEC
		959.7	Lower leg injury NOS
		959.8	Injury, multiple sites, site NEC
		996.60	Reaction, unspecified device/graft
		996.67	Reaction, internal ortho device NEC
		997.62	Infection of amputated stump
		998.3	Postop wound disruption
		998.5	Postoperative infection

REIMBURSEMENT INFORMATION

Medicare

- Follow–up Days — 0
- Assistant Surgeon — not paid
- Supply Charges — not allowed
- Outpatient Limit — applies
- Minor Surgery Rules Apply
- Fragments — 64450

CPT CODE	SERVICE
11041	Debridement; skin, full thickness

CPT NOTES

- For dermabrasions, see 15780-15791.
- For nail debridement, see 11700-11711.
- For burn(s), see 16000-16042.

ICD–9–CM

454.0	Leg varicosity w/ulcer
454.2	Varicose leg w/ulcer+inflammation
685.0	Pilonidal cyst w/abscess
686.x	Skin/Subcutaneous tissue infection
700.	Corns and callosities
701.5	Abnormal granulation tissue NEC
707.0	Decubitus ulcer
707.8	Chronic skin ulcer NEC
709.3	Degenerative skin disorders
709.4	Foreign body granuloma, skin
709.8	Skin disorders NEC
785.4	Gangrene
870.x	Open wound of ocular adnexa
873.30	Open wound of nose NOS, complicated
873.31	Open wound nasal septum, complic
873.32	Open wound nasal cavity, complic
873.39	Multiple open nose wounds, complic
873.5x	Face, complicated open wound
873.9	Open wound of head NEC, complicated
875.0	Open wound of chest
875.1	Open wound of chest, complicated
876.0	Open wound of back
876.1	Open wound of back, complicated
877.0	Open wound of buttock
877.1	Open wound of buttock, complicated
879.6	Open wound of trunk NEC
880.00	Open wound of shoulder
880.01	Open wound of scapula
880.02	Open wound of axilla
880.03	Open wound of upper arm
880.09	Multiple open wounds of shoulder
880.10	Open wound of shoulder, complicated
880.11	Open wound of scapula, complicated
880.12	Open wound of axilla, complicated
880.13	Open wound of upper arm, complic
881.00	Open wound of forearm
881.01	Open wound of elbow
881.10	Open wound of forearm, complicated
881.11	Open wound of elbow, complicated
882.0	Open wound of hand
882.1	Open wound of hand, complicated
883.0	Open wound of finger
883.1	Open wound cf finger, complicated
886.x	Traumatic finger amputation
887.0	Amputation below elbow, unilateral
887.2	Amputation above elbow, unilateral
890.0	Open wound of hip/thigh
890.1	Open wound of hip/thigh, complic
891.0	Open wound of knee/leg/ankle
891.1	Open wound of knee/leg/ankle, compl
892.0	Open wound of foot
892.1	Open wound of foot, complicated
893.0	Open wound of toe
893.1	Open wound of toe, complicated
895.x	Traumatic amputation of toe(s)
896.0	Amputation of foot, unilateral
896.1	Amputation of foot, unilat, compl

CPT CODE	SERVICE
11041 (Cont'd.)	

ICD-9-CM

897.0	Amputation below knee, unilateral
897.1	Amputate below knee, unilat, compl
897.2	Amputation above knee, unilateral
910.1	Abrasion, head, infected
911.0	Abrasion, trunk
911.1	Abrasion, trunk, infected
911.8	Superficial injury, trunk NEC
912.0	Abrasion, shoulder/arm
912.1	Abrasion, shoulder/arm, infected
913.0	Abrasion, forearm
913.1	Abrasion, forearm, infected
914.0	Abrasion, hand
914.1	Abrasion, hand, infected
916.0	Abrasion, hip/leg
916.1	Abrasion, hip/leg, infected
917.0	Abrasion, foot/toe
917.1	Abrasion, foot/toe, infected
919.0	Abrasion NEC
919.1	Abrasion NEC, infected
927.3	Crushing injury, finger
958.3	Posttraumatic wound infection NEC
958.8	Early complications of trauma NEC
959.8	Injury, multiple sites, site NEC
996.60	Reaction, unspecified device/graft
996.67	Reaction, internal ortho device NEC
997.62	Infection of amputated stump
998.3	Postop wound disruption
998.5	Postoperative infection

REIMBURSEMENT INFORMATION

Medicare

- Follow–up Days — 0
- Assistant Surgeon — not paid
- Supply Charges — not allowed
- Outpatient Limit — applies
- Minor Surgery Rules Apply
- Fragments — 11040, 64450

CPT CODE	SERVICE
11042	Debridement; skin, and subcutaneous tissue

CPT NOTES

- For dermabrasions, see 15780-15791.
- For nail debridement, see 11700-11711.
- For burn(s), see 16000-16042.

ICD–9–CM

250.00	Diabetes, uncomplicated, type II
250.01	Diabetes, uncomplicated, type I
250.7	Diabetes w/circulatory disorders
250.8	Diabetes w/manifestations
373.13	Abscess of eyelid
454.0	Leg varicosity w/ulcer
454.2	Varicose leg w/ulcer+inflammation
525.8	Dental disorder NEC
526.4	Inflammation of jaw
526.81	Exostosis of jaw
526.89	Jaw disease NEC
526.9	Jaw disease NOS
680.x	Carbuncle and furuncle
681.00	Cellulitis, finger NOS
681.10	Cellulitis, toe NOS
682.x	Cellulitis and abscess
685.0	Pilonidal cyst w/abscess
686.8	Local skin infection NEC
686.9	Local skin infection NOS
700.	Corns and callosities
707.x	Chronic ulcer of skin
709.3	Degenerative skin disorders
709.4	Foreign body granuloma, skin
709.8	Skin disorders NEC
785.4	Gangrene
870.x	Open wound of ocular adnexa
873.30	Open wound of nose NOS, complicated
873.31	Open wound nasal septum, complic
873.32	Open wound nasal cavity, complic
873.39	Multiple open nose wounds, complic
873.5x	Face, complicated open wound
873.9	Open wound of head NEC, complicated
875.0	Open wound of chest
876.0	Open wound of back
877.1	Open wound of buttock, complicated
879.6	Open wound of trunk NEC
880.00	Open wound of shoulder
880.01	Open wound of scapula
880.02	Open wound of axilla
880.03	Open wound of upper arm
880.09	Multiple open wounds of shoulder
880.13	Open wound of upper arm, complic
881.00	Open wound of forearm
881.01	Open wound of elbow
881.10	Open wound of forearm, complicated
881.11	Open wound of elbow, complicated
882.0	Open wound of hand
882.1	Open wound of hand, complicated
883.0	Open wound of finger
883.1	Open wound of finger, complicated
886.x	Traumatic finger amputation
887.0	Amputation below elbow, unilateral
887.2	Amputation above elbow, unilateral
890.0	Open wound of hip/thigh
890.1	Open wound of hip/thigh, complic
891.0	Open wound of knee/leg/ankle
891.1	Open wound of knee/leg/ankle, compl

CPT CODE	SERVICE	ICD-9-CM	
11042 (Cont'd.)		892.0	Open wound of foot
		892.1	Open wound of foot, complicated
		893.0	Open wound of toe
		893.1	Open wound of toe, complicated
		895.x	Traumatic amputation of toe(s)
		896.0	Amputation of foot, unilateral
		896.1	Amputation of foot, unilat, compl
		897.0	Amputation below knee, unilateral
		897.1	Amputate below knee, unilat, compl
		897.2	Amputation above knee, unilateral
		910.1	Abrasion, head, infected
		911.0	Abrasion, trunk
		911.1	Abrasion, trunk, infected
		912.0	Abrasion, shoulder/arm
		912.1	Abrasion, shoulder/arm, infected
		913.0	Abrasion, forearm
		913.1	Abrasion, forearm, infected
		914.0	Abrasion, hand
		914.1	Abrasion, hand, infected
		916.0	Abrasion, hip/leg
		916.1	Abrasion, hip/leg, infected
		917.0	Abrasion, foot/toe
		917.1	Abrasion, foot/toe, infected
		919.0	Abrasion NEC
		919.1	Abrasion NEC, infected
		925.1	Crushing injury to face and scalp
		925.2	Crushing injury of neck
		926.0	Crushing injury, external genitalia
		926.11	Crushing injury, back
		926.12	Crushing injury, buttock
		927.0x	Crushing injury, shoulder/upper arm
		927.3	Crushing injury, finger
		928.x	Crushing injury of lower limb
		929.x	Crushing injury, multiple sites
		941.03	Burn NOS, lip
		941.07	Burn NOS, face NEC
		958.3	Posttraumatic wound infection NEC
		958.8	Early complications of trauma NEC
		959.7	Lower leg injury NOS
		959.8	Injury, multiple sites, site NEC
		996.60	Reaction, unspecified device/graft
		996.67	Reaction, internal ortho device NEC
		997.62	Infection of amputated stump
		998.3	Postop wound disruption
		998.5	Postoperative infection

REIMBURSEMENT INFORMATION

Medicare

- Follow–up Days — 0
- Assistant Surgeon — not paid
- Supply Charges — not allowed
- Outpatient Limit — does not apply
- Minor Surgery Rules Apply
- Fragments — 11040, 11041, 64450

CPT CODE	SERVICE
11043	Debridement; skin, subcutaneous tissue, and muscle

CPT NOTES

- For dermabrasions, see 15780-15791.
- For nail debridement, see 11700-11711.
- For burn(s), see 16000-16042.

ICD–9–CM

250.00	Diabetes, uncomplicated, type II
250.01	Diabetes, uncomplicated, type I
250.7	Diabetes w/circulatory disorders
250.8	Diabetes w/manifestations
373.13	Abscess of eyelid
454.0	Leg varicosity w/ulcer
454.2	Varicose leg w/ulcer+inflammation
525.8	Dental disorder NEC
526.4	Inflammation of jaw
680.x	Carbuncle and furuncle
681.00	Cellulitis, finger NOS
681.10	Cellulitis, toe NOS
682.x	Cellulitis and abscess
685.0	Pilonidal cyst w/abscess
686.8	Local skin infection NEC
686.9	Local skin infection NOS
707.x	Chronic ulcer of skin
709.3	Degenerative skin disorders
709.4	Foreign body granuloma, skin
709.8	Skin disorders NEC
729.4	Fasciitis NOS
785.4	Gangrene
823.92	Fx tibia w/fibula NOS, open
826.1	Fx phalanx, foot, open
870.x	Open wound of ocular adnexa
873.30	Open wound of nose NOS, complicated
873.31	Open wound nasal septum, complic
873.32	Open wound nasal cavity, complic
873.39	Multiple open nose wounds, complic
873.5x	Face, complicated open wound
873.9	Open wound of head NEC, complicated
875.0	Open wound of chest
875.1	Open wound of chest, complicated
876.0	Open wound of back
876.1	Open wound of back, complicated
877.0	Open wound of buttock
877.1	Open wound of buttock, complicated
879.8	Open wound site NOS
880.00	Open wound of shoulder
880.01	Open wound of scapula
880.02	Open wound of axilla
880.03	Open wound of upper arm
880.09	Multiple open wounds of shoulder
880.10	Open wound of shoulder, complicated
880.13	Open wound of upper arm, complic
880.20	Open wound shoulder w/tendon
880.23	Open wound upper arm w/tendon
881.00	Open wound of forearm
881.01	Open wound of elbow
881.10	Open wound of forearm, complicated
881.11	Open wound of elbow, complicated
881.20	Open wound of forearm w/tendon
881.21	Open wound of elbow w/tendon
882.0	Open wound of hand
882.1	Open wound of hand, complicated
883.0	Open wound of finger
883.1	Open wound of finger, complicated

CPT CODE	SERVICE	ICD-9-CM	
11043 (Cont'd.)		886.0	Traumatic finger amputation
		887.2	Amputation above elbow, unilateral
		890.1	Open wound of hip/thigh, complic
		890.2	Open wound of hip/thigh w/tendon
		891.0	Open wound of knee/leg/ankle
		891.1	Open wound of knee/leg/ankle, compl
		891.2	Open wound knee/leg/ankle w/tendon
		892.0	Open wound of foot
		892.1	Open wound of foot, complicated
		892.2	Open wound of foot w/tendon
		893.x	Open wound of toe(s)
		895.1	Amputation of toe, complicated
		896.1	Amputation of foot, unilat, compl
		897.1	Amputate below knee, unilat, compl
		897.2	Amputation above knee, unilateral
		910.1	Abrasion, head, infected
		911.8	Superficial injury, trunk NEC
		916.1	Abrasion, hip/leg, infected
		917.1	Abrasion, foot/toe, infected
		918.0	Superficial injury periocular
		919.1	Abrasion NEC, infected
		925.1	Crushing injury to face and scalp
		925.2	Crushing injury of neck
		926.0	Crushing injury, external genitalia
		926.11	Crushing injury, back
		926.12	Crushing injury, buttock
		927.0x	Crushing injury, shoulder/upper arm
		927.3	Crushing injury, finger
		928.x	Crushing injury of lower limb
		929.x	Crushing injury, multiple sites
		958.3	Posttraumatic wound infection NEC
		958.8	Early complications of trauma NEC
		996.60	Reaction, unspecified device/graft
		996.67	Reaction, internal ortho device NEC
		997.62	Infection of amputated stump
		998.3	Postop wound disruption
		998.5	Postoperative infection

REIMBURSEMENT INFORMATION

Medicare

- Follow-up Days — 10
- Assistant Surgeon — not paid
- Supply Charges — not allowed
- Outpatient Limit — does not apply
- Minor Surgery Rules Apply
- Fragments — 11040, 11041, 11042, 64450

CPT CODE	SERVICE
11044	Debridement; skin, subcutaneous tissue, muscle, and bone

CPT NOTES

- ◆ For dermabrasions, see 15780-15791.
- ◆ For nail debridement, see 11700-11711.
- ◆ For burn(s), see 16000-16042.

ICD–9–CM

250.00	Diabetes, uncomplicated, type II
250.01	Diabetes, uncomplicated, type I
250.7	Diabetes w/circulatory disorders
250.8	Diabetes w/manifestations
454.0	Leg varicosity w/ulcer
454.2	Varicose leg w/ulcer+inflammation
526.4	Inflammation of jaw
685.0	Pilonidal cyst w/abscess
707.x	Chronic ulcer of skin
709.3	Degenerative skin disorders
709.4	Foreign body granuloma, skin
709.8	Skin disorders NEC
729.4	Fasciitis NOS
730.0x	Acute osteomyelitis
730.1x	Chronic osteomyelitis
730.2	Osteomyelitis
730.27	Osteomyelitis NOS, ankle/foot
785.4	Gangrene
873.30	Open wound of nose NOS, complicated
873.31	Open wound nasal septum, complic
873.32	Open wound nasal cavity, complic
873.39	Multiple open nose wounds, complic
873.5x	Face, complicated open wound
873.9	Open wound of head NEC, complicated
875.0	Open wound of chest
876.0	Open wound of back
877.1	Open wound of buttock, complicated
879.6	Open wound of trunk NEC
880.10	Open wound of shoulder, complicated
880.13	Open wound of upper arm, complic
880.20	Open wound shoulder w/tendon
880.23	Open wound upper arm w/tendon
881.10	Open wound of forearm, complicated
881.11	Open wound of elbow, complicated
881.20	Open wound of forearm w/tendon
881.21	Open wound of elbow w/tendon
882.0	Open wound of hand
882.1	Open wound of hand, complicated
883.0	Open wound of finger
883.1	Open wound of finger, complicated
886.x	Traumatic finger amputation
887.0	Amputation below elbow, unilateral
887.2	Amputation above elbow, unilateral
890.1	Open wound of hip/thigh, complic
890.2	Open wound of hip/thigh w/tendon
891.1	Open wound of knee/leg/ankle, compl
891.2	Open wound knee/leg/ankle w/tendon
892.1	Open wound of foot, complicated
892.2	Open wound of foot w/tendon
893.1	Open wound of toe, complicated
893.2	Open wound of toe w/tendon
895.1	Amputation of toe, complicated
896.1	Amputation of foot, unilat, compl
897.1	Amputate below knee, unilat, compl
897.2	Amputation above knee, unilateral
910.1	Abrasion, head, infected
911.8	Superficial injury, trunk NEC

CPT CODE	SERVICE	ICD-9-CM	
11044 (Cont'd.)		916.1	Abrasion, hip/leg, infected
		917.0	Abrasion, foot/toe
		919.1	Abrasion NEC, infected
		927.3	Crushing injury, finger
		958.3	Posttraumatic wound infection NEC
		958.8	Early complications of trauma NEC
		959.7	Lower leg injury NOS
		959.8	Injury, multiple sites, site NEC
		996.60	Reaction, unspecified device/graft
		996.66	Reaction, internal joint prosthesis
		996.67	Reaction, internal ortho device NEC
		997.62	Infection of amputated stump
		998.3	Postop wound disruption
		998.5	Postoperative infection

REIMBURSEMENT INFORMATION

Medicare

- Follow–up Days — 10
- Assistant Surgeon — not paid
- Supply Charges — not allowed
- Outpatient Limit — does not apply
- Minor Surgery Rules Apply
- Fragments — 11040, 11041, 11042, 11043, 64450

CPT CODE	SERVICE
11050*	Paring or curettement of benign hyperkeratotic skin lesion with or without chemical cauterization (such as verrucae or clavi) not extending through the stratum corneum (eg, callus or wart) with or without local anesthesia; single lesion
11051	Paring or curettement of benign hyperkeratotic skin lesion with or without chemical cauterization (such as verrucae or clavi) not extending through the stratum corneum (eg, callus or wart) with or without local anesthesia; two to four lesions
11052	Paring or curettement of benign hyperkeratotic skin lesion with or without chemical cauterization (such as verrucae or clavi) not extending through the stratum corneum (eg, callus or wart) with or without local anesthesia; more than four lesions

ICD–9–CM

078.0	Molluscum contagiosum
078.10	Viral warts NOS
210.0	B-Neoplasm, Lip
216.x	Benign neoplasm, Skin
370.24	Photokeratitis
373.2	Chalazion
448.1	Nevus, non-neoplastic
690.	Erythematosquamous dermatosis
691.8	Other atopic dermatitis
700.	Corns and callosities
701.1	Keratoderma, acquired
701.9	Hypertrophic/atrophic skin NOS
702.x	Other dermatosis
757.39	Skin anomaly NEC

REIMBURSEMENT INFORMATION

General

- Starred procedure. (11050)

Medicare

- Follow–up Days — 0
- Assistant Surgeon — not paid
- Supply Charges — not allowed
- Outpatient Limit — applies
- Minor Surgery Rules Apply

CPT CODE	SERVICE
11100	Biopsy of skin, subcutaneous tissue and/or mucous membrane (including simple closure), unless otherwise listed (separate procedure); single lesion

CPT NOTES

- ♦ For biopsy of conjunctiva, see 68100; eyelid, see 67810.

ICD–9–CM

140.0	M-Neoplasm, Upper lip, vermilion
140.1	M-Neoplasm, Lower lip, vermilion
140.3	M-Neoplasm, Upper lip, inner aspect
140.4	M-Neoplasm, Lower lip, inner aspect
140.5	M-Neoplasm, Lip NOS, inner NOS
140.6	M-Neoplasm, lip, commissure
140.8	M-Neoplasm, Lip NEC
140.9	M-Neoplasm, Lip/vermilion NOS
143.0	M-Neoplasm, Upper gum
143.1	M-Neoplasm, Lower gum
143.8	M-Neoplasm, Gum NEC
144.0	M-Neoplasm, Anterior floor of mouth
144.9	M-Neoplasm, Floor of mouth NOS
145.9	M-Neoplasm, Mouth NOS
149.8	M-Neoplasm, Oral cavity/pharynx NEC
171.0	M-Neoplasm, Soft tissue, head
172.x	Skin Melanoma
173.x	Malignant neoplasm, Skin
190.8	M-Neoplasm, Eye NEC
195.4	M-Neoplasm, Upper limb
195.5	M-Neoplasm, Lower limb
196.0	M-Neoplasm, Lymph head/neck/face
198.2	M2-Neoplasm, Skin
199.0	M-Neoplasm, Disseminated
202.11	Mycosis fungoides, head/neck
202.12	Mycosis fungoides, thorax
202.13	Mycosis fungoides, abdomen
202.14	Mycosis fungoides, axilla
202.15	Mycosis fungoides, inguinal
202.16	Mycosis fungoides, pelvic
210.0	B-Neoplasm, Lip
210.1	B-Neoplasm, Tongue
210.4	B-Neoplasm, Mouth NEC/NOS
214.0	Lipoma, Skin of face
216.x	Benign neoplasm, Skin
228.01	Hemangioma, Skin
230.0	CA in situ, Oral cavity/pharynx
232.0	CA in situ, Skin of lip
232.2	CA in situ, Skin of ear
232.3	CA in situ, Skin of face NEC
232.4	CA in situ, Scalp/skin of neck
232.5	CA in situ, Skin of trunk
232.6	CA in situ, Skin of arm
232.7	CA in situ, Skin of leg
235.1	UB-Neoplasm, Oral cavity/pharynx
237.71	Neurofibromatosis, type 1
238.1	UB-Neoplasm, Soft tissue
238.2	UB-Neoplasm, Skin
239.2	Bone/Skin neoplasm NOS
374.84	Cysts of eyelids
522.8	Radicular cyst
523.4	Chronic periodontitis
528.4	Oral soft tissue cyst
528.5	Diseases of lips
528.6	Leukoplakia of oral mucosa/tongue
528.7	Oral epithelium disturbance NEC
528.9	Oral soft tissue disease NEC

CPT CODE	SERVICE	ICD–9–CM	
11100 (Cont'd.)		529.0	Glossitis
		529.9	Tongue disorder NOS
		692.1	Oil & grease dermatitis
		692.79	Solar dermatitis NEC
		693.0	Drug dermatitis NOS
		694.0	Dermatitis herpetiformis
		694.5	Pemphigoid
		695.1	Erythema multiforme
		695.4	Lupus erythematosus
		696.2	Parapsoriasis
		696.5	Pityriasis NEC/NOS
		697.0	Lichen planus
		698.4	Dermatitis factitia
		701.2	Acquired acanthosis nigricans
		701.4	Keloid scar
		701.5	Abnormal granulation tissue NEC
		701.9	Hypertrophic/atrophic skin NOS
		702.0	Actinic keratosis
		702.11	Inflamed seborrheic keratosis
		709.3	Degenerative skin disorders
		709.8	Skin disorders NEC

REIMBURSEMENT INFORMATION

General

- ♦ Separate procedure rules apply.

Medicare

- ♦ Follow–up Days — 0
- ♦ Assistant Surgeon — not paid
- ♦ Supply Charges — not allowed
- ♦ Outpatient Limit — applies
- ♦ Minor Surgery Rules Apply

CPT CODE	SERVICE
11101	Biopsy of skin, subcutaneous tissue and/or mucous membrane (including simple closure), unless otherwise listed (separate procedure); each separate/additional lesion

CPT NOTES

- For biopsy of conjunctiva, see 68100; eyelid, see 67810.

ICD–9–CM

140.0	M-Neoplasm, Upper lip, vermilion
140.1	M-Neoplasm, Lower lip, vermilion
140.3	M-Neoplasm, Upper lip, inner aspect
140.4	M-Neoplasm, Lower lip, inner aspect
140.5	M-Neoplasm, Lip NOS, inner NOS
140.6	M-Neoplasm, lip, commissure
140.8	M-Neoplasm, Lip NEC
140.9	M-Neoplasm, Lip/vermilion NOS
143.0	M-Neoplasm, Upper gum
143.1	M-Neoplasm, Lower gum
143.8	M-Neoplasm, Gum NEC
144.0	M-Neoplasm, Anterior floor of mouth
144.9	M-Neoplasm, Floor of mouth NOS
145.9	M-Neoplasm, Mouth NOS
149.8	M-Neoplasm, Oral cavity/pharynx NEC
172.x	Skin Melanoma
173.x	Malignant neoplasm, Skin
195.1	M-Neoplasm, Thorax
195.4	M-Neoplasm, Upper limb
195.5	M-Neoplasm, Lower limb
198.2	M2-Neoplasm, Skin
199.0	M-Neoplasm, Disseminated
202.11	Mycosis fungoides, head/neck
202.12	Mycosis fungoides, thorax
202.13	Mycosis fungoides, abdomen
202.14	Mycosis fungoides, axilla
202.15	Mycosis fungoides, inguinal
202.16	Mycosis fungoides, pelvic
202.18	Mycosis fungoides, mult sites
210.0	B-Neoplasm, Lip
210.1	B-Neoplasm, Tongue
210.4	B-Neoplasm, Mouth NEC/NOS
214.0	Lipoma, Skin of face
216.x	Benign neoplasm, Skin
228.01	Hemangioma, Skin
230.0	CA in situ, Oral cavity/pharynx
232.0	CA in situ, Skin of lip
232.2	CA in situ, Skin of ear
232.3	CA in situ, Skin of face NEC
232.4	CA in situ, Scalp/skin of neck
232.5	CA in situ, Skin of trunk
232.6	CA in situ, Skin of arm
232.7	CA in situ, Skin of leg
235.1	UB-Neoplasm, Oral cavity/pharynx
237.71	Neurofibromatosis, type 1
238.1	UB-Neoplasm, Soft tissue
238.2	UB-Neoplasm, Skin
239.2	Bone/Skin neoplasm NOS
528.4	Oral soft tissue cyst
528.5	Diseases of lips
528.6	Leukoplakia of oral mucosa/tongue
528.7	Oral epithelium disturbance NEC
528.9	Oral soft tissue disease NEC
529.0	Glossitis
692.1	Oil & grease dermatitis
692.79	Solar dermatitis NEC
693.0	Drug dermatitis NOS

CPT CODE	SERVICE	ICD-9-CM	
11101 (Cont'd.)		694.0	Dermatitis herpetiformis
		694.5	Pemphigoid
		695.1	Erythema multiforme
		695.4	Lupus erythematosus
		696.2	Parapsoriasis
		696.5	Pityriasis NEC/NOS
		697.0	Lichen planus
		698.4	Dermatitis factitia
		701.2	Acquired acanthosis nigricans
		701.5	Abnormal granulation tissue NEC
		701.9	Hypertrophic/atrophic skin NOS
		702.0	Actinic keratosis
		702.11	Inflamed seborrheic keratosis
		709.00	Dyschromia, unspecified
		709.01	Vitiligo
		709.09	Other dyschromia
		709.3	Degenerative skin disorders
		709.8	Skin disorders NEC

REIMBURSEMENT INFORMATION

General

- Separate procedure rules apply.

Medicare

- Follow-up Days — none; falls within the global period of another procedure
- Assistant Surgeon — not paid
- Supply Charges — not allowed
- Outpatient Limit — applies
- Minor Surgery Rules Apply

CPT CODE	SERVICE
11200*	Removal of skin tags, multiple fibrocutaneous tags, any area; up to and including 15 lesions
11201	Removal of skin tags, multiple fibrocutaneous tags, any area; each additional ten lesions

CPT NOTES

- Removal by scissoring, or any sharp method or ligature strangulation including chemical or electrocauterization of wound, with or without local anesthesia.
- For electrosurgical destruction, see 17200, 17201.

ICD–9–CM

078.0	Molluscum contagiosum
078.10	Viral warts NOS
216.1	B-Neoplasm, Skin of eyelid/canthus
216.2	B-Neoplasm, Skin of ear
216.3	B-Neoplasm, Skin of face NEC
216.4	B-Neoplasm, Scalp/skin of neck
216.5	B-Neoplasm, Skin of trunk
216.6	B-Neoplasm, Skin of arm
216.7	B-Neoplasm, Skin of leg
238.2	UB-Neoplasm, Skin
239.2	Bone/Skin neoplasm NOS
455.9	Residual hemorrhoidal skin tags
701.9	Hypertrophic/atrophic skin NOS
757.39	Skin anomaly NEC

REIMBURSEMENT INFORMATION

General

- Starred procedure. (11200)

Medicare

- Follow–up Days
  11200 — 10
  11201 — none; falls within global period of another procedure
- Assistant Surgeon — not paid
- Supply Charges — not allowed
- Outpatient Limit — applies
- Minor Surgery Rules Apply
- Fragments — 12001, 12002, 12004, 12005, 12006, 12007, 12011, 12013, 12014, 12015, 12016, 12017, 12018

CPT CODE	SERVICE
11300*	Shaving of epidermal or dermal lesion, single lesion, trunk, arms or legs; lesion diameter 0.5 cm or less
11301	Shaving of epidermal or dermal lesion, single lesion, trunk, arms or legs; lesion diameter 0.6 cm to 1.0 cm
11302	Shaving of epidermal or dermal lesion, single lesion, trunk, arms or legs; lesion diameter 1.1 cm to 2.0 cm
11303	Shaving of epidermal or dermal lesion, single lesion, trunk, arms or legs; lesion diameter over 2.0 cm

CPT NOTES

- Shaving is the sharp removal by transverse incision or horizontal slicing to remove epidermal and dermal lesions without a full-thickness dermal excision. This includes local anesthesia, chemical or electrocauterization of the wound. The wound does not require suture closure.

ICD–9–CM

110.5	Dermatophytosis of body
117.x	Mycosis
214.1	Lipoma, Skin NEC
216.5	B-Neoplasm, Skin of trunk
216.6	B-Neoplasm, Skin of arm
216.7	B-Neoplasm, Skin of leg
216.8	B-Neoplasm, Skin NEC
228.01	Hemangioma, Skin
228.09	Hemangioma NEC
229.8	Benign neoplasm NEC
232.5	CA in situ, Skin of trunk
232.6	CA in situ, Skin of arm
232.7	CA in situ, Skin of leg
232.8	CA in situ, Skin NEC
237.7	UB-Neoplasm, Neurofibromatosis
238.1	UB-Neoplasm, Soft tissue
238.2	UB-Neoplasm, Skin
272.8	Lipoid metabolism disorder NEC
448.1	Nevus, non-neoplastic
686.1	Pyogenic granuloma
691.8	Other atopic dermatitis
692.70	Solar dermatitis NOS
692.79	Solar dermatitis NEC
700.	Corns and callosities
701.1	Keratoderma, acquired
701.4	Keloid scar
702.x	Other dermatosis
709.2	Scar/fibrosis of skin
709.8	Skin disorders NEC
709.9	Skin disorder NOS
757.8	Other integument anomalies
757.9	Integument anomaly NOS

REIMBURSEMENT INFORMATION

General

- Starred procedure. (11300)

Medicare

- Follow–up Days — 0
- Assistant Surgeon
  11300–11302 — by report
  11303 — paid
- Supply Charges — not allowed
- Outpatient Limit — applies
- Minor Surgery Rules Apply
- Fragments — 12001, 12002, 12004, 12005, 12006, 12007, 12011, 12013, 12014, 12015, 12016, 12017, 12018

CPT CODE	SERVICE
11305*	Shaving of epidermal or dermal lesion, single lesion, scalp, neck, hands, feet, genitalia; lesion diameter 0.5 cm or less
11306	Shaving of epidermal or dermal lesion, single lesion, scalp, neck, hands, feet, genitalia; lesion diameter 0.6 to 1.0 cm
11307	Shaving of epidermal or dermal lesion, single lesion, scalp, neck, hands, feet, genitalia; lesion diameter 1.1 to 2.0 cm
11308	Shaving of epidermal or dermal lesion, single lesion, scalp, neck, hands, feet, genitalia; lesion diameter over 2.0 cm

CPT NOTES

- Shaving is the sharp removal by transverse incision or horizontal slicing to remove epidermal and dermal lesions without a full-thickness dermal excision. This includes local anesthesia, chemical or electrocauterization of the wound. The wound does not require suture closure.

ICD–9–CM

216.4	B-Neoplasm, Scalp/skin of neck
216.6	B-Neoplasm, Skin of arm
216.7	B-Neoplasm, Skin of leg
221.2	B-Neoplasm, Vulva
222.1	B-Neoplasm, Penis
222.4	B-Neoplasm, Scrotum
228.01	Hemangioma, Skin
229.8	Benign neoplasm NEC
238.2	UB-Neoplasm, Skin
448.1	Nevus, non-neoplastic
608.4	Male genital inflammatory dis NEC
624.8	Noninflammatory disorder vulva NEC
692.70	Solar dermatitis NOS
700.	Corns and callosities
701.1	Keratoderma, acquired
701.4	Keloid scar
702.0	Actinic keratosis
702.11	Inflamed seborrheic keratosis
709.2	Scar/fibrosis of skin
709.8	Skin disorders NEC
709.9	Skin disorder NOS
738.8	Acquired deformity NEC
757.9	Integument anomaly NOS

REIMBURSEMENT INFORMATION

General

- Starred procedure. (11305)

Medicare

- Follow–up Days — 0
- Assistant Surgeon — by report
- Supply Charges — not allowed
- Outpatient Limit — applies
- Minor Surgery Rules Apply
- Fragments — 12001, 12002, 12004, 12005, 12006, 12007, 12011, 12013, 12014, 12015, 12016, 12017, 12018

CPT CODE	SERVICE
11310*	Shaving of epidermal or dermal lesion, single lesion, face, ears, eyelids, nose, lips, mucous membrane; lesion diameter 0.5 cm or less
11311	Shaving of epidermal or dermal lesion, single lesion, face, ears, eyelids, nose, lips, mucous membrane; lesion diameter 0.6 to 1.0 cm
11312	Shaving of epidermal or dermal lesion, single lesion, face, ears, eyelids, nose, lips, mucous membrane; lesion diameter 1.1 to 2.0 cm
11313	Shaving of epidermal or dermal lesion, single lesion, face, ears, eyelids, nose, lips, mucous membrane; lesion diameter over 2.0 cm

CPT NOTES

- Shaving is the sharp removal by transverse incision or horizontal slicing to remove epidermal and dermal lesions without a full-thickness dermal excision. This includes local anesthesia, chemical or electrocauterization of the wound. The wound does not require suture closure.

ICD–9–CM

210.0	B-Neoplasm, Lip
210.1	B-Neoplasm, Tongue
210.4	B-Neoplasm, Mouth NEC/NOS
214.0	Lipoma, Skin of face
214.8	Lipoma NEC
215.0	B-Neoplasm, Soft tissue, head
216.0	B-Neoplasm, Skin of lip
216.1	B-Neoplasm, Skin of eyelid/canthus
216.2	B-Neoplasm, Skin of ear
216.3	B-Neoplasm, Skin of face NEC
238.2	UB-Neoplasm, Skin
374.84	Cysts of eyelids
448.1	Nevus, non-neoplastic
692.70	Solar dermatitis NOS
702.x	Other dermatosis
709.2	Scar/fibrosis of skin
709.8	Skin disorders NEC
709.9	Skin disorder NOS

REIMBURSEMENT INFORMATION

General

- Starred procedure. (11310)

Medicare

- Follow–up Days — 0
- Assistant Surgeon — by report
- Supply Charges — not allowed
- Outpatient Limit — applies
- Minor Surgery Rules Apply
- Fragments — 12001, 12002, 12004, 12005, 12006, 12007, 12011, 12013, 12014, 12015, 12016, 12017, 12018

CPT CODE	SERVICE
11400	Excision, benign lesion, except skin tag (unless listed elsewhere), trunk, arms or legs; lesion diameter 0.5 cm or less
11401	Excision, benign lesion, except skin tag (unless listed elsewhere), trunk, arms or legs; lesion diameter 0.6 to 1.0 cm
11402	Excision, benign lesion, except skin tag (unless listed elsewhere), trunk, arms or legs; lesion diameter 1.1 to 2.0 cm
11403	Excision, benign lesion, except skin tag (unless listed elsewhere), trunk, arms or legs; lesion diameter 2.1 to 3.0 cm
11404	Excision, benign lesion, except skin tag (unless listed elsewhere), trunk, arms or legs; lesion diameter 3.1 to 4.0 cm
11406	Excision, benign lesion, except skin tag (unless listed elsewhere), trunk, arms or legs; lesion diameter over 4.0 cm

CPT NOTES

- Excision (including simple closure) of benign lesions of skin or subcutaneous tissues (e.g., cicatricial, fibrous, inflammatory, congenital, cystic lesions), including local anesthesia. See appropriate size and area below.
- Excision is defined as full–thickness (through the dermis) removal of the following lesions and includes simple (non–layered) closure. The closure of defects created by incision, excision, or trauma may require intermediate (layered) closure. Layered closure involves dermal closure with separate suture closure of at least one of the deeper layers of subcutaneous and non–muscle fascial tissues. See pages 114 and following for repair codes.
- For excision of lesions requiring more than simple closure, i.e., requiring intermediate, complex or reconstructive closure, see 12031–12057, 13100–13300, 14000–14300, 15000–15261, 15570–15770.
- For electrosurgical and other methods, see 17000 et seq.
- For unusual or complicated excision, add modifier

ICD–9–CM

214.1	Lipoma, Skin NEC
214.8	Lipoma NEC
215.2	B-Neoplasm, Soft tissue, arm
215.3	B-Neoplasm, Soft tissue, leg
215.4	B-Neoplasm, Soft tissue, thorax
215.5	B-Neoplasm, Soft tissue, abdomen
215.6	B-Neoplasm, Soft tissue, pelvis
216.5	B-Neoplasm, Skin of trunk
216.6	B-Neoplasm, Skin of arm
216.7	B-Neoplasm, Skin of leg
216.8	B-Neoplasm, Skin NEC
228.01	Hemangioma, Skin
228.09	Hemangioma NEC
229.8	Benign neoplasm NEC
237.7	UB-Neoplasm, Neurofibromatosis
238.1	UB-Neoplasm, Soft tissue
238.2	UB-Neoplasm, Skin
272.8	Lipoid metabolism disorder NEC
278.1	Localized adiposity
448.1	Nevus, non-neoplastic
610.8	Benign mammary dysplasia NEC
624.8	Noninflammatory disorder vulva NEC
686.1	Pyogenic granuloma
692.70	Solar dermatitis NOS
692.79	Solar dermatitis NEC
701.1	Keratoderma, acquired
701.4	Keloid scar
702.x	Other dermatosis
704.8	Hair diseases NEC
705.9	Sweat gland disorder NOS
706.2	Sebaceous cyst
709.2	Scar/fibrosis of skin
709.3	Degenerative skin disorders
709.4	Foreign body granuloma, skin
709.8	Skin disorders NEC
709.9	Skin disorder NOS
729.39	Panniculitis, site NEC
757.31	Congenital ectodermal dysplasia
757.32	Vascular hamartomas
757.33	Congenital skin pigment anomaly
757.8	Other integument anomalies
757.9	Integument anomaly NOS
782.2	Localized superficial swelling

REIMBURSEMENT INFORMATION

Medicare

- Follow–up Days — 10
- Assistant Surgeon — not paid
- Supply Charges — not allowed
- Outpatient Limit — applies
- Minor Surgery Rules Apply
- Fragments — 12001, 12002, 12004, 12005, 12006, 12007, 12011, 12013, 12014, 12015, 12016, 12017, 12018

CPT CODE	SERVICE
11420	Excision, benign lesion, except skin tag (unless listed elsewhere), scalp, neck, hands, feet, genitalia; lesion diameter 0.5 cm or less
11421	Excision, benign lesion, except skin tag (unless listed elsewhere), scalp, neck, hands, feet, genitalia; lesion diameter 0.6 to 1.0 cm
11422	Excision, benign lesion, except skin tag (unless listed elsewhere), scalp, neck, hands, feet, genitalia; lesion diameter 1.1 to 2.0 cm
11423	Excision, benign lesion, except skin tag (unless listed elsewhere), scalp, neck, hands, feet, genitalia; lesion diameter 2.1 to 3.0 cm
11424	Excision, benign lesion, except skin tag (unless listed elsewhere), scalp, neck, hands, feet, genitalia; lesion diameter 3.1 to 4.0 cm
11426	Excision, benign lesion, except skin tag (unless listed elsewhere), scalp, neck, hands, feet, genitalia; lesion diameter over 4.0 cm.

CPT NOTES

- Excision (including simple closure) of benign lesions of skin or subcutaneous tissues (e.g., cicatricial, fibrous, inflammatory, congenital, cystic lesions), including local anesthesia. See appropriate size and area below.
- Excision is defined as full–thickness (through the dermis) removal of the following lesions and includes simple (non–layered) closure. The closure of defects created by incision, excision, or trauma may require intermediate (layered) closure. Layered closure involves dermal closure with separate suture closure of at least one of the deeper layers of subcutaneous and non–muscle fascial tissues. See pages 114 and following for repair codes.
- For excision of lesions requiring more than simple closure, i.e., requiring intermediate, complex or reconstructive closure, see 12031–12057, 13100–13300, 14000–14300, 15000–15261, 15570–15770.
- For electrosurgical and other methods, see 17000 et seq.
- For unusual or complicated excision, add modifier "–22" or 09922.

ICD–9–CM

214.1	Lipoma, Skin NEC
214.8	Lipoma NEC
215.0	B-Neoplasm, Soft tissue, head
215.2	B-Neoplasm, Soft tissue, arm
215.3	B-Neoplasm, Soft tissue, leg
215.6	B-Neoplasm, Soft tissue, pelvis
216.4	B-Neoplasm, Scalp/skin of neck
216.6	B-Neoplasm, Skin of arm
216.7	B-Neoplasm, Skin of leg
221.2	B-Neoplasm, Vulva
222.1	B-Neoplasm, Penis
222.4	B-Neoplasm, Scrotum
228.01	Hemangioma, Skin
229.0	B-Neoplasm, Lymph nodes
229.8	Benign neoplasm NEC
238.1	UB-Neoplasm, Soft tissue
238.2	UB-Neoplasm, Skin
448.1	Nevus, non-neoplastic
608.4	Male genital inflammatory dis NEC
608.89	Male genital disorder NEC
624.8	Noninflammatory disorder vulva NEC
629.8	Female genital disorder NEC
692.70	Solar dermatitis NOS
701.1	Keratoderma, acquired
701.4	Keloid scar
702.x	Other dermatosis
704.8	Hair diseases NEC
705.9	Sweat gland disorder NOS
706.2	Sebaceous cyst
709.2	Scar/fibrosis of skin
709.8	Skin disorders NEC
709.9	Skin disorder NOS
727.43	Ganglion NOS
757.31	Congenital ectodermal dysplasia
757.32	Vascular hamartomas
757.33	Congenital skin pigment anomaly
757.8	Other integument anomalies
757.9	Integument anomaly NOS
784.2	Swelling in head/neck

REIMBURSEMENT INFORMATION

Medicare

- Follow–up Days — 10
- Assistant Surgeon — not paid
- Supply Charges — not allowed
- Outpatient Limit — applies
- Minor Surgery Rules Apply
- Fragments — 12001, 12002, 12004, 12005, 12006, 12007, 12011, 12013, 12014, 12015, 12016, 12017, 12018

CPT CODE	SERVICE
11440	Excision, other benign lesion, (unless listed elsewhere), face, ears, eyelids, nose, lips, mucous membrane; lesion diameter 0.5 cm or less
11441	Excision, other benign lesion, (unless listed elsewhere), face, ears, eyelids, nose, lips, mucous membrane; lesion diameter 0.6 to 1.0 cm
11442	Excision, other benign lesion, (unless listed elsewhere), face, ears, eyelids, nose, lips, mucous membrane; lesion diameter 1.1 to 2.0 cm
11443	Excision, other benign lesion, (unless listed elsewhere), face, ears, eyelids, nose, lips, mucous membrane; lesion diameter 2.1 to 3.0 cm
11444	Excision, other benign lesion, (unless listed elsewhere), face, ears, eyelids, nose, lips, mucous membrane; lesion diameter 3.1 to 4.0 cm
11446	Excision, other benign lesion, (unless listed elsewhere), face, ears, eyelids, nose, lips, mucous membrane; lesion diameter over 4.0 cm

CPT NOTES

- Excision (including simple closure) of benign lesions of skin or subcutaneous tissues (e.g., cicatricial, fibrous, inflammatory, congenital, cystic lesions), including local anesthesia. See appropriate size and area below.
- Excision is defined as full–thickness (through the dermis) removal of the following lesions and includes simple (non–layered) closure. The closure of defects created by incision, excision, or trauma may require intermediate (layered) closure. Layered closure involves dermal closure with separate suture closure of at least one of the deeper layers of subcutaneous and non–muscle fascial tissues. See pages 114 and following for repair codes.
- For excision of lesions requiring more than simple closure, i.e., requiring intermediate, complex or reconstructive closure, see 12031–12057, 13100–13300, 14000–14300, 15000–15261, 15570–15770.
- For electrosurgical and other methods, see 17000 et seq.
- For unusual or complicated excision, add modifier "–22" or 09922.
- For eyelids involving more than skin, see also

ICD–9–CM

078.10	Viral warts NOS
210.0	B-Neoplasm, Lip
210.1	B-Neoplasm, Tongue
210.2	B-Neoplasm, Major salivary glands
210.4	B-Neoplasm, Mouth NEC/NOS
214.0	Lipoma, Skin of face
214.8	Lipoma NEC
215.0	B-Neoplasm, Soft tissue, head
216.0	B-Neoplasm, Skin of lip
216.1	B-Neoplasm, Skin of eyelid/canthus
216.2	B-Neoplasm, Skin of ear
216.3	B-Neoplasm, Skin of face NEC
224.1	B-Neoplasm, Orbit
228.00	Hemangioma NOS
228.01	Hemangioma, Skin
235.1	UB-Neoplasm, Oral cavity/pharynx
238.1	UB-Neoplasm, Soft tissue
238.2	UB-Neoplasm, Skin
239.0	Digestive neoplasm NOS
239.2	Bone/Skin neoplasm NOS
239.8	Neoplasm NOS, site NEC
272.2	Mixed hyperlipidemia
374.51	Xanthelasma
374.52	Hyperpigmentation of eyelid
374.84	Cysts of eyelids
380.32	Acquired deformity auricle/pinna
448.1	Nevus, non-neoplastic
523.1	Chronic gingivitis
523.8	Periodontal disease NEC
526.1	Fissural cysts of jaw
527.6	Salivary gland mucocele
528.5	Diseases of lips
528.6	Leukoplakia of oral mucosa/tongue
528.7	Oral epithelium disturbance NEC
528.9	Oral soft tissue disease NEC
529.0	Glossitis
686.1	Pyogenic granuloma
692.70	Solar dermatitis NOS
694.5	Pemphigoid
702.x	Other dermatosis
704.8	Hair diseases NEC
706.2	Sebaceous cyst
709.2	Scar/fibrosis of skin
709.3	Degenerative skin disorders
709.4	Foreign body granuloma, skin
709.8	Skin disorders NEC
709.9	Skin disorder NOS
744.1	Accessory auricle
744.3	Ear anomaly NOS
757.32	Vascular hamartomas
757.33	Congenital skin pigment anomaly

CPT CODE **SERVICE**

11440–11444 (Cont'd.)

ICD–9–CM

REIMBURSEMENT INFORMATION

Medicare

- Follow–up Days — 10
- Assistant Surgeon — not paid
- Supply Charges — not allowed
- Outpatient Limit
  11404-11443 — applies
  11444–11446 — does not apply
- Minor Surgery Rules Apply
- Fragments — 12001, 12002, 12004, 12005, 12006, 12007, 12011, 12013, 12014, 12015, 12016, 12017, 12018

CPT CODE **SERVICE**

11450 Excision of skin and subcutaneous tissue for hidradenitis, axillary; with simple or intermediate repair

CPT NOTES

- Excision (including simple closure) of benign lesions of skin or subcutaneous tissues (e.g., cicatricial, fibrous, inflammatory, congenital, cystic lesions), including local anesthesia. See appropriate size and area below.
- Excision is defined as full–thickness (through the dermis) removal of the following lesions and includes simple (non–layered) closure. The closure of defects created by incision, excision, or trauma may require intermediate (layered) closure. Layered closure involves dermal closure with separate suture closure of at least one of the deeper layers of subcutaneous and non–muscle fascial tissues. See pages 114 and following for repair codes.
- For excision of lesions requiring more than simple closure, i.e., requiring intermediate, complex or reconstructive closure, see 12031–12057, 13100–13300, 14000–14300, 15000–15261, 15570–15770.
- For electrosurgical and other methods, see 17000 et seq.

ICD–9–CM

705.83 Hidradenitis

REIMBURSEMENT INFORMATION

Medicare

- Follow–up Days — 90
- Assistant Surgeon — not paid
- Supply Charges — not allowed
- Outpatient Limit — does not apply
- Major Surgery Rules Apply
- Fragments — 12001, 12002, 12004, 12005, 12006, 12007, 12011, 12013, 12014, 12015, 12016, 12017, 12018, 12031, 12032, 12034, 12035, 12036, 12037, 12041, 12042, 12044, 12045, 12046, 12047, 12051, 12052, 12053, 12054, 12055, 12057

CPT CODE	SERVICE
11451	Excision of skin and subcutaneous tissue for hidradenitis, axillary; with complex repair

CPT NOTES

- Excision (including simple closure) of benign lesions of skin or subcutaneous tissues (e.g., cicatricial, fibrous, inflammatory, congenital, cystic lesions), including local anesthesia. See appropriate size and area below.
- Excision is defined as full–thickness (through the dermis) removal of the following lesions and includes simple (non–layered) closure. The closure of defects created by incision, excision, or trauma may require intermediate (layered) closure. Layered closure involves dermal closure with separate suture closure of at least one of the deeper layers of subcutaneous and non–muscle fascial tissues. See pages 114 and following for repair codes.
- For excision of lesions requiring more than simple closure, i.e., requiring intermediate, complex or reconstructive closure, see 12031–12057, 13100–13300, 14000–14300, 15000–15261, 15570–15770.
- For electrosurgical and other methods, see 17000 et seq.

ICD–9–CM

705.83 Hidradenitis

REIMBURSEMENT INFORMATION

Medicare

- Follow–up Days — 90
- Assistant Surgeon — not paid
- Supply Charges — not allowed
- Outpatient Limit — does not apply
- Major Surgery Rules Apply
- Fragments — 12001, 12002, 12004, 12005, 12006, 12007, 12011, 12013, 12014, 12015, 12016, 12017, 12018, 12031, 12032, 12034, 12035, 12036, 12037, 12041, 12042, 12044, 12045, 12046, 12047, 12051, 12052, 12053, 12054, 12055, 12057

CPT CODE **SERVICE**

11462 Excision of skin and subcutaneous tissue for hidradenitis, inguinal; with simple or intermediate repair

CPT NOTES

- Excision (including simple closure) of benign lesions of skin or subcutaneous tissues (e.g., cicatricial, fibrous, inflammatory, congenital, cystic lesions), including local anesthesia. See appropriate size and area below.
- Excision is defined as full–thickness (through the dermis) removal of the following lesions and includes simple (non–layered) closure. The closure of defects created by incision, excision, or trauma may require intermediate (layered) closure. Layered closure involves dermal closure with separate suture closure of at least one of the deeper layers of subcutaneous and non–muscle fascial tissues. See pages 114 and following for repair codes.
- For excision of lesions requiring more than simple closure, i.e., requiring intermediate, complex or reconstructive closure, see 12031–12057, 13100–13300, 14000–14300, 15000–15261, 15570–15770.
- For electrosurgical and other methods, see 17000 et seq.

ICD–9–CM

705.83 Hidradenitis

REIMBURSEMENT INFORMATION

Medicare

- Follow–up Days — 90
- Assistant Surgeon — not paid
- Supply Charges — not allowed
- Outpatient Limit — does not apply
- Major Surgery Rules Apply
- Fragments — 12001, 12002, 12004, 12005, 12006, 12007, 12011, 12013, 12014, 12015, 12016, 12017, 12018, 12031, 12032, 12034, 12035, 12036, 12037, 12041, 12042, 12044, 12045, 12046, 12047, 12051, 12052, 12053, 12054, 12055, 12057

CPT CODE **SERVICE**

11463 Excision of skin and subcutaneous tissue for hidradenitis, inguinal; with complex repair

CPT NOTES

- Excision (including simple closure) of benign lesions of skin or subcutaneous tissues (e.g., cicatricial, fibrous, inflammatory, congenital, cystic lesions), including local anesthesia. See appropriate size and area below.
- Excision is defined as full–thickness (through the dermis) removal of the following lesions and includes simple (non–layered) closure. The closure of defects created by incision, excision, or trauma may require intermediate (layered) closure. Layered closure involves dermal closure with separate suture closure of at least one of the deeper layers of subcutaneous and non–muscle fascial tissues. See pages 114 and following for repair codes.
- For excision of lesions requiring more than simple closure, i.e., requiring intermediate, complex or reconstructive closure, see 12031–12057, 13100–13300, 14000–14300, 15000–15261, 15570–15770.
- For electrosurgical and other methods, see 17000 et seq.

ICD–9–CM

705.83 Hidradenitis

REIMBURSEMENT INFORMATION

Medicare

- Follow–up Days — 90
- Assistant Surgeon — by report
- Supply Charges — not allowed
- Outpatient Limit — does not apply
- Major Surgery Rules Apply
- Fragments — 12001, 12002, 12004, 12005, 12006, 12007, 12011, 12013, 12014, 12015, 12016, 12017, 12018, 12031, 12032, 12034, 12035, 12036, 12037, 12041, 12042, 12044, 12045, 12046, 12047, 12051, 12052, 12053, 12054, 12055, 12057, 13100, 13101, 13120, 13121, 13131, 13132, 13150, 13151, 13152, 13160, 13300

CPT CODE **SERVICE**

11470 Excision of skin and subcutaneous tissue for hidradenitis, perianal, perineal, or umbilical; with simple or intermediate repair

CPT NOTES

- Excision (including simple closure) of benign lesions of skin or subcutaneous tissues (e.g., cicatricial, fibrous, inflammatory, congenital, cystic lesions), including local anesthesia. See appropriate size and area below.
- Excision is defined as full–thickness (through the dermis) removal of the following lesions and includes simple (non–layered) closure. The closure of defects created by incision, excision, or trauma may require intermediate (layered) closure. Layered closure involves dermal closure with separate suture closure of at least one of the deeper layers of subcutaneous and non–muscle fascial tissues. See pages 114 and following for repair codes.
- For excision of lesions requiring more than simple closure, i.e., requiring intermediate, complex or reconstructive closure, see 12031–12057, 13100–13300, 14000–14300, 15000–15261, 15570–15770.
- For electrosurgical and other methods, see 17000 et seq.
- When skin graft or flap is used for closure, use appropriate procedure code in addition.
- For bilateral procedure, add modifier "-50" or 09950.

ICD–9–CM

705.83 Hidradenitis

REIMBURSEMENT INFORMATION

Medicare

- Follow–up Days — 90
- Assistant Surgeon — not paid
- Supply Charges — not allowed
- Outpatient Limit — does not apply
- Major Surgery Rules Apply
- Fragments — 12001, 12002, 12004, 12005, 12006, 12007, 12011, 12013, 12014, 12015, 12016, 12017, 12018, 12031, 12032, 12034, 12035, 12036, 12037, 12041, 12042, 12044, 12045, 12046, 12047, 12051, 12052, 12053, 12054, 12055, 12057

CPT CODE **SERVICE**

11471 Excision of skin and subcutaneous tissue for hidradenitis, perianal, perineal, or umbilical; with complex repair

CPT NOTES

- Excision (including simple closure) of benign lesions of skin or subcutaneous tissues (e.g., cicatricial, fibrous, inflammatory, congenital, cystic lesions), including local anesthesia. See appropriate size and area below.
- Excision is defined as full–thickness (through the dermis) removal of the following lesions and includes simple (non–layered) closure. The closure of defects created by incision, excision, or trauma may require intermediate (layered) closure. Layered closure involves dermal closure with separate suture closure of at least one of the deeper layers of subcutaneous and non–muscle fascial tissues. See pages 114 and following for repair codes.
- For excision of lesions requiring more than simple closure, i.e., requiring intermediate, complex or reconstructive closure, see 12031–12057, 13100–13300, 14000–14300, 15000–15261, 15570–15770.
- For electrosurgical and other methods, see 17000 et seq.
- When skin graft or flap is used for closure, use appropriate procedure code in addition.
- For bilateral procedure, add modifier "-50" or 09950.

ICD–9–CM

705.83 Hidradenitis

REIMBURSEMENT INFORMATION

Medicare

- Follow–up Days — 90
- Assistant Surgeon — not paid
- Supply Charges — not allowed
- Outpatient Limit — does not apply
- Major Surgery Rules Apply
- Fragments — 12001, 12002, 12004, 12005, 12006, 12007, 12011, 12013, 12014, 12015, 12016, 12017, 12018, 12031, 12032, 12034, 12035, 12036, 12037, 12041, 12042, 12044, 12045, 12046, 12047, 12051, 12052, 12053, 12054, 12055, 12057, 13100, 13101, 13120, 13121, 13131, 13132, 13150, 13151, 13152, 13160, 13300

CPT CODE	SERVICE
11600	Excision, malignant lesion, trunk, arms, or legs; lesion diameter 0.5 cm or less
11601	Excision, malignant lesion, trunk, arms, or legs; lesion diameter 0.6 to 1.0 cm
11602	Excision, malignant lesion, trunk, arms, or legs; lesion diameter 1.1 to 2.0 cm
11603	Excision, malignant lesion, trunk, arms, or legs; lesion diameter 2.1 to 3.0 cm
11604	Excision, malignant lesion, trunk, arms, or legs; lesion diameter 3.1 to 4.0 cm
11606	Excision, malignant lesion, trunk, arms, or legs; lesion diameter over 4.0 cm

CPT NOTES

- ♦ Excision (including simple closure) of malignant lesion of skin or subcutaneous tissues including local anesthesia, each lesion. For removal of malignant lesions of skin by any method other than excision, as defined above, see destruction codes 17000–17999.
- ♦ Excision is defined as full–thickness (through the dermis) removal of the following lesions and includes simple (non–layered) closure. The closure of defects created by incision, excision, or trauma may require intermediate (layered) closure. Layered closure involves dermal closure with separate suture closure of at least one of the deeper layers of subcutaneous and non–muscle fascial tissues.
- ♦ For excision of lesions requiring more than simple closure, i.e., requiring intermediate, complex or reconstructive repair, see 12031–12057, 13100–13300, 14000–14300, 15000–15261,

ICD–9–CM

171.2	M-Neoplasm, Soft tissue, arm
171.3	M-Neoplasm, Soft tissue, leg
171.4	M-Neoplasm, Soft tissue, thorax
171.5	M-Neoplasm, Soft tissue, abdomen
171.6	M-Neoplasm, Soft tissue, pelvis
172.5	Malignant melanoma, Trunk
172.6	Malignant melanoma, Arm
172.7	Malignant melanoma, Leg
172.8	Malignant melanoma, Skin NEC
173.5	M-Neoplasm, Skin of trunk
173.6	M-Neoplasm, Skin of arm
173.7	M-Neoplasm, Skin of leg
173.8	M-Neoplasm, Skin NEC
176.0	Kaposi's sarcoma, skin
176.1	Kaposi's sarcoma, soft tissue
195.1	M-Neoplasm, Thorax
195.4	M-Neoplasm, Upper limb
195.5	M-Neoplasm, Lower limb
195.8	M-Neoplasm, site NEC
196.3	M-Neoplasm, Lymph axilla/arm
196.5	M-Neoplasm, Lymph inguinal/leg
198.2	M2-Neoplasm, Skin
202.84	Lymphoma NEC, axilla
202.85	Lymphoma NEC, inguinal
202.88	Lymphoma NEC, mult site
232.5	CA in situ, Skin of trunk
232.6	CA in situ, Skin of arm
232.7	CA in situ, Skin of leg
232.8	CA in situ, Skin NEC
V10.82	Hx of malignant skin melanoma
V10.83	Hx of skin malignancy NEC

REIMBURSEMENT INFORMATION

Medicare

- ♦ Follow–up Days — 10
- ♦ Assistant Surgeon — not paid
- ♦ Supply Charges — not allowed
- ♦ Outpatient Limit
  11600–11603 — applies
  11604–11606 — does not apply
- ♦ Minor Surgery Rules Apply
- ♦ Fragments — 12001, 12002, 12004, 12005, 12006, 12007, 12011, 12013, 12014, 12015, 12016, 12017, 12018

CPT CODE	SERVICE
11620	Excision, malignant lesion, scalp, neck, hands, feet, genitalia; lesion diameter 0.5 cm or less
11621	Excision, malignant lesion, scalp, neck, hands, feet, genitalia; lesion diameter 0.6 to 1.0 cm
11622	Excision, malignant lesion, scalp, neck, hands, feet, genitalia; lesion diameter 1.1 to 2.0 cm
11623	Excision, malignant lesion, scalp, neck, hands, feet, genitalia; lesion diameter 2.1 cm to 3.0 cm
11624	Excision, malignant lesion, scalp, neck, hands, feet, genitalia; lesion diameter 3.1 to 4.0 cm
11626	Excision, malignant lesion, scalp, neck, hands, feet, genitalia; lesion diameter over 4.0 cm

CPT NOTES

- Excision (including simple closure) of malignant lesion of skin or subcutaneous tissues including local anesthesia, each lesion. For removal of malignant lesions of skin by any method other than excision, as defined above, see destruction codes 17000–17999.
- Excision is defined as full–thickness (through the dermis) removal of the following lesions and includes simple (non–layered) closure. The closure of defects created by incision, excision, or trauma may require intermediate (layered) closure. Layered closure involves dermal closure with separate suture closure of at least one of the deeper layers of subcutaneous and non–muscle fascial tissues.
- For excision of lesions requiring more than simple closure, i.e., requiring intermediate, complex or reconstructive repair, see 12031–12057, 13100–13300, 14000–14300, 15000–15261, 15570–15770.

ICD–9–CM

171.0	M-Neoplasm, Soft tissue, head
172.4	Malignant melanoma, Scalp/neck
172.5	Malignant melanoma, Trunk
172.6	Malignant melanoma, Arm
172.7	Malignant melanoma, Leg
173.4	M-Neoplasm, Scalp/skin neck
173.5	M-Neoplasm, Skin of trunk
173.6	M-Neoplasm, Skin of arm
173.7	M-Neoplasm, Skin of leg
176.0	Kaposi's sarcoma, skin
176.1	Kaposi's sarcoma, soft tissue
184.1	M-Neoplasm, Labia majora
184.2	M-Neoplasm, Labia minora
184.3	M-Neoplasm, Clitoris
184.4	M-Neoplasm, Vulva NOS
184.8	M-Neoplasm, Female genital NEC
187.1	M-Neoplasm, Prepuce
187.2	M-Neoplasm, Glans penis
187.3	M-Neoplasm, Penis body
187.4	M-Neoplasm, Penis NOS
187.7	M-Neoplasm, Scrotum
195.0	M-Neoplasm, Head/face/neck
195.3	M-Neoplasm, Pelvis
195.4	M-Neoplasm, Upper limb
195.5	M-Neoplasm, Lower limb
196.0	M-Neoplasm, Lymph head/neck/face
198.2	M2-Neoplasm, Skin
232.4	CA in situ, Scalp/skin of neck
232.5	CA in situ, Skin of trunk
232.6	CA in situ, Skin of arm
232.7	CA in situ, Skin of leg

REIMBURSEMENT INFORMATION

Medicare

- Follow–up Days — 10
- Assistant Surgeon — not paid
- Supply Charges — not allowed
- Outpatient Limit
  11620–11623 — applies
  11624–11626 — does not apply
- Minor Surgery Rules Apply
- Fragments — 12001, 12002, 12004, 12005, 12006, 12007, 12011, 12013, 12014, 12015, 12016, 12017, 12018

CPT CODE	SERVICE
11640	Excision, malignant lesion, face, ears, eyelids, nose, lips; lesion diameter 0.5 cm or less
11641	Excision, malignant lesion, face, ears, eyelids, nose, lips; lesion diameter 0.6 to 1.1 cm
11642	Excision, malignant lesion, face, ears, eyelids, nose, lips; lesion diameter 1.1 to 2.0 cm
11643	Excision, malignant lesion, face, ears, eyelids, nose, lips; lesion diameter 2.1 to 3.0 cm
11644	Excision, malignant lesion, face, ears, eyelids, nose, lips; lesion diameter 3.1 to 4.0 cm
11646	Excision, malignant lesion, face, ears, eyelids, nose, lips; lesion diameter over 4.0 cm

CPT NOTES

- Excision (including simple closure) of malignant lesion of skin or subcutaneous tissues including local anesthesia, each lesion. For removal of malignant lesions of skin by any method other than excision, as defined above, see destruction codes 17000–17999.
- Excision is defined as full–thickness (through the dermis) removal of the following lesions and includes simple (non–layered) closure. The closure of defects created by incision, excision, or trauma may require intermediate (layered) closure. Layered closure involves dermal closure with separate suture closure of at least one of the deeper layers of subcutaneous and non–muscle fascial tissues.
- For excision of lesions requiring more than simple closure, i.e., requiring intermediate, complex or reconstructive repair, see 12031–12057, 13100–13300, 14000–14300, 15000–15261,

ICD–9–CM

140.0	M-Neoplasm, Upper lip, vermilion
140.1	M-Neoplasm, Lower lip, vermilion
140.3	M-Neoplasm, Upper lip, inner aspect
140.4	M-Neoplasm, Lower lip, inner aspect
140.5	M-Neoplasm, Lip NOS, inner NOS
140.6	M-Neoplasm, lip, commissure
140.8	M-Neoplasm, Lip NEC
140.9	M-Neoplasm, Lip/vermilion NOS
143.0	M-Neoplasm, Upper gum
143.1	M-Neoplasm, Lower gum
143.8	M-Neoplasm, Gum NEC
144.0	M-Neoplasm, Anterior floor of mouth
144.1	M-Neoplasm, Lateral floor of mouth
144.8	M-Neoplasm, Floor of mouth NEC
144.9	M-Neoplasm, Floor of mouth NOS
145.0	M-Neoplasm, Cheek mucosa
145.1	M-Neoplasm, Mouth vestibule
145.2	M-Neoplasm, Hard palate
145.3	M-Neoplasm, Soft palate
145.4	M-Neoplasm, Uvula
145.5	M-Neoplasm, Palate NOS
145.6	M-Neoplasm, Retromolar area
145.8	M-Neoplasm, Mouth NEC
145.9	M-Neoplasm, Mouth NOS
149.8	M-Neoplasm, Oral cavity/pharynx NEC
171.0	M-Neoplasm, Soft tissue, head
172.0	Malignant melanoma, Lip
172.1	Malignant melanoma, eyelid/canthus
172.2	Malignant melanoma, Ear
172.3	Malignant melanoma, Face NEC/NOS
172.8	Malignant melanoma, Skin NEC
173.0	M-Neoplasm, Skin of lip
173.1	M-Neoplasm, Skin of eyelid/canthus
173.2	M-Neoplasm, Skin of ear
173.3	M-Neoplasm, Skin of face NEC
173.8	M-Neoplasm, Skin NEC
176.0	Kaposi's sarcoma, skin
176.1	Kaposi's sarcoma, soft tissue
176.2	Kaposi's sarcoma, palate
195.0	M-Neoplasm, Head/face/neck
230.0	CA in situ, Oral cavity/pharynx
232.0	CA in situ, Skin of lip
232.1	CA in situ, Eyelid/canthus
232.2	CA in situ, Skin of ear
232.3	CA in situ, Skin of face NEC
232.8	CA in situ, Skin NEC
238.1	UB-Neoplasm, Soft tissue
238.2	UB-Neoplasm, Skin

CPT CODE **SERVICE**

11640 (Cont'd.)

ICD–9–CM

REIMBURSEMENT INFORMATION

Medicare

- Follow–up Days — 10
- Assistant Surgeon — not paid
- Supply Charges — not allowed
- Outpatient Limit
  11640-11643 — applies
  11644-11646 — does not apply
- Minor Surgery Rules Apply
- Fragments — 12001, 12002, 12004, 12005, 12006, 12007, 12011, 12013, 12014, 12015, 12016, 12017, 12018

CPT CODE	SERVICE	ICD-9-CM

11700* Debridement of nails, manual; five or less

11701 Debridement of nails, manual; each additional five or less

CPT NOTES

- ♦ For drainage of paronychia or onychia, see 10060, 10061.

110.1	Dermatophytosis of nail
112.3	Cutaneous candidiasis
117.x	Mycosis
681.0x	Cellulitis and abscess, finger
703.x	Diseases of nail
757.5	Nail anomalies NEC
923.3	Contusion of finger
927.3	Crushing injury, finger
959.5	Finger injury NOS

REIMBURSEMENT INFORMATION

General

- ♦ Starred procedure. (11700)

Medicare

- ♦ Follow–up Days
  11700 — 0
  11701 — none; falls with global period of another procedure
- ♦ Assistant Surgeon — not paid
- ♦ Supply Charges — not allowed
- ♦ Outpatient Limit — applies
- ♦ Minor Surgery Rules Apply
- ♦ Fragments —64450

11710* Debridement of nails, electric grinder; five or less

11711 Debridement of nails, electric grinder; each additional, five or less

CPT NOTES

- ♦ For drainage of paronychia or onychia, see 10060, 10061.

110.1	Dermatophytosis of nail
112.3	Cutaneous candidiasis
117.x	Mycosis
681.0x	Cellulitis and abscess, finger
703.x	Diseases of nail
757.5	Nail anomalies NEC
923.3	Contusion of finger
927.3	Crushing injury, finger
959.5	Finger injury NOS

REIMBURSEMENT INFORMATION

General

- ♦ Starred procedure. (11710)

Medicare

- ♦ Follow–up Days
  11710 — 0
  11711 — none; falls with global period of another procedure
- ♦ Assistant Surgeon — not paid
- ♦ Supply Charges — not allowed
- ♦ Outpatient Limit — applies
- ♦ Minor Surgery Rules Apply

CPT CODE	SERVICE
11730*	Avulsion of nail plate, partial or complete, simple; single
11731	Avulsion of nail plate, partial or complete, simple; second nail plate
11732	Avulsion of nail plate, partial or complete, simple; each additional nail plate

CPT NOTES

- For drainage of paronychia or onychia, see 10060, 10061.

ICD–9–CM

110.1	Dermatophytosis of nail
112.3	Cutaneous candidiasis
117.x	Mycosis
681.x	Cellulitis/abscess of finger/toe
703.x	Diseases of nail
709.2	Scar/fibrosis of skin
883.0	Open wound of finger
883.1	Open wound of finger, complicated
893.0	Open wound of toe
893.1	Open wound of toe, complicated
906.1	Late effect, open wound extremity
906.7	Late effect of extremity burn NEC
915.8	Superficial injury, finger NEC
915.9	Superficial inj, finger NEC, infect
923.3	Contusion of finger
924.3	Contusion of toe
927.3	Crushing injury, finger
928.3	Crushing injury, toe
959.5	Finger injury NOS

REIMBURSEMENT INFORMATION

General

- Starred procedure. (11730)

Medicare

- Follow–up Days
  11730 — 0
  11731–11732 — none; falls with global period of another procedure
- Assistant Surgeon — not paid
- Supply Charges — not allowed
- Outpatient Limit — applies
- Minor Surgery Rules Apply
- Fragments —64450

CPT CODE	SERVICE	ICD-9-CM

11740 Evacuation of subungual hematoma

CPT NOTES

- For drainage of paronychia or onychia, see 10060, 10061.

ICD-9-CM

923.3	Contusion of finger
924.3	Contusion of toe
927.3	Crushing injury, finger
928.3	Crushing injury, toe
959.5	Finger injury NOS

REIMBURSEMENT INFORMATION

Medicare

- Follow–up Days — 0
- Assistant Surgeon — not paid
- Supply Charges — not allowed
- Outpatient Limit — applies
- Minor Surgery Rules Apply

11750 Excision of nail and nail matrix, partial or complete, (eg, ingrown or deformed nail) for permanent removal

CPT NOTES

- For drainage of paronychia or onychia, see 10060, 10061.
- For skin graft, if used, see 15050.

ICD-9-CM

110.1	Dermatophytosis of nail
681.0x	Cellulitis and abscess, finger
681.11	Onychia of toe
703.x	Diseases of nail
709.2	Scar/fibrosis of skin
735.8	Acquired deformities of toe NEC
736.20	Acquired finger deformity NOS
757.5	Nail anomalies NEC
883.0	Open wound of finger
883.1	Open wound of finger, complicated
893.0	Open wound of toe
893.1	Open wound of toe, complicated
906.1	Late effect, open wound extremity
906.7	Late effect of extremity burn NEC
927.3	Crushing injury, finger
959.5	Finger injury NOS

REIMBURSEMENT INFORMATION

Medicare

- Follow–up Days — 10
- Assistant Surgeon — not paid
- Supply Charges — not allowed
- Outpatient Limit — applies
- Minor Surgery Rules Apply
- Fragments —11730

CPT CODE	SERVICE	ICD-9-CM

11752 Excision of nail and nail matrix, partial or complete, (eg, ingrown or deformed nail) for permanent removal; with amputation of tuft of distal phalanx

CPT NOTES

- ◆ For drainage of paronychia or onychia, see 10060, 10061.
- ◆ For skin graft, if used, see 15050.

110.1	Dermatophytosis of nail
681.0x	Cellulitis and abscess, finger
681.11	Onychia of toe
703.x	Diseases of nail
709.2	Scar/fibrosis of skin
735.8	Acquired deformities of toe NEC
736.20	Acquired finger deformity NOS
757.5	Nail anomalies NEC
883.0	Open wound of finger
883.1	Open wound of finger, complicated
893.0	Open wound of toe
893.1	Open wound of toe, complicated
906.1	Late effect, open wound extremity
906.7	Late effect of extremity burn NEC
927.3	Crushing injury, finger
959.5	Finger injury NOS

REIMBURSEMENT INFORMATION

Medicare

- ◆ Follow-up Days — 10
- ◆ Assistant Surgeon — not paid
- ◆ Supply Charges — not allowed
- ◆ Outpatient Limit — applies
- ◆ Minor Surgery Rules Apply
- ◆ Fragments —11730, 11750

11755 Biopsy of nail unit, any method (eg, plate, bed, matrix, hyponychium, proximal and lateral nail folds) (separate procedure)

CPT NOTES

- ◆ For drainage of paronychia or onychia, see 10060, 10061.

110.1	Dermatophytosis of nail
172.6	Malignant melanoma, Arm
172.7	Malignant melanoma, Leg
173.6	M-Neoplasm, Skin of arm
173.7	M-Neoplasm, Skin of leg
198.2	M2-Neoplasm, Skin
216.6	B-Neoplasm, Skin of arm
216.7	B-Neoplasm, Skin of leg
232.6	CA in situ, Skin of arm
232.7	CA in situ, Skin of leg
238.2	UB-Neoplasm, Skin
239.2	Bone/Skin neoplasm NOS
681.0x	Cellulitis and abscess, finger
681.11	Onychia of toe
703.x	Diseases of nail

REIMBURSEMENT INFORMATION

General

- ◆ Separate procedure rules apply.

Medicare

- ◆ Follow-up Days — 0
- ◆ Assistant Surgeon — by report
- ◆ Supply Charges — not allowed
- ◆ Outpatient Limit — does not apply
- ◆ Minor Surgery Rules Apply

CPT CODE	SERVICE	ICD-9-CM

11760 Repair of nail bed

CPT NOTES

- For drainage of paronychia or onychia, see 10060, 10061.

110.1	Dermatophytosis of nail
703.x	Diseases of nail
709.2	Scar/fibrosis of skin
735.8	Acquired deformities of toe NEC
736.20	Acquired finger deformity NOS
816.12	Fx distal phalanx, hand, open
883.0	Open wound of finger
883.1	Open wound of finger, complicated
893.0	Open wound of toe
893.1	Open wound of toe, complicated
906.1	Late effect, open wound extremity
906.7	Late effect of extremity burn NEC
923.3	Contusion of finger
924.3	Contusion of toe
927.3	Crushing injury, finger
928.3	Crushing injury, toe
959.5	Finger injury NOS

REIMBURSEMENT INFORMATION

Medicare

- Follow-up Days — 10
- Assistant Surgeon — not paid
- Supply Charges — not allowed
- Outpatient Limit — applies
- Minor Surgery Rules Apply

11762 Reconstruction of nail bed with graft

CPT NOTES

- For drainage of paronychia or onychia, see 10060, 10061.

110.1	Dermatophytosis of nail
703.x	Diseases of nail
709.2	Scar/fibrosis of skin
735.8	Acquired deformities of toe NEC
736.20	Acquired finger deformity NOS
816.12	Fx distal phalanx, hand, open
883.0	Open wound of finger
883.1	Open wound of finger, complicated
893.0	Open wound of toe
893.1	Open wound of toe, complicated
906.1	Late effect, open wound extremity
906.7	Late effect of extremity burn NEC
923.3	Contusion of finger
924.3	Contusion of toe
927.3	Crushing injury, finger
928.3	Crushing injury, toe
959.5	Finger injury NOS

REIMBURSEMENT INFORMATION

Medicare

- Follow-up Days — 10
- Assistant Surgeon — not paid
- Supply Charges — not allowed
- Outpatient Limit — applies
- Minor Surgery Rules Apply

CPT CODE SERVICE	ICD-9-CM
11765 Wedge excision of skin of nail fold (eg, for ingrown toenail) **CPT NOTES** ♦ For drainage of paronychia or onychia, see 10060, 10061.	703.x Diseases of nail **REIMBURSEMENT INFORMATION** Medicare ♦ Follow-up Days — 10 ♦ Assistant Surgeon — not paid ♦ Supply Charges — not allowed ♦ Outpatient Limit — applies ♦ Minor Surgery Rules Apply
11770 Excision of pilonidal cyst or sinus; simple **11771** Excision of pilonidal cyst or sinus; extensive **11772** Excision of pilonidal cyst or sinus; complicated **CPT NOTES** ♦ For drainage of paronychia or onychia, see 10060, 10061. ♦ For incision of pilonidal cyst, see 10080, 10081.	685.0 Pilonidal cyst w/abscess 685.1 Pilonidal cyst w/o abscess **REIMBURSEMENT INFORMATION** Medicare ♦ Follow-up Days 11770 — 10 11771–11772 — 90 ♦ Assistant Surgeon — not paid ♦ Supply Charges — not allowed ♦ Outpatient Limit — does not apply ♦ Minor Surgery Rules Apply (11770) ♦ Major Surgery Rules Apply (11771, 11772)

CPT CODE	SERVICE
11900*	Injection, intralesional; up to and including seven lesions
11901*	Injection, intralesional; more than seven lesions

CPT NOTES

- For veins, see 36470, 36471.
- For intralesional chemotherapy administration, see 96405, 96406.

ICD–9–CM

210.0	B-Neoplasm, Lip
239.2	Bone/Skin neoplasm NOS
373.12	Hordeolum internum
373.2	Chalazion
375.30	Dacryocystitis NOS
446.3	Lethal midline granuloma
694.0	Dermatitis herpetiformis
695.1	Erythema multiforme
695.2	Erythema nodosum
695.4	Lupus erythematosus
695.89	Erythematous conditions NEC
696.1	Other psoriasis
696.2	Parapsoriasis
697.0	Lichen planus
698.3	Lichenification
701.4	Keloid scar
704.01	Alopecia areata
709.1	Vascular disorders of skin
709.2	Scar/fibrosis of skin

REIMBURSEMENT INFORMATION

General

- Starred procedure.

Medicare

- Follow–up Days — 0
- Assistant Surgeon — not paid
- Supply Charges — not allowed
- Outpatient Limit — applies
- Minor Surgery Rules Apply

CPT CODE SERVICE	ICD-9-CM
11920 Tattooing, intradermal introduction of insoluble opaque pigments to correct color defects of skin, including micropigmentation; 6.0 sq cm or less **11921** Tattooing, intradermal introduction of insoluble opaque pigments to correct color defects of skin, including micropigmentation; 6.1 to 20.0 sq cm **11922** Tattooing, intradermal introduction of insoluble opaque pigments to correct color defects of skin, including micropigmentation; each additional 20.0 sq cm	709.00 Dyschromia, unspecified 709.01 Vitiligo 709.09 Other dyschromia 709.1 Vascular disorders of skin 757.33 Congenital skin pigment anomaly 906.5 Late effect of head/neck burn 906.6 Late effect of wrist/hand burn 906.7 Late effect of extremity burn NEC V50.1 Plastic surgery NEC **REIMBURSEMENT INFORMATION** Medicare ◆ Follow-up Days 11920–11921 — 0 ◆ 11922 — none; falls within global period of another procedure ◆ Assistant Surgeon — by report ◆ Supply Charges — not allowed ◆ Outpatient Limit — does not apply ◆ Minor Surgery Rules Apply (11920, 11921)
11950 Subcutaneous injection of "filling" material (eg, collagen); 1 cc or less **11951** Subcutaneous injection of "filling" material (eg, collagen); 1.1 to 5 cc **11952** Subcutaneous injection of "filling" material (eg, collagen); 5.1 to 10 cc **11954** Subcutaneous injection of "filling" material (eg, collagen); over 10 cc	701.3 Striae atrophicae 701.8 Hypertrophic/atrophic skin NEC 701.9 Hypertrophic/atrophic skin NOS 706.1 Acne NEC 709.2 Scar/fibrosis of skin 709.3 Degenerative skin disorders 906.0 Late effect, open wound head/trunk 906.1 Late effect, open wound extremity 906.2 Late effect of superficial injury 906.3 Late effect of contusion 906.4 Late effect of crushing **REIMBURSEMENT INFORMATION** Medicare ◆ Follow-up Days — 0 ◆ Assistant Surgeon — by report ◆ Supply Charges — not allowed ◆ Outpatient Limit — does not apply ◆ Minor Surgery Rules Apply

CPT CODE	SERVICE
11960	Insertion of tissue expander(s) for other than breast, including subsequent expansion

CPT NOTES

- For breast reconstruction with tissue expander(s), see 19357.

ICD-9-CM

704.00	Alopecia NOS
704.01	Alopecia areata
704.09	Alopecia NEC
709.2	Scar/fibrosis of skin
870.8	Open wound of ocular adnexa NEC
870.9	Open wound of ocular adnexa NOS
872.10	Open wound, external ear NOS, compl
872.11	Open wound of auricle, complicated
873.1	Open wound of scalp, complicated
873.30	Open wound of nose NOS, complicated
873.31	Open wound nasal septum, complic
873.32	Open wound nasal cavity, complic
873.5x	Face, complicated open wound
874.9	Open wound of neck NEC, complicated
875.1	Open wound of chest, complicated
876.1	Open wound of back, complicated
877.1	Open wound of buttock, complicated
879.3	Open wound anterior abdomen, compl
879.5	Open wound lateral abdomen, compl
880.1x	Shoulder/upper arm, cplx open wound
881.1x	Elbow/forearm/wrist complex wound
882.1	Open wound of hand, complicated
883.1	Open wound of finger, complicated
884.1	Open wound of arm mult/NOS, compl
890.1	Open wound of hip/thigh, complic
891.1	Open wound of knee/leg/ankle, compl
892.1	Open wound of foot, complicated
893.1	Open wound of toe, complicated
894.1	Open wound of leg NEC, complicated
906.0	Late effect, open wound head/trunk
906.1	Late effect, open wound extremity
906.5	Late effect of head/neck burn
906.6	Late effect of wrist/hand burn
906.7	Late effect of extremity burn NEC
906.8	Late effect of burns NEC
906.9	Late effect of burns NOS
909.3	Late effect of surg/med complic
V10.82	Hx of malignant skin melanoma
V10.83	Hx of skin malignancy NEC

REIMBURSEMENT INFORMATION

Medicare

- Follow-up Days — 90
- Assistant Surgeon — not paid
- Supply Charges — not allowed
- Outpatient Limit — does not apply
- Major Surgery Rules Apply

CPT CODE	SERVICE	ICD-9-CM	
11970	Replacement of tissue expander with permanent prosthesis	611.8	Absence of breast, acquired
		709.2	Scar/fibrosis of skin
		906.0	Late effect, open wound head/trunk
		906.1	Late effect, open wound extremity
		906.5	Late effect of head/neck burn
		906.6	Late effect of wrist/hand burn
		906.7	Late effect of extremity burn NEC
		906.8	Late effect of burns NEC
		906.9	Late effect of burns NOS
		909.3	Late effect of surg/med complic
		V10.3	Hx of breast malignancy
		V51.	Aftercare w/plastic surgery

REIMBURSEMENT INFORMATION

Medicare

- Follow-up Days — 90
- Assistant Surgeon — not paid
- Supply Charges — not allowed
- Outpatient Limit — does not apply
- Major Surgery Rules Apply

CPT CODE	SERVICE	ICD-9-CM	
11971	Removal of tissue expander(s) without insertion of prosthesis	611.0	Inflammatory disease of breast
		709.2	Scar/fibrosis of skin
		906.0	Late effect, open wound head/trunk
		906.1	Late effect, open wound extremity
		906.5	Late effect of head/neck burn
		906.6	Late effect of wrist/hand burn
		906.7	Late effect of extremity burn NEC
		906.8	Late effect of burns NEC
		906.9	Late effect of burns NOS
		909.3	Late effect of surg/med complic
		V10.3	Hx of breast malignancy
		V51.	Aftercare w/plastic surgery

REIMBURSEMENT INFORMATION

Medicare

- Follow-up Days — 90
- Assistant Surgeon — not paid
- Supply Charges — not allowed
- Outpatient Limit — does not apply
- Major Surgery Rules Apply

CPT CODE	SERVICE	ICD-9-CM
11975	Insertion, implantable contraceptive capsules	V25.5 Subderm contraceptive insertion **REIMBURSEMENT INFORMATION** Medicare ♦ Follow–up Days — global concept does not apply ♦ Assistant Surgeon — by report ♦ Supply Charges — not allowed ♦ Outpatient Limit — does not apply
11976	Removal, implantable contraceptive capsules	V25.43 Subderm contraceptive surveillance **REIMBURSEMENT INFORMATION** Medicare ♦ Follow–up Days — global concept does not apply ♦ Assistant Surgeon — by report ♦ Supply Charges — not allowed ♦ Outpatient Limit — does not apply
11977	Removal with reinsertion, implantable contraceptive capsules	V25.43 Subderm contraceptive surveillance **REIMBURSEMENT INFORMATION** Medicare ♦ Follow–up Days — global concept does not apply ♦ Assistant Surgeon — by report ♦ Supply Charges — not allowed ♦ Outpatient Limit — does not apply

REPAIR (CLOSURE)

Definitions

The repair of wounds may be classified as Simple, Intermediate or Complex.

Simple repair is used when the wound is superficial; i.e., involving primarily epidermis or dermis, or subcutaneous tissues without significant involvement of deeper structures, and requires simple one layer closure/suturing. This includes local anesthesia and chemical or electrocauterization of wounds not closed.

(Closure with adhesive strips is included in appropriate E/M service.)

Intermediate repair includes the repair of wounds that, in addition to the above, require layered closure of one or more of the subcutaneous tissue and superficial (non–muscle) fascia, in addition to the skin (epidermal and dermal) closure. Single–layer closure of heavily contaminated wounds that have required extensive cleaning or removal of particulate matter also constitutes intermediate repair.

Complex repair includes the repair of wounds requiring more than layered closure, viz., scar revision, debridement (e.g., traumatic lacerations or avulsions), extensive undermining, stents or retention sutures. It may include creation of the defect and necessary preparation for repairs or the debridement and repair of complicated lacerations or avulsions.

Instructions for listing services at time of wound repair:

1. The repaired wound(s) should be measured and recorded in centimeters, whether curved, angular or stellate.
2. When multiple wounds are repaired, add together the lengths of those in the same classification (see above) and report as a single item. When more than one classification of wounds is repaired, list the more complicated as the primary procedure and the less complicated as the secondary procedure, using either modifier "–51" or 09951.
3. Decontamination and/or debridement: Debridement is considered a separate procedure only when gross contamination requires prolonged cleansing, when appreciable amounts of devitalized or contaminated tissue are removed, or when debridement is carried out separately without immediate primary closure. (For extensive debridement of soft tissue and/or bone, see 11040–11044.)
4. Involvement of nerves, blood vessels and tendons: Report under appropriate system (Nervous, Cardiovascular, Musculoskeletal) for repair of these structures. The repair of these associated wounds is included in the primary procedure unless it qualifies as a complex wound, in which case either modifier "–51" or 09951 applies.

Simple ligation of vessels in an open wound is considered as part of any wound closure.

Simple "exploration" of nerves, blood vessels or tendons exposed in an open wound is also considered part of the essential treatment of the wound and is not a separate procedure unless appreciable dissection is required.

CPT CODE	SERVICE
12001*	Simple repair of superficial wounds of scalp, neck, axillae, external genitalia, trunk and/or extremities (including hands and feet); 2.5 cm or less
12002*	Simple repair of superficial wounds of scalp, neck, axillae, external genitalia, trunk and/or extremities (including hands and feet); 2.6 cm to 7.5 cm
12004*	Simple repair of superficial wounds of scalp, neck, axillae, external genitalia, trunk and/or extremities (including hands and feet); 7.6 cm to 12.5 cm
12005	Simple repair of superficial wounds of scalp, neck, axillae, external genitalia, trunk and/or extremities (including hands and feet); 12.6 cm to 20.0 cm
12006	Simple repair of superficial wounds of scalp, neck, axillae, external genitalia, trunk and/or extremities (including hands and feet); 20.1 cm to 30.0 cm
12007	Simple repair of superficial wounds of scalp, neck, axillae, external genitalia, trunk and/or extremities (including hands and feet); over 30.0 cm

CPT NOTES

♦ Sum of lengths of repairs.

ICD–9–CM

873.0	Open wound of scalp
873.1	Open wound of scalp, complicated
873.8	Open wound of head NEC
874.8	Open wound of neck NEC
875.0	Open wound of chest
876.0	Open wound of back
877.0	Open wound of buttock
877.1	Open wound of buttock, complicated
878.0	Open wound of penis
878.2	Open wound of scrotum/testes
878.4	Open wound of vulva
878.5	Open wound of vulva, complicated
878.6	Open wound of vagina
878.7	Open wound of vagina, complicated
878.9	Open wound genital NEC, complic
879.0	Open wound of breast
879.2	Open wound of anterior abdomen
879.4	Open wound of lateral abdomen
880.00	Open wound of shoulder
880.01	Open wound of scapula
880.02	Open wound of axilla
880.03	Open wound of upper arm
880.10	Open wound of shoulder, complicated
880.11	Open wound of scapula, complicated
881.0x	Elbow/forearm/wrist open wound
882.0	Open wound of hand
882.1	Open wound of hand, complicated
883.0	Open wound of finger
883.1	Open wound of finger, complicated
884.0	Open wound of arm, mult/NOS
890.0	Open wound of hip/thigh
891.0	Open wound of knee/leg/ankle
892.0	Open wound of foot
893.0	Open wound of toe
893.1	Open wound of toe, complicated
894.0	Open wound of leg NEC
894.1	Open wound of leg NEC, complicated
910.8	Superficial injury, head NEC
917.9	Superf injury, foot/toe NEC, infect
919.6	Superficial foreign body NEC
959.0	Face and neck injury NOS
959.1	Trunk injury NOS
959.2	Shoulder/upper arm injury NOS
959.3	Elbow/forearm/wrist injury NOS
959.4	Hand injury NOS
959.5	Finger injury NOS
959.6	Hip/thigh injury NOS
959.7	Lower leg injury NOS

CPT CODE **SERVICE**

12001–12007 (Cont'd.)

ICD–9–CM

REIMBURSEMENT INFORMATION

General

- See notes on page 114.
- Starred procedure. (12001, 12002, 12004)

Medicare

- Follow–Up Days — 10
- Assistant Surgeon
  12001–12006 — not paid
  12007 — paid
- Supply Charges — not allowed
- Outpatient Limit — does not apply
- Minor Procedure Rules Apply

CPT CODE	SERVICE
12011*	Simple repair of superficial wounds of face, ears, eyelids, nose, lips and/or mucous membranes; 2.5 cm or less
12013*	Simple repair of superficial wounds of face, ears, eyelids, nose, lips and/or mucous membranes; 2.6 cm to 5.0 cm
12014	Simple repair of superficial wounds of face, ears, eyelids, nose, lips and/or mucous membranes; 5.1 cm to 7.5 cm
12015	Simple repair of superficial wounds of face, ears, eyelids, nose, lips and/or mucous membranes; 7.6 cm to 12.5 cm
12016	Simple repair of superficial wounds of face, ears, eyelids, nose, lips and/or mucous membranes; 12.6 cm to 20.0 cm
12017	Simple repair of superficial wounds of face, ears, eyelids, nose, lips and/or mucous membranes; 20.1 cm to 30.0 cm
12018	Simple repair of superficial wounds of face, ears, eyelids, nose, lips and/or mucous membranes; over 30.0 cm

CPT NOTES

- Sum of lengths of repairs.

ICD–9–CM

870.0	Laceration eyelid skin/periocular
870.1	Full-thickness laceration eyelid
870.2	Eyelid laceration inv lacrimal pas
870.8	Open wound of ocular adnexa NEC
870.9	Open wound of ocular adnexa NOS
872.00	Open wound, external ear NOS
872.01	Open wound of auricle
872.02	Open wound of auditory canal
872.8	Open wound of ear NOS
873.20	Open wound of nose NOS
873.21	Open wound of nasal septum
873.22	Open wound of nasal cavity
873.29	Multiple open nose wounds
873.30	Open wound of nose NOS, complicated
873.31	Open wound nasal septum, complic
873.32	Open wound nasal cavity, complic
873.39	Multiple open nose wounds, complic
873.4x	Face, open wound
873.5x	Face, complicated open wound
873.6x	Internal mouth structure wound
873.7x	Complex mouth structure wound
873.8	Open wound of head NEC
874.8	Open wound of neck NEC
918.0	Superficial injury periocular
959.0	Face and neck injury NOS
998.2	Accidental op laceration/puncture
998.3	Postop wound disruption

REIMBURSEMENT INFORMATION

General

- See notes on page 114.
- Starred procedure. (12011, 12013)

Medicare

- Follow–Up Days — 10
- Assistant Surgeon
  12011–12016 — not paid
  12017 — by report
  12018 — paid
- Supply Charges — not allowed
- Outpatient Limit — does not apply
- Minor Surgery Rules Apply

CPT CODE	SERVICE	ICD–9–CM

12020 Treatment of superficial wound dehiscence; simple closure

CPT NOTES

- ◆ Sum of lengths of repairs.
- ◆ For extensive or complicated secondary wound closure, see 13160.

998.3 Postop wound disruption

REIMBURSEMENT INFORMATION

General

- ◆ See notes on page 114.

Medicare

- ◆ Follow–Up Days — 10
- ◆ Assistant Surgeon — not paid
- ◆ Supply Charges — not allowed
- ◆ Outpatient Limit — does not apply
- ◆ Minor Surgery Rules Apply

12021 Treatment of superficial wound dehiscence; with packing

CPT NOTES

- ◆ Sum of lengths of repairs.
- ◆ For extensive or complicated secondary wound closure, see 13160.

682.x Cellulitis and abscess
998.3 Postop wound disruption
998.5 Postoperative infection

REIMBURSEMENT INFORMATION

General

- ◆ See notes on page 114.

Medicare

- ◆ Follow–Up Days — 10
- ◆ Assistant Surgeon — not paid
- ◆ Supply Charges — not allowed
- ◆ Outpatient Limit — does not apply
- ◆ Minor Surgery Rules Apply

CPT CODE	SERVICE
12031*	Layer closure of wounds of scalp, axillae, trunk and/or extremities (excluding hands and feet); 2.5 cm or less
12032*	Layer closure of wounds of scalp, axillae, trunk and/or extremities (excluding hands and feet); 2.6 cm to 7.5 cm
12034	Layer closure of wounds of scalp, axillae, trunk and/or extremities (excluding hands and feet); 7.6 cm to 12.5 cm
12035	Layer closure of wounds of scalp, axillae, trunk and/or extremities (excluding hands and feet); 12.6 cm to 20.0 cm
12036	Layer closure of wounds of scalp, axillae, trunk and/or extremities (excluding hands and feet); 20.1 cm to 30.0 cm
12037	Layer closure of wounds of scalp, axillae, trunk and/or extremities (excluding hands and feet); over 30.0 cm

CPT NOTES

- Sum of lengths of repairs.

ICD–9–CM

173.5	M-Neoplasm, Skin of trunk
195.5	M-Neoplasm, Lower limb
198.2	M2-Neoplasm, Skin
215.7	B-Neoplasm, Trunk NOS
232.7	CA in situ, Skin of leg
709.8	Skin disorders NEC
873.0	Open wound of scalp
873.1	Open wound of scalp, complicated
873.8	Open wound of head NEC
875.0	Open wound of chest
875.1	Open wound of chest, complicated
876.0	Open wound of back
876.1	Open wound of back, complicated
877.1	Open wound of buttock, complicated
879.0	Open wound of breast
879.1	Open wound of breast, complicated
879.2	Open wound of anterior abdomen
879.3	Open wound anterior abdomen, compl
879.4	Open wound of lateral abdomen
879.5	Open wound lateral abdomen, compl
879.6	Open wound of trunk NEC
879.7	Open wound of trunk NEC, complic
879.8	Open wound site NOS
879.9	Open wound site NOS, complicated
880.00	Open wound of shoulder
880.02	Open wound of axilla
880.03	Open wound of upper arm
880.10	Open wound of shoulder, complicated
880.11	Open wound of scapula, complicated
880.12	Open wound of axilla, complicated
880.13	Open wound of upper arm, complic
880.19	Mult open wounds of shoulder, compl
881.0x	Elbow/forearm/wrist open wound
881.1x	Elbow/forearm/wrist complex wound
890.0	Open wound of hip/thigh
890.1	Open wound of hip/thigh, complic
891.0	Open wound of knee/leg/ankle
891.1	Open wound of knee/leg/ankle, compl

REIMBURSEMENT INFORMATION

General

- See notes on page 114.
- Starred procedure. (12031, 12032)

Medicare

- Follow–Up Days — 10
- Assistant Surgeon
  12031–12036 — not paid
  12034–12037 — not paid
- Supply Charges — not allowed
- Outpatient Limit
  12031–12032 — aookues
  12034–12037 — does not apply
- Minor Surgery Rules Apply

CPT CODE	SERVICE
12041*	Layer closure of wounds of neck, hands, feet and/or external genitalia; 2.5 cm or less
12042	Layer closure of wounds of neck, hands, feet and/or external genitalia; 2.6 cm to 7.5 cm
12044	Layer closure of wounds of neck, hands, feet and/or external genitalia; 7.6 cm to 12.5 cm
12045	Layer closure of wounds of neck, hands, feet and/or external genitalia; 12.6 cm to 20.0 cm
12046	Layer closure of wounds of neck, hands, feet and/or external genitalia; 20.1 cm to 30.0 cm
12047	Layer closure of wounds of neck, hands, feet and/or external genitalia; over 30.0 cm

CPT NOTES

- Sum of lengths of repairs.

ICD-9-CM

173.4	M-Neoplasm, Scalp/skin neck
173.5	M-Neoplasm, Skin of trunk
874.8	Open wound of neck NEC
874.9	Open wound of neck NEC, complicated
878.0	Open wound of penis
878.1	Open wound of penis, complicated
878.2	Open wound of scrotum/testes
878.3	Open wound, scrotum/testes, compl
878.4	Open wound of vulva
878.5	Open wound of vulva, complicated
878.6	Open wound of vagina
878.7	Open wound of vagina, complicated
882.x	Open wound of hand
883.x	Open wound of finger(s)
885.x	Traumatic amputation of thumb
886.x	Traumatic finger amputation
892.x	Open wound of foot
893.x	Open wound of toe(s)
959.4	Hand injury NOS
998.3	Postop wound disruption

REIMBURSEMENT INFORMATION

General

- See notes on page 114.
- Starred procedure. (12041)

Medicare

- Follow-Up Days — 10
- Assistant Surgeon
  12041–12046 — not paid
  12944–12047 — paid
- Supply Charges — not allowed
- Outpatient Limit
  12041–12942 — applies
  12044–12047 — does not apply
- Minor Surgery Rules Apply

CPT CODE	SERVICE
12051*	Layer closure of wounds of face, ears, eyelids, nose, lips and/or mucous membranes; 2.5 cm or less
12052	Layer closure of wounds of face, ears, eyelids, nose, lips and/or mucous membranes; 2.6 cm to 5.0 cm

CPT NOTES

- Sum of lengths of repairs.

ICD–9–CM

140.4	M-Neoplasm, Lower lip, inner aspect
143.1	M-Neoplasm, Lower gum
172.3	Malignant melanoma, Face NEC/NOS
173.0	M-Neoplasm, Skin of lip
173.1	M-Neoplasm, Skin of eyelid/canthus
173.2	M-Neoplasm, Skin of ear
173.3	M-Neoplasm, Skin of face NEC
216.1	B-Neoplasm, Skin of eyelid/canthus
870.0	Laceration eyelid skin/periocular
870.1	Full-thickness laceration eyelid
870.2	Eyelid laceration inv lacrimal pas
870.8	Open wound of ocular adnexa NEC
872.00	Open wound, external ear NOS
872.01	Open wound of auricle
872.02	Open wound of auditory canal
872.10	Open wound, external ear NOS, compl
872.11	Open wound of auricle, complicated
872.12	Open wound, auditory canal, complic
872.8	Open wound of ear NOS
873.20	Open wound of nose NOS
873.21	Open wound of nasal septum
873.22	Open wound of nasal cavity
873.29	Multiple open nose wounds
873.30	Open wound of nose NOS, complicated
873.31	Open wound nasal septum, complic
873.32	Open wound nasal cavity, complic
873.39	Multiple open nose wounds, complic
873.4x	Face, open wound
873.5x	Face, complicated open wound
873.6x	Internal mouth structure wound
873.7x	Complex mouth structure wound
906.2	Late effect of superficial injury
959.0	Face and neck injury NOS
998.3	Postop wound disruption

REIMBURSEMENT INFORMATION

General

- See notes on page 114.
- Starred procedure. (12051)

Medicare

- Follow–Up Days — 10
- Assistant Surgeon — not paid
- Supply Charges — not allowed
- Outpatient Limit — applies
- Minor Surgery Rules Apply

CPT CODE	SERVICE
12053	Layer closure of wounds of face, ears, eyelids, nose, lips and/or mucous membranes; 5.1 cm to 7.5 cm
12054	Layer closure of wounds of face, ears, eyelids, nose, lips and/or mucous membranes; 7.6 cm to 12.5 cm

CPT NOTES

- Sum of lengths of repairs.

ICD–9–CM

143.1	M-Neoplasm, Lower gum
172.3	Malignant melanoma, Face NEC/NOS
173.0	M-Neoplasm, Skin of lip
173.1	M-Neoplasm, Skin of eyelid/canthus
173.2	M-Neoplasm, Skin of ear
173.3	M-Neoplasm, Skin of face NEC
870.0	Laceration eyelid skin/periocular
870.1	Full-thickness laceration eyelid
870.2	Eyelid laceration inv lacrimal pas
870.8	Open wound of ocular adnexa NEC
872.00	Open wound, external ear NOS
872.01	Open wound of auricle
872.02	Open wound of auditory canal
872.10	Open wound, external ear NOS, compl
872.11	Open wound of auricle, complicated
872.12	Open wound, auditory canal, complic
872.8	Open wound of ear NOS
873.20	Open wound of nose NOS
873.21	Open wound of nasal septum
873.22	Open wound of nasal cavity
873.29	Multiple open nose wounds
873.30	Open wound of nose NOS, complicated
873.31	Open wound nasal septum, complic
873.32	Open wound nasal cavity, complic
873.39	Multiple open nose wounds, complic
873.4x	Face, open wound
873.5x	Face, complicated open wound
873.6x	Internal mouth structure wound
873.7x	Complex mouth structure wound
959.0	Face and neck injury NOS
998.3	Postop wound disruption

REIMBURSEMENT INFORMATION

General

- See notes on page 114.

Medicare

- Follow–Up Days — 10
- Assistant Surgeon — not paid
- Supply Charges — not allowed
- Outpatient Limit — does not apply
- Minor Surgery Rules Apply

CPT CODE	SERVICE
12055	Layer closure of wounds of face, ears, eyelids, nose, lips and/or mucous membranes; 12.6 cm to 20.0 cm
12056	Layer closure of wounds of face, ears, eyelids, nose, lips and/or mucous membranes; 20.1 cm to 30.0 cm
12057	Layer closure of wounds of face, ears, eyelids, nose, lips and/or mucous membranes; over 30.0 cm

CPT NOTES

- Sum of lengths of repairs.

ICD–9–CM

172.3	Malignant melanoma, Face NEC/NOS
173.2	M-Neoplasm, Skin of ear
173.3	M-Neoplasm, Skin of face NEC
870.0	Laceration eyelid skin/periocular
870.1	Full-thickness laceration eyelid
870.2	Eyelid laceration inv lacrimal pas
870.8	Open wound of ocular adnexa NEC
872.00	Open wound, external ear NOS
872.01	Open wound of auricle
872.10	Open wound, external ear NOS, compl
872.11	Open wound of auricle, complicated
872.12	Open wound, auditory canal, complic
872.8	Open wound of ear NOS
873.20	Open wound of nose NOS
873.21	Open wound of nasal septum
873.22	Open wound of nasal cavity
873.29	Multiple open nose wounds
873.30	Open wound of nose NOS, complicated
873.31	Open wound nasal septum, complic
873.32	Open wound nasal cavity, complic
873.39	Multiple open nose wounds, complic
873.4x	Face, open wound
873.5x	Face, complicated open wound
873.6x	Internal mouth structure wound
873.7x	Complex mouth structure wound
959.0	Face and neck injury NOS
998.3	Postop wound disruption

REIMBURSEMENT INFORMATION

General

- See notes on page 114.

Medicare

- Follow–Up Days — 10
- Assistant Surgeon
  12055 — not paid
  12056 — by report
  12057 — paid
- Supply Charges — not allowed
- Outpatient Limit — does not apply
- Minor Surgery Rules Apply

CPT CODE	SERVICE
13100	Repair, complex, trunk; 1.1 cm to 2.5 cm
13101	Repair, complex, trunk; 2.6 cm to 7.5 cm

CPT NOTES

- Reconstructive procedures, complicated wound closure.
- Sum of lengths of repairs.
- For full thickness repair of lip or eyelid, see respective anatomical subsections.
- For 1.0 cm or less, see simple or intermediate repairs.

ICD–9–CM

172.5	Malignant melanoma, Trunk
173.5	M-Neoplasm, Skin of trunk
213.2	B-Neoplasm, Vertebrae
214.1	Lipoma, Skin NEC
216.5	B-Neoplasm, Skin of trunk
216.8	B-Neoplasm, Skin NEC
216.9	B-Neoplasm, Skin NOS
873.1	Open wound of scalp, complicated
875.0	Open wound of chest
875.1	Open wound of chest, complicated
876.0	Open wound of back
877.0	Open wound of buttock
879.0	Open wound of breast
879.1	Open wound of breast, complicated
879.2	Open wound of anterior abdomen
879.3	Open wound anterior abdomen, compl
879.4	Open wound of lateral abdomen
879.5	Open wound lateral abdomen, compl
879.6	Open wound of trunk NEC
879.7	Open wound of trunk NEC, complic
998.3	Postop wound disruption

REIMBURSEMENT INFORMATION

General

- See notes on page 114.

Medicare

- Follow–Up Days — 10
- Assistant Surgeon — not paid
- Supply Charges — not allowed
- Outpatient Limit — does not apply
- Minor Surgery Rules Apply

CPT CODE	SERVICE
13120	Repair, complex, scalp, arms, and/or legs; 1.1 cm to 2.5 cm
13121	Repair, complex, scalp, arms, and/or legs; 2.6 cm to 7.5 cm

CPT NOTES

- Reconstructive procedures, complicated wound closure.
- Sum of lengths of repairs.
- For full thickness repair of lip or eyelid, see respective anatomical subsections.
- For 1.0 cm or less, see simple or intermediate repairs.

ICD–9–CM

173.4	M-Neoplasm, Scalp/skin neck
173.6	M-Neoplasm, Skin of arm
173.7	M-Neoplasm, Skin of leg
216.4	B-Neoplasm, Scalp/skin of neck
216.6	B-Neoplasm, Skin of arm
216.7	B-Neoplasm, Skin of leg
873.0	Open wound of scalp
873.1	Open wound of scalp, complicated
880.00	Open wound of shoulder
880.01	Open wound of scapula
880.02	Open wound of axilla
880.03	Open wound of upper arm
880.09	Multiple open wounds of shoulder
880.10	Open wound of shoulder, complicated
880.11	Open wound of scapula, complicated
880.12	Open wound of axilla, complicated
880.13	Open wound of upper arm, complic
880.19	Mult open wounds of shoulder, compl
880.20	Open wound shoulder w/tendon
880.21	Open wound scapula w/tendon
880.22	Open wound axilla w/tendon
880.23	Open wound upper arm w/tendon
881.0x	Elbow/forearm/wrist open wound
881.1x	Elbow/forearm/wrist complex wound
881.2x	Elbow/forearm/wrist, tendon wound
884.x	Open wound of upper limb
890.x	Open wound of hip and thigh
891.x	Open wound of knee, leg, ankle
894.x	Open wound of lower limb
998.3	Postop wound disruption

REIMBURSEMENT INFORMATION

General

- See notes on page 114.

Medicare

- Follow–Up Days — 10
- Assistant Surgeon — not paid
- Supply Charges — not allowed
- Outpatient Limit — does not apply
- Minor Surgery Rules Apply

CPT CODE	SERVICE
13131	Repair, complex, forehead, cheeks, chin, mouth, neck, axillae, genitalia, hands and/or feet; 1.1 cm to 2.5 cm
13132	Repair, complex, forehead, cheeks, chin, mouth, neck, axillae, genitalia, hands and/or feet; 2.6 cm to 7.5 cm

CPT NOTES

- ♦ Reconstructive procedures, complicated wound closure.
- ♦ Sum of lengths of repairs.
- ♦ For full thickness repair of lip or eyelid, see respective anatomical subsections.
- ♦ For 1.0 cm or less, see simple or intermediate repairs.

ICD–9–CM

173.3	M-Neoplasm, Skin of face NEC
173.5	M-Neoplasm, Skin of trunk
214.0	Lipoma, Skin of face
215.0	B-Neoplasm, Soft tissue, head
216.3	B-Neoplasm, Skin of face NEC
216.4	B-Neoplasm, Scalp/skin of neck
216.5	B-Neoplasm, Skin of trunk
216.8	B-Neoplasm, Skin NEC
228.01	Hemangioma, Skin
701.1	Keratoderma, acquired
873.0	Open wound of scalp
873.4x	Face, open wound
873.5x	Face, complicated open wound
873.60	Open wound of mouth NOS
873.69	Open wound of mouth NEC
873.7x	Complex mouth structure wound
874.10	Open wound larynx w/trachea, compl
874.8	Open wound of neck NEC
874.9	Open wound of neck NEC, complicated
878.0	Open wound of penis
878.1	Open wound of penis, complicated
878.2	Open wound of scrotum/testes
878.3	Open wound, scrotum/testes, compl
878.4	Open wound of vulva
878.5	Open wound of vulva, complicated
878.6	Open wound of vagina
878.7	Open wound of vagina, complicated
878.9	Open wound genital NEC, complic
880.02	Open wound of axilla
880.12	Open wound of axilla, complicated
880.22	Open wound axilla w/tendon
882.x	Open wound of hand
883.x	Open wound of finger(s)
886.x	Traumatic finger amputation
892.x	Open wound of foot
893.x	Open wound of toe(s)
895.1	Amputation of toe, complicated
998.3	Postop wound disruption

REIMBURSEMENT INFORMATION

General

- ♦ See notes on page 114.

Medicare

- ♦ Follow–Up Days — 10
- ♦ Assistant Surgeon — not paid
- ♦ Supply Charges — not allowed
- ♦ Outpatient Limit — does not apply
- ♦ Minor Surgery Rules Apply

CPT CODE **SERVICE**

13150 Repair, complex, eyelids, nose, ears and/or lips; 1.0 cm or less

CPT NOTES

- Reconstructive procedures, complicated wound closure.
- Sum of lengths of repairs.
- For full thickness repair of lip or eyelid, see respective anatomical subsections.
- See also 40650-40654, 67961-67975.

ICD–9–CM

140.1	M-Neoplasm, Lower lip, vermilion
140.9	M-Neoplasm, Lip/vermilion NOS
173.0	M-Neoplasm, Skin of lip
173.1	M-Neoplasm, Skin of eyelid/canthus
173.2	M-Neoplasm, Skin of ear
173.3	M-Neoplasm, Skin of face NEC
210.0	B-Neoplasm, Lip
215.0	B-Neoplasm, Soft tissue, head
216.0	B-Neoplasm, Skin of lip
216.1	B-Neoplasm, Skin of eyelid/canthus
216.2	B-Neoplasm, Skin of ear
216.3	B-Neoplasm, Skin of face NEC
744.29	Ear anomalies NEC
744.3	Ear anomaly NOS
870.0	Laceration eyelid skin/periocular
870.1	Full-thickness laceration eyelid
870.2	Eyelid laceration inv lacrimal pas
870.8	Open wound of ocular adnexa NEC
870.9	Open wound of ocular adnexa NOS
872.10	Open wound, external ear NOS, compl
872.11	Open wound of auricle, complicated
872.12	Open wound, auditory canal, complic
873.20	Open wound of nose NOS
873.29	Multiple open nose wounds
873.30	Open wound of nose NOS, complicated
873.31	Open wound nasal septum, complic
873.32	Open wound nasal cavity, complic
873.39	Multiple open nose wounds, complic
873.43	Open wound of lip
873.53	Open wound of lip, complicated
873.59	Open wound of face NEC, complicated
998.3	Postop wound disruption

REIMBURSEMENT INFORMATION

General

- See notes on page 114.

Medicare

- Follow–Up Days — 10
- Assistant Surgeon — not paid
- Supply Charges — not allowed
- Outpatient Limit — does not apply
- Minor Surgery Rules Apply

CPT CODE	SERVICE
13151	Repair, complex, eyelids, nose, ears and/or lips; 1.1 cm to 2.5 cm
13152	Repair, complex, eyelids, nose, ears and/or lips; 2.6 cm to 7.5 cm

CPT NOTES

- Reconstructive procedures, complicated wound closure.
- Sum of lengths of repairs.
- For full thickness repair of lip or eyelid, see respective anatomical subsections.

ICD–9–CM

140.1	M-Neoplasm, Lower lip, vermilion
140.9	M-Neoplasm, Lip/vermilion NOS
171.0	M-Neoplasm, Soft tissue, head
173.0	M-Neoplasm, Skin of lip
173.1	M-Neoplasm, Skin of eyelid/canthus
173.2	M-Neoplasm, Skin of ear
173.3	M-Neoplasm, Skin of face NEC
210.0	B-Neoplasm, Lip
216.0	B-Neoplasm, Skin of lip
216.1	B-Neoplasm, Skin of eyelid/canthus
216.2	B-Neoplasm, Skin of ear
216.3	B-Neoplasm, Skin of face NEC
744.29	Ear anomalies NEC
744.3	Ear anomaly NOS
870.0	Laceration eyelid skin/periocular
870.1	Full-thickness laceration eyelid
870.2	Eyelid laceration inv lacrimal pas
870.8	Open wound of ocular adnexa NEC
870.9	Open wound of ocular adnexa NOS
872.10	Open wound, external ear NOS, compl
872.11	Open wound of auricle, complicated
872.12	Open wound, auditory canal, complic
873.20	Open wound of nose NOS
873.29	Multiple open nose wounds
873.30	Open wound of nose NOS, complicated
873.31	Open wound nasal septum, complic
873.32	Open wound nasal cavity, complic
873.39	Multiple open nose wounds, complic
873.43	Open wound of lip
873.53	Open wound of lip, complicated
873.59	Open wound of face NEC, complicated
998.3	Postop wound disruption

REIMBURSEMENT INFORMATION

General

- See notes on page 114.

Medicare

- Follow–Up Days — 10
- Assistant Surgeon — not paid
- Supply Charges — not allowed
- Outpatient Limit — does not apply
- Minor Surgery Rules Apply

CPT CODE	SERVICE
13160	Secondary closure of surgical wound or dehiscence, extensive or complicated

CPT NOTES

- ♦ Reconstructive procedures, complicated wound closure.
- ♦ Sum of lengths of repairs.
- ♦ For full thickness repair of lip or eyelid, see respective anatomical subsections.
- ♦ For packing or simple secondary wound closure, see 12020, 12021.

ICD-9-CM

173.4	M-Neoplasm, Scalp/skin neck
173.5	M-Neoplasm, Skin of trunk
195.5	M-Neoplasm, Lower limb
198.2	M2-Neoplasm, Skin
215.7	B-Neoplasm, Trunk NOS
232.7	CA in situ, Skin of leg
709.8	Skin disorders NEC
870.0	Laceration eyelid skin/periocular
870.1	Full-thickness laceration eyelid
870.2	Eyelid laceration inv lacrimal pas
870.8	Open wound of ocular adnexa NEC
870.9	Open wound of ocular adnexa NOS
872.00	Open wound, external ear NOS
872.01	Open wound of auricle
872.02	Open wound of auditory canal
872.8	Open wound of ear NOS
873.0	Open wound of scalp
873.1	Open wound of scalp, complicated
873.20	Open wound of nose NOS
873.21	Open wound of nasal septum
873.22	Open wound of nasal cavity
873.29	Multiple open nose wounds
873.30	Open wound of nose NOS, complicated
873.31	Open wound nasal septum, complic
873.32	Open wound nasal cavity, complic
873.39	Multiple open nose wounds, complic
873.4x	Face, open wound
873.5x	Face, complicated open wound
873.6x	Internal mouth structure wound
873.7x	Complex mouth structure wound
873.8	Open wound of head NEC
874.8	Open wound of neck NEC
874.9	Open wound of neck NEC, complicated
875.0	Open wound of chest
875.1	Open wound of chest, complicated
876.0	Open wound of back
876.1	Open wound of back, complicated
877.1	Open wound of buttock, complicated
878.0	Open wound of penis
878.1	Open wound of penis, complicated
878.2	Open wound of scrotum/testes
878.3	Open wound, scrotum/testes, compl
878.4	Open wound of vulva
878.5	Open wound of vulva, complicated
878.6	Open wound of vagina
878.7	Open wound of vagina, complicated
879.0	Open wound of breast
879.1	Open wound of breast, complicated
879.2	Open wound of anterior abdomen
879.3	Open wound anterior abdomen, compl
879.4	Open wound of lateral abdomen
879.5	Open wound lateral abdomen, compl
879.6	Open wound of trunk NEC
879.7	Open wound of trunk NEC, complic
879.8	Open wound site NOS
879.9	Open wound site NOS, complicated
880.00	Open wound of shoulder

CPT CODE	SERVICE	ICD-9-CM	
13160 (Cont'd.)		880.02	Open wound of axilla
		880.03	Open wound of upper arm
		880.10	Open wound of shoulder, complicated
		880.11	Open wound of scapula, complicated
		880.12	Open wound of axilla, complicated
		880.13	Open wound of upper arm, complic
		880.19	Mult open wounds of shoulder, compl
		881.0x	Elbow/forearm/wrist open wound
		881.1x	Elbow/forearm/wrist complex wound
		882.x	Open wound of hand
		883.x	Open wound of finger(s)
		885.x	Traumatic amputation of thumb
		886.x	Traumatic finger amputation
		890.0	Open wound of hip/thigh
		890.1	Open wound of hip/thigh, complic
		891.0	Open wound of knee/leg/ankle
		891.1	Open wound of knee/leg/ankle, compl
		892.0	Open wound of foot
		892.1	Open wound of foot, complicated
		893.x	Open wound of toe(s)
		918.0	Superficial injury periocular
		959.0	Face and neck injury NOS
		959.4	Hand injury NOS
		998.2	Accidental op laceration/puncture
		998.3	Postop wound disruption

REIMBURSEMENT INFORMATION

General

- See notes on page 114.

Medicare

- Follow-Up Days — 90
- Assistant Surgeon — not paid
- Supply Charges — not allowed
- Outpatient Limit — does not apply
- Major Surgery Rules Apply

CPT CODE **SERVICE**

13300 Repair, unusual, complicated, over 7.5 cm, any area

CPT NOTES

- Reconstructive procedures, complicated wound closure.
- Sum of lengths of repairs.
- For full thickness repair of lip or eyelid, see respective anatomical subsections.

ICD–9–CM

172.7	Malignant melanoma, Leg
173.3	M-Neoplasm, Skin of face NEC
173.4	M-Neoplasm, Scalp/skin neck
173.5	M-Neoplasm, Skin of trunk
195.5	M-Neoplasm, Lower limb
198.2	M2-Neoplasm, Skin
215.7	B-Neoplasm, Trunk NOS
229.0	B-Neoplasm, Lymph nodes
232.7	CA in situ, Skin of leg
709.2	Scar/fibrosis of skin
709.8	Skin disorders NEC
870.0	Laceration eyelid skin/periocular
870.1	Full-thickness laceration eyelid
870.2	Eyelid laceration inv lacrimal pas
870.8	Open wound of ocular adnexa NEC
870.9	Open wound of ocular adnexa NOS
872.00	Open wound, external ear NOS
872.01	Open wound of auricle
872.02	Open wound of auditory canal
872.8	Open wound of ear NOS
873.0	Open wound of scalp
873.1	Open wound of scalp, complicated
873.20	Open wound of nose NOS
873.21	Open wound of nasal septum
873.22	Open wound of nasal cavity
873.29	Multiple open nose wounds
873.30	Open wound of nose NOS, complicated
873.31	Open wound nasal septum, complic
873.32	Open wound nasal cavity, complic
873.39	Multiple open nose wounds, complic
873.4x	Face, open wound
873.5x	Face, complicated open wound
873.6x	Internal mouth structure wound
873.7x	Complex mouth structure wound
873.8	Open wound of head NEC
874.8	Open wound of neck NEC
874.9	Open wound of neck NEC, complicated
875.0	Open wound of chest
875.1	Open wound of chest, complicated
876.0	Open wound of back
876.1	Open wound of back, complicated
877.1	Open wound of buttock, complicated
878.0	Open wound of penis
878.1	Open wound of penis, complicated
878.2	Open wound of scrotum/testes
878.3	Open wound, scrotum/testes, compl
878.4	Open wound of vulva
878.5	Open wound of vulva, complicated
878.6	Open wound of vagina
878.7	Open wound of vagina, complicated
879.0	Open wound of breast
879.1	Open wound of breast, complicated
879.2	Open wound of anterior abdomen
879.3	Open wound anterior abdomen, compl
879.4	Open wound of lateral abdomen
879.5	Open wound lateral abdomen, compl
879.6	Open wound of trunk NEC

CPT CODE	SERVICE	ICD-9-CM	
13300 (Cont'd.)		879.7	Open wound of trunk NEC, complic
		879.8	Open wound site NOS
		879.9	Open wound site NOS, complicated
		880.00	Open wound of shoulder
		880.02	Open wound of axilla
		880.03	Open wound of upper arm
		880.10	Open wound of shoulder, complicated
		880.11	Open wound of scapula, complicated
		880.12	Open wound of axilla, complicated
		880.13	Open wound of upper arm, complic
		880.19	Mult open wounds of shoulder, compl
		881.0x	Elbow/forearm/wrist open wound
		881.1x	Elbow/forearm/wrist complex wound
		882.x	Open wound of hand
		883.x	Open wound of finger(s)
		885.x	Traumatic amputation of thumb
		886.x	Traumatic finger amputation
		890.0	Open wound of hip/thigh
		890.1	Open wound of hip/thigh, complic
		891.0	Open wound of knee/leg/ankle
		891.1	Open wound of knee/leg/ankle, compl
		892.0	Open wound of foot
		892.1	Open wound of foot, complicated
		893.x	Open wound of toe(s)
		918.0	Superficial injury periocular
		959.0	Face and neck injury NOS
		959.4	Hand injury NOS
		998.2	Accidental op laceration/puncture
		998.3	Postop wound disruption

REIMBURSEMENT INFORMATION

General

- See notes on page 114.

Medicare

- Follow–Up Days — 10
- Assistant Surgeon — not paid
- Supply Charges — not allowed
- Outpatient Limit — does not apply
- Minor Surgery Rules Apply

CPT CODE	SERVICE
14000	Adjacent tissue transfer or rearrangement, trunk; defect 10 sq cm or less
14001	Adjacent tissue transfer or rearrangement, trunk; defect 10.1 sq cm to 30.0 sq cm

CPT NOTES

- For full thickness repair of lip or eyelid, see respective anatomical subsections.
- Excision (including lesion) and/or repair by adjacent tissue transfer or rearrangement (e.g., Z-plasty, W-plasty, V-Y plasty, rotation flap, advancement flap, double pedicle flap). When applied in repairing lacerations, by procedures listed must be developed by the surgeon to accomplish the repair. They do not apply when direct closure or rearrangement of traumatic wounds incidentally result in these configurations.
- Skin graft necessary to close secondary defect is considered an additional procedure.

ICD–9–CM

172.5	Malignant melanoma, Trunk
173.5	M-Neoplasm, Skin of trunk
216.5	B-Neoplasm, Skin of trunk
232.5	CA in situ, Skin of trunk
701.4	Keloid scar
707.0	Decubitus ulcer
707.9	Chronic skin ulcer NOS
709.2	Scar/fibrosis of skin
875.0	Open wound of chest
875.1	Open wound of chest, complicated
876.0	Open wound of back
876.1	Open wound of back, complicated
877.0	Open wound of buttock
877.1	Open wound of buttock, complicated
879.0	Open wound of breast
879.1	Open wound of breast, complicated
879.2	Open wound of anterior abdomen
879.3	Open wound anterior abdomen, compl
879.4	Open wound of lateral abdomen
879.5	Open wound lateral abdomen, compl
879.7	Open wound of trunk NEC, complic
880.00	Open wound of shoulder
880.01	Open wound of scapula
880.02	Open wound of axilla
880.10	Open wound of shoulder, complicated
880.11	Open wound of scapula, complicated
880.12	Open wound of axilla, complicated
906.0	Late effect, open wound head/trunk
906.2	Late effect of superficial injury
906.4	Late effect of crushing
906.8	Late effect of burns NEC
906.9	Late effect of burns NOS
909.3	Late effect of surg/med complic
998.3	Postop wound disruption
V10.3	Hx of breast malignancy
V10.82	Hx of malignant skin melanoma
V10.83	Hx of skin malignancy NEC
V50.1	Plastic surgery NEC
V51.	Aftercare w/plastic surgery

REIMBURSEMENT INFORMATION

General

- See notes on page 114.

Medicare

- Follow–Up Days — 90
- Assistant Surgeon — not paid
- Supply Charges — not allowed
- Outpatient Limit — does not apply
- Major Surgery Rules Apply

CPT CODE	SERVICE
14020	Adjacent tissue transfer or rearrangement, scalp, arms and/or legs; defect 10 sq cm or less
14021	Adjacent tissue transfer or rearrangement, scalp, arms and/or legs; defect 10.1 sq cm to 30.0 sq cm

CPT NOTES

- ♦ For full thickness repair of lip or eyelid, see respective anatomical subsections.
- ♦ Excision (including lesion) and/or repair by adjacent tissue transfer or rearrangement (e.g., Z-plasty, W-plasty, V-Y plasty, rotation flap, advancement flap, double pedicle flap). When applied in repairing lacerations, by procedures listed must be developed by the surgeon to accomplish the repair. They do not apply when direct closure or rearrangement of traumatic wounds incidentally result in these configurations.
- ♦ Skin graft necessary to close secondary defect is considered an additional procedure.

ICD–9–CM

172.4	Malignant melanoma, Scalp/neck
172.6	Malignant melanoma, Arm
172.7	Malignant melanoma, Leg
173.4	M-Neoplasm, Scalp/skin neck
173.6	M-Neoplasm, Skin of arm
173.7	M-Neoplasm, Skin of leg
216.4	B-Neoplasm, Scalp/skin of neck
216.6	B-Neoplasm, Skin of arm
216.7	B-Neoplasm, Skin of leg
454.0	Leg varicosity w/ulcer
704.00	Alopecia NOS
704.01	Alopecia areata
704.09	Alopecia NEC
709.2	Scar/fibrosis of skin
873.0	Open wound of scalp
873.1	Open wound of scalp, complicated
880.00	Open wound of shoulder
880.01	Open wound of scapula
880.03	Open wound of upper arm
880.09	Multiple open wounds of shoulder
880.10	Open wound of shoulder, complicated
880.11	Open wound of scapula, complicated
880.13	Open wound of upper arm, complic
880.19	Mult open wounds of shoulder, compl
880.20	Open wound shoulder w/tendon
880.23	Open wound upper arm w/tendon
880.29	Mult open wound shoulder w/tendon
881.0x	Elbow/forearm/wrist open wound
881.1x	Elbow/forearm/wrist complex wound
881.2x	Elbow/forearm/wrist, tendon wound
884.0	Open wound of arm, mult/NOS
884.1	Open wound of arm mult/NOS, compl
887.x	Traumatic arm/hand amputation
890.x	Open wound of hip and thigh
891.x	Open wound of knee, leg, ankle
894.x	Open wound of lower limb
896.x	Traumatic amputation of foot
897.x	Traumatic amputation of leg(s)
905.2	Late effect, arm fracture
905.4	Late effect, leg fracture
905.9	Late effect of traumatic amputation
906.0	Late effect, open wound head/trunk
906.1	Late effect, open wound extremity
906.2	Late effect of superficial injury
906.4	Late effect of crushing
906.5	Late effect of head/neck burn
906.6	Late effect of wrist/hand burn
906.7	Late effect of extremity burn NEC
V10.82	Hx of malignant skin melanoma
V10.83	Hx of skin malignancy NEC
V50.1	Plastic surgery NEC
V51.	Aftercare w/plastic surgery

CPT CODE **SERVICE**

14020, 14021 (Cont'd.)

ICD–9–CM

REIMBURSEMENT INFORMATION

General

- See notes on page 114.

Medicare

- Follow–Up Days — 90
- Assistant Surgeon — not paid
- Supply Charges — not allowed
- Outpatient Limit — does not apply
- Major Surgery Rules Apply

CPT CODE	SERVICE
14040	Adjacent tissue transfer or rearrangement, forehead, cheeks, chin, mouth, neck, axillae, genitalia, hands and/or feet; defect 10 sq cm or less

CPT NOTES

- For full thickness repair of lip or eyelid, see respective anatomical subsections.
- Excision (including lesion) and/or repair by adjacent tissue transfer or rearrangement (e.g., Z-plasty, W-plasty, V-Y plasty, rotation flap, advancement flap, double pedicle flap). When applied in repairing lacerations, by procedures listed must be developed by the surgeon to accomplish the repair. They do not apply when direct closure or rearrangement of traumatic wounds incidentally result in these configurations.
- Skin graft necessary to close secondary defect is considered an additional procedure.

ICD–9–CM

143.1	M-Neoplasm, Lower gum
172.3	Malignant melanoma, Face NEC/NOS
173.1	M-Neoplasm, Skin of eyelid/canthus
173.3	M-Neoplasm, Skin of face NEC
216.3	B-Neoplasm, Skin of face NEC
216.4	B-Neoplasm, Scalp/skin of neck
374.30	Ptosis of eyelid NOS
374.41	Eyelid retraction or lag
701.4	Keloid scar
709.2	Scar/fibrosis of skin
873.4x	Face, open wound
873.5x	Face, complicated open wound
873.6x	Internal mouth structure wound
873.7x	Complex mouth structure wound
874.8	Open wound of neck NEC
874.9	Open wound of neck NEC, complicated
878.0	Open wound of penis
878.1	Open wound of penis, complicated
878.2	Open wound of scrotum/testes
878.3	Open wound, scrotum/testes, compl
878.4	Open wound of vulva
878.5	Open wound of vulva, complicated
878.6	Open wound of vagina
878.7	Open wound of vagina, complicated
880.02	Open wound of axilla
880.12	Open wound of axilla, complicated
880.22	Open wound axilla w/tendon
882.x	Open wound of hand
883.x	Open wound of finger(s)
885.x	Traumatic amputation of thumb
886.x	Traumatic finger amputation
887.x	Traumatic arm/hand amputation
892.x	Open wound of foot
893.x	Open wound of toe(s)
895.x	Traumatic amputation of toe(s)
896.x	Traumatic amputation of foot
906.0	Late effect, open wound head/trunk
906.1	Late effect, open wound extremity
906.2	Late effect of superficial injury
906.4	Late effect of crushing
906.5	Late effect of head/neck burn
906.6	Late effect of wrist/hand burn
906.8	Late effect of burns NEC
909.3	Late effect of surg/med complic
998.3	Postop wound disruption
V10.02	Hx of oral/pharynx malignancy NEC
V10.82	Hx of malignant skin melanoma
V10.83	Hx of skin malignancy NEC
V50.1	Plastic surgery NEC
V51.	Aftercare w/plastic surgery

CPT CODE	SERVICE	ICD-9-CM

14040 (Cont'd.)

REIMBURSEMENT INFORMATION

General

- See notes on page 114.

Medicare

- Follow-Up Days — 90
- Assistant Surgeon — not paid
- Supply Charges — not allowed
- Outpatient Limit — does not apply
- Major Surgery Rules Apply
- Fragments — 14040, 11420, 11421, 11440, 11441, 11620, 11621, 11622, 11640, 11641

CPT CODE **SERVICE**

14041 Adjacent tissue transfer or rearrangement, forehead, cheeks, chin, mouth, neck, axillae, genitalia, hands and/or feet; defect 10.1 sq cm to 30.0 sq cm

CPT NOTES

- For full thickness repair of lip or eyelid, see respective anatomical subsections.
- Excision (including lesion) and/or repair by adjacent tissue transfer or rearrangement (e.g., Z-plasty, W-plasty, V-Y plasty, rotation flap, advancement flap, double pedicle flap). When applied in repairing lacerations, by procedures listed must be developed by the surgeon to accomplish the repair. They do not apply when direct closure or rearrangement of traumatic wounds incidentally result in these configurations.
- Skin graft necessary to close secondary defect is considered an additional procedure.

ICD–9–CM

143.1	M-Neoplasm, Lower gum
172.3	Malignant melanoma, Face NEC/NOS
173.3	M-Neoplasm, Skin of face NEC
216.3	B-Neoplasm, Skin of face NEC
216.4	B-Neoplasm, Scalp/skin of neck
374.34	Blepharochalasis
701.4	Keloid scar
709.2	Scar/fibrosis of skin
873.4x	Face, open wound
873.5x	Face, complicated open wound
873.6x	Internal mouth structure wound
873.7x	Complex mouth structure wound
874.8	Open wound of neck NEC
874.9	Open wound of neck NEC, complicated
878.0	Open wound of penis
878.1	Open wound of penis, complicated
878.2	Open wound of scrotum/testes
878.3	Open wound, scrotum/testes, compl
878.4	Open wound of vulva
878.5	Open wound of vulva, complicated
878.6	Open wound of vagina
878.7	Open wound of vagina, complicated
880.02	Open wound of axilla
880.12	Open wound of axilla, complicated
880.22	Open wound axilla w/tendon
882.x	Open wound of hand
883.x	Open wound of finger(s)
885.x	Traumatic amputation of thumb
886.x	Traumatic finger amputation
887.x	Traumatic arm/hand amputation
892.x	Open wound of foot
893.x	Open wound of toe(s)
895.x	Traumatic amputation of toe(s)
896.x	Traumatic amputation of foot
906.0	Late effect, open wound head/trunk
906.1	Late effect, open wound extremity
906.2	Late effect of superficial injury
906.4	Late effect of crushing
906.5	Late effect of head/neck burn
906.6	Late effect of wrist/hand burn
906.8	Late effect of burns NEC
909.3	Late effect of surg/med complic
998.3	Postop wound disruption
V10.02	Hx of oral/pharynx malignancy NEC
V10.82	Hx of malignant skin melanoma
V10.83	Hx of skin malignancy NEC
V50.1	Plastic surgery NEC
V51.	Aftercare w/plastic surgery

CPT CODE	SERVICE	ICD–9–CM
14041 (Cont'd.)		

REIMBURSEMENT INFORMATION

General

- See notes on page 114.

Medicare

- Follow–Up Days — 90
- Assistant Surgeon — not paid
- Supply Charges — not allowed
- Outpatient Limit — does not apply
- Major Surgery Rules Apply

CPT CODE	SERVICE
14060	Adjacent tissue transfer or rearrangement, eyelids, nose, ears and/or lips; defect 10 sq cm or less

CPT NOTES

- For full thickness repair of lip or eyelid, see respective anatomical subsections.
- Excision (including lesion) and/or repair by adjacent tissue transfer or rearrangement (e.g., Z-plasty, W-plasty, V-Y plasty, rotation flap, advancement flap, double pedicle flap). When applied in repairing lacerations, by procedures listed must be developed by the surgeon to accomplish the repair. They do not apply when direct closure or rearrangement of traumatic wounds incidentally result in these configurations.
- Skin graft necessary to close secondary defect is considered an additional procedure.

ICD–9–CM

140.0	M-Neoplasm, Upper lip, vermilion
140.1	M-Neoplasm, Lower lip, vermilion
140.3	M-Neoplasm, Upper lip, inner aspect
140.4	M-Neoplasm, Lower lip, inner aspect
140.5	M-Neoplasm, Lip NOS, inner NOS
140.6	M-Neoplasm, lip, commissure
140.8	M-Neoplasm, Lip NEC
140.9	M-Neoplasm, Lip/vermilion NOS
143.1	M-Neoplasm, Lower gum
171.0	M-Neoplasm, Soft tissue, head
172.0	Malignant melanoma, Lip
172.1	Malignant melanoma, eyelid/canthus
172.2	Malignant melanoma, Ear
172.3	Malignant melanoma, Face NEC/NOS
173.0	M-Neoplasm, Skin of lip
173.1	M-Neoplasm, Skin of eyelid/canthus
173.2	M-Neoplasm, Skin of ear
173.3	M-Neoplasm, Skin of face NEC
190.8	M-Neoplasm, Eye NEC
216.0	B-Neoplasm, Skin of lip
216.1	B-Neoplasm, Skin of eyelid/canthus
216.2	B-Neoplasm, Skin of ear
216.3	B-Neoplasm, Skin of face NEC
232.0	CA in situ, Skin of lip
232.1	CA in situ, Eyelid/canthus
232.2	CA in situ, Skin of ear
232.3	CA in situ, Skin of face NEC
238.2	UB-Neoplasm, Skin
239.2	Bone/Skin neoplasm NOS
374.10	Ectropion NOS
374.11	Senile ectropion
374.14	Cicatricial ectropion
374.46	Blepharophimosis
375.56	Acquired nasolacrimal duct stenosis
709.2	Scar/fibrosis of skin
743.62	Congenital eyelid deformity
744.21	Congenital absence of ear lobe
744.22	Macrotia
744.23	Microtia
744.29	Ear anomalies NEC
744.3	Ear anomaly NOS
744.84	Microstomia
870.0	Laceration eyelid skin/periocular
870.1	Full-thickness laceration eyelid
870.2	Eyelid laceration inv lacrimal pas
872.01	Open wound of auricle
872.02	Open wound of auditory canal
872.11	Open wound of auricle, complicated
872.12	Open wound, auditory canal, complic
873.21	Open wound of nasal septum
873.22	Open wound of nasal cavity
873.31	Open wound nasal septum, complic
873.32	Open wound nasal cavity, complic
873.43	Open wound of lip
873.5x	Face, complicated open wound
873.79	Open wound of mouth NEC, complic
906.0	Late effect, open wound head/trunk

CPT CODE	SERVICE
14060 (Cont'd.)	

ICD–9–CM

906.2	Late effect of superficial injury
906.4	Late effect of crushing
906.5	Late effect of head/neck burn
918.0	Superficial injury periocular
998.3	Postop wound disruption
V50.1	Plastic surgery NEC
V51.	Aftercare w/plastic surgery

REIMBURSEMENT INFORMATION

General

- See notes on page 114.

Medicare

- Follow–Up Days — 90
- Assistant Surgeon — not paid
- Supply Charges — not allowed
- Outpatient Limit — does not apply
- Major Surgery Rules Apply
- Fragments — 11440, 11441, 11640, 11641

CPT CODE	SERVICE
14061	Adjacent tissue transfer or rearrangement, eyelids, nose, ears and/or lips; defect 10.1 sq cm to 30.0 sq cm

CPT NOTES

- For full thickness repair of lip or eyelid, see respective anatomical subsections.
- Excision (including lesion) and/or repair by adjacent tissue transfer or rearrangement (e.g., Z-plasty, W-plasty, V-Y plasty, rotation flap, advancement flap, double pedicle flap). When applied in repairing lacerations, by procedures listed must be developed by the surgeon to accomplish the repair. They do not apply when direct closure or rearrangement of traumatic wounds incidentally result in these configurations.
- Skin graft necessary to close secondary defect is considered an additional procedure.
- For eyelid, full thickness, see 67961 et seq.

ICD-9-CM

140.0	M-Neoplasm, Upper lip, vermilion
140.1	M-Neoplasm, Lower lip, vermilion
140.3	M-Neoplasm, Upper lip, inner aspect
140.4	M-Neoplasm, Lower lip, inner aspect
140.5	M-Neoplasm, Lip NOS, inner NOS
140.6	M-Neoplasm, lip, commissure
140.8	M-Neoplasm, Lip NEC
140.9	M-Neoplasm, Lip/vermilion NOS
143.1	M-Neoplasm, Lower gum
172.0	Malignant melanoma, Lip
172.1	Malignant melanoma, eyelid/canthus
172.2	Malignant melanoma, Ear
172.3	Malignant melanoma, Face NEC/NOS
173.0	M-Neoplasm, Skin of lip
173.1	M-Neoplasm, Skin of eyelid/canthus
173.2	M-Neoplasm, Skin of ear
173.3	M-Neoplasm, Skin of face NEC
216.0	B-Neoplasm, Skin of lip
216.1	B-Neoplasm, Skin of eyelid/canthus
216.2	B-Neoplasm, Skin of ear
216.3	B-Neoplasm, Skin of face NEC
232.0	CA in situ, Skin of lip
232.1	CA in situ, Eyelid/canthus
232.2	CA in situ, Skin of ear
232.3	CA in situ, Skin of face NEC
709.2	Scar/fibrosis of skin
743.62	Congenital eyelid deformity
744.21	Congenital absence of ear lobe
744.22	Macrotia
744.23	Microtia
744.29	Ear anomalies NEC
744.3	Ear anomaly NOS
744.84	Microstomia
870.0	Laceration eyelid skin/periocular
870.1	Full-thickness laceration eyelid
870.2	Eyelid laceration inv lacrimal pas
872.01	Open wound of auricle
872.02	Open wound of auditory canal
872.11	Open wound of auricle, complicated
872.12	Open wound, auditory canal, complic
873.21	Open wound of nasal septum
873.22	Open wound of nasal cavity
873.31	Open wound nasal septum, complic
873.32	Open wound nasal cavity, complic
873.43	Open wound of lip
873.5x	Face, complicated open wound
873.79	Open wound of mouth NEC, complic
906.0	Late effect, open wound head/trunk
906.2	Late effect of superficial injury
906.4	Late effect of crushing
906.5	Late effect of head/neck burn
998.3	Postop wound disruption
V10.02	Hx of oral/pharynx malignancy NEC
V10.82	Hx of malignant skin melanoma
V10.83	Hx of skin malignancy NEC

CPT CODE	SERVICE	ICD-9-CM
14061 (Cont'd.)		V50.1 Plastic surgery NEC
		V51. Aftercare w/plastic surgery

REIMBURSEMENT INFORMATION

General

- ♦ See notes on page 114.

Medicare

- ♦ Follow–Up Days — 90
- ♦ Assistant Surgeon — not paid
- ♦ Supply Charges — not allowed
- ♦ Outpatient Limit — does not apply
- ♦ Major Surgery Rules Apply

CPT CODE	SERVICE
14300	Adjacent tissue transfer or rearrangement, more than 30 sq cm, unusual or complicated, any area

CPT NOTES

- For full thickness repair of lip or eyelid, see respective anatomical subsections.
- Excision (including lesion) and/or repair by adjacent tissue transfer or rearrangement (e.g., Z-plasty, W-plasty, V-Y plasty, rotation flap, advancement flap, double pedicle flap). When applied in repairing lacerations, by procedures listed must be developed by the surgeon to accomplish the repair. They do not apply when direct closure or rearrangement of traumatic wounds incidentally result in these configurations.
- Skin graft necessary to close secondary defect is considered an additional procedure.

ICD–9–CM

140.0	M-Neoplasm, Upper lip, vermilion
140.1	M-Neoplasm, Lower lip, vermilion
140.3	M-Neoplasm, Upper lip, inner aspect
140.4	M-Neoplasm, Lower lip, inner aspect
140.5	M-Neoplasm, Lip NOS, inner NOS
140.6	M-Neoplasm, lip, commissure
140.8	M-Neoplasm, Lip NEC
140.9	M-Neoplasm, Lip/vermilion NOS
143.1	M-Neoplasm, Lower gum
171.0	M-Neoplasm, Soft tissue, head
172.0	Malignant melanoma, Lip
172.1	Malignant melanoma, eyelid/canthus
172.2	Malignant melanoma, Ear
172.3	Malignant melanoma, Face NEC/NOS
172.4	Malignant melanoma, Scalp/neck
172.5	Malignant melanoma, Trunk
172.6	Malignant melanoma, Arm
172.7	Malignant melanoma, Leg
173.0	M-Neoplasm, Skin of lip
173.1	M-Neoplasm, Skin of eyelid/canthus
173.2	M-Neoplasm, Skin of ear
173.3	M-Neoplasm, Skin of face NEC
173.4	M-Neoplasm, Scalp/skin neck
173.5	M-Neoplasm, Skin of trunk
173.6	M-Neoplasm, Skin of arm
173.7	M-Neoplasm, Skin of leg
190.8	M-Neoplasm, Eye NEC
216.x	Benign neoplasm, Skin
232.0	CA in situ, Skin of lip
232.1	CA in situ, Eyelid/canthus
232.2	CA in situ, Skin of ear
232.3	CA in situ, Skin of face NEC
232.5	CA in situ, Skin of trunk
238.2	UB-Neoplasm, Skin
239.2	Bone/Skin neoplasm NOS
374.10	Ectropion NOS
374.11	Senile ectropion
374.14	Cicatricial ectropion
374.30	Ptosis of eyelid NOS
374.41	Eyelid retraction or lag
374.46	Blepharophimosis
375.56	Acquired nasolacrimal duct stenosis
454.0	Leg varicosity w/ulcer
701.4	Keloid scar
704.00	Alopecia NOS
704.01	Alopecia areata
704.09	Alopecia NEC
707.x	Chronic ulcer of skin
709.2	Scar/fibrosis of skin
743.62	Congenital eyelid deformity
744.21	Congenital absence of ear lobe
744.22	Macrotia
744.23	Microtia
744.29	Ear anomalies NEC
744.3	Ear anomaly NOS
744.84	Microstomia

CPT CODE	SERVICE	ICD-9-CM	
14300 (Cont'd.)		870.0	Laceration eyelid skin/periocular
		870.1	Full-thickness laceration eyelid
		870.2	Eyelid laceration inv lacrimal pas
		872.01	Open wound of auricle
		872.02	Open wound of auditory canal
		872.11	Open wound of auricle, complicated
		872.12	Open wound, auditory canal, complic
		873.x	Open wound of head
		874.8	Open wound of neck NEC
		874.9	Open wound of neck NEC, complicated
		875.0	Open wound of chest
		875.1	Open wound of chest, complicated
		876.0	Open wound of back
		876.1	Open wound of back, complicated
		877.0	Open wound of buttock
		877.1	Open wound of buttock, complicated
		878.0	Open wound of penis
		878.1	Open wound of penis, complicated
		878.2	Open wound of scrotum/testes
		878.3	Open wound, scrotum/testes, compl
		878.4	Open wound of vulva
		878.5	Open wound of vulva, complicated
		878.6	Open wound of vagina
		878.7	Open wound of vagina, complicated
		879.0	Open wound of breast
		879.1	Open wound of breast, complicated
		879.2	Open wound of anterior abdomen
		879.3	Open wound anterior abdomen, compl
		879.4	Open wound of lateral abdomen
		879.5	Open wound lateral abdomen, compl
		879.7	Open wound of trunk NEC, complic
		880.00	Open wound of shoulder
		880.01	Open wound of scapula
		880.02	Open wound of axilla
		880.03	Open wound of upper arm
		880.09	Multiple open wounds of shoulder
		880.10	Open wound of shoulder, complicated
		880.11	Open wound of scapula, complicated
		880.12	Open wound of axilla, complicated
		880.13	Open wound of upper arm, complic
		880.19	Mult open wounds of shoulder, compl
		880.20	Open wound shoulder w/tendon
		880.22	Open wound axilla w/tendon
		880.23	Open wound upper arm w/tendon
		880.29	Mult open wound shoulder w/tendon
		881.0x	Elbow/forearm/wrist open wound
		881.1x	Elbow/forearm/wrist complex wound
		881.2x	Elbow/forearm/wrist, tendon wound
		882.x	Open wound of hand
		883.x	Open wound of finger(s)
		884.0	Open wound of arm, mult/NOS
		884.1	Open wound of arm mult/NOS, compl
		885.x	Traumatic amputation of thumb
		886.x	Traumatic finger amputation
		887.x	Traumatic arm/hand amputation
		890.x	Open wound of hip and thigh
		891.x	Open wound of knee, leg, ankle

CPT CODE	SERVICE	ICD-9-CM	
14300 (Cont'd.)		892.x	Open wound of foot
		893.x	Open wound of toe(s)
		894.x	Open wound of lower limb
		895.x	Traumatic amputation of toe(s)
		896.x	Traumatic amputation of foot
		897.x	Traumatic amputation of leg(s)
		905.2	Late effect, arm fracture
		905.4	Late effect, leg fracture
		905.9	Late effect of traumatic amputation
		906.0	Late effect, open wound head/trunk
		906.1	Late effect, open wound extremity
		906.2	Late effect of superficial injury
		906.4	Late effect of crushing
		906.5	Late effect of head/neck burn
		906.6	Late effect of wrist/hand burn
		906.7	Late effect of extremity burn NEC
		906.8	Late effect of burns NEC
		906.9	Late effect of burns NOS
		909.3	Late effect of surg/med complic
		918.0	Superficial injury periocular
		941.01	Burn NOS, ear
		941.03	Burn NOS, lip
		941.05	Burn NOS, nose
		941.07	Burn NOS, face NEC
		941.08	Burn NOS, neck
		941.10	1st deg burn, face/head/unspec
		941.20	2nd deg burn, face/head/unspec
		941.21	2nd deg burn, ear
		941.23	2nd deg burn, lip
		941.24	2nd deg burn, chin
		941.25	2nd deg burn, nose
		941.27	2nd deg burn, face NEC
		941.28	2nd deg burn, neck
		942.04	Burn NOS trunk, back
		947.0	Burn of mouth and pharynx
		998.3	Postop wound disruption
		V10.02	Hx of oral/pharynx malignancy NEC
		V10.3	Hx of breast malignancy
		V10.82	Hx of malignant skin melanoma
		V10.83	Hx of skin malignancy NEC
		V50.1	Plastic surgery NEC
		V51.	Aftercare w/plastic surgery

REIMBURSEMENT INFORMATION

General

- See notes on page 114.

Medicare

- Follow-Up Days — 90
- Assistant Surgeon — not paid
- Supply Charges — not allowed
- Outpatient Limit — does not apply
- Major Surgery Rules Apply

CPT CODE	SERVICE
14350	Filleted finger or toe flap, including preparation of recipient site

CPT NOTES

- For full thickness repair of lip or eyelid, see respective anatomical subsections.
- Excision (including lesion) and/or repair by adjacent tissue transfer or rearrangement (e.g., Z-plasty, W-plasty, V-Y plasty, rotation flap, advancement flap, double pedicle flap). When applied in repairing lacerations, by procedures listed must be developed by the surgeon to accomplish the repair. They do not apply when direct closure or rearrangement of traumatic wounds incidentally result in these configurations.
- Skin graft necessary to close secondary defect is considered an additional procedure.

ICD–9–CM

882.x	Open wound of hand
883.x	Open wound of finger(s)
885.x	Traumatic amputation of thumb
886.x	Traumatic finger amputation
892.x	Open wound of foot
893.x	Open wound of toe(s)
895.x	Traumatic amputation of toe(s)
927.3	Crushing injury, finger
928.3	Crushing injury, toe
944.31	3rd deg burn, finger
944.32	3rd deg burn, thumb
944.33	3rd deg burn, mult fingers
944.34	3rd deg burn, finger w/thumb
944.35	3rd deg burn, palm
944.36	3rd deg burn, back of hand

REIMBURSEMENT INFORMATION

General

- See notes on page 114.

Medicare

- Follow–Up Days — 90
- Assistant Surgeon — not paid
- Supply Charges — not allowed
- Outpatient Limit — does not apply
- Major Surgery Rules Apply

CPT CODE	SERVICE
15000	Excisional preparation or creation of recipient site by excision of essentially intact skin (including subcutaneous tissues), scar, or other lesion prior to repair with free skin graft (list as separate service in addition to skin graft)

CPT NOTES

- ♦ Identify by size and location of the defect (recipient area) and the type of graft; includes simple debridement of granulations or recent avulsion.
- ♦ When a primary procedure such as orbitectomy, radical mastectomy, or deep tumor removal requires skin graft for definitive closure, see appropriate anatomical subsection for primary procedure and this section for skin graft.
- ♦ Repair of donor site requiring skin graft or local flaps is to be added as an additional procedure.
- ♦ For appropriate skin grafts, use 15100-15261; list the free graft separately by its procedure number when the graft, immediate or delayed, is applied.

ICD–9–CM

140.0	M-Neoplasm, Upper lip, vermilion
140.1	M-Neoplasm, Lower lip, vermilion
140.3	M-Neoplasm, Upper lip, inner aspect
140.4	M-Neoplasm, Lower lip, inner aspect
140.5	M-Neoplasm, Lip NOS, inner NOS
140.6	M-Neoplasm, lip, commissure
140.8	M-Neoplasm, Lip NEC
140.9	M-Neoplasm, Lip/vermilion NOS
144.9	M-Neoplasm, Floor of mouth NOS
171.0	M-Neoplasm, Soft tissue, head
172.x	Skin Melanoma
173.x	Malignant neoplasm, Skin
184.2	M-Neoplasm, Labia minora
184.3	M-Neoplasm, Clitoris
184.4	M-Neoplasm, Vulva NOS
184.8	M-Neoplasm, Female genital NEC
195.0	M-Neoplasm, Head/face/neck
216.x	Benign neoplasm, Skin
232.0	CA in situ, Skin of lip
232.1	CA in situ, Eyelid/canthus
232.2	CA in situ, Skin of ear
232.3	CA in situ, Skin of face NEC
232.4	CA in situ, Scalp/skin of neck
232.5	CA in situ, Skin of trunk
232.6	CA in situ, Skin of arm
232.7	CA in situ, Skin of leg
232.8	CA in situ, Skin NEC
374.14	Cicatricial ectropion
454.0	Leg varicosity w/ulcer
701.4	Keloid scar
707.1	Chronic ulcer of the leg
709.2	Scar/fibrosis of skin
870.0	Laceration eyelid skin/periocular
873.30	Open wound of nose NOS, complicated
873.39	Multiple open nose wounds, complic
873.4x	Face, open wound
873.5x	Face, complicated open wound
875.0	Open wound of chest
875.1	Open wound of chest, complicated
876.0	Open wound of back
876.1	Open wound of back, complicated
877.0	Open wound of buttock
877.1	Open wound of buttock, complicated
879.0	Open wound of breast
879.1	Open wound of breast, complicated
879.2	Open wound of anterior abdomen
879.3	Open wound anterior abdomen, compl
879.4	Open wound of lateral abdomen
879.5	Open wound lateral abdomen, compl
880.00	Open wound of shoulder
880.01	Open wound of scapula
880.02	Open wound of axilla
880.03	Open wound of upper arm
880.09	Multiple open wounds of shoulder
880.10	Open wound of shoulder, complicated
880.11	Open wound of scapula, complicated

CPT CODE	SERVICE	ICD-9-CM	
15000 (Cont'd)		880.12	Open wound of axilla, complicated
		880.13	Open wound of upper arm, complic
		880.19	Mult open wounds of shoulder, compl
		881.0x	Elbow/forearm/wrist open wound
		881.1x	Elbow/forearm/wrist complex wound
		882.0	Open wound of hand
		882.1	Open wound of hand, complicated
		883.0	Open wound of finger
		883.1	Open wound of finger, complicated
		884.0	Open wound of arm, mult/NOS
		884.1	Open wound of arm mult/NOS, compl
		885.x	Traumatic amputation of thumb
		886.x	Traumatic finger amputation
		887.x	Traumatic arm/hand amputation
		890.x	Open wound of hip and thigh
		891.x	Open wound of knee, leg, ankle
		892.x	Open wound of foot
		893.x	Open wound of toe(s)
		894.x	Open wound of lower limb
		895.x	Traumatic amputation of toe(s)
		896.x	Traumatic amputation of foot
		897.x	Traumatic amputation of leg(s)
		906.0	Late effect, open wound head/trunk
		906.1	Late effect, open wound extremity
		906.2	Late effect of superficial injury
		906.3	Late effect of contusion
		906.4	Late effect of crushing
		906.5	Late effect of head/neck burn
		908.6	Late effect, trauma complications
		908.9	Late effect of injury NOS
		909.3	Late effect of surg/med complic
		940.0	Chemical burn, eyelid/periocular
		940.1	Burn, eyelid/periocular area NEC
		941.22	Blisters, epidermal loss, eye
		941.31	3rd deg burn, ear
		941.32	3rd degree burn, eye
		941.33	3rd deg burn, lip
		941.34	3rd deg burn, chin
		941.35	3rd deg burn, nose
		941.36	3rd deg burn, scalp
		941.37	3rd deg burn, face NEC
		941.38	3rd deg burn, neck
		941.42	Deep 3rd degree burn, eye
		941.52	Deep 3rd degree loss, eye
		942.31	3rd deg burn trunk, breast
		942.32	3rd deg burn trunk, chest wall
		942.33	3rd deg burn trunk, abdominal wall
		942.34	3rd deg burn trunk, back
		942.35	3rd deg burn trunk, genitalia
		943.31	3rd deg burn, forearm
		943.32	3rd deg burn, elbow
		943.33	3rd deg burn, upper arm
		943.34	3rd deg burn, axilla
		943.35	3rd deg burn, shoulder
		943.36	3rd deg burn, scapula
		943.39	3rd deg burn, arm multiple sites
		944.31	3rd deg burn, finger

CPT CODE	SERVICE	ICD–9–CM	
15000 (Cont'd.)		944.32	3rd deg burn, thumb
		944.33	3rd deg burn, mult fingers
		944.34	3rd deg burn, finger w/thumb
		944.35	3rd deg burn, palm
		944.36	3rd deg burn, back of hand
		944.37	3rd deg burn, wrist
		945.31	3rd deg burn, toe
		945.32	3rd deg burn, foot
		945.33	3rd deg burn, ankle
		945.34	3rd deg burn, lower leg
		945.35	3rd deg burn, knee
		945.36	3rd deg burn, thigh
		945.39	3rd deg burn, leg mult sites
		958.3	Posttraumatic wound infection NEC
		959.0	Face and neck injury NOS
		996.52	Other tissue graft malfunction
		996.59	Malfunction other device/graft
		V50.1	Plastic surgery NEC
		V51.	Aftercare w/plastic surgery

REIMBURSEMENT INFORMATION

General

- See notes on page 114.

Medicare

- Follow–Up Days — none; falls within global period of another procedure.
- Assistant Surgeon — not paid
- Supply Charges — not allowed
- Outpatient Limit — does not apply

CPT CODE **SERVICE**

15050 Pinch graft, single or multiple, to cover small ulcer, tip of digit, or other minimal open area (except on face), up to defect size of 2 cm diameter

CPT NOTES

- ♦ Identify by size and location of the defect (recipient area) and the type of graft; includes simple debridement of granulations or recent avulsion.
- ♦ When a primary procedure such as orbitectomy, radical mastectomy, or deep tumor removal requires skin graft for definitive closure, see appropriate anatomical subsection for primary procedure and this section for skin graft.
- ♦ Repair of donor site requiring skin graft or local flaps is to be added as an additional procedure.
- ♦ For tissue-cultured skin grafts, use 15100-15121. These codes include harvesting of keratinocytes. Procedures are coded by recipient site.

ICD-9-CM

454.0	Leg varicosity w/ulcer
707.1	Chronic ulcer of the leg
709.3	Degenerative skin disorders
883.0	Open wound of finger
883.1	Open wound of finger, complicated
886.x	Traumatic finger amputation
893.0	Open wound of toe
893.1	Open wound of toe, complicated
895.1	Amputation of toe, complicated
941.36	3rd deg burn, scalp
941.38	3rd deg burn, neck
942.3	3rd degree burn NOS, trunk
943.3	3rd degree burn NOS, upper limb
944.31	3rd deg burn, finger
944.32	3rd deg burn, thumb
944.33	3rd deg burn, mult fingers
944.34	3rd deg burn, finger w/thumb
944.35	3rd deg burn, palm
944.36	3rd deg burn, back of hand
944.37	3rd deg burn, wrist
945.3	3rd degree burn NOS, lower limb
V51.	Aftercare w/plastic surgery

REIMBURSEMENT INFORMATION

General

- ♦ See notes on page 114.

Medicare

- ♦ Follow-Up Days — 90
- ♦ Assistant Surgeon — not paid
- ♦ Supply Charges — not allowed
- ♦ Outpatient Limit — does not apply
- ♦ Major Surgery Rules Apply

CPT CODE	SERVICE
15100	Split graft, trunk, scalp, arms, legs, hands, and/or feet (except multiple digits); 100 sq cm or less, or each one percent of body area of infants and children (except 15050)
15101	Split graft, trunk, scalp, arms, legs, hands, and/or feet (except multiple digits); each additional 100 sq cm, or each one percent of body area of infants and children, or part thereof

CPT NOTES

- Identify by size and location of the defect (recipient area) and the type of graft; includes simple debridement of granulations or recent avulsion.
- When a primary procedure such as orbitectomy, radical mastectomy, or deep tumor removal requires skin graft for definitive closure, see appropriate anatomical subsection for primary procedure and this section for skin graft.
- Repair of donor site requiring skin graft or local flaps is to be added as an additional procedure.

ICD–9–CM

172.4	Malignant melanoma, Scalp/neck
172.5	Malignant melanoma, Trunk
172.6	Malignant melanoma, Arm
172.7	Malignant melanoma, Leg
173.4	M-Neoplasm, Scalp/skin neck
173.5	M-Neoplasm, Skin of trunk
173.6	M-Neoplasm, Skin of arm
173.7	M-Neoplasm, Skin of leg
216.4	B-Neoplasm, Scalp/skin of neck
216.5	B-Neoplasm, Skin of trunk
216.6	B-Neoplasm, Skin of arm
216.7	B-Neoplasm, Skin of leg
232.5	CA in situ, Skin of trunk
454.0	Leg varicosity w/ulcer
701.4	Keloid scar
707.x	Chronic ulcer of skin
709.2	Scar/fibrosis of skin
873.0	Open wound of scalp
873.1	Open wound of scalp, complicated
875.0	Open wound of chest
875.1	Open wound of chest, complicated
876.0	Open wound of back
876.1	Open wound of back, complicated
877.0	Open wound of buttock
877.1	Open wound of buttock, complicated
879.0	Open wound of breast
879.1	Open wound of breast, complicated
879.2	Open wound of anterior abdomen
879.3	Open wound anterior abdomen, compl
879.4	Open wound of lateral abdomen
879.5	Open wound lateral abdomen, compl
880.00	Open wound of shoulder
880.01	Open wound of scapula
880.03	Open wound of upper arm
880.09	Multiple open wounds of shoulder
880.10	Open wound of shoulder, complicated
880.11	Open wound of scapula, complicated
880.13	Open wound of upper arm, complic
880.19	Mult open wounds of shoulder, compl
881.0x	Elbow/forearm/wrist open wound
881.1x	Elbow/forearm/wrist complex wound
882.0	Open wound of hand
882.1	Open wound of hand, complicated
883.0	Open wound of finger
883.1	Open wound of finger, complicated
884.0	Open wound of arm, mult/NOS
884.1	Open wound of arm mult/NOS, compl
885.x	Traumatic amputation of thumb
886.x	Traumatic finger amputation
887.x	Traumatic arm/hand amputation
890.x	Open wound of hip and thigh
891.x	Open wound of knee, leg, ankle
892.x	Open wound of foot
893.x	Open wound of toe(s)
894.x	Open wound of lower limb
895.x	Traumatic amputation of toe(s)

CPT CODE	SERVICE	ICD-9-CM	
15100, 15101 (Cont'd.)		896.x	Traumatic amputation of foot
		897.x	Traumatic amputation of leg(s)
		906.0	Late effect, open wound head/trunk
		906.1	Late effect, open wound extremity
		906.5	Late effect of head/neck burn
		906.6	Late effect of wrist/hand burn
		906.7	Late effect of extremity burn NEC
		906.9	Late effect of burns NOS
		909.2	Late effect of radiation
		942.31	3rd deg burn trunk, breast
		942.32	3rd deg burn trunk, chest wall
		942.33	3rd deg burn trunk, abdominal wall
		942.34	3rd deg burn trunk, back
		942.35	3rd deg burn trunk, genitalia
		942.41	Deep 3rd deg burn trunk, breast
		942.42	Deep 3rd deg burn trunk, chest wall
		942.43	Deep 3rd deg burn trunk, abdominal
		942.44	Deep 3rd deg burn trunk, back
		942.45	Deep 3rd deg burn trunk, genitalia
		943.31	3rd deg burn, forearm
		943.32	3rd deg burn, elbow
		943.33	3rd deg burn, upper arm
		943.34	3rd deg burn, axilla
		943.35	3rd deg burn, shoulder
		943.36	3rd deg burn, scapula
		943.39	3rd deg burn, arm multiple sites
		943.41	Deep 3rd deg burn, forearm
		943.42	Deep 3rd deg burn, elbow
		943.43	Deep 3rd deg burn, upper arm
		943.44	Deep 3rd deg burn, axilla
		943.45	Deep 3rd deg burn, shoulder
		943.46	Deep 3rd deg burn, scapula
		943.49	Deep 3rd deg burn, arm mult sites
		944.31	3rd deg burn, finger
		944.32	3rd deg burn, thumb
		944.33	3rd deg burn, mult fingers
		944.34	3rd deg burn, finger w/thumb
		944.35	3rd deg burn, palm
		944.36	3rd deg burn, back of hand
		944.37	3rd deg burn, wrist
		944.41	Deep 3rd deg burn, finger
		944.42	Deep 3rd deg burn, thumb
		944.43	Deep 3rd deg burn, mult fingers
		944.44	Deep 3rd deg burn, finger w/thumb
		944.45	Deep 3rd deg burn, palm
		944.46	Deep 3rd deg burn, back of hand
		944.47	Deep 3rd deg burn, wrist
		945.31	3rd deg burn, toe
		945.32	3rd deg burn, foot
		945.33	3rd deg burn, ankle
		945.34	3rd deg burn, lower leg
		945.35	3rd deg burn, knee
		945.36	3rd deg burn, thigh
		945.39	3rd deg burn, leg mult sites
		945.41	Deep 3rd deg burn, toe
		945.42	Deep 3rd deg burn, foot
		945.43	Deep 3rd deg burn, ankle

CPT CODE	SERVICE	ICD–9–CM	
15100, 15101 (Cont'd.)		945.44	Deep 3rd deg burn, lower leg
		945.45	Deep 3rd deg burn, knee
		945.46	Deep 3rd deg burn, thigh
		945.49	Deep 3rd deg burn, leg mult sites
		V10.82	Hx of malignant skin melanoma
		V10.83	Hx of skin malignancy NEC
		V51.	Aftercare w/plastic surgery

REIMBURSEMENT INFORMATION

General

- See notes on page 114.

Medicare

- Follow–Up Days — 90
- Assistant Surgeon
  15100 — not paid
  15101 — none; falls within global period of another procedure.
- Supply Charges — not allowed
- Outpatient Limit — does not apply
- Major Surgery Rules Apply (15100)

CPT CODE	SERVICE
15120	Split graft, face, eyelids, mouth, neck, ears, orbits, genitalia, and/or multiple digits; 100 sq cm or less, or each one percent of body area of infants and children (except 15050)

CPT NOTES

- Identify by size and location of the defect (recipient area) and the type of graft; includes simple debridement of granulations or recent avulsion.
- When a primary procedure such as orbitectomy, radical mastectomy, or deep tumor removal requires skin graft for definitive closure, see appropriate anatomical subsection for primary procedure and this section for skin graft.
- Repair of donor site requiring skin graft or local flaps is to be added as an additional procedure.
- For eyelids, see also 67961 et seq.

ICD–9–CM

140.0	M-Neoplasm, Upper lip, vermilion
140.1	M-Neoplasm, Lower lip, vermilion
140.3	M-Neoplasm, Upper lip, inner aspect
140.4	M-Neoplasm, Lower lip, inner aspect
140.5	M-Neoplasm, Lip NOS, inner NOS
140.6	M-Neoplasm, lip, commissure
140.8	M-Neoplasm, Lip NEC
140.9	M-Neoplasm, Lip/vermilion NOS
143.1	M-Neoplasm, Lower gum
144.9	M-Neoplasm, Floor of mouth NOS
145.9	M-Neoplasm, Mouth NOS
170.0	M-Neoplasm, Skull/Face bone
170.1	M-Neoplasm, Mandible
171.0	M-Neoplasm, Soft tissue, head
172.0	Malignant melanoma, Lip
172.1	Malignant melanoma, eyelid/canthus
172.2	Malignant melanoma, Ear
172.3	Malignant melanoma, Face NEC/NOS
172.4	Malignant melanoma, Scalp/neck
172.5	Malignant melanoma, Trunk
172.8	Malignant melanoma, Skin NEC
173.0	M-Neoplasm, Skin of lip
173.1	M-Neoplasm, Skin of eyelid/canthus
173.2	M-Neoplasm, Skin of ear
173.3	M-Neoplasm, Skin of face NEC
173.4	M-Neoplasm, Scalp/skin neck
173.5	M-Neoplasm, Skin of trunk
184.2	M-Neoplasm, Labia minora
184.3	M-Neoplasm, Clitoris
184.4	M-Neoplasm, Vulva NOS
184.8	M-Neoplasm, Female genital NEC
190.1	M-Neoplasm, Orbit
190.8	M-Neoplasm, Eye NEC
195.0	M-Neoplasm, Head/face/neck
216.0	B-Neoplasm, Skin of lip
216.1	B-Neoplasm, Skin of eyelid/canthus
216.2	B-Neoplasm, Skin of ear
216.3	B-Neoplasm, Skin of face NEC
216.4	B-Neoplasm, Scalp/skin of neck
216.5	B-Neoplasm, Skin of trunk
216.9	B-Neoplasm, Skin NOS
228.01	Hemangioma, Skin
230.0	CA in situ, Oral cavity/pharynx
232.0	CA in situ, Skin of lip
232.1	CA in situ, Eyelid/canthus
232.2	CA in situ, Skin of ear
232.3	CA in situ, Skin of face NEC
232.4	CA in situ, Scalp/skin of neck
232.5	CA in situ, Skin of trunk
235.1	UB-Neoplasm, Oral cavity/pharynx
238.2	UB-Neoplasm, Skin
239.2	Bone/Skin neoplasm NOS
374.05	Trichiasis w/o entropion
374.10	Ectropion NOS
374.11	Senile ectropion
374.14	Cicatricial ectropion

CPT CODE	SERVICE	ICD–9–CM	
15120 (Cont'd.)		374.30	Ptosis of eyelid NOS
		374.41	Eyelid retraction or lag
		374.46	Blepharophimosis
		375.56	Acquired nasolacrimal duct stenosis
		523.2	Gingival recession
		523.4	Chronic periodontitis
		523.8	Periodontal disease NEC
		525.2	Atrophy, edentulous alveolar ridge
		526.89	Jaw disease NEC
		528.9	Oral soft tissue disease NEC
		701.4	Keloid scar
		709.2	Scar/fibrosis of skin
		743.62	Congenital eyelid deformity
		744.21	Congenital absence of ear lobe
		744.22	Macrotia
		744.23	Microtia
		744.29	Ear anomalies NEC
		744.3	Ear anomaly NOS
		744.84	Microstomia
		870.0	Laceration eyelid skin/periocular
		870.1	Full-thickness laceration eyelid
		870.2	Eyelid laceration inv lacrimal pas
		872.01	Open wound of auricle
		872.02	Open wound of auditory canal
		872.11	Open wound of auricle, complicated
		872.12	Open wound, auditory canal, complic
		873.21	Open wound of nasal septum
		873.22	Open wound of nasal cavity
		873.31	Open wound nasal septum, complic
		873.32	Open wound nasal cavity, complic
		873.4x	Face, open wound
		873.5x	Face, complicated open wound
		873.6x	Internal mouth structure wound
		873.7x	Complex mouth structure wound
		874.8	Open wound of neck NEC
		874.9	Open wound of neck NEC, complicated
		878.0	Open wound of penis
		878.1	Open wound of penis, complicated
		878.2	Open wound of scrotum/testes
		878.3	Open wound, scrotum/testes, compl
		878.4	Open wound of vulva
		878.5	Open wound of vulva, complicated
		878.6	Open wound of vagina
		878.7	Open wound of vagina, complicated
		880.02	Open wound of axilla
		880.12	Open wound of axilla, complicated
		880.22	Open wound axilla w/tendon
		882.x	Open wound of hand
		883.x	Open wound of finger(s)
		885.x	Traumatic amputation of thumb
		886.x	Traumatic finger amputation
		887.x	Traumatic arm/hand amputation
		892.x	Open wound of foot
		893.x	Open wound of toe(s)
		895.x	Traumatic amputation of toe(s)
		896.x	Traumatic amputation of foot
		906.0	Late effect, open wound head/trunk

CPT CODE	SERVICE	ICD–9–CM	
15120 (Cont'd.)		906.1	Late effect, open wound extremity
		906.2	Late effect of superficial injury
		906.4	Late effect of crushing
		906.5	Late effect of head/neck burn
		906.6	Late effect of wrist/hand burn
		906.7	Late effect of extremity burn NEC
		906.8	Late effect of burns NEC
		909.2	Late effect of radiation
		909.3	Late effect of surg/med complic
		910.8	Superficial injury, head NEC
		918.0	Superficial injury periocular
		940.0	Chemical burn, eyelid/periocular
		940.1	Burn, eyelid/periocular area NEC
		941.07	Burn NOS, face NEC
		941.10	1st deg burn, face/head/unspec
		941.20	2nd deg burn, face/head/unspec
		941.22	Blisters, epidermal loss, eye
		941.27	2nd deg burn, face NEC
		941.28	2nd deg burn, neck
		941.3	3rd degree burn NOS, face/head/neck
		941.31	3rd deg burn, ear
		941.32	3rd degree burn, eye
		941.33	3rd deg burn, lip
		941.34	3rd deg burn, chin
		941.35	3rd deg burn, nose
		941.36	3rd deg burn, scalp
		941.37	3rd deg burn, face NEC
		941.38	3rd deg burn, neck
		941.4x	Deep 3rd degree, face/head/neck
		941.5	Deep 3rd degree, face/head/neck
		941.52	Deep 3rd degree loss, eye
		947.0	Burn of mouth and pharynx
		998.3	Postop wound disruption
		V10.02	Hx of oral/pharynx malignancy NEC
		V10.82	Hx of malignant skin melanoma
		V10.83	Hx of skin malignancy NEC
		V50.1	Plastic surgery NEC
		V51.	Aftercare w/plastic surgery

REIMBURSEMENT INFORMATION

General

- See notes on page 114.

Medicare

- Follow–Up Days — 90
- Assistant Surgeon — not paid
- Supply Charges — not allowed
- Outpatient Limit — does not apply
- Major Surgery Rules Apply

CPT CODE **SERVICE**

15121 Split graft, face, eyelids, mouth, neck, ears, orbits, genitalia, and/or multiple digits; each additional 100 sq cm, or each one percent of body area of infants and children, or part thereof

CPT NOTES

- ♦ Identify by size and location of the defect (recipient area) and the type of graft; includes simple debridement of granulations or recent avulsion.
- ♦ When a primary procedure such as orbitectomy, radical mastectomy, or deep tumor removal requires skin graft for definitive closure, see appropriate anatomical subsection for primary procedure and this section for skin graft.
- ♦ Repair of donor site requiring skin graft or local flaps is to be added as an additional procedure.
- ♦ For eyelids, see also 67961 et seq.

ICD–9–CM

140.0	M-Neoplasm, Upper lip, vermilion
140.1	M-Neoplasm, Lower lip, vermilion
140.3	M-Neoplasm, Upper lip, inner aspect
140.4	M-Neoplasm, Lower lip, inner aspect
140.5	M-Neoplasm, Lip NOS, inner NOS
140.6	M-Neoplasm, lip, commissure
140.8	M-Neoplasm, Lip NEC
140.9	M-Neoplasm, Lip/vermilion NOS
143.1	M-Neoplasm, Lower gum
145.9	M-Neoplasm, Mouth NOS
170.0	M-Neoplasm, Skull/Face bone
170.1	M-Neoplasm, Mandible
171.0	M-Neoplasm, Soft tissue, head
172.0	Malignant melanoma, Lip
172.1	Malignant melanoma, eyelid/canthus
172.2	Malignant melanoma, Ear
172.3	Malignant melanoma, Face NEC/NOS
172.4	Malignant melanoma, Scalp/neck
172.5	Malignant melanoma, Trunk
172.8	Malignant melanoma, Skin NEC
173.0	M-Neoplasm, Skin of lip
173.1	M-Neoplasm, Skin of eyelid/canthus
173.2	M-Neoplasm, Skin of ear
173.3	M-Neoplasm, Skin of face NEC
173.4	M-Neoplasm, Scalp/skin neck
173.5	M-Neoplasm, Skin of trunk
184.2	M-Neoplasm, Labia minora
184.3	M-Neoplasm, Clitoris
184.4	M-Neoplasm, Vulva NOS
184.8	M-Neoplasm, Female genital NEC
190.8	M-Neoplasm, Eye NEC
195.0	M-Neoplasm, Head/face/neck
216.0	B-Neoplasm, Skin of lip
216.1	B-Neoplasm, Skin of eyelid/canthus
216.2	B-Neoplasm, Skin of ear
216.3	B-Neoplasm, Skin of face NEC
216.4	B-Neoplasm, Scalp/skin of neck
216.5	B-Neoplasm, Skin of trunk
216.9	B-Neoplasm, Skin NOS
228.01	Hemangioma, Skin
230.0	CA in situ, Oral cavity/pharynx
232.0	CA in situ, Skin of lip
232.1	CA in situ, Eyelid/canthus
232.2	CA in situ, Skin of ear
232.3	CA in situ, Skin of face NEC
232.4	CA in situ, Scalp/skin of neck
232.5	CA in situ, Skin of trunk
235.1	UB-Neoplasm, Oral cavity/pharynx
238.2	UB-Neoplasm, Skin
239.2	Bone/Skin neoplasm NOS
374.10	Ectropion NOS
374.11	Senile ectropion
374.14	Cicatricial ectropion
374.30	Ptosis of eyelid NOS
374.41	Eyelid retraction or lag
374.46	Blepharophimosis

CPT CODE	SERVICE	ICD-9-CM	
15121 (Cont.d.)		375.56	Acquired nasolacrimal duct stenosis
		523.2	Gingival recession
		523.4	Chronic periodontitis
		525.2	Atrophy, edentulous alveolar ridge
		526.89	Jaw disease NEC
		701.4	Keloid scar
		709.2	Scar/fibrosis of skin
		743.62	Congenital eyelid deformity
		744.21	Congenital absence of ear lobe
		744.22	Macrotia
		744.23	Microtia
		744.29	Ear anomalies NEC
		744.3	Ear anomaly NOS
		744.84	Microstomia
		870.0	Laceration eyelid skin/periocular
		870.1	Full-thickness laceration eyelid
		870.2	Eyelid laceration inv lacrimal pas
		872.01	Open wound of auricle
		872.02	Open wound of auditory canal
		872.11	Open wound of auricle, complicated
		872.12	Open wound, auditory canal, complic
		873.21	Open wound of nasal septum
		873.22	Open wound of nasal cavity
		873.31	Open wound nasal septum, complic
		873.32	Open wound nasal cavity, complic
		873.4x	Face, open wound
		873.5x	Face, complicated open wound
		873.6x	Internal mouth structure wound
		873.7x	Complex mouth structure wound
		874.8	Open wound of neck NEC
		874.9	Open wound of neck NEC, complicated
		878.0	Open wound of penis
		878.1	Open wound of penis, complicated
		878.2	Open wound of scrotum/testes
		878.3	Open wound, scrotum/testes, compl
		878.4	Open wound of vulva
		878.5	Open wound of vulva, complicated
		878.6	Open wound of vagina
		878.7	Open wound of vagina, complicated
		880.02	Open wound of axilla
		880.12	Open wound of axilla, complicated
		880.22	Open wound axilla w/tendon
		882.x	Open wound of hand
		883.x	Open wound of finger(s)
		885.x	Traumatic amputation of thumb
		886.x	Traumatic finger amputation
		887.x	Traumatic arm/hand amputation
		892.x	Open wound of foot
		893.x	Open wound of toe(s)
		895.x	Traumatic amputation of toe(s)
		896.x	Traumatic amputation of foot
		906.0	Late effect, open wound head/trunk
		906.1	Late effect, open wound extremity
		906.2	Late effect of superficial injury
		906.4	Late effect of crushing
		906.5	Late effect of head/neck burn
		906.6	Late effect of wrist/hand burn

CPT CODE	SERVICE	ICD–9–CM	
15121 (Cont'd.)		906.7	Late effect of extremity burn NEC
		906.8	Late effect of burns NEC
		909.2	Late effect of radiation
		909.3	Late effect of surg/med complic
		910.8	Superficial injury, head NEC
		918.0	Superficial injury periocular
		941.07	Burn NOS, face NEC
		941.10	1st deg burn, face/head/unspec
		941.20	2nd deg burn, face/head/unspec
		941.27	2nd deg burn, face NEC
		941.28	2nd deg burn, neck
		941.31	3rd deg burn, ear
		941.32	3rd degree burn, eye
		941.33	3rd deg burn, lip
		941.34	3rd deg burn, chin
		941.35	3rd deg burn, nose
		941.36	3rd deg burn, scalp
		941.37	3rd deg burn, face NEC
		941.38	3rd deg burn, neck
		941.41	Deep 3rd deg burn, ear
		941.42	Deep 3rd degree burn, eye
		941.43	Deep 3rd deg burn, lip
		941.44	Deep 3rd deg burn, chin
		941.45	Deep 3rd deg burn, nose
		941.46	Deep 3rd deg burn, scalp
		941.47	Deep 3rd deg burn, face NEC
		941.48	Deep 3rd deg burn, neck
		947.0	Burn of mouth and pharynx
		998.3	Postop wound disruption
		V10.02	Hx of oral/pharynx malignancy NEC
		V10.82	Hx of malignant skin melanoma
		V10.83	Hx of skin malignancy NEC
		V50.1	Plastic surgery NEC
		V51.	Aftercare w/plastic surgery

REIMBURSEMENT INFORMATION

General

- ♦ See notes on page 114.

Medicare

- ♦ Follow–Up Days — none; falls within global period of another procedure.
- ♦ Assistant Surgeon — paid
- ♦ Supply Charges — not allowed
- ♦ Outpatient Limit — does not apply

CPT CODE	SERVICE
15200	Full thickness graft, free, including direct closure of donor site, trunk; 20 sq cm or less
15201	Full thickness graft, free, including direct closure of donor site, trunk; each additional 20 sq cm

CPT NOTES

- ♦ Identify by size and location of the defect (recipient area) and the type of graft; includes simple debridement of granulations or recent avulsion.
- ♦ When a primary procedure such as orbitectomy, radical mastectomy, or deep tumor removal requires skin graft for definitive closure, see appropriate anatomical subsection for primary procedure and this section for skin graft.
- ♦ Repair of donor site requiring skin graft or local flaps is to be added as an additional procedure.

ICD–9–CM

172.5	Malignant melanoma, Trunk
173.5	M-Neoplasm, Skin of trunk
216.5	B-Neoplasm, Skin of trunk
232.5	CA in situ, Skin of trunk
701.4	Keloid scar
707.0	Decubitus ulcer
707.9	Chronic skin ulcer NOS
709.2	Scar/fibrosis of skin
875.0	Open wound of chest
875.1	Open wound of chest, complicated
876.0	Open wound of back
876.1	Open wound of back, complicated
877.0	Open wound of buttock
877.1	Open wound of buttock, complicated
879.0	Open wound of breast
879.1	Open wound of breast, complicated
879.2	Open wound of anterior abdomen
879.3	Open wound anterior abdomen, compl
879.4	Open wound of lateral abdomen
879.5	Open wound lateral abdomen, compl
879.7	Open wound of trunk NEC, complic
880.00	Open wound of shoulder
880.01	Open wound of scapula
880.02	Open wound of axilla
880.10	Open wound of shoulder, complicated
880.11	Open wound of scapula, complicated
880.12	Open wound of axilla, complicated
906.0	Late effect, open wound head/trunk
906.2	Late effect of superficial injury
906.4	Late effect of crushing
906.8	Late effect of burns NEC
906.9	Late effect of burns NOS
909.3	Late effect of surg/med complic
942.31	3rd deg burn trunk, breast
942.32	3rd deg burn trunk, chest wall
942.33	3rd deg burn trunk, abdominal wall
942.34	3rd deg burn trunk, back
942.35	3rd deg burn trunk, genitalia
942.41	Deep 3rd deg burn trunk, breast
942.42	Deep 3rd deg burn trunk, chest wall
942.43	Deep 3rd deg burn trunk, abdominal
942.44	Deep 3rd deg burn trunk, back
942.45	Deep 3rd deg burn trunk, genitalia
942.51	Deep 3rd deg loss trunk, breast
942.52	Deep 3rd deg loss trunk, chest wall
942.53	Deep 3rd deg loss trunk, abdominal
942.54	Deep 3rd deg loss trunk, back
942.55	Deep 3rd deg loss trunk, genitalia
998.3	Postop wound disruption
V10.3	Hx of breast malignancy
V10.82	Hx of malignant skin melanoma
V10.83	Hx of skin malignancy NEC
V50.1	Plastic surgery NEC
V51.	Aftercare w/plastic surgery

CPT CODE	SERVICE	ICD-9-CM

15200, 15201 (Cont'd.)

REIMBURSEMENT INFORMATION

General

- See notes on page 114.

Medicare

- Follow-Up Days
  15200 — 90
  15201 — none; falls within global period of another procedure
- Assistant Surgeon — not paid
- Supply Charges — not allowed
- Outpatient Limit — does not apply
- Major Surgery Rules Apply (15200)

CPT CODE	SERVICE
15220	Full thickness graft, free, including direct closure of donor site, scalp, arms, and/or legs; 20 sq cm or less
15221	Full thickness graft, free, including direct closure of donor site, scalp, arms, and/or legs; each additional 20 sq cm

CPT NOTES

- ♦ Identify by size and location of the defect (recipient area) and the type of graft; includes simple debridement of granulations or recent avulsion.
- ♦ When a primary procedure such as orbitectomy, radical mastectomy, or deep tumor removal requires skin graft for definitive closure, see appropriate anatomical subsection for primary procedure and this section for skin graft.
- ♦ Repair of donor site requiring skin graft or local flaps is to be added as an additional procedure.

ICD-9-CM

172.4	Malignant melanoma, Scalp/neck
172.6	Malignant melanoma, Arm
172.7	Malignant melanoma, Leg
173.4	M-Neoplasm, Scalp/skin neck
173.6	M-Neoplasm, Skin of arm
173.7	M-Neoplasm, Skin of leg
216.4	B-Neoplasm, Scalp/skin of neck
216.6	B-Neoplasm, Skin of arm
216.7	B-Neoplasm, Skin of leg
232.4	CA in situ, Scalp/skin of neck
232.6	CA in situ, Skin of arm
232.7	CA in situ, Skin of leg
454.0	Leg varicosity w/ulcer
704.00	Alopecia NOS
704.01	Alopecia areata
704.09	Alopecia NEC
709.2	Scar/fibrosis of skin
873.0	Open wound of scalp
873.1	Open wound of scalp, complicated
880.00	Open wound of shoulder
880.01	Open wound of scapula
880.03	Open wound of upper arm
880.09	Multiple open wounds of shoulder
880.10	Open wound of shoulder, complicated
880.11	Open wound of scapula, complicated
880.13	Open wound of upper arm, complic
880.19	Mult open wounds of shoulder, compl
880.20	Open wound shoulder w/tendon
880.23	Open wound upper arm w/tendon
880.29	Mult open wound shoulder w/tendon
881.0x	Elbow/forearm/wrist open wound
881.1x	Elbow/forearm/wrist complex wound
881.2x	Elbow/forearm/wrist, tendon wound
884.0	Open wound of arm, mult/NOS
884.1	Open wound of arm mult/NOS, compl
887.x	Traumatic arm/hand amputation
890.x	Open wound of hip and thigh
891.x	Open wound of knee, leg, ankle
894.x	Open wound of lower limb
896.x	Traumatic amputation of foot
897.x	Traumatic amputation of leg(s)
905.2	Late effect, arm fracture
905.4	Late effect, leg fracture
905.9	Late effect of traumatic amputation
906.0	Late effect, open wound head/trunk
906.1	Late effect, open wound extremity
906.2	Late effect of superficial injury
906.4	Late effect of crushing
906.5	Late effect of head/neck burn
906.6	Late effect of wrist/hand burn
906.7	Late effect of extremity burn NEC
906.9	Late effect of burns NOS
943.31	3rd deg burn, forearm
943.32	3rd deg burn, elbow
943.33	3rd deg burn, upper arm
943.34	3rd deg burn, axilla
943.35	3rd deg burn, shoulder

CPT CODE **SERVICE**

15220, 15221 (Cont'd.)

ICD–9–CM

943.36	3rd deg burn, scapula
943.39	3rd deg burn, arm multiple sites
943.41	Deep 3rd deg burn, forearm
943.42	Deep 3rd deg burn, elbow
943.43	Deep 3rd deg burn, upper arm
943.44	Deep 3rd deg burn, axilla
943.45	Deep 3rd deg burn, shoulder
943.46	Deep 3rd deg burn, scapula
943.49	Deep 3rd deg burn, arm mult sites
943.51	Deep 3rd deg loss, forearm
943.52	Deep 3rd deg loss, elbow
943.53	Deep 3rd deg loss, upper arm
943.54	Deep 3rd deg loss, axilla
943.55	Deep 3rd deg loss, shoulder
943.56	Deep 3rd deg loss, scapula
943.59	Deep 3rd deg loss, arm mult sites
V10.82	Hx of malignant skin melanoma
V10.83	Hx of skin malignancy NEC
V50.1	Plastic surgery NEC
V51.	Aftercare w/plastic surgery

REIMBURSEMENT INFORMATION

General

- See notes on page 114.

Medicare

- Follow–Up Days
  15220 — 90
  15221 — none; falls within global period of another procedure
- Assistant Surgeon — not paid
- Supply Charges — not allowed
- Outpatient Limit — does not apply
- Major Surgery Rules Apply (15220)

CPT CODE	SERVICE
15240	Full thickness graft, free, including direct closure of donor site, forehead, cheeks, chin, mouth, neck, axillae, genitalia, hands, and/or feet; 20 sq cm or less
15241	Full thickness graft, free, including direct closure of donor site, forehead, cheeks, chin, mouth, neck, axillae, genitalia, hands, and/or feet; each additional 20 sq cm

CPT NOTES

- Identify by size and location of the defect (recipient area) and the type of graft; includes simple debridement of granulations or recent avulsion.
- When a primary procedure such as orbitectomy, radical mastectomy, or deep tumor removal requires skin graft for definitive closure, see appropriate anatomical subsection for primary procedure and this section for skin graft.
- Repair of donor site requiring skin graft or local flaps is to be added as an additional procedure.
- For finger tip graft, see 15050.
- For repair of syndactyly, fingers, see 26560-26562.

ICD–9–CM

145.9	M-Neoplasm, Mouth NOS
170.0	M-Neoplasm, Skull/Face bone
170.1	M-Neoplasm, Mandible
172.3	Malignant melanoma, Face NEC/NOS
172.4	Malignant melanoma, Scalp/neck
172.5	Malignant melanoma, Trunk
172.8	Malignant melanoma, Skin NEC
173.3	M-Neoplasm, Skin of face NEC
173.4	M-Neoplasm, Scalp/skin neck
173.5	M-Neoplasm, Skin of trunk
184.2	M-Neoplasm, Labia minora
184.3	M-Neoplasm, Clitoris
184.4	M-Neoplasm, Vulva NOS
184.8	M-Neoplasm, Female genital NEC
195.0	M-Neoplasm, Head/face/neck
216.3	B-Neoplasm, Skin of face NEC
216.4	B-Neoplasm, Scalp/skin of neck
216.5	B-Neoplasm, Skin of trunk
216.9	B-Neoplasm, Skin NOS
228.01	Hemangioma, Skin
230.0	CA in situ, Oral cavity/pharynx
232.3	CA in situ, Skin of face NEC
232.5	CA in situ, Skin of trunk
235.1	UB-Neoplasm, Oral cavity/pharynx
238.2	UB-Neoplasm, Skin
239.2	Bone/Skin neoplasm NOS
523.2	Gingival recession
523.4	Chronic periodontitis
525.2	Atrophy, edentulous alveolar ridge
526.89	Jaw disease NEC
709.2	Scar/fibrosis of skin
873.4x	Face, open wound
873.5x	Face, complicated open wound
873.70	Open wound of mouth NOS, complic
874.8	Open wound of neck NEC
874.9	Open wound of neck NEC, complicated
878.0	Open wound of penis
878.1	Open wound of penis, complicated
878.2	Open wound of scrotum/testes
878.3	Open wound, scrotum/testes, compl
878.4	Open wound of vulva
878.5	Open wound of vulva, complicated
878.6	Open wound of vagina
878.7	Open wound of vagina, complicated
880.02	Open wound of axilla
880.12	Open wound of axilla, complicated
880.22	Open wound axilla w/tendon
882.0	Open wound of hand
882.1	Open wound of hand, complicated
883.0	Open wound of finger
883.1	Open wound of finger, complicated
885.x	Traumatic amputation of thumb
886.x	Traumatic finger amputation
887.x	Traumatic arm/hand amputation
892.x	Open wound of foot
893.x	Open wound of toe(s)

CPT CODE	SERVICE	ICD-9-CM	
15240, 15241 (Cont'd.)		895.x	Traumatic amputation of toe(s)
		896.x	Traumatic amputation of foot
		905.9	Late effect of traumatic amputation
		906.0	Late effect, open wound head/trunk
		906.1	Late effect, open wound extremity
		906.5	Late effect of head/neck burn
		906.6	Late effect of wrist/hand burn
		910.8	Superficial injury, head NEC
		941.07	Burn NOS, face NEC
		941.10	1st deg burn, face/head/unspec
		941.20	2nd deg burn, face/head/unspec
		941.27	2nd deg burn, face NEC
		941.28	2nd deg burn, neck
		941.34	3rd deg burn, chin
		941.37	3rd deg burn, face NEC
		941.38	3rd deg burn, neck
		941.44	Deep 3rd deg burn, chin
		941.47	Deep 3rd deg burn, face NEC
		941.48	Deep 3rd deg burn, neck
		941.54	Deep 3rd deg loss, chin
		941.57	Deep 3rd deg loss, face NEC
		941.58	Deep 3rd deg loss, neck
		942.35	3rd deg burn trunk, genitalia
		942.45	Deep 3rd deg burn trunk, genitalia
		942.55	Deep 3rd deg loss trunk, genitalia
		943.35	3rd deg burn, shoulder
		943.45	Deep 3rd deg burn, shoulder
		943.55	Deep 3rd deg loss, shoulder
		944.31	3rd deg burn, finger
		944.32	3rd deg burn, thumb
		944.33	3rd deg burn, mult fingers
		944.34	3rd deg burn, finger w/thumb
		944.35	3rd deg burn, palm
		944.36	3rd deg burn, back of hand
		944.37	3rd deg burn, wrist
		944.41	Deep 3rd deg burn, finger
		944.42	Deep 3rd deg burn, thumb
		944.43	Deep 3rd deg burn, mult fingers
		944.44	Deep 3rd deg burn, finger w/thumb
		944.45	Deep 3rd deg burn, palm
		944.46	Deep 3rd deg burn, back of hand
		944.47	Deep 3rd deg burn, wrist
		944.51	Deep 3rd deg loss, finger
		944.52	Deep 3rd deg loss, thumb
		944.53	Deep 3rd deg loss, mult fingers
		944.54	Deep 3rd deg loss, finger w/thumb
		944.55	Deep 3rd deg loss, palm
		944.56	Deep 3rd deg loss, back of hand
		944.57	Deep 3rd deg loss, wrist
		945.31	3rd deg burn, toe
		945.32	3rd deg burn, foot
		945.41	Deep 3rd deg burn, toe
		945.42	Deep 3rd deg burn, foot
		945.51	Deep 3rd deg loss, toe
		945.52	Deep 3rd deg loss, foot
		947.0	Burn of mouth and pharynx
		V10.02	Hx of oral/pharynx malignancy NEC

CPT CODE	SERVICE	ICD–9–CM

15240, 15241 (Cont'd.)

V10.82 Hx of malignant skin melanoma
V10.83 Hx of skin malignancy NEC
V51. Aftercare w/plastic surgery

REIMBURSEMENT INFORMATION

General

- See notes on page 114.

Medicare

- Follow–Up Days
  15240 — 90
  15241 — none; falls within global period of another procedure
- Assistant Surgeon — not paid
- Supply Charges — not allowed
- Outpatient Limit — does not apply
- Major Surgery Rules Apply (15240)

CPT CODE	SERVICE
15260	Full thickness graft, free, including direct closure of donor site, nose, ears, eyelids, and/or lips; 20 sq cm or less

CPT NOTES

- ♦ Identify by size and location of the defect (recipient area) and the type of graft; includes simple debridement of granulations or recent avulsion.
- ♦ When a primary procedure such as orbitectomy, radical mastectomy, or deep tumor removal requires skin graft for definitive closure, see appropriate anatomical subsection for primary procedure and this section for skin graft.
- ♦ Repair of donor site requiring skin graft or local flaps is to be added as an additional procedure.
- ♦ For eyelids, see also 67961 et seq.
- ♦ Repair of donor site requiring skin graft or local flaps, to be added as additional separate procedure.

ICD–9–CM

140.0	M-Neoplasm, Upper lip, vermilion
140.1	M-Neoplasm, Lower lip, vermilion
140.3	M-Neoplasm, Upper lip, inner aspect
140.4	M-Neoplasm, Lower lip, inner aspect
140.5	M-Neoplasm, Lip NOS, inner NOS
140.6	M-Neoplasm, lip, commissure
140.8	M-Neoplasm, Lip NEC
140.9	M-Neoplasm, Lip/vermilion NOS
171.0	M-Neoplasm, Soft tissue, head
172.0	Malignant melanoma, Lip
172.1	Malignant melanoma, eyelid/canthus
172.2	Malignant melanoma, Ear
172.3	Malignant melanoma, Face NEC/NOS
172.8	Malignant melanoma, Skin NEC
173.0	M-Neoplasm, Skin of lip
173.1	M-Neoplasm, Skin of eyelid/canthus
173.2	M-Neoplasm, Skin of ear
173.3	M-Neoplasm, Skin of face NEC
195.0	M-Neoplasm, Head/face/neck
216.0	B-Neoplasm, Skin of lip
216.1	B-Neoplasm, Skin of eyelid/canthus
216.2	B-Neoplasm, Skin of ear
216.3	B-Neoplasm, Skin of face NEC
232.0	CA in situ, Skin of lip
232.1	CA in situ, Eyelid/canthus
232.2	CA in situ, Skin of ear
232.3	CA in situ, Skin of face NEC
239.2	Bone/Skin neoplasm NOS
374.01	Senile entropion
374.05	Trichiasis w/o entropion
374.10	Ectropion NOS
374.14	Cicatricial ectropion
374.22	Mechanical lagophthalmos
374.23	Cicatricial lagophthalmos
374.41	Eyelid retraction or lag
374.84	Cysts of eyelids
709.2	Scar/fibrosis of skin
709.9	Skin disorder NOS
744.23	Microtia
744.3	Ear anomaly NOS
870.0	Laceration eyelid skin/periocular
872.01	Open wound of auricle
872.11	Open wound of auricle, complicated
873.21	Open wound of nasal septum
873.31	Open wound nasal septum, complic
873.43	Open wound of lip
873.53	Open wound of lip, complicated
906.0	Late effect, open wound head/trunk
906.2	Late effect of superficial injury
906.4	Late effect of crushing
906.5	Late effect of head/neck burn
918.0	Superficial injury periocular
940.0	Chemical burn, eyelid/periocular
940.1	Burn, eyelid/periocular area NEC
941.22	Blisters, epidermal loss, eye
941.31	3rd deg burn, ear
941.32	3rd degree burn, eye

CPT CODE	SERVICE	ICD–9–CM
15260 (Cont'd.)		

941.33 3rd deg burn, lip
941.34 3rd deg burn, chin
941.35 3rd deg burn, nose
941.41 Deep 3rd deg burn, ear
941.42 Deep 3rd degree burn, eye
941.43 Deep 3rd deg burn, lip
941.44 Deep 3rd deg burn, chin
941.45 Deep 3rd deg burn, nose
941.51 Deep 3rd deg loss, ear
941.52 Deep 3rd degree loss, eye
941.53 Deep 3rd deg loss, lip
941.54 Deep 3rd deg loss, chin
941.55 Deep 3rd deg loss, nose
V10.02 Hx of oral/pharynx malignancy NEC
V10.82 Hx of malignant skin melanoma
V10.83 Hx of skin malignancy NEC

REIMBURSEMENT INFORMATION

General

- See notes on page 114.

Medicare

- Follow–Up Days — 90
- Assistant Surgeon — not paid
- Supply Charges — not allowed
- Outpatient Limit — does not apply
- Major Surgery Rules Apply

CPT CODE	SERVICE
15261	Full thickness graft, free, including direct closure of donor site, nose, ears, eyelids, and/or lips; each additional 20 sq cm

CPT NOTES

- ♦ Identify by size and location of the defect (recipient area) and the type of graft; includes simple debridement of granulations or recent avulsion.
- ♦ When a primary procedure such as orbitectomy, radical mastectomy, or deep tumor removal requires skin graft for definitive closure, see appropriate anatomical subsection for primary procedure and this section for skin graft.
- ♦ Repair of donor site requiring skin graft or local flaps is to be added as an additional procedure.
- ♦ For eyelids, see also 67961 et seq.
- ♦ Repair of donor site requiring skin graft or local flaps, to be added as additional separate procedure.

ICD–9–CM

140.0	M-Neoplasm, Upper lip, vermilion
140.1	M-Neoplasm, Lower lip, vermilion
140.3	M-Neoplasm, Upper lip, inner aspect
140.4	M-Neoplasm, Lower lip, inner aspect
140.5	M-Neoplasm, Lip NOS, inner NOS
140.6	M-Neoplasm, lip, commissure
140.8	M-Neoplasm, Lip NEC
140.9	M-Neoplasm, Lip/vermilion NOS
171.0	M-Neoplasm, Soft tissue, head
172.0	Malignant melanoma, Lip
172.1	Malignant melanoma, eyelid/canthus
172.2	Malignant melanoma, Ear
172.3	Malignant melanoma, Face NEC/NOS
172.8	Malignant melanoma, Skin NEC
173.0	M-Neoplasm, Skin of lip
173.1	M-Neoplasm, Skin of eyelid/canthus
173.2	M-Neoplasm, Skin of ear
173.3	M-Neoplasm, Skin of face NEC
195.0	M-Neoplasm, Head/face/neck
216.0	B-Neoplasm, Skin of lip
216.1	B-Neoplasm, Skin of eyelid/canthus
216.2	B-Neoplasm, Skin of ear
216.3	B-Neoplasm, Skin of face NEC
232.0	CA in situ, Skin of lip
232.1	CA in situ, Eyelid/canthus
232.2	CA in situ, Skin of ear
232.3	CA in situ, Skin of face NEC
239.2	Bone/Skin neoplasm NOS
709.2	Scar/fibrosis of skin
744.23	Microtia
744.3	Ear anomaly NOS
870.0	Laceration eyelid skin/periocular
872.01	Open wound of auricle
872.11	Open wound of auricle, complicated
873.21	Open wound of nasal septum
873.31	Open wound nasal septum, complic
873.43	Open wound of lip
873.53	Open wound of lip, complicated
906.0	Late effect, open wound head/trunk
906.2	Late effect of superficial injury
906.4	Late effect of crushing
906.5	Late effect of head/neck burn
940.0	Chemical burn, eyelid/periocular
940.1	Burn, eyelid/periocular area NEC
941.22	Blisters, epidermal loss, eye
941.31	3rd deg burn, ear
941.32	3rd degree burn, eye
941.33	3rd deg burn, lip
941.34	3rd deg burn, chin
941.35	3rd deg burn, nose
941.41	Deep 3rd deg burn, ear
941.42	Deep 3rd degree burn, eye
941.43	Deep 3rd deg burn, lip
941.44	Deep 3rd deg burn, chin
941.45	Deep 3rd deg burn, nose
941.51	Deep 3rd deg loss, ear
941.52	Deep 3rd degree loss, eye

CPT CODE	SERVICE	ICD–9–CM
15261 (Cont'd.)		

941.53	Deep 3rd deg loss, lip
941.54	Deep 3rd deg loss, chin
941.55	Deep 3rd deg loss, nose
V10.02	Hx of oral/pharynx malignancy NEC
V10.82	Hx of malignant skin melanoma
V10.83	Hx of skin malignancy NEC

REIMBURSEMENT INFORMATION

General

- ♦ See notes on page 114.

Medicare

- ♦ Follow–Up Days — none; falls within global period of another procedure
- ♦ Assistant Surgeon — not paid
- ♦ Supply Charges — not allowed
- ♦ Outpatient Limit — does not apply

CPT CODE **SERVICE**

15350 Application of allograft (homograft), skin

CPT NOTES

- Identify by size and location of the defect (recipient area) and the type of graft; includes simple debridement of granulations or recent avulsion.
- When a primary procedure such as orbitectomy, radical mastectomy, or deep tumor removal requires skin graft for definitive closure, see appropriate anatomical subsection for primary procedure and this section for skin graft.
- Repair of donor site requiring skin graft or local flaps is to be added as an additional procedure.

ICD–9–CM

172.x	Skin Melanoma
173.x	Malignant neoplasm, Skin
216.x	Benign neoplasm, Skin
232.x	Carcinoma in situ, Skin
701.4	Keloid scar
707.1	Chronic ulcer of the leg
870.0	Laceration eyelid skin/periocular
873.30	Open wound of nose NOS, complicated
873.39	Multiple open nose wounds, complic
873.4x	Face, open wound
873.5x	Face, complicated open wound
875.0	Open wound of chest
875.1	Open wound of chest, complicated
876.0	Open wound of back
876.1	Open wound of back, complicated
877.0	Open wound of buttock
877.1	Open wound of buttock, complicated
879.0	Open wound of breast
879.1	Open wound of breast, complicated
879.2	Open wound of anterior abdomen
879.3	Open wound anterior abdomen, compl
879.4	Open wound of lateral abdomen
879.5	Open wound lateral abdomen, compl
880.00	Open wound of shoulder
880.01	Open wound of scapula
880.02	Open wound of axilla
880.03	Open wound of upper arm
880.09	Multiple open wounds of shoulder
880.10	Open wound of shoulder, complicated
880.11	Open wound of scapula, complicated
880.12	Open wound of axilla, complicated
880.13	Open wound of upper arm, complic
880.19	Mult open wounds of shoulder, compl
881.0x	Elbow/forearm/wrist open wound
881.1x	Elbow/forearm/wrist complex wound
882.0	Open wound of hand
882.1	Open wound of hand, complicated
883.0	Open wound of finger
883.1	Open wound of finger, complicated
884.0	Open wound of arm, mult/NOS
884.1	Open wound of arm mult/NOS, compl
885.x	Traumatic amputation of thumb
886.x	Traumatic finger amputation
887.x	Traumatic arm/hand amputation
890.x	Open wound of hip and thigh
891.x	Open wound of knee, leg, ankle
892.x	Open wound of foot
893.x	Open wound of toe(s)
894.x	Open wound of lower limb
895.x	Traumatic amputation of toe(s)
896.x	Traumatic amputation of foot
897.x	Traumatic amputation of leg(s)
906.5	Late effect of head/neck burn
906.6	Late effect of wrist/hand burn
906.7	Late effect of extremity burn NEC
941.31	3rd deg burn, ear
941.32	3rd degree burn, eye

CPT CODE	SERVICE	ICD-9-CM
15350 (Cont'd.)		941.33 3rd deg burn, lip
		941.34 3rd deg burn, chin
		941.35 3rd deg burn, nose
		941.36 3rd deg burn, scalp
		941.37 3rd deg burn, face NEC
		941.38 3rd deg burn, neck
		942.31 3rd deg burn trunk, breast
		942.32 3rd deg burn trunk, chest wall
		942.33 3rd deg burn trunk, abdominal wall
		942.34 3rd deg burn trunk, back
		942.35 3rd deg burn trunk, genitalia
		943.31 3rd deg burn, forearm
		943.32 3rd deg burn, elbow
		943.33 3rd deg burn, upper arm
		943.34 3rd deg burn, axilla
		943.35 3rd deg burn, shoulder
		943.36 3rd deg burn, scapula
		943.39 3rd deg burn, arm multiple sites
		944.31 3rd deg burn, finger
		944.32 3rd deg burn, thumb
		944.33 3rd deg burn, mult fingers
		944.34 3rd deg burn, finger w/thumb
		944.35 3rd deg burn, palm
		944.36 3rd deg burn, back of hand
		944.37 3rd deg burn, wrist
		945.31 3rd deg burn, toe
		945.32 3rd deg burn, foot
		945.33 3rd deg burn, ankle
		945.34 3rd deg burn, lower leg
		945.35 3rd deg burn, knee
		945.36 3rd deg burn, thigh
		945.39 3rd deg burn, leg mult sites

REIMBURSEMENT INFORMATION

General

- See notes on page 114.

Medicare

- Follow–Up Days — 90
- Assistant Surgeon — not paid
- Supply Charges — not allowed
- Outpatient Limit — does not apply
- Major Surgery Rules Apply

CPT CODE	SERVICE
15400	Application of xenograft (heterograft), skin

CPT NOTES

- Identify by size and location of the defect (recipient area) and the type of graft; includes simple debridement of granulations or recent avulsion.
- When a primary procedure such as orbitectomy, radical mastectomy, or deep tumor removal requires skin graft for definitive closure, see appropriate anatomical subsection for primary procedure and this section for skin graft.
- Repair of donor site requiring skin graft or local flaps is to be added as an additional procedure.

ICD–9–CM

172.x	Skin Melanoma
173.x	Malignant neoplasm, Skin
216.x	Benign neoplasm, Skin
232.x	Carcinoma in situ, Skin
701.4	Keloid scar
707.1	Chronic ulcer of the leg
870.0	Laceration eyelid skin/periocular
873.30	Open wound of nose NOS, complicated
873.39	Multiple open nose wounds, complic
873.4x	Face, open wound
873.5x	Face, complicated open wound
875.0	Open wound of chest
875.1	Open wound of chest, complicated
876.0	Open wound of back
876.1	Open wound of back, complicated
877.0	Open wound of buttock
877.1	Open wound of buttock, complicated
879.0	Open wound of breast
879.1	Open wound of breast, complicated
879.2	Open wound of anterior abdomen
879.3	Open wound anterior abdomen, compl
879.4	Open wound of lateral abdomen
879.5	Open wound lateral abdomen, compl
880.00	Open wound of shoulder
880.01	Open wound of scapula
880.02	Open wound of axilla
880.03	Open wound of upper arm
880.09	Multiple open wounds of shoulder
880.10	Open wound of shoulder, complicated
880.11	Open wound of scapula, complicated
880.12	Open wound of axilla, complicated
880.13	Open wound of upper arm, complic
880.19	Mult open wounds of shoulder, compl
881.0x	Elbow/forearm/wrist open wound
881.1x	Elbow/forearm/wrist complex wound
882.0	Open wound of hand
882.1	Open wound of hand, complicated
883.0	Open wound of finger
883.1	Open wound of finger, complicated
884.0	Open wound of arm, mult/NOS
884.1	Open wound of arm mult/NOS, compl
885.x	Traumatic amputation of thumb
886.x	Traumatic finger amputation
887.x	Traumatic arm/hand amputation
890.x	Open wound of hip and thigh
891.x	Open wound of knee, leg, ankle
892.x	Open wound of foot
893.x	Open wound of toe(s)
894.x	Open wound of lower limb
895.x	Traumatic amputation of toe(s)
896.x	Traumatic amputation of foot
897.x	Traumatic amputation of leg(s)
906.5	Late effect of head/neck burn
906.6	Late effect of wrist/hand burn
906.7	Late effect of extremity burn NEC
941.31	3rd deg burn, ear
941.32	3rd degree burn, eye

CPT CODE	SERVICE	ICD–9–CM
15400 (Cont'd.)		941.33 3rd deg burn, lip
		941.34 3rd deg burn, chin
		941.35 3rd deg burn, nose
		941.36 3rd deg burn, scalp
		941.37 3rd deg burn, face NEC
		941.38 3rd deg burn, neck
		942.31 3rd deg burn trunk, breast
		942.32 3rd deg burn trunk, chest wall
		942.33 3rd deg burn trunk, abdominal wall
		942.34 3rd deg burn trunk, back
		942.35 3rd deg burn trunk, genitalia
		943.31 3rd deg burn, forearm
		943.32 3rd deg burn, elbow
		943.33 3rd deg burn, upper arm
		943.34 3rd deg burn, axilla
		943.35 3rd deg burn, shoulder
		943.36 3rd deg burn, scapula
		943.39 3rd deg burn, arm multiple sites
		944.31 3rd deg burn, finger
		944.32 3rd deg burn, thumb
		944.33 3rd deg burn, mult fingers
		944.34 3rd deg burn, finger w/thumb
		944.35 3rd deg burn, palm
		944.36 3rd deg burn, back of hand
		944.37 3rd deg burn, wrist
		945.31 3rd deg burn, toe
		945.32 3rd deg burn, foot
		945.33 3rd deg burn, ankle
		945.34 3rd deg burn, lower leg
		945.35 3rd deg burn, knee
		945.36 3rd deg burn, thigh
		945.39 3rd deg burn, leg mult sites

REIMBURSEMENT INFORMATION

General

- See notes on page 114.

Medicare

- Follow–Up Days — 90
- Assistant Surgeon — not paid
- Supply Charges — not allowed
- Outpatient Limit — does not apply
- Major Surgery Rules Apply

CPT CODE	SERVICE
15570	Formation of direct or tubed pedicle, with or without transfer; trunk

CPT NOTES

- Regions listed refer to recipient area (not donor site) when flap is being attached in transfer or to final site.
- Regions listed refer to donor site when tube is formed for later or when "delay" of flap is prior to transfer.
- Procedures 15570-15738 do not include extensive immobilization (e.g., large plaster casts and other immobilizing devices are considered additional separate procedures).
- Repair of donor site requiring skin graft or local flap is considered an additional separate procedure.

ICD–9–CM

172.5	Malignant melanoma, Trunk
173.5	M-Neoplasm, Skin of trunk
216.5	B-Neoplasm, Skin of trunk
232.5	CA in situ, Skin of trunk
707.0	Decubitus ulcer
707.8	Chronic skin ulcer NEC
875.0	Open wound of chest
875.1	Open wound of chest, complicated
876.0	Open wound of back
876.1	Open wound of back, complicated
877.0	Open wound of buttock
877.1	Open wound of buttock, complicated
879.0	Open wound of breast
879.1	Open wound of breast, complicated
879.2	Open wound of anterior abdomen
879.3	Open wound anterior abdomen, compl
879.4	Open wound of lateral abdomen
879.5	Open wound lateral abdomen, compl
879.7	Open wound of trunk NEC, complic
879.8	Open wound site NOS
879.9	Open wound site NOS, complicated
880.00	Open wound of shoulder
880.01	Open wound of scapula
880.02	Open wound of axilla
906.0	Late effect, open wound head/trunk
906.8	Late effect of burns NEC
942.31	3rd deg burn trunk, breast
942.32	3rd deg burn trunk, chest wall
942.33	3rd deg burn trunk, abdominal wall
942.34	3rd deg burn trunk, back
942.35	3rd deg burn trunk, genitalia
942.41	Deep 3rd deg burn trunk, breast
942.42	Deep 3rd deg burn trunk, chest wall
942.43	Deep 3rd deg burn trunk, abdominal
942.44	Deep 3rd deg burn trunk, back
942.45	Deep 3rd deg burn trunk, genitalia
942.51	Deep 3rd deg loss trunk, breast
942.52	Deep 3rd deg loss trunk, chest wall
942.53	Deep 3rd deg loss trunk, abdominal
942.54	Deep 3rd deg loss trunk, back
942.55	Deep 3rd deg loss trunk, genitalia
998.3	Postop wound disruption
V10.3	Hx of breast malignancy
V10.82	Hx of malignant skin melanoma
V10.83	Hx of skin malignancy NEC
V50.1	Plastic surgery NEC
V51.	Aftercare w/plastic surgery

CPT CODE **SERVICE**

15570 (Cont'd.)

ICD–9–CM

REIMBURSEMENT INFORMATION

General

- See notes on page 114.

Medicare

- Follow–Up Days — 90
- Assistant Surgeon — not paid
- Supply Charges — not allowed
- Outpatient Limit — does not apply
- Major Surgery Rules Apply

CPT CODE	SERVICE
15572	Formation of direct or tubed pedicle, with or without transfer; scalp, arms, or legs

CPT NOTES

- Regions listed refer to recipient area (not donor site) when flap is being attached in transfer or to final site.
- Regions listed refer to donor site when tube is formed for later or when "delay" of flap is prior to transfer.
- Procedures 15570-15738 do not include extensive immobilization (e.g., large plaster casts and other immobilizing devices are considered additional separate procedures).
- Repair of donor site requiring skin graft or local flap is considered an additional separate procedure.

ICD-9-CM

172.4	Malignant melanoma, Scalp/neck
172.6	Malignant melanoma, Arm
172.7	Malignant melanoma, Leg
173.4	M-Neoplasm, Scalp/skin neck
173.6	M-Neoplasm, Skin of arm
173.7	M-Neoplasm, Skin of leg
216.4	B-Neoplasm, Scalp/skin of neck
216.6	B-Neoplasm, Skin of arm
216.7	B-Neoplasm, Skin of leg
232.4	CA in situ, Scalp/skin of neck
232.6	CA in situ, Skin of arm
232.7	CA in situ, Skin of leg
707.1	Chronic ulcer of the leg
873.0	Open wound of scalp
873.1	Open wound of scalp, complicated
880.00	Open wound of shoulder
880.01	Open wound of scapula
880.03	Open wound of upper arm
880.09	Multiple open wounds of shoulder
880.10	Open wound of shoulder, complicated
880.11	Open wound of scapula, complicated
880.13	Open wound of upper arm, complic
880.19	Mult open wounds of shoulder, compl
880.20	Open wound shoulder w/tendon
880.23	Open wound upper arm w/tendon
880.29	Mult open wound shoulder w/tendon
881.0x	Elbow/forearm/wrist open wound
881.1x	Elbow/forearm/wrist complex wound
884.0	Open wound of arm, mult/NOS
884.1	Open wound of arm mult/NOS, compl
887.x	Traumatic arm/hand amputation
890.0	Open wound of hip/thigh
890.1	Open wound of hip/thigh, complic
891.0	Open wound of knee/leg/ankle
891.1	Open wound of knee/leg/ankle, compl
894.0	Open wound of leg NEC
894.1	Open wound of leg NEC, complicated
896.x	Traumatic amputation of foot
897.x	Traumatic amputation of leg(s)
906.1	Late effect, open wound extremity
906.2	Late effect of superficial injury
906.3	Late effect of contusion
906.4	Late effect of crushing
906.6	Late effect of wrist/hand burn
906.7	Late effect of extremity burn NEC
943.31	3rd deg burn, forearm
943.32	3rd deg burn, elbow
943.33	3rd deg burn, upper arm
943.34	3rd deg burn, axilla
943.35	3rd deg burn, shoulder
943.36	3rd deg burn, scapula
943.39	3rd deg burn, arm multiple sites
943.41	Deep 3rd deg burn, forearm
943.42	Deep 3rd deg burn, elbow
943.43	Deep 3rd deg burn, upper arm
943.44	Deep 3rd deg burn, axilla

CPT CODE	SERVICE	ICD-9-CM	
15572 (Cont'd.)		943.45	Deep 3rd deg burn, shoulder
		943.46	Deep 3rd deg burn, scapula
		943.49	Deep 3rd deg burn, arm mult sites
		943.51	Deep 3rd deg loss, forearm
		943.52	Deep 3rd deg loss, elbow
		943.53	Deep 3rd deg loss, upper arm
		943.54	Deep 3rd deg loss, axilla
		943.55	Deep 3rd deg loss, shoulder
		943.56	Deep 3rd deg loss, scapula
		943.59	Deep 3rd deg loss, arm mult sites
		944.31	3rd deg burn, finger
		944.32	3rd deg burn, thumb
		944.33	3rd deg burn, mult fingers
		944.34	3rd deg burn, finger w/thumb
		944.35	3rd deg burn, palm
		944.36	3rd deg burn, back of hand
		944.37	3rd deg burn, wrist
		944.41	Deep 3rd deg burn, finger
		944.42	Deep 3rd deg burn, thumb
		944.43	Deep 3rd deg burn, mult fingers
		944.44	Deep 3rd deg burn, finger w/thumb
		944.45	Deep 3rd deg burn, palm
		944.46	Deep 3rd deg burn, back of hand
		944.47	Deep 3rd deg burn, wrist
		944.51	Deep 3rd deg loss, finger
		944.52	Deep 3rd deg loss, thumb
		944.53	Deep 3rd deg loss, mult fingers
		944.54	Deep 3rd deg loss, finger w/thumb
		944.55	Deep 3rd deg loss, palm
		944.56	Deep 3rd deg loss, back of hand
		944.57	Deep 3rd deg loss, wrist
		945.31	3rd deg burn, toe
		945.32	3rd deg burn, foot
		945.33	3rd deg burn, ankle
		945.34	3rd deg burn, lower leg
		945.35	3rd deg burn, knee
		945.36	3rd deg burn, thigh
		945.39	3rd deg burn, leg mult sites
		945.41	Deep 3rd deg burn, toe
		945.42	Deep 3rd deg burn, foot
		945.43	Deep 3rd deg burn, ankle
		945.44	Deep 3rd deg burn, lower leg
		945.45	Deep 3rd deg burn, knee
		945.46	Deep 3rd deg burn, thigh
		945.49	Deep 3rd deg burn, leg mult sites
		945.51	Deep 3rd deg loss, toe
		945.52	Deep 3rd deg loss, foot
		945.53	Deep 3rd deg loss, ankle
		945.54	Deep 3rd deg loss, lower leg
		945.55	Deep 3rd deg loss, knee
		945.56	Deep 3rd deg loss, thigh
		945.59	Deep 3rd deg loss, leg mult sites
		V10.82	Hx of malignant skin melanoma
		V10.83	Hx of skin malignancy NEC
		V50.1	Plastic surgery NEC

CPT CODE	SERVICE	ICD–9–CM
15572 (Cont'd.)		V51. Aftercare w/plastic surgery

REIMBURSEMENT INFORMATION

General

- ♦ See notes on page 114.

Medicare

- ♦ Follow–Up Days — 90
- ♦ Assistant Surgeon — not paid
- ♦ Supply Charges — not allowed
- ♦ Outpatient Limit — does not apply
- ♦ Major Surgery Rules Apply

CPT CODE	SERVICE
15574	Formation of direct or tubed pedicle, with or without transfer; forehead, cheeks, chin, mouth, neck, axillae, genitalia, hands, or feet

CPT NOTES

- ♦ Regions listed refer to recipient area (not donor site) when flap is being attached in transfer or to final site.
- ♦ Regions listed refer to donor site when tube is formed for later or when "delay" of flap is prior to transfer.
- ♦ Procedures 15570-15738 do not include extensive immobilization (e.g., large plaster casts and other immobilizing devices are considered additional separate procedures).
- ♦ Repair of donor site requiring skin graft or local flap is considered an additional separate procedure.

ICD-9-CM

144.9	M-Neoplasm, Floor of mouth NOS
172.3	Malignant melanoma, Face NEC/NOS
172.4	Malignant melanoma, Scalp/neck
173.3	M-Neoplasm, Skin of face NEC
173.4	M-Neoplasm, Scalp/skin neck
216.3	B-Neoplasm, Skin of face NEC
216.4	B-Neoplasm, Scalp/skin of neck
523.4	Chronic periodontitis
526.8	Jaw disease
526.89	Jaw disease NEC
526.9	Jaw disease NOS
873.41	Open wound of cheek
873.42	Open wound of forehead
873.49	Open wound of face NEC
873.51	Open wound of cheek, complicated
873.52	Open wound of forehead, complicated
873.59	Open wound of face NEC, complicated
873.60	Open wound of mouth NOS
878.0	Open wound of penis
878.1	Open wound of penis, complicated
878.2	Open wound of scrotum/testes
878.3	Open wound, scrotum/testes, compl
878.4	Open wound of vulva
878.5	Open wound of vulva, complicated
878.6	Open wound of vagina
878.7	Open wound of vagina, complicated
880.02	Open wound of axilla
880.12	Open wound of axilla, complicated
882.0	Open wound of hand
882.1	Open wound of hand, complicated
883.0	Open wound of finger
883.1	Open wound of finger, complicated
885.x	Traumatic amputation of thumb
886.x	Traumatic finger amputation
887.x	Traumatic arm/hand amputation
892.x	Open wound of foot
893.x	Open wound of toe(s)
895.x	Traumatic amputation of toe(s)
896.x	Traumatic amputation of foot
941.34	3rd deg burn, chin
941.37	3rd deg burn, face NEC
941.38	3rd deg burn, neck
941.44	Deep 3rd deg burn, chin
941.47	Deep 3rd deg burn, face NEC
941.48	Deep 3rd deg burn, neck
941.54	Deep 3rd deg loss, chin
941.57	Deep 3rd deg loss, face NEC
941.58	Deep 3rd deg loss, neck
942.35	3rd deg burn trunk, genitalia
942.45	Deep 3rd deg burn trunk, genitalia
942.55	Deep 3rd deg loss trunk, genitalia
943.35	3rd deg burn, shoulder
943.45	Deep 3rd deg burn, shoulder
943.55	Deep 3rd deg loss, shoulder
944.31	3rd deg burn, finger
944.32	3rd deg burn, thumb

CPT CODE	SERVICE	ICD-9-CM
15574 (Cont'd.)		
		944.33 3rd deg burn, mult fingers
		944.34 3rd deg burn, finger w/thumb
		944.35 3rd deg burn, palm
		944.36 3rd deg burn, back of hand
		944.37 3rd deg burn, wrist
		944.41 Deep 3rd deg burn, finger
		944.42 Deep 3rd deg burn, thumb
		944.43 Deep 3rd deg burn, mult fingers
		944.44 Deep 3rd deg burn, finger w/thumb
		944.45 Deep 3rd deg burn, palm
		944.46 Deep 3rd deg burn, back of hand
		944.47 Deep 3rd deg burn, wrist
		944.51 Deep 3rd deg loss, finger
		944.52 Deep 3rd deg loss, thumb
		944.53 Deep 3rd deg loss, mult fingers
		944.54 Deep 3rd deg loss, finger w/thumb
		944.55 Deep 3rd deg loss, palm
		944.56 Deep 3rd deg loss, back of hand
		944.57 Deep 3rd deg loss, wrist
		945.31 3rd deg burn, toe
		945.32 3rd deg burn, foot
		945.41 Deep 3rd deg burn, toe
		945.42 Deep 3rd deg burn, foot
		945.51 Deep 3rd deg loss, toe
		945.52 Deep 3rd deg loss, foot
		V10.02 Hx of oral/pharynx malignancy NEC
		V10.82 Hx of malignant skin melanoma
		V10.83 Hx of skin malignancy NEC

REIMBURSEMENT INFORMATION

General

- ◆ See notes on page 114.

Medicare

- ◆ Follow–Up Days — 90
- ◆ Assistant Surgeon — not paid
- ◆ Supply Charges — not allowed
- ◆ Outpatient Limit — does not apply
- ◆ Major Surgery Rules Apply

CPT CODE	SERVICE
15576	Formation of direct or tubed pedicle, with or without transfer; eyelids, nose, ears, lips, or intraoral

CPT NOTES

- Regions listed refer to recipient area (not donor site) when flap is being attached in transfer or to final site.
- Regions listed refer to donor site when tube is formed for later or when "delay" of flap is prior to transfer.
- Procedures 15570-15738 do not include extensive immobilization (e.g., large plaster casts and other immobilizing devices are considered additional separate procedures).
- Repair of donor site requiring skin graft or local flap is considered an additional separate procedure.

ICD–9–CM

140.0	M-Neoplasm, Upper lip, vermilion
140.1	M-Neoplasm, Lower lip, vermilion
140.3	M-Neoplasm, Upper lip, inner aspect
140.4	M-Neoplasm, Lower lip, inner aspect
140.5	M-Neoplasm, Lip NOS, inner NOS
140.6	M-Neoplasm, lip, commissure
140.8	M-Neoplasm, Lip NEC
140.9	M-Neoplasm, Lip/vermilion NOS
171.0	M-Neoplasm, Soft tissue, head
172.0	Malignant melanoma, Lip
172.1	Malignant melanoma, eyelid/canthus
172.2	Malignant melanoma, Ear
172.3	Malignant melanoma, Face NEC/NOS
173.0	M-Neoplasm, Skin of lip
173.1	M-Neoplasm, Skin of eyelid/canthus
173.2	M-Neoplasm, Skin of ear
173.3	M-Neoplasm, Skin of face NEC
195.0	M-Neoplasm, Head/face/neck
216.0	B-Neoplasm, Skin of lip
216.1	B-Neoplasm, Skin of eyelid/canthus
216.2	B-Neoplasm, Skin of ear
216.3	B-Neoplasm, Skin of face NEC
232.0	CA in situ, Skin of lip
232.1	CA in situ, Eyelid/canthus
232.2	CA in situ, Skin of ear
232.3	CA in situ, Skin of face NEC
709.2	Scar/fibrosis of skin
744.23	Microtia
744.3	Ear anomaly NOS
870.0	Laceration eyelid skin/periocular
872.01	Open wound of auricle
872.11	Open wound of auricle, complicated
873.21	Open wound of nasal septum
873.31	Open wound nasal septum, complic
873.43	Open wound of lip
873.53	Open wound of lip, complicated
940.0	Chemical burn, eyelid/periocular
940.1	Burn, eyelid/periocular area NEC
941.22	Blisters, epidermal loss, eye
941.31	3rd deg burn, ear
941.32	3rd degree burn, eye
941.33	3rd deg burn, lip
941.34	3rd deg burn, chin
941.35	3rd deg burn, nose
941.41	Deep 3rd deg burn, ear
941.42	Deep 3rd degree burn, eye
941.43	Deep 3rd deg burn, lip
941.44	Deep 3rd deg burn, chin
941.45	Deep 3rd deg burn, nose
941.51	Deep 3rd deg loss, ear
941.52	Deep 3rd degree loss, eye
941.53	Deep 3rd deg loss, lip
941.54	Deep 3rd deg loss, chin
941.55	Deep 3rd deg loss, nose

CPT CODE	SERVICE	ICD-9-CM

15576 (Cont'd.)

REIMBURSEMENT INFORMATION

General

- See notes on page 114.

Medicare

- Follow-Up Days — 90
- Assistant Surgeon — not paid
- Supply Charges — not allowed
- Outpatient Limit — does not apply
- Major Surgery Rules Apply

15580 Cross finger flap, including free graft to donor site

CPT NOTES

- For major debridement or excisional preparation of recipient area at the time of attachment of pedicle flap, see 15570-15576.
- Regions listed refer to recipient area (not donor site) when flap is being attached in transfer or to final site.
- Regions listed refer to donor site when tube is formed for later or when "delay" of flap is prior to transfer.
- Procedures 15570-15738 do not include extensive immobilization (e.g., large plaster casts and other immobilizing devices are considered additional separate procedures).
- Repair of donor site requiring skin graft or local flap is considered an additional separate procedure.

882.0	Open wound of hand
882.1	Open wound of hand, complicated
883.0	Open wound of finger
883.1	Open wound of finger, complicated
885.x	Traumatic amputation of thumb
886.x	Traumatic finger amputation
893.0	Open wound of toe
893.1	Open wound of toe, complicated
895.x	Traumatic amputation of toe(s)
927.3	Crushing injury, finger
928.3	Crushing injury, toe
944.31	3rd deg burn, finger
944.32	3rd deg burn, thumb
944.33	3rd deg burn, mult fingers
944.34	3rd deg burn, finger w/thumb
944.41	Deep 3rd deg burn, finger
944.42	Deep 3rd deg burn, thumb
944.43	Deep 3rd deg burn, mult fingers
944.44	Deep 3rd deg burn, finger w/thumb
944.51	Deep 3rd deg loss, finger
944.52	Deep 3rd deg loss, thumb
944.53	Deep 3rd deg loss, mult fingers
944.54	Deep 3rd deg loss, finger w/thumb
V50.1	Plastic surgery NEC
V51.	Aftercare w/plastic surgery

REIMBURSEMENT INFORMATION

General

- See notes on page 114.

Medicare

- Follow-Up Days — 90
- Assistant Surgeon — not paid
- Supply Charges — not allowed
- Outpatient Limit — does not apply
- Major Surgery Rules Apply

CPT CODE	SERVICE
15600	Delay of flap or sectioning of flap (division and inset); at trunk

CPT NOTES

- ♦ Regions listed refer to recipient area (not donor site) when flap is being attached in transfer or to final site.
- ♦ Regions listed refer to donor site when tube is formed for later or when "delay" of flap is prior to transfer.
- ♦ Procedures 15570-15738 do not include extensive immobilization (e.g., large plaster casts and other immobilizing devices are considered additional separate procedures).
- ♦ Repair of donor site requiring skin graft or local flap is considered an additional separate procedure.

ICD-9-CM

172.5	Malignant melanoma, Trunk
173.5	M-Neoplasm, Skin of trunk
216.5	B-Neoplasm, Skin of trunk
232.5	CA in situ, Skin of trunk
611.8	Absence of breast, acquired
707.0	Decubitus ulcer
707.8	Chronic skin ulcer NEC
738.3	Acquired chest/rib deformity
738.9	Acquired deformity NOS
875.0	Open wound of chest
875.1	Open wound of chest, complicated
876.0	Open wound of back
876.1	Open wound of back, complicated
877.0	Open wound of buttock
877.1	Open wound of buttock, complicated
879.0	Open wound of breast
879.1	Open wound of breast, complicated
879.2	Open wound of anterior abdomen
879.3	Open wound anterior abdomen, compl
879.4	Open wound of lateral abdomen
879.5	Open wound lateral abdomen, compl
942.31	3rd deg burn trunk, breast
942.32	3rd deg burn trunk, chest wall
942.33	3rd deg burn trunk, abdominal wall
942.34	3rd deg burn trunk, back
942.35	3rd deg burn trunk, genitalia
942.41	Deep 3rd deg burn trunk, breast
942.42	Deep 3rd deg burn trunk, chest wall
942.43	Deep 3rd deg burn trunk, abdominal
942.44	Deep 3rd deg burn trunk, back
942.45	Deep 3rd deg burn trunk, genitalia
942.51	Deep 3rd deg loss trunk, breast
942.52	Deep 3rd deg loss trunk, chest wall
942.53	Deep 3rd deg loss trunk, abdominal
942.54	Deep 3rd deg loss trunk, back
942.55	Deep 3rd deg loss trunk, genitalia
V50.1	Plastic surgery NEC
V51.	Aftercare w/plastic surgery

REIMBURSEMENT INFORMATION

General

- ♦ See notes on page 114.

Medicare

- ♦ Follow-Up Days — 90
- ♦ Assistant Surgeon — not paid
- ♦ Supply Charges — not allowed
- ♦ Outpatient Limit — does not apply
- ♦ Major Surgery Rules Apply

CPT CODE	SERVICE
15610	Delay of flap or sectioning of flap (division and inset); at scalp, arms or legs

CPT NOTES

- ♦ Regions listed refer to recipient area (not donor site) when flap is being attached in transfer or to final site.
- ♦ Regions listed refer to donor site when tube is formed for later or when "delay" of flap is prior to transfer.
- ♦ Procedures 15570-15738 do not include extensive immobilization (e.g., large plaster casts and other immobilizing devices are considered additional separate procedures).
- ♦ Repair of donor site requiring skin graft or local flap is considered an additional separate procedure.

ICD–9–CM

172.4	Malignant melanoma, Scalp/neck
172.6	Malignant melanoma, Arm
172.7	Malignant melanoma, Leg
173.4	M-Neoplasm, Scalp/skin neck
173.6	M-Neoplasm, Skin of arm
173.7	M-Neoplasm, Skin of leg
216.4	B-Neoplasm, Scalp/skin of neck
216.6	B-Neoplasm, Skin of arm
216.7	B-Neoplasm, Skin of leg
232.4	CA in situ, Scalp/skin of neck
232.6	CA in situ, Skin of arm
232.7	CA in situ, Skin of leg
707.1	Chronic ulcer of the leg
736.89	Other acquired limb deformity
738.10	Acquired head deformity NOS
873.0	Open wound of scalp
873.1	Open wound of scalp, complicated
880.00	Open wound of shoulder
880.01	Open wound of scapula
880.03	Open wound of upper arm
880.09	Multiple open wounds of shoulder
880.10	Open wound of shoulder, complicated
880.11	Open wound of scapula, complicated
880.13	Open wound of upper arm, complic
880.19	Mult open wounds of shoulder, compl
881.0x	Elbow/forearm/wrist open wound
881.1x	Elbow/forearm/wrist complex wound
884.0	Open wound of arm, mult/NOS
884.1	Open wound of arm mult/NOS, compl
887.x	Traumatic arm/hand amputation
890.0	Open wound of hip/thigh
890.1	Open wound of hip/thigh, complic
891.0	Open wound of knee/leg/ankle
891.1	Open wound of knee/leg/ankle, compl
894.0	Open wound of leg NEC
894.1	Open wound of leg NEC, complicated
896.x	Traumatic amputation of foot
897.x	Traumatic amputation of leg(s)
943.31	3rd deg burn, forearm
943.32	3rd deg burn, elbow
943.33	3rd deg burn, upper arm
943.34	3rd deg burn, axilla
943.35	3rd deg burn, shoulder
943.36	3rd deg burn, scapula
943.39	3rd deg burn, arm multiple sites
943.41	Deep 3rd deg burn, forearm
943.42	Deep 3rd deg burn, elbow
943.43	Deep 3rd deg burn, upper arm
943.44	Deep 3rd deg burn, axilla
943.45	Deep 3rd deg burn, shoulder
943.46	Deep 3rd deg burn, scapula
943.49	Deep 3rd deg burn, arm mult sites
943.51	Deep 3rd deg loss, forearm
943.52	Deep 3rd deg loss, elbow
943.53	Deep 3rd deg loss, upper arm
943.54	Deep 3rd deg loss, axilla

CPT CODE	SERVICE	ICD-9-CM	
15610 (Cont'd.)		943.55	Deep 3rd deg loss, shoulder
		943.56	Deep 3rd deg loss, scapula
		943.59	Deep 3rd deg loss, arm mult sites
		944.31	3rd deg burn, finger
		944.32	3rd deg burn, thumb
		944.33	3rd deg burn, mult fingers
		944.34	3rd deg burn, finger w/thumb
		944.35	3rd deg burn, palm
		944.36	3rd deg burn, back of hand
		944.37	3rd deg burn, wrist
		944.41	Deep 3rd deg burn, finger
		944.42	Deep 3rd deg burn, thumb
		944.43	Deep 3rd deg burn, mult fingers
		944.44	Deep 3rd deg burn, finger w/thumb
		944.45	Deep 3rd deg burn, palm
		944.46	Deep 3rd deg burn, back of hand
		944.47	Deep 3rd deg burn, wrist
		944.51	Deep 3rd deg loss, finger
		944.52	Deep 3rd deg loss, thumb
		944.53	Deep 3rd deg loss, mult fingers
		944.54	Deep 3rd deg loss, finger w/thumb
		944.55	Deep 3rd deg loss, palm
		944.56	Deep 3rd deg loss, back of hand
		944.57	Deep 3rd deg loss, wrist
		945.31	3rd deg burn, toe
		945.32	3rd deg burn, foot
		945.33	3rd deg burn, ankle
		945.34	3rd deg burn, lower leg
		945.35	3rd deg burn, knee
		945.36	3rd deg burn, thigh
		945.39	3rd deg burn, leg mult sites
		945.41	Deep 3rd deg burn, toe
		945.42	Deep 3rd deg burn, foot
		945.43	Deep 3rd deg burn, ankle
		945.44	Deep 3rd deg burn, lower leg
		945.45	Deep 3rd deg burn, knee
		945.46	Deep 3rd deg burn, thigh
		945.49	Deep 3rd deg burn, leg mult sites
		945.51	Deep 3rd deg loss, toe
		945.52	Deep 3rd deg loss, foot
		945.53	Deep 3rd deg loss, ankle
		945.54	Deep 3rd deg loss, lower leg
		945.55	Deep 3rd deg loss, knee
		945.56	Deep 3rd deg loss, thigh
		945.59	Deep 3rd deg loss, leg mult sites
		V50.1	Plastic surgery NEC
		V51.	Aftercare w/plastic surgery

CPT CODE	SERVICE	ICD–9–CM
15610 (Cont'd.)		

REIMBURSEMENT INFORMATION

General

- ◆ See notes on page 114.

Medicare

- ◆ Follow–Up Days — 90
- ◆ Assistant Surgeon — not paid
- ◆ Supply Charges — not allowed
- ◆ Outpatient Limit — does not apply
- ◆ Major Surgery Rules Apply

CPT CODE	SERVICE
15620	Delay of flap or sectioning of flap (division and inset); at forehead, cheeks, chin, neck, axillae, genitalia, hands (except 15625), or feet

CPT NOTES

- Regions listed refer to recipient area (not donor site) when flap is being attached in transfer or to final site.
- Regions listed refer to donor site when tube is formed for later or when "delay" of flap is prior to transfer.
- Procedures 15570-15738 do not include extensive immobilization (e.g., large plaster casts and other immobilizing devices are considered additional separate procedures).
- Repair of donor site requiring skin graft or local flap is considered an additional separate procedure.

ICD–9–CM

172.3	Malignant melanoma, Face NEC/NOS
172.4	Malignant melanoma, Scalp/neck
173.3	M-Neoplasm, Skin of face NEC
173.4	M-Neoplasm, Scalp/skin neck
216.3	B-Neoplasm, Skin of face NEC
216.4	B-Neoplasm, Scalp/skin of neck
738.10	Acquired head deformity NOS
873.41	Open wound of cheek
873.42	Open wound of forehead
873.49	Open wound of face NEC
873.51	Open wound of cheek, complicated
873.52	Open wound of forehead, complicated
873.59	Open wound of face NEC, complicated
878.0	Open wound of penis
878.1	Open wound of penis, complicated
878.2	Open wound of scrotum/testes
878.3	Open wound, scrotum/testes, compl
878.4	Open wound of vulva
878.5	Open wound of vulva, complicated
878.6	Open wound of vagina
878.7	Open wound of vagina, complicated
880.02	Open wound of axilla
880.12	Open wound of axilla, complicated
882.0	Open wound of hand
882.1	Open wound of hand, complicated
883.0	Open wound of finger
883.1	Open wound of finger, complicated
885.x	Traumatic amputation of thumb
886.x	Traumatic finger amputation
887.x	Traumatic arm/hand amputation
892.x	Open wound of foot
893.x	Open wound of toe(s)
895.x	Traumatic amputation of toe(s)
896.x	Traumatic amputation of foot
941.34	3rd deg burn, chin
941.37	3rd deg burn, face NEC
941.38	3rd deg burn, neck
941.44	Deep 3rd deg burn, chin
941.47	Deep 3rd deg burn, face NEC
941.48	Deep 3rd deg burn, neck
941.54	Deep 3rd deg loss, chin
941.57	Deep 3rd deg loss, face NEC
941.58	Deep 3rd deg loss, neck
942.35	3rd deg burn trunk, genitalia
942.45	Deep 3rd deg burn trunk, genitalia
942.55	Deep 3rd deg loss trunk, genitalia
943.35	3rd deg burn, shoulder
943.45	Deep 3rd deg burn, shoulder
943.55	Deep 3rd deg loss, shoulder
944.31	3rd deg burn, finger
944.32	3rd deg burn, thumb
944.33	3rd deg burn, mult fingers
944.34	3rd deg burn, finger w/thumb
944.35	3rd deg burn, palm
944.36	3rd deg burn, back of hand
944.37	3rd deg burn, wrist

CPT CODE **SERVICE**

15620 (Cont'd.)

ICD-9-CM

944.41 Deep 3rd deg burn, finger
944.42 Deep 3rd deg burn, thumb
944.43 Deep 3rd deg burn, mult fingers
944.44 Deep 3rd deg burn, finger w/thumb
944.45 Deep 3rd deg burn, palm
944.46 Deep 3rd deg burn, back of hand
944.47 Deep 3rd deg burn, wrist
944.51 Deep 3rd deg loss, finger
944.52 Deep 3rd deg loss, thumb
944.53 Deep 3rd deg loss, mult fingers
944.54 Deep 3rd deg loss, finger w/thumb
944.55 Deep 3rd deg loss, palm
944.56 Deep 3rd deg loss, back of hand
944.57 Deep 3rd deg loss, wrist
945.31 3rd deg burn, toe
945.32 3rd deg burn, foot
945.41 Deep 3rd deg burn, toe
945.42 Deep 3rd deg burn, foot
945.51 Deep 3rd deg loss, toe
945.52 Deep 3rd deg loss, foot

REIMBURSEMENT INFORMATION

General

- See notes on page 114.

Medicare

- Follow-Up Days — 90
- Assistant Surgeon — not paid
- Supply Charges — not allowed
- Outpatient Limit — does not apply
- Major Surgery Rules Apply

CPT CODE	SERVICE
15625	Delay of flap or sectioning of flap (division and inset); section pedicle of cross finger flap

CPT NOTES

- ♦ Regions listed refer to recipient area (not donor site) when flap is being attached in transfer or to final site.
- ♦ Regions listed refer to donor site when tube is formed for later or when "delay" of flap is prior to transfer.
- ♦ Procedures 15570-15738 do not include extensive immobilization (e.g., large plaster casts and other immobilizing devices are considered additional separate procedures).
- ♦ Repair of donor site requiring skin graft or local flap is considered an additional separate procedure.

ICD-9-CM

882.0	Open wound of hand
882.1	Open wound of hand, complicated
883.0	Open wound of finger
883.1	Open wound of finger, complicated
885.x	Traumatic amputation of thumb
886.x	Traumatic finger amputation
887.x	Traumatic arm/hand amputation
892.x	Open wound of foot
893.x	Open wound of toe(s)
895.x	Traumatic amputation of toe(s)
896.x	Traumatic amputation of foot
927.3	Crushing injury, finger
928.3	Crushing injury, toe
944.31	3rd deg burn, finger
944.32	3rd deg burn, thumb
944.33	3rd deg burn, mult fingers
944.34	3rd deg burn, finger w/thumb
944.35	3rd deg burn, palm
944.36	3rd deg burn, back of hand
944.37	3rd deg burn, wrist
944.41	Deep 3rd deg burn, finger
944.42	Deep 3rd deg burn, thumb
944.43	Deep 3rd deg burn, mult fingers
944.44	Deep 3rd deg burn, finger w/thumb
944.45	Deep 3rd deg burn, palm
944.46	Deep 3rd deg burn, back of hand
944.47	Deep 3rd deg burn, wrist
944.51	Deep 3rd deg loss, finger
944.52	Deep 3rd deg loss, thumb
944.53	Deep 3rd deg loss, mult fingers
944.54	Deep 3rd deg loss, finger w/thumb
944.55	Deep 3rd deg loss, palm
944.56	Deep 3rd deg loss, back of hand
944.57	Deep 3rd deg loss, wrist
V50.1	Plastic surgery NEC
V51.	Aftercare w/plastic surgery

REIMBURSEMENT INFORMATION

General

- ♦ See notes on page 114.

Medicare

- ♦ Follow–Up Days — 90
- ♦ Assistant Surgeon — paid
- ♦ Supply Charges — not allowed
- ♦ Outpatient Limit — does not apply
- ♦ Major Surgery Rules Apply

CPT CODE	SERVICE	ICD-9-CM	
15630	Delay of flap or sectioning of flap (division and inset); at eyelids, nose, ears, or lips	140.0	M-Neoplasm, Upper lip, vermilion
		140.1	M-Neoplasm, Lower lip, vermilion
		140.3	M-Neoplasm, Upper lip, inner aspect
		140.4	M-Neoplasm, Lower lip, inner aspect
		140.5	M-Neoplasm, Lip NOS, inner NOS
		140.6	M-Neoplasm, lip, commissure
		140.8	M-Neoplasm, Lip NEC
		140.9	M-Neoplasm, Lip/vermilion NOS
		171.0	M-Neoplasm, Soft tissue, head
		172.0	Malignant melanoma, Lip
		172.1	Malignant melanoma, eyelid/canthus
		172.2	Malignant melanoma, Ear
		172.3	Malignant melanoma, Face NEC/NOS
		173.0	M-Neoplasm, Skin of lip
		173.1	M-Neoplasm, Skin of eyelid/canthus
		173.2	M-Neoplasm, Skin of ear
		173.3	M-Neoplasm, Skin of face NEC
		195.0	M-Neoplasm, Head/face/neck
		216.0	B-Neoplasm, Skin of lip
		216.1	B-Neoplasm, Skin of eyelid/canthus
		216.2	B-Neoplasm, Skin of ear
		216.3	B-Neoplasm, Skin of face NEC
		232.0	CA in situ, Skin of lip
		232.1	CA in situ, Eyelid/canthus
		232.2	CA in situ, Skin of ear
		232.3	CA in situ, Skin of face NEC
		709.2	Scar/fibrosis of skin
		744.23	Microtia
		744.3	Ear anomaly NOS
		870.0	Laceration eyelid skin/periocular
		872.01	Open wound of auricle
		872.11	Open wound of auricle, complicated
		873.21	Open wound of nasal septum
		873.31	Open wound nasal septum, complic
		873.43	Open wound of lip
		873.53	Open wound of lip, complicated
		940.0	Chemical burn, eyelid/periocular
		940.1	Burn, eyelid/periocular area NEC
		941.22	Blisters, epidermal loss, eye
		941.31	3rd deg burn, ear
		941.32	3rd degree burn, eye
		941.33	3rd deg burn, lip
		941.34	3rd deg burn, chin
		941.35	3rd deg burn, nose
		941.41	Deep 3rd deg burn, ear
		941.42	Deep 3rd degree burn, eye
		941.43	Deep 3rd deg burn, lip
		941.44	Deep 3rd deg burn, chin
		941.45	Deep 3rd deg burn, nose
		941.51	Deep 3rd deg loss, ear
		941.52	Deep 3rd degree loss, eye
		941.53	Deep 3rd deg loss, lip
		941.54	Deep 3rd deg loss, chin
		941.55	Deep 3rd deg loss, nose

CPT NOTES

- ◆ Regions listed refer to recipient area (not donor site) when flap is being attached in transfer or to final site.
- ◆ Regions listed refer to donor site when tube is formed for later or when "delay" of flap is prior to transfer.
- ◆ Procedures 15570-15738 do not include extensive immobilization (e.g., large plaster casts and other immobilizing devices are considered additional separate procedures).
- ◆ Repair of donor site requiring skin graft or local flap is considered an additional separate procedure.

CPT CODE	SERVICE	ICD-9-CM
15630 (Cont'd.)		

REIMBURSEMENT INFORMATION

General

- See notes on page 114.

Medicare

- Follow-Up Days — 90
- Assistant Surgeon — not paid
- Supply Charges — not allowed
- Outpatient Limit — does not apply
- Major Surgery Rules Apply

CPT CODE	SERVICE
15650	Transfer, intermediate, of any pedicle flap (eg, abdomen to wrist, 'Walking' tube), any location

CPT NOTES

- Regions listed refer to recipient area (not donor site) when flap is being attached in transfer or to final site.
- Regions listed refer to donor site when tube is formed for later or when "delay" of flap is prior to transfer.
- Procedures 15570-15738 do not include extensive immobilization (e.g., large plaster casts and other immobilizing devices are considered additional separate procedures).
- Repair of donor site requiring skin graft or local flap is considered an additional separate procedure.
- For eyelids, nose, ears, or lips, see also anatomical area.
- For revision, defatting or rearranging of transferred pedicle flap or skin grafts, see 13100-14300.

ICD–9–CM

873.0	Open wound of scalp
873.1	Open wound of scalp, complicated
875.0	Open wound of chest
875.1	Open wound of chest, complicated
876.0	Open wound of back
876.1	Open wound of back, complicated
877.0	Open wound of buttock
877.1	Open wound of buttock, complicated
880.00	Open wound of shoulder
880.01	Open wound of scapula
880.02	Open wound of axilla
880.03	Open wound of upper arm
880.09	Multiple open wounds of shoulder
880.10	Open wound of shoulder, complicated
880.11	Open wound of scapula, complicated
880.12	Open wound of axilla, complicated
880.13	Open wound of upper arm, complic
880.19	Mult open wounds of shoulder, compl
881.00	Open wound of forearm
881.01	Open wound of elbow
881.10	Open wound of forearm, complicated
881.11	Open wound of elbow, complicated
882.0	Open wound of hand
882.1	Open wound of hand, complicated
883.0	Open wound of finger
883.1	Open wound of finger, complicated
884.0	Open wound of arm, mult/NOS
884.1	Open wound of arm mult/NOS, compl
885.x	Traumatic amputation of thumb
886.x	Traumatic finger amputation
887.x	Traumatic arm/hand amputation
890.x	Open wound of hip and thigh
891.x	Open wound of knee, leg, ankle
892.x	Open wound of foot
893.x	Open wound of toe(s)
894.x	Open wound of lower limb
895.x	Traumatic amputation of toe(s)
896.x	Traumatic amputation of foot
897.x	Traumatic amputation of leg(s)
942.41	Deep 3rd deg burn trunk, breast
942.42	Deep 3rd deg burn trunk, chest wall
942.43	Deep 3rd deg burn trunk, abdominal
942.44	Deep 3rd deg burn trunk, back
942.45	Deep 3rd deg burn trunk, genitalia
942.51	Deep 3rd deg loss trunk, breast
942.52	Deep 3rd deg loss trunk, chest wall
942.53	Deep 3rd deg loss trunk, abdominal
942.54	Deep 3rd deg loss trunk, back
942.55	Deep 3rd deg loss trunk, genitalia
943.31	3rd deg burn, forearm
943.32	3rd deg burn, elbow
943.33	3rd deg burn, upper arm
943.34	3rd deg burn, axilla
943.35	3rd deg burn, shoulder
943.36	3rd deg burn, scapula
943.39	3rd deg burn, arm multiple sites

CPT CODE	SERVICE	ICD-9-CM	
15650 (Cont'd.)		943.41	Deep 3rd deg burn, forearm
		943.42	Deep 3rd deg burn, elbow
		943.43	Deep 3rd deg burn, upper arm
		943.44	Deep 3rd deg burn, axilla
		943.45	Deep 3rd deg burn, shoulder
		943.46	Deep 3rd deg burn, scapula
		943.49	Deep 3rd deg burn, arm mult sites
		943.51	Deep 3rd deg loss, forearm
		943.52	Deep 3rd deg loss, elbow
		943.53	Deep 3rd deg loss, upper arm
		943.54	Deep 3rd deg loss, axilla
		943.55	Deep 3rd deg loss, shoulder
		943.56	Deep 3rd deg loss, scapula
		943.59	Deep 3rd deg loss, arm mult sites
		944.31	3rd deg burn, finger
		944.32	3rd deg burn, thumb
		944.33	3rd deg burn, mult fingers
		944.34	3rd deg burn, finger w/thumb
		944.35	3rd deg burn, palm
		944.36	3rd deg burn, back of hand
		944.37	3rd deg burn, wrist
		944.41	Deep 3rd deg burn, finger
		944.42	Deep 3rd deg burn, thumb
		944.43	Deep 3rd deg burn, mult fingers
		944.44	Deep 3rd deg burn, finger w/thumb
		944.45	Deep 3rd deg burn, palm
		944.46	Deep 3rd deg burn, back of hand
		944.47	Deep 3rd deg burn, wrist
		944.51	Deep 3rd deg loss, finger
		944.52	Deep 3rd deg loss, thumb
		944.53	Deep 3rd deg loss, mult fingers
		944.54	Deep 3rd deg loss, finger w/thumb
		944.55	Deep 3rd deg loss, palm
		944.56	Deep 3rd deg loss, back of hand
		944.57	Deep 3rd deg loss, wrist
		945.31	3rd deg burn, toe
		945.32	3rd deg burn, foot
		945.33	3rd deg burn, ankle
		945.34	3rd deg burn, lower leg
		945.35	3rd deg burn, knee
		945.36	3rd deg burn, thigh
		945.39	3rd deg burn, leg mult sites
		945.41	Deep 3rd deg burn, toe
		945.42	Deep 3rd deg burn, foot
		945.43	Deep 3rd deg burn, ankle
		945.44	Deep 3rd deg burn, lower leg
		945.45	Deep 3rd deg burn, knee
		945.46	Deep 3rd deg burn, thigh
		945.49	Deep 3rd deg burn, leg mult sites
		945.51	Deep 3rd deg loss, toe
		945.52	Deep 3rd deg loss, foot
		945.53	Deep 3rd deg loss, ankle
		945.54	Deep 3rd deg loss, lower leg
		945.55	Deep 3rd deg loss, knee
		945.56	Deep 3rd deg loss, thigh
		945.59	Deep 3rd deg loss, leg mult sites

CPT CODE	SERVICE	ICD–9–CM
15650 (Cont'd.)		V50.1 Plastic surgery NEC V51. Aftercare w/plastic surgery

REIMBURSEMENT INFORMATION

General

- ◆ See notes on page 114.

Medicare

- ◆ Follow–Up Days — 90
- ◆ Assistant Surgeon — not paid
- ◆ Supply Charges — not allowed
- ◆ Outpatient Limit — does not apply
- ◆ Major Surgery Rules Apply

CPT CODE	SERVICE
15732	Muscle, myocutaneous, or fasciocutaneous flap; head and neck (eg, temporalis, masseter, sternocleidomastoid, levator scapulae)

CPT NOTES

- ♦ Regions listed refer to recipient area (not donor site) when flap is being attached in transfer or to final site.
- ♦ Regions listed refer to donor site when tube is formed for later or when "delay" of flap is prior to transfer.
- ♦ Procedures 15570-15738 do not include extensive immobilization (e.g., large plaster casts and other immobilizing devices are considered additional separate procedures).
- ♦ Repair of donor site requiring skin graft or local flap is considered an additional separate procedure.
- ♦ Procedures 15732-15738 are described by donor site of the muscle, myocutaneous, or fasciocutaneous flap.

ICD–9–CM

171.0	M-Neoplasm, Soft tissue, head
172.3	Malignant melanoma, Face NEC/NOS
172.4	Malignant melanoma, Scalp/neck
173.1	M-Neoplasm, Skin of eyelid/canthus
173.3	M-Neoplasm, Skin of face NEC
173.4	M-Neoplasm, Scalp/skin neck
216.1	B-Neoplasm, Skin of eyelid/canthus
216.3	B-Neoplasm, Skin of face NEC
216.4	B-Neoplasm, Scalp/skin of neck
232.1	CA in situ, Eyelid/canthus
238.8	Uncertain behavior, neoplasm NEC
374.11	Senile ectropion
374.41	Eyelid retraction or lag
374.84	Cysts of eyelids
873.41	Open wound of cheek
873.42	Open wound of forehead
873.49	Open wound of face NEC
873.51	Open wound of cheek, complicated
873.52	Open wound of forehead, complicated
873.59	Open wound of face NEC, complicated
905.0	Late effect, skull/face fracture
906.5	Late effect of head/neck burn
925.	Crushing injury, face/scalp/neck
941.34	3rd deg burn, chin
941.37	3rd deg burn, face NEC
941.38	3rd deg burn, neck
941.44	Deep 3rd deg burn, chin
941.47	Deep 3rd deg burn, face NEC
941.48	Deep 3rd deg burn, neck
941.54	Deep 3rd deg loss, chin
941.57	Deep 3rd deg loss, face NEC
941.58	Deep 3rd deg loss, neck
952.2	Lumbar spinal cord injury
V51.	Aftercare w/plastic surgery

REIMBURSEMENT INFORMATION

General

- ♦ See notes on page 114.

Medicare

- ♦ Follow–Up Days — 90
- ♦ Assistant Surgeon — paid
- ♦ Supply Charges — not allowed
- ♦ Outpatient Limit — does not apply
- ♦ Major Surgery Rules Apply

CPT CODE	SERVICE
15734	Muscle, myocutaneous, or fasciocutaneous flap; trunk

CPT NOTES

- Regions listed refer to recipient area (not donor site) when flap is being attached in transfer or to final site.
- Regions listed refer to donor site when tube is formed for later or when "delay" of flap is prior to transfer.
- Procedures 15570-15738 do not include extensive immobilization (e.g., large plaster casts and other immobilizing devices are considered additional separate procedures).
- Repair of donor site requiring skin graft or local flap is considered an additional separate procedure.
- Procedures 15732-15738 are described by donor site of the muscle, myocutaneous, or fasciocutaneous flap.

ICD–9–CM

172.5	Malignant melanoma, Trunk
173.5	M-Neoplasm, Skin of trunk
216.5	B-Neoplasm, Skin of trunk
232.5	CA in situ, Skin of trunk
553.21	Incisional hernia
553.29	Ventral hernia NEC
553.8	Hernia NEC
707.0	Decubitus ulcer
707.8	Chronic skin ulcer NEC
875.0	Open wound of chest
875.1	Open wound of chest, complicated
876.0	Open wound of back
876.1	Open wound of back, complicated
877.0	Open wound of buttock
877.1	Open wound of buttock, complicated
879.0	Open wound of breast
879.1	Open wound of breast, complicated
879.2	Open wound of anterior abdomen
879.3	Open wound anterior abdomen, compl
879.4	Open wound of lateral abdomen
879.5	Open wound lateral abdomen, compl
879.6	Open wound of trunk NEC
879.7	Open wound of trunk NEC, complic
926.11	Crushing injury, back
926.12	Crushing injury, buttock
926.19	Crushing injury, trunk NEC
926.8	Multiple crushing injuries, trunk
942.31	3rd deg burn trunk, breast
942.32	3rd deg burn trunk, chest wall
942.33	3rd deg burn trunk, abdominal wall
942.34	3rd deg burn trunk, back
942.35	3rd deg burn trunk, genitalia
942.41	Deep 3rd deg burn trunk, breast
942.42	Deep 3rd deg burn trunk, chest wall
942.43	Deep 3rd deg burn trunk, abdominal
942.44	Deep 3rd deg burn trunk, back
942.45	Deep 3rd deg burn trunk, genitalia
942.51	Deep 3rd deg loss trunk, breast
942.52	Deep 3rd deg loss trunk, chest wall
942.53	Deep 3rd deg loss trunk, abdominal
942.54	Deep 3rd deg loss trunk, back
942.55	Deep 3rd deg loss trunk, genitalia
V51.	Aftercare w/plastic surgery

REIMBURSEMENT INFORMATION

General

- See notes on page 114.

Medicare

- Follow–Up Days — 90
- Assistant Surgeon — paid
- Supply Charges — not allowed
- Outpatient Limit — does not apply
- Major Surgery Rules Apply

CPT CODE	SERVICE
15736	Muscle, myocutaneous, or fasciocutaneous flap; upper extremity

CPT NOTES

- ♦ Regions listed refer to recipient area (not donor site) when flap is being attached in transfer or to final site.
- ♦ Regions listed refer to donor site when tube is formed for later or when "delay" of flap is prior to transfer.
- ♦ Procedures 15570-15738 do not include extensive immobilization (e.g., large plaster casts and other immobilizing devices are considered additional separate procedures).
- ♦ Repair of donor site requiring skin graft or local flap is considered an additional separate procedure.
- ♦ Procedures 15732-15738 are described by donor site of the muscle, myocutaneous, or fasciocutaneous flap.

ICD–9–CM

172.6	Malignant melanoma, Arm
173.6	M-Neoplasm, Skin of arm
216.6	B-Neoplasm, Skin of arm
232.6	CA in situ, Skin of arm
880.00	Open wound of shoulder
880.01	Open wound of scapula
880.03	Open wound of upper arm
880.09	Multiple open wounds of shoulder
880.10	Open wound of shoulder, complicated
880.11	Open wound of scapula, complicated
880.13	Open wound of upper arm, complic
880.19	Mult open wounds of shoulder, compl
881.0x	Elbow/forearm/wrist open wound
881.1x	Elbow/forearm/wrist complex wound
884.0	Open wound of arm, mult/NOS
884.1	Open wound of arm mult/NOS, compl
887.x	Traumatic arm/hand amputation
905.2	Late effect, arm fracture
906.1	Late effect, open wound extremity
906.6	Late effect of wrist/hand burn
906.7	Late effect of extremity burn NEC
927.0x	Crushing injury, shoulder/upper arm
927.1x	Crushing injury, elbow and forearm
943.31	3rd deg burn, forearm
943.32	3rd deg burn, elbow
943.33	3rd deg burn, upper arm
943.34	3rd deg burn, axilla
943.35	3rd deg burn, shoulder
943.36	3rd deg burn, scapula
943.39	3rd deg burn, arm multiple sites
943.41	Deep 3rd deg burn, forearm
943.42	Deep 3rd deg burn, elbow
943.43	Deep 3rd deg burn, upper arm
943.44	Deep 3rd deg burn, axilla
943.45	Deep 3rd deg burn, shoulder
943.46	Deep 3rd deg burn, scapula
943.49	Deep 3rd deg burn, arm mult sites
943.51	Deep 3rd deg loss, forearm
943.52	Deep 3rd deg loss, elbow
943.53	Deep 3rd deg loss, upper arm
943.54	Deep 3rd deg loss, axilla
943.55	Deep 3rd deg loss, shoulder
943.56	Deep 3rd deg loss, scapula
943.59	Deep 3rd deg loss, arm mult sites
944.31	3rd deg burn, finger
944.32	3rd deg burn, thumb
944.33	3rd deg burn, mult fingers
944.34	3rd deg burn, finger w/thumb
944.35	3rd deg burn, palm
944.36	3rd deg burn, back of hand
944.37	3rd deg burn, wrist
944.41	Deep 3rd deg burn, finger
944.42	Deep 3rd deg burn, thumb
944.43	Deep 3rd deg burn, mult fingers
944.44	Deep 3rd deg burn, finger w/thumb
944.45	Deep 3rd deg burn, palm

CPT CODE	SERVICE	ICD–9–CM	
15736 (Cont'd.)		944.46	Deep 3rd deg burn, back of hand
		944.47	Deep 3rd deg burn, wrist
		944.51	Deep 3rd deg loss, finger
		944.52	Deep 3rd deg loss, thumb
		944.53	Deep 3rd deg loss, mult fingers
		944.54	Deep 3rd deg loss, finger w/thumb
		944.55	Deep 3rd deg loss, palm
		944.56	Deep 3rd deg loss, back of hand
		944.57	Deep 3rd deg loss, wrist
		V51.	Aftercare w/plastic surgery

REIMBURSEMENT INFORMATION

General

- See notes on page 114.

Medicare

- Follow–Up Days — 90
- Assistant Surgeon — paid
- Supply Charges — not allowed
- Outpatient Limit — does not apply
- Major Surgery Rules Apply

CPT CODE	SERVICE
15738	Muscle, myocutaneous, or fasciocutaneous flap; lower extremity

CPT NOTES

- Regions listed refer to recipient area (not donor site) when flap is being attached in transfer or to final site.
- Regions listed refer to donor site when tube is formed for later or when "delay" of flap is prior to transfer.
- Procedures 15570-15738 do not include extensive immobilization (e.g., large plaster casts and other immobilizing devices are considered additional separate procedures).
- Repair of donor site requiring skin graft or local flap is considered an additional separate procedure.
- Procedures 15732-15738 are described by donor site of the muscle, myocutaneous, or fasciocutaneous flap.

ICD–9–CM

172.7	Malignant melanoma, Leg
173.7	M-Neoplasm, Skin of leg
216.7	B-Neoplasm, Skin of leg
232.7	CA in situ, Skin of leg
707.1	Chronic ulcer of the leg
890.0	Open wound of hip/thigh
890.1	Open wound of hip/thigh, complic
891.0	Open wound of knee/leg/ankle
891.1	Open wound of knee/leg/ankle, compl
894.0	Open wound of leg NEC
894.1	Open wound of leg NEC, complicated
896.x	Traumatic amputation of foot
897.x	Traumatic amputation of leg(s)
905.4	Late effect, leg fracture
906.1	Late effect, open wound extremity
906.4	Late effect of crushing
906.7	Late effect of extremity burn NEC
945.31	3rd deg burn, toe
945.32	3rd deg burn, foot
945.33	3rd deg burn, ankle
945.34	3rd deg burn, lower leg
945.35	3rd deg burn, knee
945.36	3rd deg burn, thigh
945.39	3rd deg burn, leg mult sites
945.41	Deep 3rd deg burn, toe
945.42	Deep 3rd deg burn, foot
945.43	Deep 3rd deg burn, ankle
945.44	Deep 3rd deg burn, lower leg
945.45	Deep 3rd deg burn, knee
945.46	Deep 3rd deg burn, thigh
945.49	Deep 3rd deg burn, leg mult sites
945.51	Deep 3rd deg loss, toe
945.52	Deep 3rd deg loss, foot
945.53	Deep 3rd deg loss, ankle
945.54	Deep 3rd deg loss, lower leg
945.55	Deep 3rd deg loss, knee
945.56	Deep 3rd deg loss, thigh
945.59	Deep 3rd deg loss, leg mult sites
V51.	Aftercare w/plastic surgery

REIMBURSEMENT INFORMATION

General

- See notes on page 114.

Medicare

- Follow–Up Days — 90
- Assistant Surgeon — paid
- Supply Charges — not allowed
- Outpatient Limit — does not apply
- Major Surgery Rules Apply

CPT CODE	SERVICE	ICD–9–CM	
15740	Flap; island pedicle	140.0	M-Neoplasm, Upper lip, vermilion
		140.1	M-Neoplasm, Lower lip, vermilion
15750	Flap; neurovascular pedicle	140.3	M-Neoplasm, Upper lip, inner aspect
		140.4	M-Neoplasm, Lower lip, inner aspect
		140.5	M-Neoplasm, Lip NOS, inner NOS
		140.6	M-Neoplasm, lip, commissure
		140.8	M-Neoplasm, Lip NEC
		140.9	M-Neoplasm, Lip/vermilion NOS
		172.x	Skin Melanoma
		173.x	Malignant neoplasm, Skin
		216.x	Benign neoplasm, Skin
		232.x	Carcinoma in situ, Skin
		707.x	Chronic ulcer of skin
		709.2	Scar/fibrosis of skin
		744.23	Microtia
		744.3	Ear anomaly NOS
		870.0	Laceration eyelid skin/periocular
		872.01	Open wound of auricle
		872.11	Open wound of auricle, complicated
		873.0	Open wound of scalp
		873.1	Open wound of scalp, complicated
		873.21	Open wound of nasal septum
		873.31	Open wound nasal septum, complic
		873.4x	Face, open wound
		873.5x	Face, complicated open wound
		875.0	Open wound of chest
		875.1	Open wound of chest, complicated
		876.0	Open wound of back
		876.1	Open wound of back, complicated
		877.0	Open wound of buttock
		877.1	Open wound of buttock, complicated
		878.0	Open wound of penis
		878.1	Open wound of penis, complicated
		878.2	Open wound of scrotum/testes
		878.3	Open wound, scrotum/testes, compl
		878.4	Open wound of vulva
		878.5	Open wound of vulva, complicated
		878.6	Open wound of vagina
		878.7	Open wound of vagina, complicated
		879.0	Open wound of breast
		879.1	Open wound of breast, complicated
		879.2	Open wound of anterior abdomen
		879.3	Open wound anterior abdomen, compl
		879.4	Open wound of lateral abdomen
		879.5	Open wound lateral abdomen, compl
		880.00	Open wound of shoulder
		880.01	Open wound of scapula
		880.02	Open wound of axilla
		880.03	Open wound of upper arm
		880.09	Multiple open wounds of shoulder
		880.10	Open wound of shoulder, complicated
		880.11	Open wound of scapula, complicated
		880.12	Open wound of axilla, complicated
		880.13	Open wound of upper arm, complic
		880.19	Mult open wounds of shoulder, compl
		881.0x	Elbow/forearm/wrist open wound

CPT NOTES

- ♦ Repair of donor site requiring skin graft or local flaps should be reported as an additional procedure.

CPT CODE	SERVICE	ICD-9-CM	
15740, 15750	(Cont'd.)	881.1x	Elbow/forearm/wrist complex wound
		882.0	Open wound of hand
		882.1	Open wound of hand, complicated
		883.0	Open wound of finger
		883.1	Open wound of finger, complicated
		884.0	Open wound of arm, mult/NOS
		884.1	Open wound of arm mult/NOS, compl
		885.x	Traumatic amputation of thumb
		886.x	Traumatic finger amputation
		887.x	Traumatic arm/hand amputation
		890.x	Open wound of hip and thigh
		891.x	Open wound of knee, leg, ankle
		892.x	Open wound of foot
		893.x	Open wound of toe(s)
		894.x	Open wound of lower limb
		895.x	Traumatic amputation of toe(s)
		896.x	Traumatic amputation of foot
		897.x	Traumatic amputation of leg(s)
		V50.1	Plastic surgery NEC
		V51.	Aftercare w/plastic surgery

REIMBURSEMENT INFORMATION

General

- See notes on page 114.

Medicare

- Follow-Up Days — 90
- Assistant Surgeon — not paid
- Supply Charges — not allowed
- Outpatient Limit — does not apply
- Major Surgery Rules Apply

CPT CODE	SERVICE
15755	Free flap (microvascular transfer)

CPT NOTES

- ♦ Repair of donor site requiring skin graft or local flaps should be reported as an additional procedure.

ICD-9-CM

140.0	M-Neoplasm, Upper lip, vermilion
140.1	M-Neoplasm, Lower lip, vermilion
140.3	M-Neoplasm, Upper lip, inner aspect
140.4	M-Neoplasm, Lower lip, inner aspect
140.5	M-Neoplasm, Lip NOS, inner NOS
140.6	M-Neoplasm, lip, commissure
140.8	M-Neoplasm, Lip NEC
140.9	M-Neoplasm, Lip/vermilion NOS
172.x	Skin Melanoma
173.x	Malignant neoplasm, Skin
216.x	Benign neoplasm, Skin
232.x	Carcinoma in situ, Skin
701.0	Circumscribed scleroderma
707.x	Chronic ulcer of skin
709.2	Scar/fibrosis of skin
744.23	Microtia
744.3	Ear anomaly NOS
870.0	Laceration eyelid skin/periocular
872.01	Open wound of auricle
872.11	Open wound of auricle, complicated
873.0	Open wound of scalp
873.1	Open wound of scalp, complicated
873.21	Open wound of nasal septum
873.31	Open wound nasal septum, complic
873.4x	Face, open wound
873.5x	Face, complicated open wound
875.0	Open wound of chest
875.1	Open wound of chest, complicated
876.0	Open wound of back
876.1	Open wound of back, complicated
877.0	Open wound of buttock
877.1	Open wound of buttock, complicated
878.0	Open wound of penis
878.1	Open wound of penis, complicated
878.2	Open wound of scrotum/testes
878.3	Open wound, scrotum/testes, compl
878.4	Open wound of vulva
878.5	Open wound of vulva, complicated
878.6	Open wound of vagina
878.7	Open wound of vagina, complicated
879.0	Open wound of breast
879.1	Open wound of breast, complicated
879.2	Open wound of anterior abdomen
879.3	Open wound anterior abdomen, compl
879.4	Open wound of lateral abdomen
879.5	Open wound lateral abdomen, compl
880.00	Open wound of shoulder
880.01	Open wound of scapula
880.02	Open wound of axilla
880.03	Open wound of upper arm
880.09	Multiple open wounds of shoulder
880.10	Open wound of shoulder, complicated
880.11	Open wound of scapula, complicated
880.12	Open wound of axilla, complicated
880.13	Open wound of upper arm, complic
880.19	Mult open wounds of shoulder, compl

CPT CODE	SERVICE	ICD-9-CM
15755 (Cont'd.)		

881.0x	Elbow/forearm/wrist open wound
881.1x	Elbow/forearm/wrist complex wound
881.20	Open wound of forearm w/tendon
882.0	Open wound of hand
882.1	Open wound of hand, complicated
883.0	Open wound of finger
883.1	Open wound of finger, complicated
884.0	Open wound of arm, mult/NOS
884.1	Open wound of arm mult/NOS, compl
885.x	Traumatic amputation of thumb
886.x	Traumatic finger amputation
887.x	Traumatic arm/hand amputation
890.x	Open wound of hip and thigh
891.x	Open wound of knee, leg, ankle
892.x	Open wound of foot
893.x	Open wound of toe(s)
894.x	Open wound of lower limb
895.x	Traumatic amputation of toe(s)
896.x	Traumatic amputation of foot
897.x	Traumatic amputation of leg(s)
905.0	Late effect, skull/face fracture
905.2	Late effect, arm fracture
905.4	Late effect, leg fracture
906.0	Late effect, open wound head/trunk
906.1	Late effect, open wound extremity
906.4	Late effect of crushing
906.5	Late effect of head/neck burn
906.6	Late effect of wrist/hand burn
906.7	Late effect of extremity burn NEC
906.8	Late effect of burns NEC
V50.1	Plastic surgery NEC
V51.	Aftercare w/plastic surgery

REIMBURSEMENT INFORMATION

General

- See notes on page 114.

Medicare

- Follow–Up Days — 90
- Assistant Surgeon — paid
- Supply Charges — not allowed
- Outpatient Limit — does not apply
- Major Surgery Rules Apply

CPT CODE	SERVICE
15760	Graft; composite (full thickness of external ear or nasal ala), including primary closure, donor area

CPT NOTES

- Repair of donor site requiring skin graft or local flaps should be reported as an additional procedure.

ICD–9–CM

872.01	Open wound of auricle
872.02	Open wound of auditory canal
872.11	Open wound of auricle, complicated
872.12	Open wound, auditory canal, complic
873.21	Open wound of nasal septum
873.22	Open wound of nasal cavity
873.31	Open wound nasal septum, complic
873.32	Open wound nasal cavity, complic

REIMBURSEMENT INFORMATION

General

- See notes on page 114.

Medicare

- Follow–Up Days — 90
- Assistant Surgeon — not paid
- Supply Charges — not allowed
- Outpatient Limit — does not apply
- Major Surgery Rules Apply

CPT CODE	SERVICE
15770	Graft; derma-fat-fascia

CPT NOTES

- ◆ Repair of donor site requiring skin graft or local flaps should be reported as an additional procedure.

ICD–9–CM

215.3	B-Neoplasm, Soft tissue, leg
350.8	Trigeminal nerve disorder NEC
374.10	Ectropion NOS
374.14	Cicatricial ectropion
374.41	Eyelid retraction or lag
384.21	Cent perforate tympanic membrane
384.22	Attic perforate tympanic membrane
384.23	Marginal perf tympanic membrane NEC
384.24	Multiple perfs tympanic membrane
384.25	Total perforate tympanic membrane
385.01	Tympanosclerosis, tympanic membrane
385.02	Tympanosclerosis, tympanic/ossicle
385.03	Tympanosclerosis, all parts
385.09	Tympanosclerosis, other site comb
385.31	Cholesteatoma of attic
385.32	Cholesteatoma of middle ear
385.33	Cholesteatoma, middle ear/mastoid
528.9	Oral soft tissue disease NEC
701.0	Circumscribed scleroderma
709.2	Scar/fibrosis of skin
722.10	Lumbar disc displacement
736.89	Other acquired limb deformity
738.0	Acquired nose deformity
738.10	Acquired head deformity NOS
744.9	Congenital face/neck anomaly NOS
754.0	Congen skull/face/jaw deformity
V48.6	Disfigurements of head
V48.7	Disfigurements of neck/trunk

REIMBURSEMENT INFORMATION

General

- ◆ See notes on page 114.

Medicare

- ◆ Follow–Up Days — 90
- ◆ Assistant Surgeon — paid
- ◆ Supply Charges — not allowed
- ◆ Outpatient Limit — does not apply
- ◆ Major Surgery Rules Apply

CPT CODE	SERVICE	ICD–9–CM	
15775	Punch graft for hair transplant; 1 to 15 punch grafts	704.00	Alopecia NOS
		704.01	Alopecia areata
		704.09	Alopecia NEC
15776	Punch graft for hair transplant; more than 15 punch grafts	906.5	Late effect of head/neck burn
		V50.0	Hair transplant
		V50.1	Plastic surgery NEC

CPT NOTES

- ♦ For strip transplant, use 15220.
- ♦ Repair of donor site requiring skin graft or local flaps should be reported as an additional procedure.

REIMBURSEMENT INFORMATION

General

- ♦ See notes on page 114.

Medicare

- ♦ Follow–Up Days — 0
- ♦ Assistant Surgeon — by report
- ♦ Supply Charges — not allowed
- ♦ Outpatient Limit — does not apply
- ♦ Minor Surgery Rules Apply

CPT CODE	SERVICE	ICD–9–CM	
15780	Dermabrasion; total face (eg, for acne scarring, fine wrinkling, rhytids, general keratosis)	692.79	Solar dermatitis NEC
		701.1	Keratoderma, acquired
		701.4	Keloid scar
15781	Dermabrasion; segmental, face	701.8	Hypertrophic/atrophic skin NEC
		706.1	Acne NEC
		709.00	Dyschromia, unspecified
		709.01	Vitiligo
		709.09	Other dyschromia
		709.2	Scar/fibrosis of skin
		V50.1	Plastic surgery NEC

REIMBURSEMENT INFORMATION

General

- ♦ See notes on page 114.

Medicare

- ♦ Follow–Up Days — 90
- ♦ Assistant Surgeon — not paid
- ♦ Supply Charges — not allowed
- ♦ Outpatient Limit — applies
- ♦ Major Surgery Rules Apply

CPT CODE	SERVICE	ICD–9–CM
15782	Dermabrasion; regional, other than face	692.79 Solar dermatitis NEC 701.1 Keratoderma, acquired 701.8 Hypertrophic/atrophic skin NEC 709.00 Dyschromia, unspecified 709.01 Vitiligo 709.09 Other dyschromia 709.2 Scar/fibrosis of skin V50.1 Plastic surgery NEC **REIMBURSEMENT INFORMATION** General ♦ See notes on page 114. Medicare ♦ Follow–Up Days — 90 ♦ Assistant Surgeon — not paid ♦ Supply Charges — not allowed ♦ Outpatient Limit — applies ♦ Major Surgery Rules Apply
15783	Dermabrasion; superficial, any site, (eg, tattoo removal)	701.1 Keratoderma, acquired 701.8 Hypertrophic/atrophic skin NEC 709.00 Dyschromia, unspecified 709.01 Vitiligo 709.09 Other dyschromia 709.2 Scar/fibrosis of skin **REIMBURSEMENT INFORMATION** General ♦ See notes on page 114. Medicare ♦ Follow–Up Days — 90 ♦ Assistant Surgeon — by report ♦ Supply Charges — not allowed ♦ Outpatient Limit — applies ♦ Major Surgery Rules Apply

CPT CODE	SERVICE	ICD–9–CM
15786*	Abrasion; single lesion (eg, keratosis, scar)	370.24 Photokeratitis 528.6 Leukoplakia of oral mucosa/tongue 700. Corns and callosities 701.1 Keratoderma, acquired 701.4 Keloid scar 701.8 Hypertrophic/atrophic skin NEC 709.00 Dyschromia, unspecified 709.01 Vitiligo 709.09 Other dyschromia 709.2 Scar/fibrosis of skin

REIMBURSEMENT INFORMATION

General

- ♦ See notes on page 114.
- ♦ Starred procedure.

Medicare

- ♦ Follow–Up Days — 10
- ♦ Assistant Surgeon — not paid
- ♦ Supply Charges — not allowed
- ♦ Outpatient Limit — applies
- ♦ Minor Surgery Rules Apply

CPT CODE	SERVICE	ICD–9–CM
15787	Abrasion; each additional four lesions or less	701.1 Keratoderma, acquired 701.4 Keloid scar 701.8 Hypertrophic/atrophic skin NEC 709.00 Dyschromia, unspecified 709.01 Vitiligo 709.09 Other dyschromia 709.2 Scar/fibrosis of skin V50.1 Plastic surgery NEC

REIMBURSEMENT INFORMATION

General

- ♦ See notes on page 114.

Medicare

- ♦ Follow–Up Days — none; falls within global period of another procedure
- ♦ Assistant Surgeon — not paid
- ♦ Supply Charges — not allowed
- ♦ Outpatient Limit — applies

CPT CODE	SERVICE	ICD-9-CM
15788	Chemical peel, facial; epidermal	701.8 Hypertrophic/atrophic skin NEC 702.x Other dermatosis 706.1 Acne NEC 709.00 Dyschromia, unspecified 709.01 Vitiligo 709.09 Other dyschromia 709.2 Scar/fibrosis of skin V50.1 Plastic surgery NEC
15789	Chemical peel, facial; dermal	

REIMBURSEMENT INFORMATION

General

- ♦ See notes on page 114.

Medicare

- ♦ Follow–Up Days — 90
- ♦ Assistant Surgeon — not paid
- ♦ Supply Charges — not allowed
- ♦ Outpatient Limit — does not apply
- ♦ Major Surgery Rules Apply

CPT CODE	SERVICE	ICD-9-CM
15792	Chemical peel, nonfacial; epidermal	701.8 Hypertrophic/atrophic skin NEC 702.x Other dermatosis 706.1 Acne NEC 709.00 Dyschromia, unspecified 709.01 Vitiligo 709.09 Other dyschromia 709.2 Scar/fibrosis of skin V50.1 Plastic surgery NEC
15793	Chemical peel, nonfacial; dermal	

REIMBURSEMENT INFORMATION

General

- ♦ See notes on page 114.

Medicare

- ♦ Follow–Up Days — 90
- ♦ Assistant Surgeon — not paid
- ♦ Supply Charges — not allowed
- ♦ Outpatient Limit — does not apply
- ♦ Major Surgery Rules Apply

CPT CODE	SERVICE
15820	Blepharoplasty, lower eyelid

ICD–9–CM

351.0	Bell's palsy
374.01	Senile entropion
374.02	Mechanical entropion
374.03	Spastic entropion
374.04	Cicatricial entropion
374.10	Ectropion NOS
374.11	Senile ectropion
374.14	Cicatricial ectropion
374.30	Ptosis of eyelid NOS
374.31	Paralytic ptosis
374.32	Myogenic ptosis
374.33	Mechanical ptosis
374.34	Blepharochalasis
374.41	Eyelid retraction or lag
374.46	Blepharophimosis
374.87	Dermatochalasis
701.8	Hypertrophic/atrophic skin NEC
743.62	Congenital eyelid deformity
V50.1	Plastic surgery NEC

REIMBURSEMENT INFORMATION

General

- See notes on page 114.

Medicare

- Follow–Up Days — 90
- Assistant Surgeon — not paid
- Supply Charges — not allowed
- Outpatient Limit — does not apply
- Major Surgery Rules Apply

CPT CODE	SERVICE
15821	Blepharoplasty, lower eyelid; with extensive herniated fat pad

ICD–9–CM

351.0	Bell's palsy
374.01	Senile entropion
374.02	Mechanical entropion
374.03	Spastic entropion
374.04	Cicatricial entropion
374.10	Ectropion NOS
374.11	Senile ectropion
374.14	Cicatricial ectropion
374.30	Ptosis of eyelid NOS
374.31	Paralytic ptosis
374.32	Myogenic ptosis
374.33	Mechanical ptosis
374.34	Blepharochalasis
374.87	Dermatochalasis
701.8	Hypertrophic/atrophic skin NEC
V50.1	Plastic surgery NEC

REIMBURSEMENT INFORMATION

General

- See notes on page 114.

Medicare

- Follow–Up Days — 90
- Assistant Surgeon — not paid
- Supply Charges — not allowed
- Outpatient Limit — does not apply
- Major Surgery Rules Apply

CPT CODE	SERVICE
15822	Blepharoplasty, upper eyelid

CPT NOTES

- For bilateral blepharoplasty, add modifier "-50" or 09950.
- See also 67916, 67917, 67923, 97924.

ICD–9–CM

173.1	M-Neoplasm, Skin of eyelid/canthus
351.0	Bell's palsy
368.40	Visual field defect NOS
370.34	Exposure keratoconjunctivitis
374.00	Entropion NOS
374.01	Senile entropion
374.02	Mechanical entropion
374.03	Spastic entropion
374.04	Cicatricial entropion
374.10	Ectropion NOS
374.11	Senile ectropion
374.12	Mechanical ectropion
374.13	Spastic ectropion
374.14	Cicatricial ectropion
374.30	Ptosis of eyelid NOS
374.31	Paralytic ptosis
374.32	Myogenic ptosis
374.33	Mechanical ptosis
374.34	Blepharochalasis
374.41	Eyelid retraction or lag
374.87	Dermatochalasis
701.8	Hypertrophic/atrophic skin NEC
709.2	Scar/fibrosis of skin
757.39	Skin anomaly NEC
V50.1	Plastic surgery NEC

REIMBURSEMENT INFORMATION

General

- See notes on page 114.

Medicare

- Follow–Up Days — 90
- Assistant Surgeon — not paid
- Supply Charges — not allowed
- Outpatient Limit — does not apply
- Major Surgery Rules Apply

CPT CODE **SERVICE**

15823 Blepharoplasty, upper eyelid; with excessive skin weighing down lid

CPT NOTES

- For bilateral blepharoplasty, add modifier "-50" or 09950.
- See also 67916, 67917, 67923, 97924.

ICD–9–CM

173.1	M-Neoplasm, Skin of eyelid/canthus
351.0	Bell's palsy
368.40	Visual field defect NOS
370.34	Exposure keratoconjunctivitis
374.00	Entropion NOS
374.01	Senile entropion
374.02	Mechanical entropion
374.03	Spastic entropion
374.04	Cicatricial entropion
374.10	Ectropion NOS
374.11	Senile ectropion
374.12	Mechanical ectropion
374.13	Spastic ectropion
374.14	Cicatricial ectropion
374.30	Ptosis of eyelid NOS
374.31	Paralytic ptosis
374.32	Myogenic ptosis
374.33	Mechanical ptosis
374.34	Blepharochalasis
374.41	Eyelid retraction or lag
374.87	Dermatochalasis
701.8	Hypertrophic/atrophic skin NEC
743.62	Congenital eyelid deformity
756.83	Ehlers-Danlos syndrome
V50.1	Plastic surgery NEC

REIMBURSEMENT INFORMATION

General

- See notes on page 114.

Medicare

- Follow–Up Days — 90
- Assistant Surgeon — not paid
- Supply Charges — not allowed
- Outpatient Limit — does not apply
- Major Surgery Rules Apply
- Fragments — 15822

CPT CODE SERVICE	ICD–9–CM
15824 Rhytidectomy; forehead **CPT NOTES** ◆ For repair of brow ptosis, see 67900. ◆ For bilateral rhytidectomy, add modifier "-50" or 09950.	351.0 Bell's palsy 374.30 Ptosis of eyelid NOS 374.33 Mechanical ptosis 701.8 Hypertrophic/atrophic skin NEC 951.4 Injury to facial nerve V50.1 Plastic surgery NEC **REIMBURSEMENT INFORMATION** General ◆ See notes on page 114. Medicare ◆ Follow–Up Days — global concept does not apply ◆ Assistant Surgeon — by report ◆ Supply Charges — not allowed ◆ Outpatient Limit — does not apply
15825 Rhytidectomy; neck with platysmal tightening (platysmal flap, 'P-flap') **CPT NOTES** ◆ For bilateral rhytidectomy, add modifier "-50" or 09950.	701.3 Striae atrophicae 701.8 Hypertrophic/atrophic skin NEC 701.9 Hypertrophic/atrophic skin NOS 709.2 Scar/fibrosis of skin 951.4 Injury to facial nerve V50.1 Plastic surgery NEC **REIMBURSEMENT INFORMATION** General ◆ See notes on page 114. Medicare ◆ Follow–Up Days — global concept does not apply ◆ Assistant Surgeon — by report ◆ Supply Charges — not allowed ◆ Outpatient Limit — does not apply
15826 Rhytidectomy; glabellar frown lines **CPT NOTES** ◆ For bilateral rhytidectomy, add modifier "-50" or 09950.	701.3 Striae atrophicae 701.8 Hypertrophic/atrophic skin NEC 701.9 Hypertrophic/atrophic skin NOS 951.4 Injury to facial nerve V50.1 Plastic surgery NEC **REIMBURSEMENT INFORMATION** General ◆ See notes on page 114. Medicare ◆ Follow–Up Days — global concept does not apply ◆ Assistant Surgeon — by report ◆ Supply Charges — not allowed ◆ Outpatient Limit — does not apply

CPT CODE	SERVICE	ICD-9-CM

15828 Rhytidectomy; cheek, chin, and neck

CPT NOTES

- For bilateral rhytidectomy, add modifier "-50" or 09950.

ICD-9-CM

272.6	Lipodystrophy
351.0	Bell's palsy
701.3	Striae atrophicae
701.8	Hypertrophic/atrophic skin NEC
701.9	Hypertrophic/atrophic skin NOS
906.0	Late effect, open wound head/trunk
951.4	Injury to facial nerve
V50.1	Plastic surgery NEC

REIMBURSEMENT INFORMATION

General

- See notes on page 114.

Medicare

- Follow–Up Days — global concept does not apply
- Assistant Surgeon — by report
- Supply Charges — not allowed
- Outpatient Limit — does not apply

15829 Rhytidectomy; superficial musculoaponeurotic system (SMAS) flap

CPT NOTES

- For bilateral rhytidectomy, add modifier "-50" or 09950.

272.6	Lipodystrophy
351.0	Bell's palsy
701.3	Striae atrophicae
701.8	Hypertrophic/atrophic skin NEC
701.9	Hypertrophic/atrophic skin NOS
906.0	Late effect, open wound head/trunk
951.4	Injury to facial nerve
V50.1	Plastic surgery NEC

REIMBURSEMENT INFORMATION

General

- See notes on page 114.

Medicare

- Follow–Up Days — global concept does not apply
- Assistant Surgeon — by report
- Supply Charges — not allowed
- Outpatient Limit — does not apply

CPT CODE	SERVICE	ICD–9–CM	
15831	Excision, excessive skin and subcutaneous tissue (including lipectomy); abdomen (abdominoplasty)	272.6	Lipodystrophy
		278.1	Localized adiposity
		701.3	Striae atrophicae
		701.8	Hypertrophic/atrophic skin NEC
15832	Excision, excessive skin and subcutaneous tissue (including lipectomy); thigh	701.9	Hypertrophic/atrophic skin NOS
		724.8	Other back symptoms
		729.30	Panniculitis, site unspecified
		729.39	Panniculitis, site NEC
		906.0	Late effect, open wound head/trunk
		V50.1	Plastic surgery NEC

CPT NOTES

- ♦ For bilateral procedure, add modifier "-50" or 09950.

REIMBURSEMENT INFORMATION

General

- ♦ See notes on page 114.

Medicare

- ♦ Follow–Up Days — 90
- ♦ Assistant Surgeon — paid
- ♦ Supply Charges — not allowed
- ♦ Outpatient Limit — does not apply
- ♦ Major Surgery Rules Apply

CPT CODE	SERVICE	ICD–9–CM	
15833	Excision, excessive skin and subcutaneous tissue (including lipectomy); leg	272.6	Lipodystrophy
		278.1	Localized adiposity
		701.3	Striae atrophicae
		701.8	Hypertrophic/atrophic skin NEC
		701.9	Hypertrophic/atrophic skin NOS
		729.31	Hypertrophy of fat pad, knee
		729.39	Panniculitis, site NEC
		V50.1	Plastic surgery NEC

CPT NOTES

- ♦ For bilateral procedure, add modifier "-50" or 09950.

REIMBURSEMENT INFORMATION

General

- ♦ See notes on page 114.

Medicare

- ♦ Follow–Up Days — 90
- ♦ Assistant Surgeon — by report
- ♦ Supply Charges — not allowed
- ♦ Outpatient Limit — does not apply
- ♦ Major Surgery Rules Apply

CPT CODE	SERVICE	ICD-9-CM	
15834	Excision, excessive skin and subcutaneous tissue (including lipectomy); hip	272.6	Lipodystrophy
		278.1	Localized adiposity
		701.3	Striae atrophicae
		701.8	Hypertrophic/atrophic skin NEC
		701.9	Hypertrophic/atrophic skin NOS
		729.39	Panniculitis, site NEC
		V50.1	Plastic surgery NEC

CPT NOTES

- ♦ For bilateral procedure, add modifier "-50" or 09950.

REIMBURSEMENT INFORMATION

General

- ♦ See notes on page 114.

Medicare

- ♦ Follow–Up Days — 90
- ♦ Assistant Surgeon — by report
- ♦ Supply Charges — not allowed
- ♦ Outpatient Limit — does not apply
- ♦ Major Surgery Rules Apply

CPT CODE	SERVICE	ICD-9-CM	
15835	Excision, excessive skin and subcutaneous tissue (including lipectomy); buttock	272.6	Lipodystrophy
15836	Excision, excessive skin and subcutaneous tissue (including lipectomy); arm	278.1	Localized adiposity
15837	Excision, excessive skin and subcutaneous tissue (including lipectomy); forearm or hand	701.3	Striae atrophicae
		701.8	Hypertrophic/atrophic skin NEC
		701.9	Hypertrophic/atrophic skin NOS
		729.39	Panniculitis, site NEC
		V50.1	Plastic surgery NEC

CPT NOTES

- ♦ For bilateral procedure, add modifier "-50" or 09950.

REIMBURSEMENT INFORMATION

General

- ♦ See notes on page 114.

Medicare

- ♦ Follow–Up Days — 90
- ♦ Assistant Surgeon — by report
- ♦ Supply Charges — not allowed
- ♦ Outpatient Limit — does not apply
- ♦ Major Surgery Rules Apply

CPT CODE	SERVICE	ICD-9-CM

15838 Excision, excessive skin and subcutaneous tissue (including lipectomy); submental fat pad

CPT NOTES

- For bilateral procedure, add modifier "-50" or 09950.

ICD-9-CM

272.6	Lipodystrophy
278.1	Localized adiposity
701.8	Hypertrophic/atrophic skin NEC
729.39	Panniculitis, site NEC
V50.1	Plastic surgery NEC

REIMBURSEMENT INFORMATION

General

- See notes on page 114.

Medicare

- Follow–Up Days — 90
- Assistant Surgeon — by report
- Supply Charges — not allowed
- Outpatient Limit — does not apply
- Major Surgery Rules Apply

15839 Excision, excessive skin and subcutaneous tissue (including lipectomy); other area

CPT NOTES

- For bilateral procedure, add modifier "-50" or 09950.

ICD-9-CM

272.6	Lipodystrophy
278.1	Localized adiposity
701.8	Hypertrophic/atrophic skin NEC
V50.1	Plastic surgery NEC

REIMBURSEMENT INFORMATION

General

- See notes on page 114.

Medicare

- Follow–Up Days — 90
- Assistant Surgeon — not paid
- Supply Charges — not allowed
- Outpatient Limit — does not apply
- Major Surgery Rules Apply

15840 Graft for facial nerve paralysis; free fascia graft (including obtaining fascia)

CPT NOTES

- For bilateral procedure, add modifier "-50" or 09950.
- For intravenous fluorescein examination of blood flow in graft or flap, see 15860.
- For nerve transfers, decompression, or repair, see 64830-64876, 64905, 64907, 69720, 69725, 69740, 69745, 69955.

ICD-9-CM

351.0	Bell's palsy
352.6	Multiple cranial nerve palsy
767.5	Facial nerve injury at birth
951.4	Injury to facial nerve
V48.6	Disfigurements of head

REIMBURSEMENT INFORMATION

General

- See notes on page 114.

Medicare

- Follow–Up Days — 90
- Assistant Surgeon — paid
- Supply Charges — not allowed
- Outpatient Limit — does not apply
- Major Surgery Rules Apply

CPT CODE	SERVICE	ICD–9–CM

15841 Graft for facial nerve paralysis; free muscle graft (including obtaining graft)

CPT NOTES

- For intravenous fluorescein examination of blood flow in graft or flap, see 15860.
- For nerve transfers, decompression, or repair, see 64830-64876, 64905, 64907, 69720, 69725, 69740, 69745, 69955.

351.0	Bell's palsy
352.6	Multiple cranial nerve palsy
374.12	Mechanical ectropion
767.5	Facial nerve injury at birth
951.4	Injury to facial nerve
V48.6	Disfigurements of head

REIMBURSEMENT INFORMATION

General

- See notes on page 114.

Medicare

- Follow–Up Days — 90
- Assistant Surgeon — paid
- Supply Charges — not allowed
- Outpatient Limit — does not apply
- Major Surgery Rules Apply

15842 Graft for facial nerve paralysis; free muscle graft by microsurgical technique

CPT NOTES

- For intravenous fluorescein examination of blood flow in graft or flap, see 15860.
- For nerve transfers, decompression, or repair, see 64830-64876, 64905, 64907, 69720, 69725, 69740, 69745, 69955.

351.0	Bell's palsy
352.6	Multiple cranial nerve palsy
767.5	Facial nerve injury at birth
951.4	Injury to facial nerve
V48.6	Disfigurements of head

REIMBURSEMENT INFORMATION

General

- See notes on page 114.

Medicare

- Follow–Up Days — 90
- Assistant Surgeon — paid
- Supply Charges — not allowed
- Outpatient Limit — does not apply
- Major Surgery Rules Apply

15845 Graft for facial nerve paralysis; regional muscle transfer

CPT NOTES

- For intravenous fluorescein examination of blood flow in graft or flap, see 15860.
- For nerve transfers, decompression, or repair, see 64830-64876, 64905, 64907, 69720, 69725, 69740, 69745, 69955.

351.0	Bell's palsy
374.12	Mechanical ectropion
767.5	Facial nerve injury at birth

REIMBURSEMENT INFORMATION

General

- See notes on page 114.

Medicare

- Follow–Up Days — 90
- Assistant Surgeon — paid
- Supply Charges — not allowed
- Outpatient Limit — does not apply
- Major Surgery Rules Apply

CPT CODE	SERVICE	ICD–9–CM
15850	Removal of sutures under anesthesia (other than local), same surgeon	V58.3 Attention to surg dressing/suture
15851	Removal of sutures under anesthesia (other than local), other surgeon	

REIMBURSEMENT INFORMATION

General

- See notes on page 114.

Medicare

- Follow–Up Days — global concept does not apply
- Assistant Surgeon — not paid
- Supply Charges — not allowed
- Outpatient Limit — does not apply

CPT CODE	SERVICE	ICD-9-CM	
15852	Dressing change (for other than burns) under anesthesia (other than local)	140.0	M-Neoplasm, Upper lip, vermilion
		140.1	M-Neoplasm, Lower lip, vermilion
		140.3	M-Neoplasm, Upper lip, inner aspect
		140.4	M-Neoplasm, Lower lip, inner aspect
		140.5	M-Neoplasm, Lip NOS, inner NOS
		140.6	M-Neoplasm, lip, commissure
		140.8	M-Neoplasm, Lip NEC
		140.9	M-Neoplasm, Lip/vermilion NOS
		172.x	Skin Melanoma
		173.x	Malignant neoplasm, Skin
		216.x	Benign neoplasm, Skin
		232.x	Carcinoma in situ, Skin
		707.x	Chronic ulcer of skin
		709.2	Scar/fibrosis of skin
		744.23	Microtia
		744.3	Ear anomaly NOS
		870.0	Laceration eyelid skin/periocular
		872.01	Open wound of auricle
		872.11	Open wound of auricle, complicated
		873.0	Open wound of scalp
		873.1	Open wound of scalp, complicated
		873.21	Open wound of nasal septum
		873.31	Open wound nasal septum, complic
		873.4x	Face, open wound
		873.5x	Face, complicated open wound
		875.0	Open wound of chest
		875.1	Open wound of chest, complicated
		876.0	Open wound of back
		876.1	Open wound of back, complicated
		877.0	Open wound of buttock
		877.1	Open wound of buttock, complicated
		878.0	Open wound of penis
		878.1	Open wound of penis, complicated
		878.2	Open wound of scrotum/testes
		878.3	Open wound, scrotum/testes, compl
		878.4	Open wound of vulva
		878.5	Open wound of vulva, complicated
		878.6	Open wound of vagina
		878.7	Open wound of vagina, complicated
		879.0	Open wound of breast
		879.1	Open wound of breast, complicated
		879.2	Open wound of anterior abdomen
		879.3	Open wound anterior abdomen, compl
		879.4	Open wound of lateral abdomen
		879.5	Open wound lateral abdomen, compl
		879.6	Open wound of trunk NEC
		879.7	Open wound of trunk NEC, complic
		880.00	Open wound of shoulder
		880.01	Open wound of scapula
		880.02	Open wound of axilla
		880.03	Open wound of upper arm
		880.09	Multiple open wounds of shoulder
		880.10	Open wound of shoulder, complicated
		880.11	Open wound of scapula, complicated
		880.12	Open wound of axilla, complicated
		880.13	Open wound of upper arm, complic

CPT CODE	SERVICE	ICD-9-CM
15852 (Cont'd.)		

880.19	Mult open wounds of shoulder, compl
881.0x	Elbow/forearm/wrist open wound
881.1x	Elbow/forearm/wrist complex wound
882.0	Open wound of hand
882.1	Open wound of hand, complicated
883.0	Open wound of finger
883.1	Open wound of finger, complicated
884.0	Open wound of arm, mult/NOS
884.1	Open wound of arm mult/NOS, compl
885.x	Traumatic amputation of thumb
886.x	Traumatic finger amputation
887.x	Traumatic arm/hand amputation
890.x	Open wound of hip and thigh
891.x	Open wound of knee, leg, ankle
892.x	Open wound of foot
893.x	Open wound of toe(s)
894.x	Open wound of lower limb
895.x	Traumatic amputation of toe(s)
896.x	Traumatic amputation of foot
897.x	Traumatic amputation of leg(s)
V50.1	Plastic surgery NEC
V51.	Aftercare w/plastic surgery
V58.3	Attention to surg dressing/suture

REIMBURSEMENT INFORMATION

General

- See notes on page 114.

Medicare

- Follow–Up Days — 0
- Assistant Surgeon — not paid
- Supply Charges — not allowed
- Outpatient Limit — applies
- Minor Surgery Rules Apply

CPT CODE	SERVICE	ICD-9-CM	
15860	Intravenous injection of agent (eg, fluorescein) to test blood flow in flap or graft	140.0	M-Neoplasm, Upper lip, vermilion
		140.1	M-Neoplasm, Lower lip, vermilion
		140.3	M-Neoplasm, Upper lip, inner aspect
		140.4	M-Neoplasm, Lower lip, inner aspect
		140.5	M-Neoplasm, Lip NOS, inner NOS
		140.6	M-Neoplasm, lip, commissure
		140.8	M-Neoplasm, Lip NEC
		140.9	M-Neoplasm, Lip/vermilion NOS
		172.x	Skin Melanoma
		173.x	Malignant neoplasm, Skin
		216.x	Benign neoplasm, Skin
		232.x	Carcinoma in situ, Skin
		707.x	Chronic ulcer of skin
		709.2	Scar/fibrosis of skin
		744.23	Microtia
		744.3	Ear anomaly NOS
		870.0	Laceration eyelid skin/periocular
		872.01	Open wound of auricle
		872.11	Open wound of auricle, complicated
		873.0	Open wound of scalp
		873.1	Open wound of scalp, complicated
		873.21	Open wound of nasal septum
		873.31	Open wound nasal septum, complic
		873.4x	Face, open wound
		873.5x	Face, complicated open wound
		875.0	Open wound of chest
		875.1	Open wound of chest, complicated
		876.0	Open wound of back
		876.1	Open wound of back, complicated
		877.0	Open wound of buttock
		877.1	Open wound of buttock, complicated
		878.0	Open wound of penis
		878.1	Open wound of penis, complicated
		878.2	Open wound of scrotum/testes
		878.3	Open wound, scrotum/testes, compl
		878.4	Open wound of vulva
		878.5	Open wound of vulva, complicated
		878.6	Open wound of vagina
		878.7	Open wound of vagina, complicated
		879.0	Open wound of breast
		879.1	Open wound of breast, complicated
		879.2	Open wound of anterior abdomen
		879.3	Open wound anterior abdomen, compl
		879.4	Open wound of lateral abdomen
		879.5	Open wound lateral abdomen, compl
		880.00	Open wound of shoulder
		880.01	Open wound of scapula
		880.02	Open wound of axilla
		880.03	Open wound of upper arm
		880.09	Multiple open wounds of shoulder
		880.10	Open wound of shoulder, complicated
		880.11	Open wound of scapula, complicated
		880.12	Open wound of axilla, complicated
		880.13	Open wound of upper arm, complic
		880.19	Mult open wounds of shoulder, compl
		881.0x	Elbow/forearm/wrist open wound

CPT CODE	SERVICE	ICD–9–CM	
15860 (Cont'd.)		881.1x	Elbow/forearm/wrist complex wound
		882.0	Open wound of hand
		882.1	Open wound of hand, complicated
		883.0	Open wound of finger
		883.1	Open wound of finger, complicated
		884.0	Open wound of arm, mult/NOS
		884.1	Open wound of arm mult/NOS, compl
		885.x	Traumatic amputation of thumb
		886.x	Traumatic finger amputation
		887.x	Traumatic arm/hand amputation
		890.x	Open wound of hip and thigh
		891.x	Open wound of knee, leg, ankle
		892.x	Open wound of foot
		893.x	Open wound of toe(s)
		894.x	Open wound of lower limb
		895.x	Traumatic amputation of toe(s)
		896.x	Traumatic amputation of foot
		897.x	Traumatic amputation of leg(s)
		V50.1	Plastic surgery NEC
		V51.	Aftercare w/plastic surgery
		V58.3	Attention to surg dressing/suture

REIMBURSEMENT INFORMATION

General

- See notes on page 114.

Medicare

- Follow–Up Days — 0
- Assistant Surgeon — not paid
- Supply Charges — not allowed
- Outpatient Limit — does not apply
- Minor Surgery Rules Apply

CPT CODE	SERVICE	ICD–9–CM
15876	Suction assisted lipectomy; head and neck	214.0 Lipoma, Skin of face 272.6 Lipodystrophy 278.0 Obesity 278.1 Localized adiposity 738.10 Acquired head deformity NOS 738.19 Acquired head deformity NEC 738.2 Acquired neck deformity

REIMBURSEMENT INFORMATION

General

- ♦ See notes on page 114.

Medicare

- ♦ Follow–Up Days — global concept does not apply
- ♦ Assistant Surgeon — by report
- ♦ Supply Charges — not allowed
- ♦ Outpatient Limit — does not apply

CPT CODE	SERVICE	ICD–9–CM
15877	Suction assisted lipectomy; trunk	214.1 Lipoma, Skin NEC 272.6 Lipodystrophy 278.0 Obesity 278.1 Localized adiposity 738.3 Acquired chest/rib deformity 738.5 Other acquired back/spine deformity 738.6 Acquired pelvic deformity

REIMBURSEMENT INFORMATION

General

- ♦ See notes on page 114.

Medicare

- ♦ Follow–Up Days — global concept does not apply
- ♦ Assistant Surgeon — by report
- ♦ Supply Charges — not allowed
- ♦ Outpatient Limit — does not apply

CPT CODE	SERVICE	ICD-9-CM
15878 **15879**	Suction assisted lipectomy; upper extremity Suction assisted lipectomy; lower extremity	214.1 Lipoma, Skin NEC 272.6 Lipodystrophy 278.0 Obesity 278.1 Localized adiposity **REIMBURSEMENT INFORMATION** General ◆ See notes on page 114. Medicare ◆ Follow–Up Days — global concept does not apply ◆ Assistant Surgeon — by report ◆ Supply Charges — not allowed ◆ Outpatient Limit — does not apply
15920 **15922**	Excision, coccygeal pressure ulcer, with coccygectomy; with primary suture Excision, coccygeal pressure ulcer, with coccygectomy; with flap closure	707.0 Decubitus ulcer 707.8 Chronic skin ulcer NEC 730.05 Acute osteomyelitis, pelvis/thigh 730.15 Chronic osteomyelitis, pelvis/thigh **REIMBURSEMENT INFORMATION** General ◆ See notes on page 114. Medicare ◆ Follow–Up Days — 90 ◆ Assistant Surgeon — not paid ◆ Supply Charges — not allowed ◆ Outpatient Limit — does not apply ◆ Major Surgery Rules Apply
15931	Excision, sacral pressure ulcer, with primary suture	707.0 Decubitus ulcer 707.8 Chronic skin ulcer NEC **REIMBURSEMENT INFORMATION** General ◆ See notes on page 114. Medicare ◆ Follow–Up Days — 90 ◆ Assistant Surgeon — not paid ◆ Supply Charges — not allowed ◆ Outpatient Limit — does not apply ◆ Major Surgery Rules Apply

CPT CODE	SERVICE	ICD–9–CM
15933	Excision, sacral pressure ulcer, with primary suture; with ostectomy	707.0 Decubitus ulcer 707.8 Chronic skin ulcer NEC 730.05 Acute osteomyelitis, pelvis/thigh 730.15 Chronic osteomyelitis, pelvis/thigh **REIMBURSEMENT INFORMATION** General ◆ See notes on page 114. Medicare ◆ Follow–Up Days — 90 ◆ Assistant Surgeon — by report ◆ Supply Charges — not allowed ◆ Outpatient Limit — does not apply ◆ Major Surgery Rules Apply
15934	Excision, sacral pressure ulcer, with skin flap closure	707.0 Decubitus ulcer 707.8 Chronic skin ulcer NEC **REIMBURSEMENT INFORMATION** General ◆ See notes on page 114. Medicare ◆ Follow–Up Days — 90 ◆ Assistant Surgeon — not paid ◆ Supply Charges — not allowed ◆ Outpatient Limit — does not apply ◆ Major Surgery Rules Apply
15935	Excision, sacral pressure ulcer, with skin flap closure; with ostectomy	707.0 Decubitus ulcer 707.8 Chronic skin ulcer NEC 730.05 Acute osteomyelitis, pelvis/thigh 730.15 Chronic osteomyelitis, pelvis/thigh **REIMBURSEMENT INFORMATION** General ◆ See notes on page 114. Medicare ◆ Follow–Up Days — 90 ◆ Assistant Surgeon — paid ◆ Supply Charges — not allowed ◆ Outpatient Limit — does not apply ◆ Major Surgery Rules Apply

CPT CODE	SERVICE	ICD-9-CM	
15936	Excision, sacral pressure ulcer, with muscle or myocutaneous flap closure	707.0	Decubitus ulcer
		707.8	Chronic skin ulcer NEC

CPT NOTES

- To identify muscle or myocutaneous flap closure, use also code number for specific flap.

REIMBURSEMENT INFORMATION

General

- See notes on page 114.

Medicare

- Follow-Up Days — 90
- Assistant Surgeon — paid
- Supply Charges — not allowed
- Outpatient Limit — does not apply
- Major Surgery Rules Apply

CPT CODE	SERVICE	ICD-9-CM	
15937	Excision, sacral pressure ulcer, with muscle or myocutaneous flap closure; with ostectomy	707.0	Decubitus ulcer
		707.8	Chronic skin ulcer NEC
		730.05	Acute osteomyelitis, pelvis/thigh
		730.15	Chronic osteomyelitis, pelvis/thigh

CPT NOTES

- To identify muscle or myocutaneous flap closure, use also code number for specific flap.

REIMBURSEMENT INFORMATION

General

- See notes on page 114.

Medicare

- Follow-Up Days — 90
- Assistant Surgeon — paid
- Supply Charges — not allowed
- Outpatient Limit — does not apply
- Major Surgery Rules Apply

CPT CODE	SERVICE	ICD-9-CM	
15940	Excision, ischial pressure ulcer, with primary suture	707.0	Decubitus ulcer
		707.8	Chronic skin ulcer NEC

REIMBURSEMENT INFORMATION

General

- See notes on page 114.

Medicare

- Follow-Up Days — 90
- Assistant Surgeon — not paid
- Supply Charges — not allowed
- Outpatient Limit — does not apply
- Major Surgery Rules Apply

CPT CODE	SERVICE	ICD–9–CM
15941	Excision, ischial pressure ulcer, with primary suture; with ostectomy (ischiectomy)	707.0 Decubitus ulcer 707.8 Chronic skin ulcer NEC 730.05 Acute osteomyelitis, pelvis/thigh 730.15 Chronic osteomyelitis, pelvis/thigh **REIMBURSEMENT INFORMATION** <u>General</u> ♦ See notes on page 114. <u>Medicare</u> ♦ Follow–Up Days — 90 ♦ Assistant Surgeon — not paid ♦ Supply Charges — not allowed ♦ Outpatient Limit — does not apply ♦ Major Surgery Rules Apply
15944	Excision, ischial pressure ulcer, with skin flap closure	707.0 Decubitus ulcer 707.8 Chronic skin ulcer NEC **REIMBURSEMENT INFORMATION** <u>General</u> ♦ See notes on page 114. <u>Medicare</u> ♦ Follow–Up Days — 90 ♦ Assistant Surgeon — paid ♦ Supply Charges — not allowed ♦ Outpatient Limit — does not apply ♦ Major Surgery Rules Apply
15945	Excision, ischial pressure ulcer, with skin flap closure; with ostectomy	707.0 Decubitus ulcer 707.8 Chronic skin ulcer NEC 730.05 Acute osteomyelitis, pelvis/thigh 730.15 Chronic osteomyelitis, pelvis/thigh **REIMBURSEMENT INFORMATION** <u>General</u> ♦ See notes on page 114. <u>Medicare</u> ♦ Follow–Up Days — 90 ♦ Assistant Surgeon — paid ♦ Supply Charges — not allowed ♦ Outpatient Limit — does not apply ♦ Major Surgery Rules Apply

CPT CODE	SERVICE	ICD-9-CM
15946	Excision, ischial pressure ulcer, with ostectomy, with muscle or myocutaneous flap closure **CPT NOTES** ◆ To identify muscle or myocutaneous flap closure, use also code number for specific flap.	707.0 Decubitus ulcer 707.8 Chronic skin ulcer NEC 730.05 Acute osteomyelitis, pelvis/thigh 730.15 Chronic osteomyelitis, pelvis/thigh **REIMBURSEMENT INFORMATION** General ◆ See notes on page 114. Medicare ◆ Follow–Up Days — 90 ◆ Assistant Surgeon — paid ◆ Supply Charges — not allowed ◆ Outpatient Limit — does not apply ◆ Major Surgery Rules Apply
15950	Excision, trochanteric pressure ulcer, with primary suture	707.0 Decubitus ulcer 707.8 Chronic skin ulcer NEC **REIMBURSEMENT INFORMATION** General ◆ See notes on page 114. Medicare ◆ Follow–Up Days — 90 ◆ Assistant Surgeon — not paid ◆ Supply Charges — not allowed ◆ Outpatient Limit — does not apply ◆ Major Surgery Rules Apply
15951	Excision, trochanteric pressure ulcer, with primary suture; with ostectomy	707.0 Decubitus ulcer 707.8 Chronic skin ulcer NEC 730.05 Acute osteomyelitis, pelvis/thigh 730.15 Chronic osteomyelitis, pelvis/thigh **REIMBURSEMENT INFORMATION** General ◆ See notes on page 114. Medicare ◆ Follow–Up Days — 90 ◆ Assistant Surgeon — paid ◆ Supply Charges — not allowed ◆ Outpatient Limit — does not apply ◆ Major Surgery Rules Apply

CPT CODE	SERVICE	ICD-9-CM
15952	Excision, trochanteric pressure ulcer, with skin flap closure	707.0 Decubitus ulcer 707.8 Chronic skin ulcer NEC **REIMBURSEMENT INFORMATION** General ♦ See notes on page 114. Medicare ♦ Follow–Up Days — 90 ♦ Assistant Surgeon — paid ♦ Supply Charges — not allowed ♦ Outpatient Limit — does not apply ♦ Major Surgery Rules Apply
15953	Excision, trochanteric pressure ulcer, with skin flap closure; with ostectomy	707.0 Decubitus ulcer 707.8 Chronic skin ulcer NEC 730.05 Acute osteomyelitis, pelvis/thigh 730.15 Chronic osteomyelitis, pelvis/thigh **REIMBURSEMENT INFORMATION** General ♦ See notes on page 114. Medicare ♦ Follow–Up Days — 90 ♦ Assistant Surgeon — paid ♦ Supply Charges — not allowed ♦ Outpatient Limit — does not apply ♦ Major Surgery Rules Apply
15956	Excision, trochanteric pressure ulcer, with muscle or myocutaneous flap closure **CPT NOTES** ♦ To identify muscle or myocutaneous flap closure, use also code number for specific flap.	707.0 Decubitus ulcer 707.8 Chronic skin ulcer NEC **REIMBURSEMENT INFORMATION** General ♦ See notes on page 114. Medicare ♦ Follow–Up Days — 90 ♦ Assistant Surgeon — paid ♦ Supply Charges — not allowed ♦ Outpatient Limit — does not apply ♦ Major Surgery Rules Apply

CPT CODE	SERVICE	ICD-9-CM

15958 Excision, trochanteric pressure ulcer, with muscle or myocutaneous flap closure; with ostectomy

CPT NOTES

- ◆ To identify muscle or myocutaneous flap closure, use also code number for specific flap.

707.0	Decubitus ulcer
707.8	Chronic skin ulcer NEC
730.05	Acute osteomyelitis, pelvis/thigh
730.15	Chronic osteomyelitis, pelvis/thigh

REIMBURSEMENT INFORMATION

General

- ◆ See notes on page 114.

Medicare

- ◆ Follow–Up Days — 90
- ◆ Assistant Surgeon — paid
- ◆ Supply Charges — not allowed
- ◆ Outpatient Limit — does not apply
- ◆ Major Surgery Rules Apply

15999 Unlisted procedure, excision pressure ulcer

CPT NOTES

- ◆ For free skin graft to close ulcer or donor site, see 15000 et seq.

707.0	Decubitus ulcer
707.8	Chronic skin ulcer NEC
730.05	Acute osteomyelitis, pelvis/thigh
730.15	Chronic osteomyelitis, pelvis/thigh

REIMBURSEMENT INFORMATION

General

- ◆ See notes on page 114.

Medicare

- ◆ Follow–Up Days — determined by local carrier
- ◆ Assistant Surgeon — paid
- ◆ Supply Charges — determined by local carrier
- ◆ Outpatient Limit — determined by local carrier

CPT CODE	SERVICE
16000	Initial treatment, first degree burn, when no more than local treatment is required

CPT NOTES

- Procedure refers to local treatment of burned surface only.
- List percentage of body surface involved and depth of burn.
- For necessary related medical services, (e.g., hospital visits, detention) in management of burned patients, see appropriate services in Evaluation and Management and Medicine sections.
- For skin grafts, see 15100-15650.

ICD–9–CM

940.0	Chemical burn, eyelid/periocular
940.1	Burn, eyelid/periocular area NEC
940.9	Burn of eye/adnexa NOS
941.10	1st deg burn, face/head/unspec
941.11	1st deg burn, ear
941.12	Erythema, eye
941.13	1st deg burn, lip
941.14	1st deg burn, chin
941.15	1st deg burn, nose
941.16	1st deg burn, scalp
941.17	1st deg burn, face NEC
941.18	1st deg burn, neck
941.19	1st deg burn, head multiple sites
942.10	1st deg burn trunk NOS
942.11	1st deg burn trunk, breast
942.12	1st deg burn trunk, chest wall
942.13	1st deg burn trunk, abdominal wall
942.14	1st deg burn trunk, back
942.15	1st deg burn trunk, genitalia
942.19	1st deg burn trunk NEC
943.10	1st deg burn, arm NOS
943.11	1st deg burn, forearm
943.12	1st deg burn, elbow
943.13	1st deg burn, upper arm
943.14	1st deg burn, axilla
943.15	1st deg burn, shoulder
943.16	1st deg burn, scapula
943.19	1st deg burn, arm multiple sites
944.10	1st deg burn, hand NOS
944.11	1st deg burn, finger
944.12	1st deg burn, thumb
944.13	1st deg burn, mult fingers
944.14	1st deg burn, finger w/thumb
944.15	1st deg burn, palm
944.16	1st deg burn, back of hand
944.17	1st deg burn, wrist
944.18	1st deg burn, hand mult sites
945.10	1st deg burn, leg NOS
945.11	1st deg burn, toe
945.12	1st deg burn, foot
945.13	1st deg burn, ankle
945.14	1st deg burn, lower leg
945.15	1st deg burn, knee
945.16	1st deg burn, thigh
945.19	1st deg burn, leg mult sites
946.1	1st deg burn, multiple sites
949.1	1st degree burn NOS

CPT CODE	SERVICE	ICD–9–CM
16000 (Cont'd.)		

REIMBURSEMENT INFORMATION

General

- See notes on page 114.

Medicare

- Follow–Up Days — 0
- Assistant Surgeon — not paid
- Supply Charges — not allowed
- Outpatient Limit — applies
- Minor Surgery Rules Apply

CPT CODE	SERVICE	ICD-9-CM

16010 Dressings and/or debridement, initial or subsequent; under anesthesia, small

CPT NOTES

- Procedure refers to local treatment of burned surface only.
- List percentage of body surface involved and depth of burn.
- For necessary related medical services, (e.g., hospital visits, detention) in management of burned patients, see appropriate services in Evaluation and Management and Medicine sections.
- For skin grafts, see 15100-15650.

ICD-9-CM

940.x Burn confined to eye and adnexa
941.x Burn of face, head and neck
942.x Burn of trunk
943.x Burn of upper limb
944.x Burn of wrist and hand
945.x Burn of lower limb
946.x Burns of multiple sites
947.x Burn of internal organs
948.x Burns according to surface extent
949.x Burn NOS

REIMBURSEMENT INFORMATION

General

- See notes on page 114.

Medicare

- Follow-Up Days — 0
- Assistant Surgeon — not paid
- Supply Charges — not allowed
- Outpatient Limit — applies
- Minor Surgery Rules Apply

16015 Dressings and/or debridement, initial or subsequent; under anesthesia, medium or large with major debridement

CPT NOTES

- Procedure refers to local treatment of burned surface only.
- List percentage of body surface involved and depth of burn.
- For necessary related medical services, (e.g., hospital visits, detention) in management of burned patients, see appropriate services in Evaluation and Management and Medicine sections.
- For skin grafts, see 15100-15650.

ICD-9-CM

906.5 Late effect of head/neck burn
906.6 Late effect of wrist/hand burn
906.7 Late effect of extremity burn NEC
906.8 Late effect of burns NEC
940.x Burn confined to eye and adnexa
941.x Burn of face, head and neck
942.x Burn of trunk
943.x Burn of upper limb
944.x Burn of wrist and hand
945.x Burn of lower limb
946.x Burns of multiple sites
947.x Burn of internal organs
948.x Burns according to surface extent
949.x Burn NOS

REIMBURSEMENT INFORMATION

General

- See notes on page 114.

Medicare

- Follow-Up Days — 0
- Assistant Surgeon — not paid
- Supply Charges — not allowed
- Outpatient Limit — does not apply
- Minor Surgery Rules Apply

CPT CODE	SERVICE
16020*	Dressings and/or debridement, initial or subsequent; without anesthesia, office or hospital, small

CPT NOTES

- Procedure refers to local treatment of burned surface only.
- List percentage of body surface involved and depth of burn.
- For necessary related medical services, (e.g., hospital visits, detention) in management of burned patients, see appropriate services in Evaluation and Management and Medicine sections.
- For skin grafts, see 15100-15650.

ICD–9–CM

906.5	Late effect of head/neck burn
906.6	Late effect of wrist/hand burn
906.7	Late effect of extremity burn NEC
906.8	Late effect of burns NEC
940.0	Chemical burn, eyelid/periocular
940.x	Burn confined to eye and adnexa
941.x	Burn of face, head and neck
942.x	Burn of trunk
943.x	Burn of upper limb
944.x	Burn of wrist and hand
945.x	Burn of lower limb
946.x	Burns of multiple sites
947.x	Burn of internal organs
948.x	Burns according to surface extent
949.x	Burn NOS

REIMBURSEMENT INFORMATION

General

- See notes on page 114.
- Starred procedure.

Medicare

- Follow–Up Days — 0
- Assistant Surgeon — not paid
- Supply Charges — not allowed
- Outpatient Limit — applies
- Minor Surgery Rules Apply

CPT CODE / SERVICE	ICD-9-CM
16025* Dressings and/or debridement, initial or subsequent; without anesthesia, medium (eg, whole face or whole extremity) **16030** Dressings and/or debridement, initial or subsequent; without anesthesia, large (eg, more than one extremity) **CPT NOTES** ♦ Procedure refers to local treatment of burned surface only. ♦ List percentage of body surface involved and depth of burn. ♦ For necessary related medical services, (e.g., hospital visits, detention) in management of burned patients, see appropriate services in Evaluation and Management and Medicine sections. ♦ For skin grafts, see 15100-15650.	906.5 Late effect of head/neck burn 906.6 Late effect of wrist/hand burn 906.7 Late effect of extremity burn NEC 906.8 Late effect of burns NEC 940.x Burn confined to eye and adnexa 941.x Burn of face, head and neck 942.x Burn of trunk 943.x Burn of upper limb 944.x Burn of wrist and hand 945.x Burn of lower limb 946.x Burns of multiple sites 947.x Burn of internal organs 948.x Burns according to surface extent 949.x Burn NOS **REIMBURSEMENT INFORMATION** General ♦ See notes on page 114. ♦ Starred procedure. (16025) Medicare ♦ Follow–Up Days — 0 ♦ Assistant Surgeon — not paid ♦ Supply Charges — not allowed ♦ Outpatient Limit — applies ♦ Minor Surgery Rules Apply
16035 Escharotomy **CPT NOTES** ♦ Procedure refers to local treatment of burned surface only. ♦ List percentage of body surface involved and depth of burn. ♦ For necessary related medical services, (e.g., hospital visits, detention) in management of burned patients, see appropriate services in Evaluation and Management and Medicine sections. ♦ For skin grafts, see 15100-15650.	940.x Burn confined to eye and adnexa 941.x Burn of face, head and neck 942.x Burn of trunk 943.x Burn of upper limb 944.x Burn of wrist and hand 945.x Burn of lower limb 946.x Burns of multiple sites 947.x Burn of internal organs 948.x Burns according to surface extent 949.x Burn NOS **REIMBURSEMENT INFORMATION** General ♦ See notes on page 114. Medicare ♦ Follow–Up Days — 90 ♦ Assistant Surgeon — not paid ♦ Supply Charges — not allowed ♦ Outpatient Limit — does not apply ♦ Major Surgery Rules Apply

CPT CODE	SERVICE	ICD–9–CM

16040 Excision burn wound, without skin grafting, employing alloplastic dressing (eg, synthetic mesh), any anatomic site; less than one percent total body surface area

16041 Excision burn wound, without skin grafting, employing alloplastic dressing (eg, synthetic mesh), any anatomic site; greater than one percent and less than nine percent total body surface area

CPT NOTES

- Procedure refers to local treatment of burned surface only.
- List percentage of body surface involved and depth of burn.
- For necessary related medical services, (e.g., hospital visits, detention) in management of burned patients, see appropriate services in Evaluation and Management and Medicine sections.
- For skin grafts, see 15100-15650.
- For debridement, curettement of burn wound, see 16010-16030.

ICD–9–CM

906.5	Late effect of head/neck burn
906.6	Late effect of wrist/hand burn
906.7	Late effect of extremity burn NEC
906.8	Late effect of burns NEC
940.x	Burn confined to eye and adnexa
941.x	Burn of face, head and neck
942.x	Burn of trunk
943.x	Burn of upper limb
944.x	Burn of wrist and hand
945.x	Burn of lower limb
946.x	Burns of multiple sites
947.x	Burn of internal organs
948.00	Burn, 0-10% surface, 0-9% 3rd deg
949.x	Burn NOS

REIMBURSEMENT INFORMATION

General

- See notes on page 114.

Medicare

- Follow–Up Days — 0
- Assistant Surgeon — by report
- Supply Charges — not allowed
- Outpatient Limit — does not apply
- Minor Surgery Rules Apply

16042 Excision burn wound, without skin grafting, employing alloplastic dressing (eg, synthetic mesh), any anatomic site; each additional nine percent total body surface area, or part thereof

CPT NOTES

- Procedure refers to local treatment of burned surface only.
- List percentage of body surface involved and depth of burn.
- For necessary related medical services, (e.g., hospital visits, detention) in management of burned patients, see appropriate services in Evaluation and Management and Medicine sections.
- For skin grafts, see 15100-15650.
- For debridement, curettement of burn wound, see 16010-16030.

906.5	Late effect of head/neck burn
906.6	Late effect of wrist/hand burn
906.7	Late effect of extremity burn NEC
906.8	Late effect of burns NEC
940.x	Burn confined to eye and adnexa
941.x	Burn of face, head and neck
942.x	Burn of trunk
943.x	Burn of upper limb
944.x	Burn of wrist and hand
945.x	Burn of lower limb
946.x	Burns of multiple sites
947.x	Burn of internal organs
948.x	Burns according to surface extent
949.x	Burn NOS

REIMBURSEMENT INFORMATION

General

- See notes on page 114.

Medicare

- Follow–Up Days — 0
- Assistant Surgeon — by report
- Supply Charges — not allowed
- Outpatient Limit — does not apply
- Minor Surgery Rules Apply

CPT CODE **SERVICE**

17000* Destruction by any method, including laser, with or without surgical curettement, all benign facial lesions or premalignant lesions in any location, or benign lesions other than cutaneous vascular proliferative lesions, including local anesthesia; one lesion

CPT NOTES

- Destruction means the ablation of benign, premalignant or malignant tissues by any method, with or without curettement, including local anesthesia, and not usually requiring closure. Any method includes electrocautery, electrodesiccation, cryosurgery, laser and chemical treatment. Lesions include condylomata, papillomata, molluscum contagiosum, herpetic lesions, flat (plane, juvenile) warts, milia, or other benign, pre-malignant, or malignant lesions.
- For sharp removal of skin tags and fibrocutaneous lesions, see codes 11200, 11201.
- For electrosurgical destruction of skin tags, see codes 17200, 17201.
- For destruction of malignant skin lesions, see 17260-17286.
- For cryotherapy of acne, use 17340.

ICD-9-CM

078.10	Viral warts NOS
210.0	B-Neoplasm, Lip
215.0	B-Neoplasm, Soft tissue, head
215.6	B-Neoplasm, Soft tissue, pelvis
216.0	B-Neoplasm, Skin of lip
216.1	B-Neoplasm, Skin of eyelid/canthus
216.2	B-Neoplasm, Skin of ear
216.3	B-Neoplasm, Skin of face NEC
216.5	B-Neoplasm, Skin of trunk
221.2	B-Neoplasm, Vulva
228.1	Lymphangioma, any site
232.0	CA in situ, Skin of lip
232.1	CA in situ, Eyelid/canthus
232.3	CA in situ, Skin of face NEC
232.4	CA in situ, Scalp/skin of neck
232.5	CA in situ, Skin of trunk
232.6	CA in situ, Skin of arm
232.7	CA in situ, Skin of leg
232.8	CA in situ, Skin NEC
235.1	UB-Neoplasm, Oral cavity/pharynx
238.2	UB-Neoplasm, Skin
239.2	Bone/Skin neoplasm NOS
373.2	Chalazion
374.05	Trichiasis w/o entropion
374.84	Cysts of eyelids
448.1	Nevus, non-neoplastic
528.5	Diseases of lips
528.9	Oral soft tissue disease NEC
690.	Erythematosquamous dermatosis
692.70	Solar dermatitis NOS
692.79	Solar dermatitis NEC
695.3	Rosacea
698.3	Lichenification
701.4	Keloid scar
702.x	Other dermatosis
709.2	Scar/fibrosis of skin
709.3	Degenerative skin disorders
709.8	Skin disorders NEC
709.9	Skin disorder NOS

REIMBURSEMENT INFORMATION

General

- Starred procedure.

Medicare

- Follow–Up Days — 10
- Assistant Surgeon — not paid
- Supply Charges — not allowed
- Outpatient Limit — applies
- Minor Surgery Rules Apply

CPT CODE	SERVICE
17001	Destruction by any method, including laser, with or without surgical curettement, all benign facial lesions or premalignant lesions in any location, or benign lesions other than cutaneous vascular proliferative lesions, including local anesthesia; second and third lesions, each

CPT NOTES

- Destruction means the ablation of benign, premalignant or malignant tissues by any method, with or without curettement, including local anesthesia, and not usually requiring closure. Any method includes electrocautery, electrodesiccation, cryosurgery, laser and chemical treatment. Lesions include condylomata, papillomata, molluscum contagiosum, herpetic lesions, flat (plane, juvenile) warts, milia, or other benign, pre-malignant, or malignant lesions.
- For sharp removal of skin tags and fibrocutaneous lesions, see codes 11200, 11201.
- For electrosurgical destruction of skin tags, see codes 17200, 17201.
- For destruction of malignant skin lesions, see 17260-17286.
- For cryotherapy of acne, use 17340.

ICD–9–CM

078.10	Viral warts NOS
210.0	B-Neoplasm, Lip
215.0	B-Neoplasm, Soft tissue, head
215.6	B-Neoplasm, Soft tissue, pelvis
216.0	B-Neoplasm, Skin of lip
216.1	B-Neoplasm, Skin of eyelid/canthus
216.2	B-Neoplasm, Skin of ear
216.3	B-Neoplasm, Skin of face NEC
216.5	B-Neoplasm, Skin of trunk
221.2	B-Neoplasm, Vulva
228.1	Lymphangioma, any site
232.0	CA in situ, Skin of lip
232.1	CA in situ, Eyelid/canthus
232.2	CA in situ, Skin of ear
232.3	CA in situ, Skin of face NEC
232.5	CA in situ, Skin of trunk
232.6	CA in situ, Skin of arm
232.7	CA in situ, Skin of leg
232.8	CA in situ, Skin NEC
235.1	UB-Neoplasm, Oral cavity/pharynx
238.2	UB-Neoplasm, Skin
239.2	Bone/Skin neoplasm NOS
374.84	Cysts of eyelids
448.1	Nevus, non-neoplastic
528.5	Diseases of lips
528.9	Oral soft tissue disease NEC
690.	Erythematosquamous dermatosis
692.70	Solar dermatitis NOS
692.79	Solar dermatitis NEC
695.3	Rosacea
698.3	Lichenification
701.1	Keratoderma, acquired
701.4	Keloid scar
702.x	Other dermatosis
709.2	Scar/fibrosis of skin
709.3	Degenerative skin disorders
709.8	Skin disorders NEC
709.9	Skin disorder NOS

REIMBURSEMENT INFORMATION

Medicare

- Follow–Up Days — none; falls within global period of another procedure
- Assistant Surgeon — not paid
- Supply Charges — not allowed
- Outpatient Limit — applies

CPT CODE	SERVICE
17002	Destruction by any method, including laser, with or without surgical curettement, all benign facial lesions or premalignant lesions in any location, or benign lesions other than cutaneous vascular proliferative lesions, including local anesthesia; over three lesions, each additional

CPT NOTES

- Destruction means the ablation of benign, premalignant or malignant tissues by any method, with or without curettement, including local anesthesia, and not usually requiring closure. Any method includes electrocautery, electrodesiccation, cryosurgery, laser and chemical treatment. Lesions include condylomata, papillomata, molluscum contagiosum, herpetic lesions, flat (plane, juvenile) warts, milia, or other benign, pre-malignant, or malignant lesions.
- For sharp removal of skin tags and fibrocutaneous lesions, see codes 11200, 11201.
- For electrosurgical destruction of skin tags, see codes 17200, 17201.
- For destruction of malignant skin lesions, see 17260-17286.
- For cryotherapy of acne, use 17340.

ICD–9–CM

078.10	Viral warts NOS
210.0	B-Neoplasm, Lip
215.0	B-Neoplasm, Soft tissue, head
215.6	B-Neoplasm, Soft tissue, pelvis
216.0	B-Neoplasm, Skin of lip
216.1	B-Neoplasm, Skin of eyelid/canthus
216.2	B-Neoplasm, Skin of ear
216.3	B-Neoplasm, Skin of face NEC
216.5	B-Neoplasm, Skin of trunk
221.2	B-Neoplasm, Vulva
228.1	Lymphangioma, any site
232.0	CA in situ, Skin of lip
232.1	CA in situ, Eyelid/canthus
232.3	CA in situ, Skin of face NEC
232.4	CA in situ, Scalp/skin of neck
232.5	CA in situ, Skin of trunk
232.6	CA in situ, Skin of arm
232.7	CA in situ, Skin of leg
232.8	CA in situ, Skin NEC
235.1	UB-Neoplasm, Oral cavity/pharynx
238.2	UB-Neoplasm, Skin
239.2	Bone/Skin neoplasm NOS
448.1	Nevus, non-neoplastic
528.5	Diseases of lips
528.9	Oral soft tissue disease NEC
690.	Erythematosquamous dermatosis
692.70	Solar dermatitis NOS
692.79	Solar dermatitis NEC
695.3	Rosacea
698.3	Lichenification
701.1	Keratoderma, acquired
701.4	Keloid scar
702.x	Other dermatosis
709.2	Scar/fibrosis of skin
709.3	Degenerative skin disorders
709.8	Skin disorders NEC
709.9	Skin disorder NOS

REIMBURSEMENT INFORMATION

Medicare

- Follow–Up Days — none; falls within global period of another procedure
- Assistant Surgeon — not paid
- Supply Charges — not allowed
- Outpatient Limit — applies

CPT CODE	SERVICE
17010	Destruction by any method, including laser, with or without surgical curettement, all benign facial lesions or premalignant lesions in any location, or benign lesions other than cutaneous vascular proliferative lesions, including local anesthesia; complicated lesion(s)

CPT NOTES

- Destruction means the ablation of benign, premalignant or malignant tissues by any method, with or without curettement, including local anesthesia, and not usually requiring closure. Any method includes electrocautery, electrodesiccation, cryosurgery, laser and chemical treatment. Lesions include condylomata, papillomata, molluscum contagiosum, herpetic lesions, flat (plane, juvenile) warts, milia, or other benign, pre-malignant, or malignant lesions.
- For sharp removal of skin tags and fibrocutaneous lesions, see codes 11200, 11201.
- For electrosurgical destruction of skin tags, see codes 17200, 17201.
- For destruction of malignant skin lesions, see 17260-17286.
- For cryotherapy of acne, use 17340.

ICD–9–CM

210.0	B-Neoplasm, Lip
215.0	B-Neoplasm, Soft tissue, head
215.6	B-Neoplasm, Soft tissue, pelvis
216.0	B-Neoplasm, Skin of lip
216.1	B-Neoplasm, Skin of eyelid/canthus
216.2	B-Neoplasm, Skin of ear
216.3	B-Neoplasm, Skin of face NEC
216.5	B-Neoplasm, Skin of trunk
221.2	B-Neoplasm, Vulva
228.1	Lymphangioma, any site
232.0	CA in situ, Skin of lip
232.1	CA in situ, Eyelid/canthus
232.3	CA in situ, Skin of face NEC
232.4	CA in situ, Scalp/skin of neck
232.5	CA in situ, Skin of trunk
232.6	CA in situ, Skin of arm
232.7	CA in situ, Skin of leg
232.8	CA in situ, Skin NEC
235.1	UB-Neoplasm, Oral cavity/pharynx
238.2	UB-Neoplasm, Skin
239.2	Bone/Skin neoplasm NOS
375.56	Acquired nasolacrimal duct stenosis
448.1	Nevus, non-neoplastic
528.5	Diseases of lips
528.9	Oral soft tissue disease NEC
690.	Erythematosquamous dermatosis
692.70	Solar dermatitis NOS
692.79	Solar dermatitis NEC
695.3	Rosacea
698.3	Lichenification
701.1	Keratoderma, acquired
702.x	Other dermatosis
709.2	Scar/fibrosis of skin
709.3	Degenerative skin disorders
709.8	Skin disorders NEC
709.9	Skin disorder NOS

REIMBURSEMENT INFORMATION

Medicare

- Follow–Up Days — 10
- Assistant Surgeon — not paid
- Supply Charges — not allowed
- Outpatient Limit — applies
- Minor Surgery Rules Apply

CPT CODE **SERVICE**

17100* Destruction by any method, including laser, of benign skin lesions other than cutaneous vascular proliferative lesions on any area other than the face, including local anesthesia; one lesion

CPT NOTES

- Destruction means the ablation of benign, premalignant or malignant tissues by any method, with or without curettement, including local anesthesia, and not usually requiring closure. Any method includes electrocautery, electrodesiccation, cryosurgery, laser and chemical treatment. Lesions include condylomata, papillomata, molluscum contagiosum, herpetic lesions, flat (plane, juvenile) warts, milia, or other benign, pre-malignant, or malignant lesions.
- For sharp removal of skin tags and fibrocutaneous lesions, see codes 11200, 11201.
- For electrosurgical destruction of skin tags, see codes 17200, 17201.
- For destruction of malignant skin lesions, see 17260-17286.
- For cryotherapy of acne, use 17340.

ICD–9–CM

078.10	Viral warts NOS
091.3	Secondary syphilis, skin
111.0	Pityriasis versicolor
216.1	B-Neoplasm, Skin of eyelid/canthus
216.4	B-Neoplasm, Scalp/skin of neck
216.5	B-Neoplasm, Skin of trunk
216.6	B-Neoplasm, Skin of arm
216.7	B-Neoplasm, Skin of leg
216.8	B-Neoplasm, Skin NEC
216.9	B-Neoplasm, Skin NOS
232.7	CA in situ, Skin of leg
239.2	Bone/Skin neoplasm NOS
370.24	Photokeratitis
686.1	Pyogenic granuloma
690.	Erythematosquamous dermatosis
691.8	Other atopic dermatitis
695.3	Rosacea
698.3	Lichenification
701.4	Keloid scar
702.x	Other dermatosis
706.1	Acne NEC
709.8	Skin disorders NEC
757.39	Skin anomaly NEC
757.9	Integument anomaly NOS

REIMBURSEMENT INFORMATION

General

- Starred procedure.

Medicare

- Follow–Up Days — 10
- Assistant Surgeon — not paid
- Supply Charges — not allowed
- Outpatient Limit — applies
- Minor Surgery Rules Apply

CPT CODE	SERVICE
17101	Destruction by any method, including laser, of benign skin lesions other than cutaneous vascular proliferative lesions on any area other than the face, including local anesthesia; second lesion
17102	Destruction by any method, including laser, of benign skin lesions other than cutaneous vascular proliferative lesions on any area other than the face, including local anesthesia; over two lesions, each additional lesion up to 15 lesions
17104	Destruction by any method, including laser, of benign skin lesions other than cutaneous vascular proliferative lesions on any area other than the face, including local anesthesia; 15 or more lesions
17105	Destruction by any method, including laser, of benign skin lesions other than cutaneous vascular proliferative lesions on any area other than the face, including local anesthesia; complicated or extensive lesions

CPT NOTES

- Destruction means the ablation of benign, premalignant or malignant tissues by any method, with or without curettement, including local anesthesia, and not usually requiring closure. Any method includes electrocautery, electrodesiccation, cryosurgery, laser and chemical treatment. Lesions include condylomata, papillomata, molluscum contagiosum, herpetic lesions, flat (plane, juvenile) warts, milia, or other benign, pre-malignant, or malignant lesions.
- For sharp removal of skin tags and fibrocutaneous lesions, see codes 11200, 11201.
- For electrosurgical destruction of skin tags, see codes 17200, 17201.
- For destruction of malignant skin lesions, see 17260-17286.
- For cryotherapy of acne, use 17340.

ICD–9–CM

091.3	Secondary syphilis, skin
111.0	Pityriasis versicolor
215.7	B-Neoplasm, Trunk NOS
216.4	B-Neoplasm, Scalp/skin of neck
216.5	B-Neoplasm, Skin of trunk
216.6	B-Neoplasm, Skin of arm
216.7	B-Neoplasm, Skin of leg
216.8	B-Neoplasm, Skin NEC
216.9	B-Neoplasm, Skin NOS
229.8	Benign neoplasm NEC
232.7	CA in situ, Skin of leg
370.24	Photokeratitis
690.	Erythematosquamous dermatosis
691.8	Other atopic dermatitis
695.3	Rosacea
698.3	Lichenification
701.4	Keloid scar
702.x	Other dermatosis
706.1	Acne NEC
709.8	Skin disorders NEC
709.9	Skin disorder NOS
757.39	Skin anomaly NEC
757.9	Integument anomaly NOS

REIMBURSEMENT INFORMATION

Medicare

- Follow–Up Days — none; falls within global period of another procedure
- Assistant Surgeon — not paid
- Supply Charges — not allowed
- Outpatient Limit — applies

CPT CODE	SERVICE	ICD-9-CM
17106	Destruction of cutaneous vascular proliferative lesions (eg, laser technique); less than 10 sq cm	228.00 Hemangioma NOS 228.01 Hemangioma, Skin 228.1 Lymphangioma, any site 448.1 Nevus, non-neoplastic 448.9 Capillary disease NEC/NOS 757.32 Vascular hamartomas
17107	Destruction of cutaneous vascular proliferative lesions (eg, laser technique); 10.0 - 50.0 sq cm	
17108	Destruction of cutaneous vascular proliferative lesions (eg, laser technique); over 50.0 sq cm	

CPT NOTES

- Destruction means the ablation of benign, premalignant or malignant tissues by any method, with or without curettement, including local anesthesia, and not usually requiring closure. Any method includes electrocautery, electrodesiccation, cryosurgery, laser and chemical treatment. Lesions include condylomata, papillomata, molluscum contagiosum, herpetic lesions, flat (plane, juvenile) warts, milia, or other benign, pre-malignant, or malignant lesions.
- For sharp removal of skin tags and fibrocutaneous lesions, see codes 11200, 11201.
- For electrosurgical destruction of skin tags, see codes 17200, 17201.
- For destruction of malignant skin lesions, see 17260-17286.
- For cryotherapy of acne, use 17340.

REIMBURSEMENT INFORMATION

Medicare

- Follow-Up Days — 90
- Assistant Surgeon — not paid
- Supply Charges — not allowed
- Outpatient Limit — applies
- Major Surgery Rules Apply

CPT CODE	SERVICE	ICD-9-CM
17110*	Destruction by any method of flat (plane, juvenile) warts or molluscum contagiosum, milia, up to 15 lesions	078.0 Molluscum contagiosum 078.10 Viral warts NOS 374.84 Cysts of eyelids

CPT NOTES

- Destruction means the ablation of benign, premalignant or malignant tissues by any method, with or without curettement, including local anesthesia, and not usually requiring closure. Any method includes electrocautery, electrodesiccation, cryosurgery, laser and chemical treatment. Lesions include condylomata, papillomata, molluscum contagiosum, herpetic lesions, flat (plane, juvenile) warts, milia, or other benign, pre-malignant, or malignant lesions.
- For sharp removal of skin tags and fibrocutaneous lesions, see codes 11200, 11201.
- For electrosurgical destruction of skin tags, see codes 17200, 17201.
- For destruction of malignant skin lesions, see 17260-17286.
- For cryotherapy of acne, use 17340.
- Retreatment same as office visit.

REIMBURSEMENT INFORMATION

General

- Starred procedure.

Medicare

- Follow-Up Days — 10
- Assistant Surgeon — not paid
- Supply Charges — not allowed
- Outpatient Limit — applies
- Minor Surgery Rules Apply

CPT CODE	SERVICE
17200*	Electrosurgical destruction of multiple fibrocutaneous tags; up to 15 lesions
17201	Electrosurgical destruction of multiple fibrocutaneous tags; each additional ten lesions

CPT NOTES

- Destruction means the ablation of benign, premalignant or malignant tissues by any method, with or without curettement, including local anesthesia, and not usually requiring closure. Any method includes electrocautery, electrodesiccation, cryosurgery, laser and chemical treatment. Lesions include condylomata, papillomata, molluscum contagiosum, herpetic lesions, flat (plane, juvenile) warts, milia, or other benign, pre-malignant, or malignant lesions.
- For sharp removal of skin tags and fibrocutaneous lesions, see codes 11200, 11201.
- For electrosurgical destruction of skin tags, see codes 17200, 17201.
- For destruction of malignant skin lesions, see 17260-17286.
- For cryotherapy of acne, use 17340.
- For excision of fibrocutaneous tags, see 11200, 11201.

ICD–9–CM

216.1	B-Neoplasm, Skin of eyelid/canthus
216.2	B-Neoplasm, Skin of ear
216.3	B-Neoplasm, Skin of face NEC
216.4	B-Neoplasm, Scalp/skin of neck
216.5	B-Neoplasm, Skin of trunk
216.6	B-Neoplasm, Skin of arm
216.7	B-Neoplasm, Skin of leg
216.8	B-Neoplasm, Skin NEC
216.9	B-Neoplasm, Skin NOS
701.1	Keratoderma, acquired
701.2	Acquired acanthosis nigricans
701.8	Hypertrophic/atrophic skin NEC
701.9	Hypertrophic/atrophic skin NOS
709.9	Skin disorder NOS
757.39	Skin anomaly NEC

REIMBURSEMENT INFORMATION

General

- Starred procedure. (17200)

Medicare

- Follow–Up Days
  17200 — 10
  17201 — none; falls within global period of another procedure
- Assistant Surgeon — not paid
- Supply Charges — not allowed
- Outpatient Limit — applies
- Minor Surgery Rules Apply (17200)

CPT CODE **SERVICE**

17250* Chemical cauterization of granulation tissue (proud flesh, sinus or fistula)

CPT NOTES

- Destruction means the ablation of benign, premalignant or malignant tissues by any method, with or without curettement, including local anesthesia, and not usually requiring closure. Any method includes electrocautery, electrodesiccation, cryosurgery, laser and chemical treatment. Lesions include condylomata, papillomata, molluscum contagiosum, herpetic lesions, flat (plane, juvenile) warts, milia, or other benign, pre-malignant, or malignant lesions.
- For sharp removal of skin tags and fibrocutaneous lesions, see codes 11200, 11201.
- For electrosurgical destruction of skin tags, see codes 17200, 17201.
- For destruction of malignant skin lesions, see 17260-17286.
- For cryotherapy of acne, use 17340.
- Not to be used with removal or excision codes.

ICD–9–CM

078.10	Viral warts NOS
454.0	Leg varicosity w/ulcer
527.4	Salivary gland fistula
528.9	Oral soft tissue disease NEC
565.1	Anal fistula
685.1	Pilonidal cyst w/o abscess
686.1	Pyogenic granuloma
709.4	Foreign body granuloma, skin
822.0	Fracture of patella, closed
998.5	Postoperative infection
998.8	Surgical complications NEC

REIMBURSEMENT INFORMATION

General

- Starred procedure.

Medicare

- Follow–Up Days — 0
- Assistant Surgeon — not paid
- Supply Charges — not allowed
- Outpatient Limit — applies
- Minor Surgery Rules Apply

CPT CODE	SERVICE
17260*	Destruction, malignant lesion, any method, trunk, arms or legs; lesion diameter 0.5 cm or less
17261	Destruction, malignant lesion, any method, trunk, arms or legs; lesion diameter 0.6 to 1.0 cm
17262	Destruction, malignant lesion, any method, trunk, arms or legs; lesion diameter 1.1 to 2.0 cm
17263	Destruction, malignant lesion, any method, trunk, arms or legs; lesion diameter 2.1 to 3.0 cm
17264	Destruction, malignant lesion, any method, trunk, arms or legs; lesion diameter 3.1 to 4.0 cm
17266	Destruction, malignant lesion, any method, trunk, arms or legs; lesion diameter over 4.0 cm

CPT NOTES

- Destruction means the ablation of benign, premalignant or malignant tissues by any method, with or without curettement, including local anesthesia, and not usually requiring closure. Any method includes electrocautery, electrodesiccation, cryosurgery, laser and chemical treatment. Lesions include condylomata, papillomata, molluscum contagiosum, herpetic lesions, flat (plane, juvenile) warts, milia, or other benign, pre-malignant, or malignant lesions.
- For sharp removal of skin tags and fibrocutaneous lesions, see codes 11200, 11201.
- For electrosurgical destruction of skin tags, see codes 17200, 17201.
- For destruction of malignant skin lesions, see 17260-17286.
- For cryotherapy of acne, use 17340.

ICD–9–CM

172.5	Malignant melanoma, Trunk
172.6	Malignant melanoma, Arm
172.7	Malignant melanoma, Leg
172.8	Malignant melanoma, Skin NEC
173.5	M-Neoplasm, Skin of trunk
173.6	M-Neoplasm, Skin of arm
173.7	M-Neoplasm, Skin of leg
173.8	M-Neoplasm, Skin NEC
173.9	M-Neoplasm, Skin NOS
174.0	M-Neoplasm, Female nipple
174.1	M-Neoplasm, Female breast, central
174.2	M-Neoplasm, Female breast, up/inner
174.3	M-Neoplasm, Female breast low/inner
174.4	M-Neoplasm, Female breast, up/outer
174.5	M-Neoplasm, Female breast low/outer
174.6	M-Neoplasm, Female breast, axillary
174.8	M-Neoplasm, Female breast NEC
175.0	M-Neoplasm, Male nipple
175.9	M-Neoplasm, Male breast NOS
176.0	Kaposi's sarcoma, skin
176.1	Kaposi's sarcoma, soft tissue

REIMBURSEMENT INFORMATION

General

- Starred procedure. (17260)

Medicare

- Follow–Up Days — 10
- Assistant Surgeon — not paid
- Supply Charges — not allowed
- Outpatient Limit — applies
- Minor Surgery Rules Apply

CPT CODE	SERVICE
17270*	Destruction, malignant lesion, any method, scalp, neck, hands, feet, genitalia; lesion diameter 0.5 cm or less
17271	Destruction, malignant lesion, any method, scalp, neck, hands, feet, genitalia; lesion diameter 0.6 to 1.0 cm
17272	Destruction, malignant lesion, any method, scalp, neck, hands, feet, genitalia; lesion diameter 1.1 to 2.0 cm
17273	Destruction, malignant lesion, any method, scalp, neck, hands, feet, genitalia; lesion diameter 2.1 to 3.0 cm
17274	Destruction, malignant lesion, any method, scalp, neck, hands, feet, genitalia; lesion diameter 3.1 to 4.0 cm
17276	Destruction, malignant lesion, any method, scalp, neck, hands, feet, genitalia; lesion diameter over 4.0 cm

CPT NOTES

- ♦ Destruction means the ablation of benign, premalignant or malignant tissues by any method, with or without curettement, including local anesthesia, and not usually requiring closure. Any method includes electrocautery, electrodesiccation, cryosurgery, laser and chemical treatment. Lesions include condylomata, papillomata, molluscum contagiosum, herpetic lesions, flat (plane, juvenile) warts, milia, or other benign, pre-malignant, or malignant lesions.
- ♦ For sharp removal of skin tags and fibrocutaneous lesions, see codes 11200, 11201.
- ♦ For electrosurgical destruction of skin tags, see codes 17200, 17201.
- ♦ For destruction of malignant skin lesions, see 17260-17286.
- ♦ For cryotherapy of acne, use 17340.

ICD-9-CM

172.4	Malignant melanoma, Scalp/neck
172.5	Malignant melanoma, Trunk
172.6	Malignant melanoma, Arm
172.7	Malignant melanoma, Leg
172.8	Malignant melanoma, Skin NEC
173.4	M-Neoplasm, Scalp/skin neck
173.5	M-Neoplasm, Skin of trunk
173.6	M-Neoplasm, Skin of arm
173.7	M-Neoplasm, Skin of leg
173.8	M-Neoplasm, Skin NEC
184.2	M-Neoplasm, Labia minora
184.3	M-Neoplasm, Clitoris
184.4	M-Neoplasm, Vulva NOS
184.8	M-Neoplasm, Female genital NEC
187.1	M-Neoplasm, Prepuce
187.2	M-Neoplasm, Glans penis
187.3	M-Neoplasm, Penis body
187.4	M-Neoplasm, Penis NOS
187.5	M-Neoplasm, Epididymis
187.6	M-Neoplasm, Spermatic cord
187.7	M-Neoplasm, Scrotum
187.8	M-Neoplasm, Male genital NEC

REIMBURSEMENT INFORMATION

General

- ♦ Starred procedure. (17270)

Medicare

- ♦ Follow–Up Days — 10
- ♦ Assistant Surgeon — not paid
- ♦ Supply Charges — not allowed
- ♦ Outpatient Limit — applies
- ♦ Minor Surgery Rules Apply

CPT CODE	SERVICE
17280*	Destruction, malignant lesion, any method, face, ears, eyelids, nose, lips, mucous membrane; lesion diameter 0.5 cm or less

CPT NOTES

- Destruction means the ablation of benign, premalignant or malignant tissues by any method, with or without curettement, including local anesthesia, and not usually requiring closure. Any method includes electrocautery, electrodesiccation, cryosurgery, laser and chemical treatment. Lesions include condylomata, papillomata, molluscum contagiosum, herpetic lesions, flat (plane, juvenile) warts, milia, or other benign, pre-malignant, or malignant lesions.
- For sharp removal of skin tags and fibrocutaneous lesions, see codes 11200, 11201.
- For electrosurgical destruction of skin tags, see codes 17200, 17201.
- For destruction of malignant skin lesions, see 17260-17286.
- For cryotherapy of acne, use 17340.

ICD–9–CM

140.0	M-Neoplasm, Upper lip, vermilion
140.1	M-Neoplasm, Lower lip, vermilion
140.3	M-Neoplasm, Upper lip, inner aspect
140.4	M-Neoplasm, Lower lip, inner aspect
140.5	M-Neoplasm, Lip NOS, inner NOS
140.6	M-Neoplasm, lip, commissure
140.8	M-Neoplasm, Lip NEC
140.9	M-Neoplasm, Lip/vermilion NOS
141.x	Malignant neoplasm of tongue
143.x	Malignant neoplasm, Gum
144.x	Malignant neoplasm, Floor of mouth
145.x	Malignant neoplasm, Mouth NOS
172.0	Malignant melanoma, Lip
172.1	Malignant melanoma, eyelid/canthus
172.2	Malignant melanoma, Ear
172.3	Malignant melanoma, Face NEC/NOS
173.0	M-Neoplasm, Skin of lip
173.1	M-Neoplasm, Skin of eyelid/canthus
173.2	M-Neoplasm, Skin of ear
173.3	M-Neoplasm, Skin of face NEC

REIMBURSEMENT INFORMATION

General

- Starred procedure.

Medicare

- Follow–Up Days — 10
- Assistant Surgeon — not paid
- Supply Charges — not allowed
- Outpatient Limit — applies
- Minor Surgery Rules Apply

CPT CODE	SERVICE
17281	Destruction, malignant lesion, any method, face, ears, eyelids, nose, lips, mucous membrane; lesion diameter 0.6 to 1.0 cm
17282	Destruction, malignant lesion, any method, face, ears, eyelids, nose, lips, mucous membrane; lesion diameter 1.1 to 2.0 cm
17283	Destruction, malignant lesion, any method, face, ears, eyelids, nose, lips, mucous membrane; lesion diameter 2.1 to 3.0 cm
17284	Destruction, malignant lesion, any method, face, ears, eyelids, nose, lips, mucous membrane; lesion diameter 3.1 to 4.0 cm
17286	Destruction, malignant lesion, any method, face, ears, eyelids, nose, lips, mucous membrane; lesion diameter over 4.0 cm

CPT NOTES

- Destruction means the ablation of benign, premalignant or malignant tissues by any method, with or without curettement, including local anesthesia, and not usually requiring closure. Any method includes electrocautery, electrodesiccation, cryosurgery, laser and chemical treatment. Lesions include condylomata, papillomata, molluscum contagiosum, herpetic lesions, flat (plane, juvenile) warts, milia, or other benign, pre-malignant, or malignant lesions.
- For sharp removal of skin tags and fibrocutaneous lesions, see codes 11200, 11201.
- For electrosurgical destruction of skin tags, see codes 17200, 17201.
- For destruction of malignant skin lesions, see 17260-17286.
- For cryotherapy of acne, use 17340.

ICD–9–CM

140.x	Malignant neoplasm of lip
141.x	Malignant neoplasm of tongue
143.x	Malignant neoplasm, Gum
144.x	Malignant neoplasm, Floor of mouth
145.x	Malignant neoplasm, Mouth NOS
172.0	Malignant melanoma, Lip
172.1	Malignant melanoma, eyelid/canthus
172.2	Malignant melanoma, Ear
172.3	Malignant melanoma, Face NEC/NOS
173.0	M-Neoplasm, Skin of lip
173.1	M-Neoplasm, Skin of eyelid/canthus
173.2	M-Neoplasm, Skin of ear
173.3	M-Neoplasm, Skin of face NEC

REIMBURSEMENT INFORMATION

Medicare

- Follow–Up Days — 10
- Assistant Surgeon — not paid
- Supply Charges — not allowed
- Outpatient Limit — applies
- Minor Surgery Rules Apply

CPT CODE	SERVICE
▲ 17304	Chemosurgery (Mohs' micrographic technique); including removal of all gross tumor, surgical excision of tissue specimens, mapping, color coding of specimens, microscopic examination of specimens by the surgeon, and complete histopathologic preparation; first stage, fresh tissue technique, up to 5 specimens

CPT NOTES

- Destruction means the ablation of benign, premalignant or malignant tissues by any method, with or without curettement, including local anesthesia, and not usually requiring closure. Any method includes electrocautery, electrodesiccation, cryosurgery, laser and chemical treatment. Lesions include condylomata, papillomata, molluscum contagiosum, herpetic lesions, flat (plane, juvenile) warts, milia, or other benign, pre-malignant, or malignant lesions.
- For sharp removal of skin tags and fibrocutaneous lesions, see codes 11200, 11201.
- For electrosurgical destruction of skin tags, see codes 17200, 17201.
- For destruction of malignant skin lesions, see 17260-17286.
- For cryotherapy of acne, use 17340.
- Mohs' micrographic surgery, for the removal of complex or ill-defined skin cancer, requires a single physician to act in two integrated, but separate and distinct capacities: surgeon and pathologist. If either of these responsibilities are delegated to another physician who reports his services separately, these codes are not appropriate. If repair is performed, use separate repair, flap or graft codes.
- For initiation or follow-up care of topical chemotherapy (e.g., 5-FU or similar agents), see appropriate office visits.

ICD–9–CM

140.0	M-Neoplasm, Upper lip, vermilion
140.1	M-Neoplasm, Lower lip, vermilion
140.3	M-Neoplasm, Upper lip, inner aspect
140.4	M-Neoplasm, Lower lip, inner aspect
140.5	M-Neoplasm, Lip NOS, inner NOS
140.6	M-Neoplasm, lip, commissure
140.8	M-Neoplasm, Lip NEC
140.9	M-Neoplasm, Lip/vermilion NOS
171.0	M-Neoplasm, Soft tissue, head
172.x	Skin Melanoma
173.x	Malignant neoplasm, Skin
195.x	Malignant neoplasm, ill-defined
216.3	B-Neoplasm, Skin of face NEC
239.2	Bone/Skin neoplasm NOS
702.	Other dermatosis

REIMBURSEMENT INFORMATION

General

- Description changed in 1995 CPT.

Medicare

- Follow–Up Days — 0
- Assistant Surgeon — not paid
- Supply Charges — not allowed
- Outpatient Limit — applies
- Minor Surgery Rules Apply
- Fragments — 88300, 88302, 88304, 88305, 88307, 88309, 88331, 88332

CPT CODE	SERVICE
▲ 17305	Chemosurgery (Mohs' micrographic technique); including removal of all gross tumor, surgical excision of tissue specimens, mapping, color coding of specimens, microscopic examination of specimens by the surgeon, and complete histopathologic preparation; second stage, fixed or fresh tissue, up to 5 specimens
▲ 17306	Chemosurgery (Mohs' micrographic technique); including removal of all gross tumor, surgical excision of tissue specimens, mapping, color coding of specimens, microscopic examination of specimens by the surgeon, and complete histopathologic preparation; third stage, fixed or fresh tissue, up to 5 specimens
▲ 17307	Chemosurgery (Mohs' micrographic technique); including removal of all gross tumor, surgical excision of tissue specimens, mapping, color coding of specimens, microscopic examination of specimens by the surgeon, and complete histopathologic preparation; additional stage(s), up to 5 specimens, each stage
▲ 17310	Chemosurgery (Mohs' micrographic technique); including removal of all gross tumor, surgical excision of tissue specimens, mapping, color coding of specimens, microscopic examination of specimens by the surgeon, and complete histopathologic preparation; more than 5 specimens, fixed or fresh tissue, any stage

CPT NOTES

- Destruction means the ablation of benign, premalignant or malignant tissues by any method, with or without curettement, including local anesthesia, and not usually requiring closure. Any method includes electrocautery, electrodesiccation, cryosurgery, laser and chemical treatment. Lesions include condylomata, papillomata, molluscum contagiosum, herpetic lesions, flat (plane, juvenile) warts, milia, or other benign, pre-malignant, or malignant lesions.
- For sharp removal of skin tags and fibrocutaneous lesions, see codes 11200, 11201.
- For electrosurgical destruction of skin tags, see codes 17200, 17201.
- For destruction of malignant skin lesions, see 17260-17286.
- For cryotherapy of acne, use 17340.

(Cont'd. on next page.)

ICD–9–CM

140.0	M-Neoplasm, Upper lip, vermilion
140.1	M-Neoplasm, Lower lip, vermilion
140.3	M-Neoplasm, Upper lip, inner aspect
140.4	M-Neoplasm, Lower lip, inner aspect
140.5	M-Neoplasm, Lip NOS, inner NOS
140.6	M-Neoplasm, lip, commissure
140.8	M-Neoplasm, Lip NEC
140.9	M-Neoplasm, Lip/vermilion NOS
172.x	Skin Melanoma
173.x	Malignant neoplasm, Skin
195.x	Malignant neoplasm, ill-defined

REIMBURSEMENT INFORMATION

General

- Description changed in 1995 CPT.

Medicare

- Follow–Up Days — 0
- Assistant Surgeon — not paid
- Supply Charges — not allowed
- Outpatient Limit — applies
- Minor Surgery Rules Apply
- Fragments — 88300, 88302, 88304, 88305, 88307, 88309, 88331, 88332

CPT CODE SERVICE	ICD-9-CM
17305–17310 (Cont'd..) **CPT NOTES** (Cont'd. from previous page.) ♦ Mohs' micrographic surgery, for the removal of complex or ill-defined skin cancer, requires a single physician to act in two integrated, but separate and distinct capacities: surgeon and pathologist. If either of these responsibilities are delegated to another physician who reports his services separately, these codes are not appropriate. If repair is performed, use separate repair, flap or graft codes. ♦ For initiation or follow-up care of topical chemotherapy (e.g., 5-FU or similar agents), see appropriate office visits.	
17340* Cryotherapy (CO2 slush, liquid N2) for acne **CPT NOTES** ♦ Destruction means the ablation of benign, premalignant or malignant tissues by any method, with or without curettement, including local anesthesia, and not usually requiring closure. Any method includes electrocautery, electrodesiccation, cryosurgery, laser and chemical treatment. Lesions include condylomata, papillomata, molluscum contagiosum, herpetic lesions, flat (plane, juvenile) warts, milia, or other benign, pre-malignant, or malignant lesions. ♦ For sharp removal of skin tags and fibrocutaneous lesions, see codes 11200, 11201. ♦ For electrosurgical destruction of skin tags, see codes 17200, 17201. ♦ For destruction of malignant skin lesions, see 17260-17286. ♦ For cryotherapy of acne, use 17340.	695.3 Rosacea 706.0 Acne varioliformis 706.1 Acne NEC **REIMBURSEMENT INFORMATION** <u>General</u> ♦ Starred procedure. <u>Medicare</u> ♦ Follow-Up Days — 10 ♦ Assistant Surgeon — not paid ♦ Supply Charges — not allowed ♦ Outpatient Limit — applies ♦ Minor Surgery Rules Apply

CPT CODE	SERVICE	ICD–9–CM

17360* Chemical exfoliation for acne (eg, acne paste, acid)

CPT NOTES

- ♦ Destruction means the ablation of benign, premalignant or malignant tissues by any method, with or without curettement, including local anesthesia, and not usually requiring closure. Any method includes electrocautery, electrodesiccation, cryosurgery, laser and chemical treatment. Lesions include condylomata, papillomata, molluscum contagiosum, herpetic lesions, flat (plane, juvenile) warts, milia, or other benign, pre-malignant, or malignant lesions.
- ♦ For sharp removal of skin tags and fibrocutaneous lesions, see codes 11200, 11201.
- ♦ For electrosurgical destruction of skin tags, see codes 17200, 17201.
- ♦ For destruction of malignant skin lesions, see 17260-17286.
- ♦ For cryotherapy of acne, use 17340.

695.3 Rosacea
706.0 Acne varioliformis
706.1 Acne NEC

REIMBURSEMENT INFORMATION

General

- ♦ Starred procedure.

Medicare

- ♦ Follow–Up Days — 10
- ♦ Assistant Surgeon — not paid
- ♦ Supply Charges — not allowed
- ♦ Outpatient Limit — applies
- ♦ Minor Surgery Rules Apply

17380* Electrolysis epilation, each 1/2 hour

CPT NOTES

- ♦ Destruction means the ablation of benign, premalignant or malignant tissues by any method, with or without curettement, including local anesthesia, and not usually requiring closure. Any method includes electrocautery, electrodesiccation, cryosurgery, laser and chemical treatment. Lesions include condylomata, papillomata, molluscum contagiosum, herpetic lesions, flat (plane, juvenile) warts, milia, or other benign, pre-malignant, or malignant lesions.
- ♦ For sharp removal of skin tags and fibrocutaneous lesions, see codes 11200, 11201.
- ♦ For electrosurgical destruction of skin tags, see codes 17200, 17201.
- ♦ For destruction of malignant skin lesions, see 17260-17286.
- ♦ For cryotherapy of acne, use 17340.
- ♦ For actinotherapy, see 96900.

374.05 Trichiasis w/o entropion
704.1 Hirsutism

REIMBURSEMENT INFORMATION

General

- ♦ Starred procedure.

Medicare

- ♦ Follow–Up Days — global concept does not apply
- ♦ Assistant Surgeon — by report
- ♦ Supply Charges — not allowed
- ♦ Outpatient Limit — does not apply

CPT CODE	SERVICE	ICD-9-CM
17999	Unlisted procedure, skin, mucous membrane and subcutaneous tissue	448.1 Nevus, non-neoplastic 701.8 Hypertrophic/atrophic skin NEC 873.51 Open wound of cheek, complicated

CPT NOTES

- Destruction means the ablation of benign, premalignant or malignant tissues by any method, with or without curettement, including local anesthesia, and not usually requiring closure. Any method includes electrocautery, electrodesiccation, cryosurgery, laser and chemical treatment. Lesions include condylomata, papillomata, molluscum contagiosum, herpetic lesions, flat (plane, juvenile) warts, milia, or other benign, pre-malignant, or malignant lesions.
- For sharp removal of skin tags and fibrocutaneous lesions, see codes 11200, 11201.
- For electrosurgical destruction of skin tags, see codes 17200, 17201.
- For destruction of malignant skin lesions, see 17260-17286.
- For cryotherapy of acne, use 17340.

REIMBURSEMENT INFORMATION

Medicare

- Follow-Up Days — determined by local carrier
- Assistant Surgeon — determined by local carrier
- Supply Charges — determined by local carrier
- Outpatient Limit — determined by local carrier

19000* Puncture aspiration of cyst of breast

19001 Puncture aspiration of cyst of breast; each additional cyst

ICD-9-CM	
610.0	Solitary cyst of breast
610.1	Diffuse cystic mastopathy
610.2	Fibroadenosis of breast
610.3	Fibrosclerosis of breast
610.4	Mammary duct ectasia
610.8	Benign mammary dysplasia NEC
610.9	Benign mammary dysplasia NOS
611.3	Fat necrosis of breast
611.5	Galactocele
611.72	Lump or mass in breast
611.8	Absence of breast, acquired
793.8	Abnormal finding, breast
V10.3	Hx of breast malignancy
V16.3	Family Hx, breast malignancy

REIMBURSEMENT INFORMATION

General

- Starred procedure. (19000)

Medicare

- Follow-Up Days
  19000 — 0
  19001 — none; falls within global period of another procedure
- Assistant Surgeon — not paid
- Supply Charges — not allowed
- Outpatient Limit — applies
- Minor Surgery Rules Apply (19000)

CPT CODE	SERVICE	ICD-9-CM
19020	Mastotomy with exploration or drainage of abscess, deep	451.89 Thrombophlebitis NEC 611.0 Inflammatory disease of breast 611.72 Lump or mass in breast 675.10 Breast abscess preg, unspecified 675.11 Breast abscess preg, delivered 675.12 Breast abscess preg, delivered w/PP 675.13 Breast abscess preg, antepartum 675.14 Breast abscess preg, postpartum 998.5 Postoperative infection

REIMBURSEMENT INFORMATION

Medicare

- Follow–Up Days — 90
- Assistant Surgeon — not paid
- Supply Charges — not allowed
- Outpatient Limit — does not apply
- Major Surgery Rules Apply

CPT CODE	SERVICE	ICD-9-CM
19030	Injection procedure only for mammary ductogram or galactogram	611.5 Galactocele 611.6 Galactorrhea, non-obstetric 611.71 Mastodynia 611.72 Lump or mass in breast V76.1 Screening, malig neop, breast

CPT NOTES

- For radiological supervision and interpretation, see 76086, 76088.

REIMBURSEMENT INFORMATION

Medicare

- Follow–Up Days — 0
- Assistant Surgeon — not paid
- Supply Charges — not allowed
- Outpatient Limit — does not apply
- Minor Surgery Rules Apply

CPT CODE	SERVICE
19100*	Biopsy of breast; needle core (separate procedure)

CPT NOTES

- To report bilateral procedures, add modifier "-50" or 09950.
- For fine needle aspiration, use 88170.

ICD–9–CM

174.0	M-Neoplasm, Female nipple
174.1	M-Neoplasm, Female breast, central
174.2	M-Neoplasm, Female breast, up/inner
174.3	M-Neoplasm, Female breast low/inner
174.4	M-Neoplasm, Female breast, up/outer
174.5	M-Neoplasm, Female breast low/outer
174.6	M-Neoplasm, Female breast, axillary
174.8	M-Neoplasm, Female breast NEC
175.0	M-Neoplasm, Male nipple
175.9	M-Neoplasm, Male breast NOS
198.81	M2-Neoplasm, Breast
217.	Benign neoplasm, Breast
233.0	CA in situ, Breast
238.3	UB-Neoplasm, Breast
239.3	Breast Neoplasm NOS
610.0	Solitary cyst of breast
610.1	Diffuse cystic mastopathy
610.2	Fibroadenosis of breast
610.3	Fibrosclerosis of breast
610.4	Mammary duct ectasia
610.8	Benign mammary dysplasia NEC
610.9	Benign mammary dysplasia NOS
611.0	Inflammatory disease of breast
611.3	Fat necrosis of breast
611.5	Galactocele
611.6	Galactorrhea, non-obstetric
611.72	Lump or mass in breast
611.8	Absence of breast, acquired
611.9	Breast disorder NOS
793.8	Abnormal finding, breast
793.9	Abnormal finding, body struct NEC
V10.3	Hx of breast malignancy
V16.3	Family Hx, breast malignancy

REIMBURSEMENT INFORMATION

General

- Starred procedure.
- Separate procedure rules apply.

Medicare

- Follow–Up Days — 0
- Assistant Surgeon — not paid
- Supply Charges — not allowed
- Outpatient Limit — does not apply
- Minor Surgery Rules Apply

CPT CODE	SERVICE
19101	Biopsy of breast; incisional

CPT NOTES

- To report bilateral procedures, add modifier "-50" or 09950.

ICD–9–CM

174.0	M-Neoplasm, Female nipple
174.1	M-Neoplasm, Female breast, central
174.2	M-Neoplasm, Female breast, up/inner
174.3	M-Neoplasm, Female breast low/inner
174.4	M-Neoplasm, Female breast, up/outer
174.5	M-Neoplasm, Female breast low/outer
174.6	M-Neoplasm, Female breast, axillary
174.8	M-Neoplasm, Female breast NEC
175.0	M-Neoplasm, Male nipple
175.9	M-Neoplasm, Male breast NOS
198.81	M2-Neoplasm, Breast
217.	Benign neoplasm, Breast
233.0	CA in situ, Breast
238.3	UB-Neoplasm, Breast
239.3	Breast Neoplasm NOS
610.0	Solitary cyst of breast
610.1	Diffuse cystic mastopathy
610.2	Fibroadenosis of breast
610.3	Fibrosclerosis of breast
610.4	Mammary duct ectasia
610.8	Benign mammary dysplasia NEC
610.9	Benign mammary dysplasia NOS
611.0	Inflammatory disease of breast
611.3	Fat necrosis of breast
611.5	Galactocele
611.6	Galactorrhea, non-obstetric
611.72	Lump or mass in breast
611.8	Absence of breast, acquired
611.9	Breast disorder NOS
793.8	Abnormal finding, breast
793.9	Abnormal finding, body struct NEC
V10.3	Hx of breast malignancy
V16.3	Family Hx, breast malignancy

REIMBURSEMENT INFORMATION

Medicare

- Follow–Up Days — 10
- Assistant Surgeon — not paid
- Supply Charges — allowed
- Outpatient Limit — does not apply
- Minor Surgery Rules Apply

CPT CODE	SERVICE	ICD-9-CM
19110	Nipple exploration, with or without excision of a solitary lactiferous duct or a papilloma lactiferous duct	611.0 Inflammatory disease of breast 611.5 Galactocele 611.72 Lump or mass in breast V10.3 Hx of breast malignancy V16.3 Family Hx, breast malignancy

CPT NOTES

- To report bilateral procedures, add modifier "-50" or 09950.

REIMBURSEMENT INFORMATION

Medicare

- Follow-Up Days — 90
- Assistant Surgeon — not paid
- Supply Charges — not allowed
- Outpatient Limit — does not apply
- Major Surgery Rules Apply

CPT CODE	SERVICE	ICD-9-CM
19112	Excision of lactiferous duct fistula	611.0 Inflammatory disease of breast 675.1 Abscess of breast, childbirth

CPT NOTES

- To report bilateral procedures, add modifier "-50" or 09950.

REIMBURSEMENT INFORMATION

Medicare

- Follow-Up Days — 90
- Assistant Surgeon — by report
- Supply Charges — not allowed
- Outpatient Limit — does not apply
- Major Surgery Rules Apply

CPT CODE	SERVICE
19120	Excision of cyst, fibroadenoma, or other benign or malignant tumor aberrant breast tissue, duct lesion or nipple lesion (except 19140), male or female, one or more lesions

CPT NOTES

- To report bilateral procedures, add modifier "-50" or 09950.

ICD-9-CM

174.0	M-Neoplasm, Female nipple
174.1	M-Neoplasm, Female breast, central
174.2	M-Neoplasm, Female breast, up/inner
174.3	M-Neoplasm, Female breast low/inner
174.4	M-Neoplasm, Female breast, up/outer
174.5	M-Neoplasm, Female breast low/outer
174.6	M-Neoplasm, Female breast, axillary
174.8	M-Neoplasm, Female breast NEC
175.0	M-Neoplasm, Male nipple
175.9	M-Neoplasm, Male breast NOS
198.81	M2-Neoplasm, Breast
217.	Benign neoplasm, Breast
233.0	CA in situ, Breast
238.3	UB-Neoplasm, Breast
239.3	Breast Neoplasm NOS
610.0	Solitary cyst of breast
610.1	Diffuse cystic mastopathy
610.2	Fibroadenosis of breast
610.3	Fibrosclerosis of breast
610.4	Mammary duct ectasia
610.8	Benign mammary dysplasia NEC
610.9	Benign mammary dysplasia NOS
611.1	Hypertrophy of breast
611.3	Fat necrosis of breast
611.72	Lump or mass in breast
611.79	Signs/symptoms in breast NEC
757.6	Breast anomalies NEC
V10.3	Hx of breast malignancy
V16.3	Family Hx, breast malignancy

REIMBURSEMENT INFORMATION

Medicare

- Follow–Up Days — 90
- Assistant Surgeon — not paid
- Supply Charges — allowed
- Outpatient Limit — does not apply
- Major Surgery Rules Apply
- Fragments — 19100, 19101

CPT CODE	SERVICE
19125	Excision of breast lesion identified by pre-operative placement of radiological marker; single lesion

CPT NOTES

- To report bilateral procedures, add modifier "-50" or 09950.

ICD–9–CM

174.0	M-Neoplasm, Female nipple
174.1	M-Neoplasm, Female breast, central
174.2	M-Neoplasm, Female breast, up/inner
174.3	M-Neoplasm, Female breast low/inner
174.4	M-Neoplasm, Female breast, up/outer
174.5	M-Neoplasm, Female breast low/outer
174.6	M-Neoplasm, Female breast, axillary
174.8	M-Neoplasm, Female breast NEC
175.0	M-Neoplasm, Male nipple
175.9	M-Neoplasm, Male breast NOS
198.81	M2-Neoplasm, Breast
217.	Benign neoplasm, Breast
233.0	CA in situ, Breast
238.3	UB-Neoplasm, Breast
239.3	Breast Neoplasm NOS
610.0	Solitary cyst of breast
610.1	Diffuse cystic mastopathy
610.2	Fibroadenosis of breast
610.3	Fibrosclerosis of breast
610.4	Mammary duct ectasia
610.8	Benign mammary dysplasia NEC
610.9	Benign mammary dysplasia NOS
611.1	Hypertrophy of breast
611.3	Fat necrosis of breast
611.72	Lump or mass in breast
611.79	Signs/symptoms in breast NEC
V10.3	Hx of breast malignancy
V16.3	Family Hx, breast malignancy

REIMBURSEMENT INFORMATION

Medicare

- Follow–Up Days — 0
- Assistant Surgeon — not paid
- Supply Charges — allowed
- Outpatient Limit — does not apply
- Minor Surgery Rules Apply

CPT CODE	SERVICE	ICD-9-CM

19126 Excision of breast lesion identified by pre-operative placement of radiological marker; each additional lesion separately identified by a radiological marker

CPT NOTES

- To report bilateral procedures, add modifier "-50" or 09950.

ICD-9-CM

174.0	M-Neoplasm, Female nipple
174.1	M-Neoplasm, Female breast, central
174.2	M-Neoplasm, Female breast, up/inner
174.3	M-Neoplasm, Female breast low/inner
174.4	M-Neoplasm, Female breast, up/outer
174.5	M-Neoplasm, Female breast low/outer
174.6	M-Neoplasm, Female breast, axillary
174.8	M-Neoplasm, Female breast NEC
175.0	M-Neoplasm, Male nipple
175.9	M-Neoplasm, Male breast NOS
198.81	M2-Neoplasm, Breast
217.	Benign neoplasm, Breast
233.0	CA in situ, Breast
238.3	UB-Neoplasm, Breast
239.3	Breast Neoplasm NOS
610.0	Solitary cyst of breast
610.1	Diffuse cystic mastopathy
610.2	Fibroadenosis of breast
610.3	Fibrosclerosis of breast
610.4	Mammary duct ectasia
610.8	Benign mammary dysplasia NEC
610.9	Benign mammary dysplasia NOS
611.1	Hypertrophy of breast
611.72	Lump or mass in breast
V10.3	Hx of breast malignancy
V16.3	Family Hx, breast malignancy

REIMBURSEMENT INFORMATION

Medicare

- Follow-Up Days — none; falls within global period of another procedure
- Assistant Surgeon — not paid
- Supply Charges — allowed
- Outpatient Limit — does not apply

19140 Mastectomy for gynecomastia

CPT NOTES

- To report bilateral procedures, add modifier "-50" or 09950.

611.1	Hypertrophy of breast
611.72	Lump or mass in breast

REIMBURSEMENT INFORMATION

Medicare

- Follow-Up Days — 90
- Assistant Surgeon — not paid
- Supply Charges — not allowed
- Outpatient Limit — does not apply
- Major Surgery Rules Apply

CPT CODE	SERVICE
19160	Mastectomy, partial

CPT NOTES

- To report bilateral procedures, add modifier "-50" or 09950.

ICD–9–CM

174.0	M-Neoplasm, Female nipple
174.1	M-Neoplasm, Female breast, central
174.2	M-Neoplasm, Female breast, up/inner
174.3	M-Neoplasm, Female breast low/inner
174.4	M-Neoplasm, Female breast, up/outer
174.5	M-Neoplasm, Female breast low/outer
174.6	M-Neoplasm, Female breast, axillary
174.8	M-Neoplasm, Female breast NEC
174.9	M-Neoplasm, Female breast NOS
175.0	M-Neoplasm, Male nipple
175.9	M-Neoplasm, Male breast NOS
233.0	CA in situ, Breast
238.3	UB-Neoplasm, Breast
239.3	Breast Neoplasm NOS
610.1	Diffuse cystic mastopathy
610.2	Fibroadenosis of breast
610.3	Fibrosclerosis of breast
610.4	Mammary duct ectasia
611.72	Lump or mass in breast
V10.3	Hx of breast malignancy
V16.3	Family Hx, breast malignancy
V50.41	Prophylactic breast removal

REIMBURSEMENT INFORMATION

Medicare

- Follow–Up Days — 90
- Assistant Surgeon — by report
- Supply Charges — not allowed
- Outpatient Limit — does not apply
- Major Surgery Rules Apply
- Fragments — 19100, 19101, 19120

CPT CODE **SERVICE**

19162 Mastectomy, partial; with axillary lymphadenectomy

CPT NOTES

- To report bilateral procedures, add modifier "-50" or 09950.

ICD–9–CM

174.1	M-Neoplasm, Female breast, central
174.2	M-Neoplasm, Female breast, up/inner
174.3	M-Neoplasm, Female breast low/inner
174.4	M-Neoplasm, Female breast, up/outer
174.5	M-Neoplasm, Female breast low/outer
174.6	M-Neoplasm, Female breast, axillary
174.8	M-Neoplasm, Female breast NEC
174.9	M-Neoplasm, Female breast NOS
175.0	M-Neoplasm, Male nipple
175.9	M-Neoplasm, Male breast NOS
196.3	M-Neoplasm, Lymph axilla/arm
233.0	CA in situ, Breast
238.3	UB-Neoplasm, Breast
239.3	Breast Neoplasm NOS
610.1	Diffuse cystic mastopathy
610.2	Fibroadenosis of breast
610.3	Fibrosclerosis of breast
610.4	Mammary duct ectasia
611.72	Lump or mass in breast
V10.3	Hx of breast malignancy
V16.3	Family Hx, breast malignancy
V50.41	Prophylactic breast removal

REIMBURSEMENT INFORMATION

Medicare

- Follow–Up Days — 90
- Assistant Surgeon — paid
- Supply Charges — not allowed
- Outpatient Limit — does not apply
- Major Surgery Rules Apply
- Fragments — 19100, 19101, 19120, 19160, 38525, 38755

CPT CODE	SERVICE
19180	Mastectomy, simple, complete

CPT NOTES

- To report bilateral procedures, add modifier "-50" or 09950.
- For immediate or delayed insertion of implant, use 19340 or 19342.
- For gynecomastia, see 19140.

ICD–9–CM

174.0	M-Neoplasm, Female nipple
174.1	M-Neoplasm, Female breast, central
174.2	M-Neoplasm, Female breast, up/inner
174.3	M-Neoplasm, Female breast low/inner
174.4	M-Neoplasm, Female breast, up/outer
174.5	M-Neoplasm, Female breast low/outer
174.6	M-Neoplasm, Female breast, axillary
174.8	M-Neoplasm, Female breast NEC
174.9	M-Neoplasm, Female breast NOS
175.0	M-Neoplasm, Male nipple
175.9	M-Neoplasm, Male breast NOS
198.81	M2-Neoplasm, Breast
233.0	CA in situ, Breast
238.3	UB-Neoplasm, Breast
239.3	Breast Neoplasm NOS
610.1	Diffuse cystic mastopathy
610.2	Fibroadenosis of breast
610.3	Fibrosclerosis of breast
610.4	Mammary duct ectasia
611.72	Lump or mass in breast
V10.3	Hx of breast malignancy
V16.3	Family Hx, breast malignancy
V50.41	Prophylactic breast removal

REIMBURSEMENT INFORMATION

Medicare

- Follow–Up Days — 90
- Assistant Surgeon — paid
- Supply Charges — not allowed
- Outpatient Limit — does not apply
- Major Surgery Rules Apply

CPT CODE	SERVICE
19182	Mastectomy, subcutaneous

CPT NOTES

- To report bilateral procedures, add modifier "-50" or 09950.

ICD–9–CM

174.0	M-Neoplasm, Female nipple
174.1	M-Neoplasm, Female breast, central
174.2	M-Neoplasm, Female breast, up/inner
174.3	M-Neoplasm, Female breast low/inner
174.4	M-Neoplasm, Female breast, up/outer
174.5	M-Neoplasm, Female breast low/outer
174.6	M-Neoplasm, Female breast, axillary
174.8	M-Neoplasm, Female breast NEC
174.9	M-Neoplasm, Female breast NOS
175.0	M-Neoplasm, Male nipple
175.9	M-Neoplasm, Male breast NOS
198.81	M2-Neoplasm, Breast
233.0	CA in situ, Breast
238.3	UB-Neoplasm, Breast
239.3	Breast Neoplasm NOS
610.0	Solitary cyst of breast
610.2	Fibroadenosis of breast
610.3	Fibrosclerosis of breast
610.4	Mammary duct ectasia
611.72	Lump or mass in breast
V10.3	Hx of breast malignancy
V16.3	Family Hx, breast malignancy
V50.41	Prophylactic breast removal

REIMBURSEMENT INFORMATION

Medicare

- Follow–Up Days — 90
- Assistant Surgeon — paid
- Supply Charges — not allowed
- Outpatient Limit — does not apply
- Major Surgery Rules Apply

CPT CODE **SERVICE**

19200 Mastectomy, radical, including pectoral muscles, axillary lymph nodes

CPT NOTES

- To report bilateral procedures, add modifier "-50" or 09950.

ICD–9–CM

174.0	M-Neoplasm, Female nipple
174.1	M-Neoplasm, Female breast, central
174.2	M-Neoplasm, Female breast, up/inner
174.3	M-Neoplasm, Female breast low/inner
174.4	M-Neoplasm, Female breast, up/outer
174.5	M-Neoplasm, Female breast low/outer
174.6	M-Neoplasm, Female breast, axillary
174.8	M-Neoplasm, Female breast NEC
174.9	M-Neoplasm, Female breast NOS
175.0	M-Neoplasm, Male nipple
175.9	M-Neoplasm, Male breast NOS
196.3	M-Neoplasm, Lymph axilla/arm
198.81	M2-Neoplasm, Breast
233.0	CA in situ, Breast
238.3	UB-Neoplasm, Breast
239.3	Breast Neoplasm NOS
610.1	Diffuse cystic mastopathy
610.2	Fibroadenosis of breast
610.3	Fibrosclerosis of breast
610.4	Mammary duct ectasia
611.72	Lump or mass in breast
V10.3	Hx of breast malignancy
V16.3	Family Hx, breast malignancy
V50.41	Prophylactic breast removal

REIMBURSEMENT INFORMATION

Medicare

- Follow–Up Days — 90
- Assistant Surgeon — paid
- Supply Charges — not allowed
- Outpatient Limit — does not apply
- Major Surgery Rules Apply

CPT CODE	SERVICE
19220	Mastectomy, radical, including pectoral muscles, axillary and internal mammary lymph nodes (Urban type operation)

CPT NOTES

- To report bilateral procedures, add modifier "-50" or 09950.

ICD-9-CM

174.0	M-Neoplasm, Female nipple
174.1	M-Neoplasm, Female breast, central
174.2	M-Neoplasm, Female breast, up/inner
174.3	M-Neoplasm, Female breast low/inner
174.4	M-Neoplasm, Female breast, up/outer
174.5	M-Neoplasm, Female breast low/outer
174.6	M-Neoplasm, Female breast, axillary
174.8	M-Neoplasm, Female breast NEC
174.9	M-Neoplasm, Female breast NOS
175.0	M-Neoplasm, Male nipple
175.9	M-Neoplasm, Male breast NOS
196.1	M-Neoplasm, Lymph intrathoracic
196.3	M-Neoplasm, Lymph axilla/arm
198.81	M2-Neoplasm, Breast
233.0	CA in situ, Breast
238.9	Uncertain behavior, neoplasm NOS
239.3	Breast Neoplasm NOS
610.1	Diffuse cystic mastopathy
610.2	Fibroadenosis of breast
610.3	Fibrosclerosis of breast
610.4	Mammary duct ectasia
611.72	Lump or mass in breast
V10.3	Hx of breast malignancy
V16.3	Family Hx, breast malignancy
V50.41	Prophylactic breast removal

REIMBURSEMENT INFORMATION

Medicare

- Follow–Up Days — 90
- Assistant Surgeon — paid
- Supply Charges — not allowed
- Outpatient Limit — does not apply
- Major Surgery Rules Apply

CPT CODE	SERVICE
19240	Mastectomy, modified radical, including axillary lymph nodes, with or without pectoralis minor muscle, but excluding pectoralis major muscle

CPT NOTES

- To report bilateral procedures, add modifier "-50" or 09950.

ICD-9-CM

174.0	M-Neoplasm, Female nipple
174.1	M-Neoplasm, Female breast, central
174.2	M-Neoplasm, Female breast, up/inner
174.3	M-Neoplasm, Female breast low/inner
174.4	M-Neoplasm, Female breast, up/outer
174.5	M-Neoplasm, Female breast low/outer
174.6	M-Neoplasm, Female breast, axillary
174.8	M-Neoplasm, Female breast NEC
174.9	M-Neoplasm, Female breast NOS
175.0	M-Neoplasm, Male nipple
175.9	M-Neoplasm, Male breast NOS
196.3	M-Neoplasm, Lymph axilla/arm
198.81	M2-Neoplasm, Breast
233.0	CA in situ, Breast
238.3	UB-Neoplasm, Breast
239.3	Breast Neoplasm NOS
610.1	Diffuse cystic mastopathy
610.2	Fibroadenosis of breast
610.3	Fibrosclerosis of breast
610.4	Mammary duct ectasia
611.72	Lump or mass in breast
V10.3	Hx of breast malignancy
V16.3	Family Hx, breast malignancy
V50.41	Prophylactic breast removal

REIMBURSEMENT INFORMATION

Medicare

- Follow–Up Days — 90
- Assistant Surgeon — paid
- Supply Charges — not allowed
- Outpatient Limit — does not apply
- Major Surgery Rules Apply
- Fragments — 19100, 19101, 19120, 19160, 19180, 38525,

CPT CODE	SERVICE	ICD-9-CM

19260 Excision of chest wall tumor including ribs

CPT NOTES

- To report bilateral procedures, add modifier "-50" or 09950.

ICD-9-CM

170.3	M-Neoplasm, Ribs/Sternum/Clavicle
171.4	M-Neoplasm, Soft tissue, thorax
171.7	M-Neoplasm, Trunk NOS
171.8	M-Neoplasm, Soft tissue NEC
171.9	M-Neoplasm, Soft tissue NOS
172.5	Malignant melanoma, Trunk
173.5	M-Neoplasm, Skin of trunk

REIMBURSEMENT INFORMATION

Medicare

- Follow-Up Days — 90
- Assistant Surgeon — paid
- Supply Charges — not allowed
- Outpatient Limit — does not apply
- Major Surgery Rules Apply

19271 Excision of chest wall tumor involving ribs, with plastic reconstruction; without mediastinal lymphadenectomy

19272 Excision of chest wall tumor involving ribs, with plastic reconstruction; with mediastinal lymphadenectomy

CPT NOTES

- To report bilateral procedures, add modifier "-50" or 09950.

ICD-9-CM

170.3	M-Neoplasm, Ribs/Sternum/Clavicle
171.0	M-Neoplasm, Soft tissue, head
171.4	M-Neoplasm, Soft tissue, thorax
171.7	M-Neoplasm, Trunk NOS
171.8	M-Neoplasm, Soft tissue NEC
171.9	M-Neoplasm, Soft tissue NOS
172.5	Malignant melanoma, Trunk
173.5	M-Neoplasm, Skin of trunk

REIMBURSEMENT INFORMATION

Medicare

- Follow-Up Days — 90
- Assistant Surgeon — paid
- Supply Charges — not allowed
- Outpatient Limit — does not apply
- Major Surgery Rules Apply

CPT CODE	SERVICE
19290	Preoperative placement of needle localization wire, breast
19291	Preoperative placement of needle localization wire, breast; each additional lesion

CPT NOTES

- For radiological supervision and interpretation, see 76096.

ICD–9–CM

174.0	M-Neoplasm, Female nipple
174.1	M-Neoplasm, Female breast, central
174.2	M-Neoplasm, Female breast, up/inner
174.3	M-Neoplasm, Female breast low/inner
174.4	M-Neoplasm, Female breast, up/outer
174.5	M-Neoplasm, Female breast low/outer
174.6	M-Neoplasm, Female breast, axillary
174.8	M-Neoplasm, Female breast NEC
174.9	M-Neoplasm, Female breast NOS
175.0	M-Neoplasm, Male nipple
175.9	M-Neoplasm, Male breast NOS
198.81	M2-Neoplasm, Breast
233.0	CA in situ, Breast
238.9	Uncertain behavior, neoplasm NOS
239.3	Breast Neoplasm NOS
610.1	Diffuse cystic mastopathy
610.2	Fibroadenosis of breast
610.3	Fibrosclerosis of breast
610.4	Mammary duct ectasia
611.72	Lump or mass in breast
V10.3	Hx of breast malignancy
V16.3	Family Hx, breast malignancy
V50.41	Prophylactic breast removal
V51.	Aftercare w/plastic surgery

REIMBURSEMENT INFORMATION

Medicare

- Follow–Up Days
  19290 — 0
  19291 — none; falls within global period of another procedure
- Assistant Surgeon — paid
- Supply Charges — not allowed
- Outpatient Limit — does not apply
- Minor Surgery Rules Apply (19290)

CPT CODE **SERVICE**

19316 Mastopexy

CPT NOTES

- To report bilateral procedures, add modifier "-50" or 09950.

ICD-9-CM

611.1	Hypertrophy of breast
611.4	Atrophy of breast
611.8	Absence of breast, acquired
757.6	Breast anomalies NEC
V50.1	Plastic surgery NEC
V51.	Aftercare w/plastic surgery

REIMBURSEMENT INFORMATION

Medicare

- Follow-Up Days — 90
- Assistant Surgeon — paid
- Supply Charges — not allowed
- Outpatient Limit — does not apply
- Major Surgery Rules Apply

19318 Reduction mammaplasty

CPT NOTES

- To report bilateral procedures, add modifier "-50" or 09950.

611.1	Hypertrophy of breast
611.71	Mastodynia
611.8	Absence of breast, acquired
645.8	Breast disorders NOS
695.89	Erythematous conditions NEC
709.8	Skin disorders NEC
719.41	Pain in joint, shoulder
723.1	Cervicalgia
723.9	Neck disorder/symptom NOS
724.1	Pain in thoracic spine
724.5	Backache NOS
757.6	Breast anomalies NEC
V50.1	Plastic surgery NEC

REIMBURSEMENT INFORMATION

Medicare

- Follow-Up Days — 90
- Assistant Surgeon — paid
- Supply Charges — not allowed
- Outpatient Limit — does not apply
- Major Surgery Rules Apply

CPT CODE	SERVICE	ICD–9–CM

19324 Mammaplasty, augmentation; without prosthetic implant

CPT NOTES

- To report bilateral procedures, add modifier "-50" or 09950.
- For flap or graft, use also appropriate number.

ICD–9–CM

611.4	Atrophy of breast
611.8	Absence of breast, acquired
757.6	Breast anomalies NEC
V50.1	Plastic surgery NEC

REIMBURSEMENT INFORMATION

Medicare

- Follow–Up Days — 90
- Assistant Surgeon — by report
- Supply Charges — not allowed
- Outpatient Limit — does not apply
- Major Surgery Rules Apply

19325 Mammaplasty, augmentation; with prosthetic implant

CPT NOTES

- To report bilateral procedures, add modifier "-50" or 09950.
- For flap or graft, use also appropriate number.

ICD–9–CM

611.4	Atrophy of breast
611.8	Absence of breast, acquired
757.6	Breast anomalies NEC
V50.1	Plastic surgery NEC
V51.	Aftercare w/plastic surgery

REIMBURSEMENT INFORMATION

Medicare

- Follow–Up Days — 90
- Assistant Surgeon — by report
- Supply Charges — not allowed
- Outpatient Limit — does not apply
- Major Surgery Rules Apply

19328 Removal of intact mammary implant

CPT NOTES

- To report bilateral procedures, add modifier "-50" or 09950.

ICD–9–CM

611.0	Inflammatory disease of breast
611.71	Mastodynia
709.3	Degenerative skin disorders
879.1	Open wound of breast, complicated
996.54	Breast prosthesis malfunction
996.69	Reaction, intern prosth device NEC
998.1	Hemorrhage complicating a procedure
998.5	Postoperative infection
V51.	Aftercare w/plastic surgery

REIMBURSEMENT INFORMATION

Medicare

- Follow–Up Days — 90
- Assistant Surgeon — not paid
- Supply Charges — not allowed
- Outpatient Limit — does not apply
- Major Surgery Rules Apply

CPT CODE	SERVICE	ICD–9–CM

19330 Removal of mammary implant material

CPT NOTES

- To report bilateral procedures, add modifier "-50" or 09950.

611.0	Inflammatory disease of breast
611.71	Mastodynia
709.3	Degenerative skin disorders
879.1	Open wound of breast, complicated
996.54	Breast prosthesis malfunction
996.69	Reaction, intern prosth device NEC
998.1	Hemorrhage complicating a procedure
998.5	Postoperative infection
V51.	Aftercare w/plastic surgery

REIMBURSEMENT INFORMATION

Medicare

- Follow–Up Days — 90
- Assistant Surgeon — not paid
- Supply Charges — not allowed
- Outpatient Limit — does not apply
- Major Surgery Rules Apply

19340 Immediate insertion of breast prosthesis following mastopexy, mastectomy or in reconstruction

CPT NOTES

- To report bilateral procedures, add modifier "-50" or 09950.

174.0	M-Neoplasm, Female nipple
174.1	M-Neoplasm, Female breast, central
174.2	M-Neoplasm, Female breast, up/inner
174.3	M-Neoplasm, Female breast low/inner
174.4	M-Neoplasm, Female breast, up/outer
174.5	M-Neoplasm, Female breast low/outer
174.8	M-Neoplasm, Female breast NEC
233.0	CA in situ, Breast
611.8	Absence of breast, acquired
757.6	Breast anomalies NEC
V10.3	Hx of breast malignancy
V16.3	Family Hx, breast malignancy
V50.1	Plastic surgery NEC
V51.	Aftercare w/plastic surgery

REIMBURSEMENT INFORMATION

Medicare

- Follow–Up Days — none; falls within global period of another procedure
- Assistant Surgeon — paid
- Supply Charges — not allowed
- Outpatient Limit — does not apply

CPT CODE	SERVICE	ICD-9-CM
19342	Delayed insertion of breast prosthesis following mastopexy, mastectomy or in reconstruction	174.0 M-Neoplasm, Female nipple 174.1 M-Neoplasm, Female breast, central 174.2 M-Neoplasm, Female breast, up/inner 174.3 M-Neoplasm, Female breast low/inner 174.4 M-Neoplasm, Female breast, up/outer 174.5 M-Neoplasm, Female breast low/outer 174.8 M-Neoplasm, Female breast NEC 233.0 CA in situ, Breast 611.8 Absence of breast, acquired 757.6 Breast anomalies NEC 998.5 Postoperative infection V10.3 Hx of breast malignancy V16.3 Family Hx, breast malignancy V50.1 Plastic surgery NEC V51. Aftercare w/plastic surgery

CPT NOTES

- To report bilateral procedures, add modifier "-50" or 09950.
- For supply of implant, use 99070.
- For preparation of custom breast implant, see 19396.

REIMBURSEMENT INFORMATION

Medicare

- Follow-Up Days — 90
- Assistant Surgeon — paid
- Supply Charges — not allowed
- Outpatient Limit — does not apply
- Major Surgery Rules Apply

CPT CODE	SERVICE	ICD-9-CM
19350	Nipple/areola reconstruction	174.0 M-Neoplasm, Female nipple 174.1 M-Neoplasm, Female breast, central 174.2 M-Neoplasm, Female breast, up/inner 174.4 M-Neoplasm, Female breast, up/outer 174.5 M-Neoplasm, Female breast low/outer 174.8 M-Neoplasm, Female breast NEC 233.0 CA in situ, Breast 611.8 Absence of breast, acquired 996.70 Complication, unspec device/graft V10.3 Hx of breast malignancy V51. Aftercare w/plastic surgery

CPT NOTES

- To report bilateral procedures, add modifier "-50" or 09950.

REIMBURSEMENT INFORMATION

Medicare

- Follow-Up Days — 90
- Assistant Surgeon — not paid
- Supply Charges — not allowed
- Outpatient Limit — does not apply
- Major Surgery Rules Apply

CPT CODE	SERVICE	ICD–9–CM

19355 Correction of inverted nipples

CPT NOTES

- ♦ To report bilateral procedures, add modifier "-50" or 09950.

611.79	Signs/symptoms in breast NEC
757.6	Breast anomalies NEC

REIMBURSEMENT INFORMATION

Medicare

- ♦ Follow–Up Days — 90
- ♦ Assistant Surgeon — by report
- ♦ Supply Charges — not allowed
- ♦ Outpatient Limit — does not apply
- ♦ Major Surgery Rules Apply

19357 Breast reconstruction, immediate or delayed, with tissue expander, including subsequent expansion

CPT NOTES

- ♦ To report bilateral procedures, add modifier "-50" or 09950.

174.0	M-Neoplasm, Female nipple
174.1	M-Neoplasm, Female breast, central
174.2	M-Neoplasm, Female breast, up/inner
174.3	M-Neoplasm, Female breast low/inner
174.4	M-Neoplasm, Female breast, up/outer
174.5	M-Neoplasm, Female breast low/outer
174.6	M-Neoplasm, Female breast, axillary
174.8	M-Neoplasm, Female breast NEC
175.0	M-Neoplasm, Male nipple
175.9	M-Neoplasm, Male breast NOS
198.81	M2-Neoplasm, Breast
233.0	CA in situ, Breast
611.8	Absence of breast, acquired
V10.3	Hx of breast malignancy
V16.3	Family Hx, breast malignancy
V50.1	Plastic surgery NEC
V51.	Aftercare w/plastic surgery

REIMBURSEMENT INFORMATION

Medicare

- ♦ Follow–Up Days — 90
- ♦ Assistant Surgeon — paid
- ♦ Supply Charges — not allowed
- ♦ Outpatient Limit — does not apply
- ♦ Major Surgery Rules Apply

CPT CODE	SERVICE
19361	Breast reconstruction with latissimus dorsi flap, with or without prosthetic implant

CPT NOTES

- To report bilateral procedures, add modifier "-50" or 09950.

ICD–9–CM

174.0	M-Neoplasm, Female nipple
174.1	M-Neoplasm, Female breast, central
174.2	M-Neoplasm, Female breast, up/inner
174.3	M-Neoplasm, Female breast low/inner
174.4	M-Neoplasm, Female breast, up/outer
174.5	M-Neoplasm, Female breast low/outer
174.6	M-Neoplasm, Female breast, axillary
174.8	M-Neoplasm, Female breast NEC
175.0	M-Neoplasm, Male nipple
175.9	M-Neoplasm, Male breast NOS
198.81	M2-Neoplasm, Breast
233.0	CA in situ, Breast
611.8	Absence of breast, acquired
V10.3	Hx of breast malignancy
V16.3	Family Hx, breast malignancy
V50.1	Plastic surgery NEC
V51.	Aftercare w/plastic surgery

REIMBURSEMENT INFORMATION

Medicare

- Follow–Up Days — 90
- Assistant Surgeon — paid
- Supply Charges — not allowed
- Outpatient Limit — does not apply
- Major Surgery Rules Apply

CPT CODE	SERVICE
19364	Breast reconstruction with free flap

CPT NOTES

- To report bilateral procedures, add modifier "-50" or 09950.
- Use also code number for specific flap.

ICD–9–CM

174.0	M-Neoplasm, Female nipple
174.1	M-Neoplasm, Female breast, central
174.2	M-Neoplasm, Female breast, up/inner
174.3	M-Neoplasm, Female breast low/inner
174.4	M-Neoplasm, Female breast, up/outer
174.5	M-Neoplasm, Female breast low/outer
174.6	M-Neoplasm, Female breast, axillary
174.8	M-Neoplasm, Female breast NEC
175.0	M-Neoplasm, Male nipple
175.9	M-Neoplasm, Male breast NOS
198.81	M2-Neoplasm, Breast
233.0	CA in situ, Breast
611.8	Absence of breast, acquired
996.54	Breast prosthesis malfunction
V10.3	Hx of breast malignancy
V16.3	Family Hx, breast malignancy
V50.1	Plastic surgery NEC
V51.	Aftercare w/plastic surgery

REIMBURSEMENT INFORMATION

Medicare

- Follow–Up Days — 90
- Assistant Surgeon — paid
- Supply Charges — not allowed
- Outpatient Limit — does not apply
- Major Surgery Rules Apply

CPT CODE	SERVICE	ICD–9–CM

19366 Breast reconstruction with other technique

CPT NOTES

- ♦ To report bilateral procedures, add modifier "-50" or 09950.
- ♦ For microsurgical technique, add modifier "-20" or 09920.
- ♦ For insertion of prosthesis, use also 19340 or 19342.

174.0	M-Neoplasm, Female nipple
174.1	M-Neoplasm, Female breast, central
174.2	M-Neoplasm, Female breast, up/inner
174.3	M-Neoplasm, Female breast low/inner
174.4	M-Neoplasm, Female breast, up/outer
174.5	M-Neoplasm, Female breast low/outer
174.8	M-Neoplasm, Female breast NEC
175.0	M-Neoplasm, Male nipple
175.9	M-Neoplasm, Male breast NOS
198.81	M2-Neoplasm, Breast
233.0	CA in situ, Breast
611.8	Absence of breast, acquired
996.54	Breast prosthesis malfunction
V10.3	Hx of breast malignancy
V16.3	Family Hx, breast malignancy
V50.1	Plastic surgery NEC
V51.	Aftercare w/plastic surgery

REIMBURSEMENT INFORMATION

Medicare

- ♦ Follow–Up Days — 90
- ♦ Assistant Surgeon — paid
- ♦ Supply Charges — not allowed
- ♦ Outpatient Limit — does not apply
- ♦ Major Surgery Rules Apply

● **19367** Breast reconstruction with transverse rectus abdominis myocutaneous flap (TRAM), single pedicle, including closure of donor site

● **19368** Breast reconstruction with transverse rectus abdominis myocutaneous flap (TRAM), single pedicle, including closure of donor site; with microvascular anastomosis (supercharging)

● **19369** Breast reconstruction with transverse rectus abdominis myocutaneous flap (TRAM), double pedicle, including closure of donor site

CPT NOTES

- ♦ To report bilateral procedures, add modifier "-50" or 09950.

611.8	Absence of breast, acquired
V10.3	Hx of breast malignancy
V51.	Aftercare w/plastic surgery

REIMBURSEMENT INFORMATION

General

- ♦ New procedure, 1995 CPT.

Medicare

- ♦ Follow–Up Days — 90
- ♦ Assistant Surgeon — paid
- ♦ Supply Charges — not allowed
- ♦ Outpatient Limit — does not apply
- ♦ Major Surgery Rules Apply

CPT CODE	SERVICE	ICD–9–CM

19370 Open periprosthetic capsulotomy, breast

CPT NOTES

- To report bilateral procedures, add modifier "-50" or 09950.

611.71	Mastodynia
611.8	Absence of breast, acquired
709.2	Scar/fibrosis of skin
996.54	Breast prosthesis malfunction
996.69	Reaction, intern prosth device NEC
998.1	Hemorrhage complicating a procedure
998.5	Postoperative infection
V51.	Aftercare w/plastic surgery

REIMBURSEMENT INFORMATION

Medicare

- Follow–Up Days — 90
- Assistant Surgeon — not paid
- Supply Charges — not allowed
- Outpatient Limit — does not apply
- Major Surgery Rules Apply

19371 Periprosthetic capsulectomy, breast

CPT NOTES

- To report bilateral procedures, add modifier "-50" or 09950.

611.71	Mastodynia
611.8	Absence of breast, acquired
709.2	Scar/fibrosis of skin
996.54	Breast prosthesis malfunction
996.69	Reaction, intern prosth device NEC
998.1	Hemorrhage complicating a procedure
998.5	Postoperative infection
V51.	Aftercare w/plastic surgery

REIMBURSEMENT INFORMATION

Medicare

- Follow–Up Days — 90
- Assistant Surgeon — not paid
- Supply Charges — not allowed
- Outpatient Limit — does not apply
- Major Surgery Rules Apply

CPT CODE	SERVICE	ICD-9-CM
19380	Revision of reconstructed breast	174.0 M-Neoplasm, Female nipple 174.1 M-Neoplasm, Female breast, central 174.2 M-Neoplasm, Female breast, up/inner 174.3 M-Neoplasm, Female breast low/inner 174.4 M-Neoplasm, Female breast, up/outer 174.5 M-Neoplasm, Female breast low/outer 174.8 M-Neoplasm, Female breast NEC 175.0 M-Neoplasm, Male nipple 175.9 M-Neoplasm, Male breast NOS 198.81 M2-Neoplasm, Breast 233.0 CA in situ, Breast 611.71 Mastodynia 611.8 Absence of breast, acquired 709.2 Scar/fibrosis of skin 909.3 Late effect of surg/med complic 996.54 Breast prosthesis malfunction 996.69 Reaction, intern prosth device NEC 998.1 Hemorrhage complicating a procedure 998.5 Postoperative infection V10.3 Hx of breast malignancy V51. Aftercare w/plastic surgery

CPT NOTES

- To report bilateral procedures, add modifier "-50" or 09950.

REIMBURSEMENT INFORMATION

Medicare

- Follow-Up Days — 90
- Assistant Surgeon — not paid
- Supply Charges — not allowed
- Outpatient Limit — does not apply
- Major Surgery Rules Apply

CPT CODE	SERVICE	ICD-9-CM
19396	Preparation of moulage for custom breast implant	611.8 Absence of breast, acquired 757.6 Breast anomalies NEC V10.3 Hx of breast malignancy V50.1 Plastic surgery NEC V51. Aftercare w/plastic surgery

CPT NOTES

- To report bilateral procedures, add modifier "-50" or 09950.

REIMBURSEMENT INFORMATION

Medicare

- Follow-Up Days — 0
- Assistant Surgeon — by report
- Supply Charges — not allowed
- Outpatient Limit — does not apply
- Minor Surgery Rules Apply

CPT CODE	SERVICE	ICD–9–CM	
19499	Unlisted procedure, breast	174.8	M-Neoplasm, Female breast NEC
		611.72	Lump or mass in breast
		611.8	Absence of breast, acquired
		V10.3	Hx of breast malignancy
		V16.3	Family Hx, breast malignancy
		V50.1	Plastic surgery NEC

REIMBURSEMENT INFORMATION

Medicare

- Follow–Up Days — determined by local carrier
- Assistant Surgeon — determined by local carrier
- Supply Charges — determined by local carrier
- Outpatient Limit — determined by local carrier

MUSCULOSKELETAL SYSTEM

Cast and strapping procedures appear at the end of the section. The services listed include the application and removal of the first cast or traction device only. Subsequent replacement of cast and/or traction device may require an additional listing.

Definitions

The terms "closed treatment," "open treatment," and "percutaneous skeletal fixation" have been carefully chosen to accurately reflect current orthopaedic procedural treatments.

Closed treatment. "Closed treatment" specifically means that the fracture site is not surgically opened (exposed to the external environment and directly visualized). This terminology is used to describe procedures that treat fractures by three methods: 1) without manipulation 2) with manipulation 3) with or without traction.

Open treatment. "Open treatment" is used when the fracture is surgically opened (exposed to the external environment). In this instance, the fracture (bone ends) is visualized and internal fixation may be used.

Percutaneous skeletal fixation. "Percutaneous skeletal fixation" describes fracture treatment which is neither open nor closed. In this procedure, the fracture fragments are not visualized, but fixation (e.g., pins) is placed across the fracture site, usually under x-ray imaging.

The type of fracture (e.g., open, compound, closed) does not have any coding correlation with the type of treatment (e.g., closed, open, or percutaneous) provided.

The codes for treatment of fractures and joint injuries (dislocations) are categorized by the type of manipulation (reduction) and stabilization (fixation or immobilization). These codes can apply to either open (compound) or closed fractures or joint injuries.

Skeletal traction is the application of a force (distracting or traction force) to a limb segment through a wire, pin, screw, or clamp that is attached (e.g., penetrates) to bone.

Skin traction is the application of a force (longitudinal) to a limb using felt or strapping applied directly to skin only.

External fixation is the usage of skeletal pins plus an attaching mechanism/device used for temporary or definitive treatment of acute or chronic bony deformity.

Codes for obtaining autogenous bone grafts, cartilage, tendon fascia lata grafts or other tissues, through separate incisions are to be used only when the graft is not already listed as part of the basic procedure.

Re-reduction of a fracture and/or dislocation performed by the primary physician may be identified by either the addition of the modifier "-76" to the usual procedure number or by use of modifier code 09976 to indicate "Repeat Procedure by Same Physician." (See Surgery Guidelines in your CPT.)

Codes for external fixation are to be used only when external fixation is not already listed as part of the basic procedure.

All codes for suction irrigation have been deleted. To report, list only the primary surgical procedure performed (e.g., sequestrectomy, deep incision).

Manipulation. The term manipulation is used throughout the musculoskeletal fracture and dislocation subsections to specifically mean the attempted reduction or restoration of a fracture or joint dislocation to its normal anatomic alignment by the application of manually applied forces.

CPT CODE	SERVICE
20000*	Incision of soft tissue abscess (eg, secondary to osteomyelitis); superficial
20005	Incision of soft tissue abscess (eg, secondary to osteomyelitis); deep or complicated

ICD–9–CM

383.20	Petrositis NOS
383.21	Acute petrositis
383.22	Chronic petrositis
526.0	Developmental odontogenic cysts
526.1	Fissural cysts of jaw
526.2	Jaw cysts NEC
526.4	Inflammation of jaw
526.5	Alveolitis of jaw
528.3	Cellulitis/abscess of mouth
528.6	Leukoplakia of oral mucosa/tongue
682.x	Cellulitis and abscess
730.0x	Acute osteomyelitis
730.1x	Chronic osteomyelitis
730.2x	Osteomyelitis
730.3x	Periostitis
730.9x	Infection of bone NOS

REIMBURSEMENT INFORMATION

General

- See notes on page 286.
- Starred procedure. (20000)

Medicare

- Follow–up Days — 10
- Assistant Surgeon — not paid
- Supply Charges — not allowed
- Outpatient Limit — applies
- Minor Surgery Rules Apply

CPT CODE	SERVICE
20200	Biopsy, muscle; superficial
20205	Biopsy, muscle; deep

CPT NOTES

- ♦ For aspiration of bone marrow, see 85095.

ICD–9–CM

171.0	M-Neoplasm, Soft tissue, head
171.2	M-Neoplasm, Soft tissue, arm
171.3	M-Neoplasm, Soft tissue, leg
171.4	M-Neoplasm, Soft tissue, thorax
171.5	M-Neoplasm, Soft tissue, abdomen
171.6	M-Neoplasm, Soft tissue, pelvis
171.7	M-Neoplasm, Trunk NOS
171.8	M-Neoplasm, Soft tissue NEC
171.9	M-Neoplasm, Soft tissue NOS
195.0	M-Neoplasm, Head/face/neck
198.89	M2-Neoplasm NEC
215.0	B-Neoplasm, Soft tissue, head
215.2	B-Neoplasm, Soft tissue, arm
215.3	B-Neoplasm, Soft tissue, leg
215.4	B-Neoplasm, Soft tissue, thorax
215.5	B-Neoplasm, Soft tissue, abdomen
215.6	B-Neoplasm, Soft tissue, pelvis
215.7	B-Neoplasm, Trunk NOS
215.8	B-Neoplasm, Soft tissue NEC
215.9	B-Neoplasm, Soft tissue NOS
238.1	UB-Neoplasm, Soft tissue
244.0	Postsurgical hypothyroidism
244.1	Postablative hypothyroidism NEC
244.2	Iodine hypothyroidism
244.3	Iatrogenic hypothyroidism NEC
244.8	Acquired hypothyroidism NEC
244.9	Hypothyroidism NOS
253.2	Panhypopituitarism
255.0	Cushing's syndrome
255.4	Corticoadrenal insufficiency
335.20	Amyotrophic lateral sclerosis
335.21	Progressive muscular atrophy
335.22	Progressive bulbar palsy
335.23	Pseudobulbar palsy
335.24	Primary lateral sclerosis
359.0	Congen hered muscular dystrophy
359.1	Hered prog muscular dystrophy
359.2	Myotonic disorders
359.3	Familial periodic paralysis
359.4	Toxic myopathy
359.8	Myopathy NEC
359.9	Myopathy NOS
446.0	Polyarteritis nodosa
710.0	Systemic lupus erythematosus
710.1	Systemic sclerosis
710.2	Sicca syndrome
728.0	Infective myositis
728.1x	Muscular calcification/ossification
728.2	Muscular disuse atrophy NEC
728.3	Muscle disorders NEC
728.81	Interstitial myositis
728.82	Foreign body granuloma of muscle
728.9	Muscle/ligament disorder NOS

CPT CODE **SERVICE**

20200, 20205 (Cont'd.)

ICD–9–CM

729.1 Myalgia and myositis NOS

REIMBURSEMENT INFORMATION

General

- See notes on page 286.

Medicare

- Follow–up Days — 0
- Assistant Surgeon — not paid
- Supply Charges — allowed
- Outpatient Limit — does not apply
- Minor Surgery Rules Apply

CPT CODE	SERVICE
20206*	Biopsy, muscle, percutaneous needle

CPT NOTES

- For aspiration of bone marrow, see 85095.
- For radiological supervision and interpretation, see 76360, 76942.
- For fine needle aspiration, preparation, and interpretation of smears, see 88170-88173.
- For excision of muscle tumor, deep, see specific anatomic section.

ICD–9–CM

171.0	M-Neoplasm, Soft tissue, head
171.2	M-Neoplasm, Soft tissue, arm
171.3	M-Neoplasm, Soft tissue, leg
171.4	M-Neoplasm, Soft tissue, thorax
171.5	M-Neoplasm, Soft tissue, abdomen
171.6	M-Neoplasm, Soft tissue, pelvis
171.7	M-Neoplasm, Trunk NOS
171.8	M-Neoplasm, Soft tissue NEC
171.9	M-Neoplasm, Soft tissue NOS
195.0	M-Neoplasm, Head/face/neck
198.89	M2-Neoplasm NEC
215.0	B-Neoplasm, Soft tissue, head
215.2	B-Neoplasm, Soft tissue, arm
215.3	B-Neoplasm, Soft tissue, leg
215.4	B-Neoplasm, Soft tissue, thorax
215.5	B-Neoplasm, Soft tissue, abdomen
215.6	B-Neoplasm, Soft tissue, pelvis
215.7	B-Neoplasm, Trunk NOS
215.8	B-Neoplasm, Soft tissue NEC
215.9	B-Neoplasm, Soft tissue NOS
238.1	UB-Neoplasm, Soft tissue
244.0	Postsurgical hypothyroidism
244.1	Postablative hypothyroidism NEC
244.2	Iodine hypothyroidism
244.3	Iatrogenic hypothyroidism NEC
244.8	Acquired hypothyroidism NEC
244.9	Hypothyroidism NOS
253.2	Panhypopituitarism
255.0	Cushing's syndrome
255.4	Corticoadrenal insufficiency
335.20	Amyotrophic lateral sclerosis
335.21	Progressive muscular atrophy
335.22	Progressive bulbar palsy
335.23	Pseudobulbar palsy
335.24	Primary lateral sclerosis
359.0	Congen hered muscular dystrophy
359.1	Hered prog muscular dystrophy
359.2	Myotonic disorders
359.3	Familial periodic paralysis
359.4	Toxic myopathy
359.8	Myopathy NEC
359.9	Myopathy NOS
446.0	Polyarteritis nodosa
710.0	Systemic lupus erythematosus
710.1	Systemic sclerosis
710.2	Sicca syndrome
728.0	Infective myositis
728.1x	Muscular calcification/ossification
728.2	Muscular disuse atrophy NEC
728.3	Muscle disorders NEC
728.81	Interstitial myositis
728.82	Foreign body granuloma of muscle
728.9	Muscle/ligament disorder NOS

CPT CODE	SERVICE	ICD–9–CM
20206* (Cont'd.)		729.1 Myalgia and myositis NOS

REIMBURSEMENT INFORMATION

General

- ♦ See notes on page 286.
- ♦ Starred procedure.

Medicare

- ♦ Follow–up Days — 0
- ♦ Assistant Surgeon — not paid
- ♦ Supply Charges — not allowed
- ♦ Outpatient Limit — does not apply
- ♦ Minor Surgery Rules Apply

CPT CODE	SERVICE
20220	Biopsy, bone, trocar or needle; superficial (eg, ilium, sternum, spinous process, ribs)

CPT NOTES

- For aspiration of bone marrow, see 85095.
- For bone marrow biopsy, use 85102.

ICD–9–CM

170.0	M-Neoplasm, Skull/Face bone
170.1	M-Neoplasm, Mandible
170.2	M-Neoplasm, Vertebrae
170.3	M-Neoplasm, Ribs/Sternum/Clavicle
170.4	M-Neoplasm, Long arm bones
170.5	M-Neoplasm, Wrist/Hand bones
170.6	M-Neoplasm, Pelvic girdle
170.7	M-Neoplasm, Long bones, lower limb
170.8	M-Neoplasm, Short bones, lower limb
170.9	M-Neoplasm, Bone/cartilage NOS
198.5	M2-Neoplasm, Bone and bone marrow
210.4	B-Neoplasm, Mouth NEC/NOS
213.0	B-Neoplasm, Skull/Face bone
213.1	B-Neoplasm, Lower jaw bone
213.2	B-Neoplasm, Vertebrae
213.3	B-Neoplasm, Ribs/Sternum/Clavicle
213.4	B-Neoplasm, Long bones, arm
213.5	B-Neoplasm, Wrist/Hand bones
213.6	B-Neoplasm, Pelvic girdle
213.7	B-Neoplasm, Long bones, lower limb
213.8	B-Neoplasm, Short bones, lower limb
213.9	B-Neoplasm, Bone/cartilage NOS
238.0	UB-Neoplasm, Bone
239.2	Bone/Skin neoplasm NOS
526.89	Jaw disease NEC
730.0x	Acute osteomyelitis
730.1x	Chronic osteomyelitis
733.20	Cyst of bone NOS
733.21	Solitary bone cyst
733.22	Aneurysmal bone cyst
733.29	Bone cyst NEC
733.9x	Disorders of bone and cartilage NOS
756.54	Polyostotic fibrous bone dysplasia
756.59	Osteodystrophy NEC
759.89	Specified congenital anomaly NEC

REIMBURSEMENT INFORMATION

General

- See notes on page 286.

Medicare

- Follow–up Days — 0
- Assistant Surgeon — not paid
- Supply Charges — allowed
- Outpatient Limit — does not apply
- Minor Surgery Rules Apply

CPT CODE	SERVICE
20225	Biopsy, bone, trocar or needle; deep (vertebral body, femur)

CPT NOTES

- For aspiration of bone marrow, see 85095.
- For bone marrow biopsy, use 85102.

ICD–9–CM

170.0	M-Neoplasm, Skull/Face bone
170.1	M-Neoplasm, Mandible
170.2	M-Neoplasm, Vertebrae
170.3	M-Neoplasm, Ribs/Sternum/Clavicle
170.4	M-Neoplasm, Long arm bones
170.5	M-Neoplasm, Wrist/Hand bones
170.6	M-Neoplasm, Pelvic girdle
170.7	M-Neoplasm, Long bones, lower limb
170.8	M-Neoplasm, Short bones, lower limb
170.9	M-Neoplasm, Bone/cartilage NOS
195.0	M-Neoplasm, Head/face/neck
198.5	M2-Neoplasm, Bone and bone marrow
213.0	B-Neoplasm, Skull/Face bone
213.1	B-Neoplasm, Lower jaw bone
213.2	B-Neoplasm, Vertebrae
213.3	B-Neoplasm, Ribs/Sternum/Clavicle
213.4	B-Neoplasm, Long bones, arm
213.5	B-Neoplasm, Wrist/Hand bones
213.6	B-Neoplasm, Pelvic girdle
213.7	B-Neoplasm, Long bones, lower limb
213.8	B-Neoplasm, Short bones, lower limb
213.9	B-Neoplasm, Bone/cartilage NOS
238.0	UB-Neoplasm, Bone
526.89	Jaw disease NEC
730.0x	Acute osteomyelitis
730.1x	Chronic osteomyelitis
733.29	Bone cyst NEC
756.54	Polyostotic fibrous bone dysplasia
756.59	Osteodystrophy NEC
759.89	Specified congenital anomaly NEC

REIMBURSEMENT INFORMATION

General

- See notes on page 286.

Medicare

- Follow–up Days — 0
- Assistant Surgeon — not paid
- Supply Charges — allowed
- Outpatient Limit — does not apply
- Minor Surgery Rules Apply

CPT CODE	SERVICE
20240	Biopsy, excisional; superficial (eg, ilium, sternum, spinous process, ribs, trochanter of femur)

CPT NOTES

- ♦ For aspiration of bone marrow, see 85095.

ICD–9–CM

170.0	M-Neoplasm, Skull/Face bone
170.1	M-Neoplasm, Mandible
170.2	M-Neoplasm, Vertebrae
170.3	M-Neoplasm, Ribs/Sternum/Clavicle
170.4	M-Neoplasm, Long arm bones
170.5	M-Neoplasm, Wrist/Hand bones
170.6	M-Neoplasm, Pelvic girdle
170.7	M-Neoplasm, Long bones, lower limb
170.8	M-Neoplasm, Short bones, lower limb
170.9	M-Neoplasm, Bone/cartilage NOS
198.5	M2-Neoplasm, Bone and bone marrow
213.0	B-Neoplasm, Skull/Face bone
213.1	B-Neoplasm, Lower jaw bone
213.2	B-Neoplasm, Vertebrae
213.3	B-Neoplasm, Ribs/Sternum/Clavicle
213.4	B-Neoplasm, Long bones, arm
213.5	B-Neoplasm, Wrist/Hand bones
213.6	B-Neoplasm, Pelvic girdle
213.7	B-Neoplasm, Long bones, lower limb
213.8	B-Neoplasm, Short bones, lower limb
213.9	B-Neoplasm, Bone/cartilage NOS
238.0	UB-Neoplasm, Bone
239.2	Bone/Skin neoplasm NOS
522.8	Radicular cyst
526.2	Jaw cysts NEC
526.4	Inflammation of jaw
526.89	Jaw disease NEC
730.0x	Acute osteomyelitis
730.1x	Chronic osteomyelitis
733.20	Cyst of bone NOS
733.21	Solitary bone cyst
733.22	Aneurysmal bone cyst
733.29	Bone cyst NEC
756.54	Polyostotic fibrous bone dysplasia
756.59	Osteodystrophy NEC
759.89	Specified congenital anomaly NEC

REIMBURSEMENT INFORMATION

General

- ♦ See notes on page 286.

Medicare

- ♦ Follow–up Days — 10
- ♦ Assistant Surgeon — not paid
- ♦ Supply Charges — allowed
- ♦ Outpatient Limit — does not apply
- ♦ Minor Surgery Rules Apply

20245 Biopsy, excisional; deep (eg, humerus, ischium, femur)

CPT NOTES

- For aspiration of bone marrow, see 85095.

170.0	M-Neoplasm, Skull/Face bone
170.1	M-Neoplasm, Mandible
170.2	M-Neoplasm, Vertebrae
170.3	M-Neoplasm, Ribs/Sternum/Clavicle
170.4	M-Neoplasm, Long arm bones
170.5	M-Neoplasm, Wrist/Hand bones
170.6	M-Neoplasm, Pelvic girdle
170.7	M-Neoplasm, Long bones, lower limb
170.8	M-Neoplasm, Short bones, lower limb
170.9	M-Neoplasm, Bone/cartilage NOS
198.5	M2-Neoplasm, Bone and bone marrow
213.0	B-Neoplasm, Skull/Face bone
213.1	B-Neoplasm, Lower jaw bone
213.2	B-Neoplasm, Vertebrae
213.3	B-Neoplasm, Ribs/Sternum/Clavicle
213.4	B-Neoplasm, Long bones, arm
213.5	B-Neoplasm, Wrist/Hand bones
213.6	B-Neoplasm, Pelvic girdle
213.7	B-Neoplasm, Long bones, lower limb
213.8	B-Neoplasm, Short bones, lower limb
213.9	B-Neoplasm, Bone/cartilage NOS
238.0	UB-Neoplasm, Bone
239.2	Bone/Skin neoplasm NOS
526.89	Jaw disease NEC
730.0x	Acute osteomyelitis
730.1x	Chronic osteomyelitis
733.20	Cyst of bone NOS
733.21	Solitary bone cyst
733.22	Aneurysmal bone cyst
733.29	Bone cyst NEC
756.54	Polyostotic fibrous bone dysplasia
756.59	Osteodystrophy NEC
759.89	Specified congenital anomaly NEC

REIMBURSEMENT INFORMATION

General

- See notes on page 286.

Medicare

- Follow–up Days — 10
- Assistant Surgeon — not paid
- Supply Charges — not allowed
- Outpatient Limit — does not apply
- Minor Surgery Rules Apply

CPT CODE	SERVICE
20520*	Removal of foreign body in muscle or tendon sheath; simple
20525	Removal of foreign body in muscle or tendon sheath; deep or complicated

CPT NOTES

- ◆ For injection procedure for arthrography, see anatomical area.

ICD-9-CM

728.82	Foreign body granuloma of muscle
729.6	Old foreign body in soft tissue
874.9	Open wound of neck NEC, complicated
875.1	Open wound of chest, complicated
876.1	Open wound of back, complicated
877.1	Open wound of buttock, complicated
879.1	Open wound of breast, complicated
879.3	Open wound anterior abdomen, compl
879.5	Open wound lateral abdomen, compl
879.7	Open wound of trunk NEC, complic
879.9	Open wound site NOS, complicated
880.10	Open wound of shoulder, complicated
880.11	Open wound of scapula, complicated
880.12	Open wound of axilla, complicated
880.13	Open wound of upper arm, complic
880.19	Mult open wounds of shoulder, compl
880.2	Shoulder/upper arm, w/tendon
881.1x	Elbow/forearm/wrist complex wound
881.2	Elbow/forearm/wrist, tendon wound
882.1	Open wound of hand, complicated
882.2	Open wound of hand, w/tendon
883.1	Open wound of finger, complicated
883.2	Open wound of finger w/tendon
884.1	Open wound of arm mult/NOS, compl
884.2	Open wound of arm NOS w/tendon
885.1	Traumatic thumb amputation, compl
890.1	Open wound of hip/thigh, complic
890.2	Open wound of hip/thigh w/tendon
891.1	Open wound of knee/leg/ankle, compl
891.2	Open wound knee/leg/ankle w/tendon
892.1	Open wound of foot, complicated
892.2	Open wound of foot w/tendon
893.1	Open wound of toe, complicated
893.2	Open wound of toe w/tendon
894.1	Open wound of leg NEC, complicated
930.1	Foreign body in conjunctival sac

REIMBURSEMENT INFORMATION

General

- ◆ See notes on page 286.
- ◆ Starred procedure. (20520)

Medicare

- ◆ Follow-up Days — 10
- ◆ Assistant Surgeon — not paid
- ◆ Supply Charges — not allowed
- ◆ Outpatient Limit
  20520 — applies
  20525 — does not apply
- ◆ Minor Procedure Rules

CPT CODE **SERVICE**

20550* Injection, tendon sheath, ligament, trigger points or ganglion cyst

CPT NOTES

- For injection procedure for arthrography, see anatomical area.

ICD–9–CM

350.1	Trigeminal neuralgia
350.2	Atypical face pain
524.60	TMJ disorders NOS
715.18	Loc prim osteoarthritis NEC
725.	Polymyalgia rheumatica
726.0	Adhesive capsulitis of shoulder
726.12	Bicipital tenosynovitis
726.31	Medial epicondylitis
726.32	Lateral epicondylitis
726.33	Olecranon bursitis
726.4	Enthesopathy of wrist/carpus
726.5	Enthesopathy of hip
726.6x	Enthesopathy of knee
726.7x	Enthesopathy of ankle and tarsus
727.00	Synovitis NOS
727.02	Giant cell tumor of tendon sheath
727.03	Trigger finger
727.04	Radial styloid tenosynovitis
727.05	Tenosynovitis of hand/wrist NEC
727.06	Tenosynovitis of foot/ankle
727.09	Synovitis NEC
727.1	Bunion
727.2	Occupational bursitis
727.3	Bursitis NOS
727.4x	Ganglion/cyst synovium/tendon/bursa
727.50	Rupture of synovium NOS
727.51	Popliteal synovial cyst
727.59	Rupture of synovium NEC
727.81	Contracture of tendon
727.82	Calcium deposits in tendon/bursa
727.89	Synovium/tendon/bursa disorder NEC
727.9	Synovium/tendon/bursa disorder NOS
728.89	Muscle/ligament disorder NEC
830.0	Dislocation jaw, closed

REIMBURSEMENT INFORMATION

General

- See notes on page 286.
- Starred procedure.

Medicare

- Follow–up Days — 0
- Assistant Surgeon — not paid
- Supply Charges — not allowed
- Outpatient Limit — applies
- Minor Procedure Rules
- Fragments — 10160, 64450

CPT CODE	SERVICE
20600*	Arthrocentesis, aspiration and/or injection; small joint, bursa or ganglion cyst (eg, fingers, toes)

CPT NOTES

- ♦ For injection procedure for arthrography, see anatomical area.

ICD–9–CM

274.0	Gouty arthropathy
274.9	Gout NOS
275.4	Disorders of calcium metabolism
711.0	Pyogenic arthritis
711.9	Infective arthritis NOS
712.10	Dicalc phosphate cryst, unspecified
712.14	Dicalc phosphate cryst, hand
712.19	Dicalc phosphate cryst, mult sites
712.20	Pyrophosphate cryst, unspecified
712.24	Pyrophosphate cryst, hand
712.27	Pyrophosphate cryst, ankle/foot
712.29	Pyrophosphate cryst, multiple sites
714.0	Rheumatoid arthritis
715.14	Loc prim osteoarthritis, hand
715.17	Loc prim osteoarthritis, ankle/foot
715.24	Loc 2nd osteoarthritis, hand
715.27	Loc 2nd osteoarthritis, ankle/foot
715.34	Loc osteoarthritis NOS, hand
715.37	Loc osteoarthritis NOS, ankle/foot
716.14	Traumatic arthropathy, hand
716.17	Traumatic arthropathy, ankle/foot
718.04	Articular cartilage dis, hand
718.07	Articular cartilage dis, ankle/foot
718.14	Loose body in joint, hand
718.17	Loose body in joint, ankle/foot
718.24	Pathologic dislocation, hand
718.27	Pathologic dislocation, ankle/foot
718.34	Recurrent dislocation, hand
718.37	Recurrent dislocation, ankle/foot
719.04	Joint effusion, hand
719.07	Joint effusion, ankle/foot
719.54	Joint stiffness NEC, hand
719.57	Joint stiffness NEC, ankle/foot
727.00	Synovitis NOS
727.03	Trigger finger
727.05	Tenosynovitis of hand/wrist NEC
727.06	Tenosynovitis of foot/ankle
727.1	Bunion
727.2	Occupational bursitis
727.89	Synovium/tendon/bursa disorder NEC
727.9	Synovium/tendon/bursa disorder NOS
905.2	Late effect, arm fracture
905.4	Late effect, leg fracture
905.6	Late effect of dislocation
905.7	Late effect of sprain/strain
905.8	Late effect of tendon injury
959.5	Finger injury NOS
959.7	Lower leg injury NOS

CPT CODE	SERVICE	ICD-9-CM

20600* (Cont'd.)

REIMBURSEMENT INFORMATION

General

- ♦ See notes on page 286.
- ♦ Starred procedure.

Medicare

- ♦ Follow-up Days — 0
- ♦ Assistant Surgeon — not paid
- ♦ Supply Charges — not allowed
- ♦ Outpatient Limit — applies
- ♦ Minor Procedure Rules
- ♦ Fragments — 10160, 64450

CPT CODE	SERVICE
20605*	Arthrocentesis, aspiration and/or injection; intermediate joint, bursa or ganglion cyst (eg, temporomandibular, acromioclavicular, wrist, elbow or ankle, olecranon bursa)

CPT NOTES

- For injection procedure for arthrography, see anatomical area.

ICD-9-CM

274.0	Gouty arthropathy
274.9	Gout NOS
275.4	Disorders of calcium metabolism
524.6	Temporomandibular joint disorder
526.4	Inflammation of jaw
711.0	Pyogenic arthritis
711.9	Infective arthritis NOS
712.10	Dicalc phosphate cryst, unspecified
712.12	Dicalc phosphate cryst, upper arm
712.13	Dicalc phosphate cryst, forearm
712.14	Dicalc phosphate cryst, hand
712.16	Dicalc phosphate cryst, lower leg
712.17	Dicalc phosphate cryst, ankle/foot
712.18	Dicalc phosphate cryst, other site
712.20	Pyrophosphate cryst, unspecified
712.22	Pyrophosphate cryst, upper arm
712.23	Pyrophosphate cryst, forearm
712.24	Pyrophosphate cryst, hand
712.26	Pyrophosphate cryst, lower leg
712.27	Pyrophosphate cryst, ankle/foot
712.28	Pyrophosphate cryst, other site
714.0	Rheumatoid arthritis
715.11	Loc prim osteoarthritis, shoulder
715.12	Loc prim osteoarthritis, upper arm
715.13	Loc prim osteoarthritis, forearm
715.16	Loc prim osteoarthritis, lower leg
715.17	Loc prim osteoarthritis, ankle/foot
715.18	Loc prim osteoarthritis NEC
715.21	Loc 2nd osteoarthritis, shoulder
715.22	Loc 2nd osteoarthritis, upper arm
715.23	Loc 2nd osteoarthritis, forearm
715.26	Loc 2nd osteoarthritis, lower leg
715.27	Loc 2nd osteoarthritis, ankle/foot
715.28	Loc 2nd osteoarthritis NEC
715.31	Loc osteoarthritis NOS, shoulder
715.32	Loc osteoarthritis NOS, upper arm
715.33	Loc osteoarthritis NOS, forearm
715.36	Loc osteoarthritis NOS, lower leg
715.37	Loc osteoarthritis NOS, ankle/foot
715.38	Loc osteoarthritis NOS, site NEC
716.11	Traumatic arthropathy, shoulder
716.12	Traumatic arthropathy, upper arm
716.13	Traumatic arthropathy, forearm
716.16	Traumatic arthropathy, lower leg
716.17	Traumatic arthropathy, ankle/foot
716.18	Traumatic arthropathy NEC
718.01	Articular cartilage dis, shoulder
718.02	Articular cartilage dis, upper arm
718.03	Articular cartilage dis, forearm
718.07	Articular cartilage dis, ankle/foot
718.08	Articular cartilage dis, joint NEC
718.09	Articular cartilage dis, mult joint
718.11	Loose body in joint, shoulder
718.12	Loose body in joint, upper arm
718.13	Loose body in joint, forearm

CPT CODE	SERVICE	ICD-9-CM	
20605* (Cont'd.)		718.17	Loose body in joint, ankle/foot
		718.18	Loose body in joint, joint NEC
		718.19	Loose body in joint, mult joints
		718.21	Pathologic dislocation, shoulder
		718.22	Pathologic dislocation, upper arm
		718.23	Pathologic dislocation, forearm
		718.27	Pathologic dislocation, ankle/foot
		718.28	Pathologic dislocation, joint NEC
		718.29	Pathologic dislocation, mult joints
		718.31	Recurrent dislocation, shoulder
		718.32	Recurrent dislocation, upper arm
		718.33	Recurrent dislocation, forearm
		718.37	Recurrent dislocation, ankle/foot
		718.38	Recurrent dislocation, joint NEC
		718.39	Recurrent dislocation, mult joints
		719.01	Joint effusion, shoulder
		719.02	Joint effusion, upper arm
		719.03	Joint effusion, forearm
		719.07	Joint effusion, ankle/foot
		719.08	Joint effusion, joint NEC
		719.09	Joint effusion, multiple joints
		719.51	Joint stiffness NEC, shoulder
		719.52	Joint stiffness NEC, upper arm
		719.53	Joint stiffness NEC, forearm
		719.57	Joint stiffness NEC, ankle/foot
		719.58	Joint stiffness NEC, other joint
		719.59	Joint stiffness NEC, mult joints
		726.30	Elbow enthesopathy NOS
		726.31	Medial epicondylitis
		726.32	Lateral epicondylitis
		726.33	Olecranon bursitis
		726.39	Elbow enthesopathy NEC
		726.4	Enthesopathy of wrist/carpus
		726.7x	Enthesopathy of ankle and tarsus
		726.8	Peripheral enthesopathy NEC
		727.00	Synovitis NOS
		727.2	Occupational bursitis
		727.3	Bursitis NOS
		727.4x	Ganglion/cyst synovium/tendon/bursa
		727.89	Synovium/tendon/bursa disorder NEC
		727.9	Synovium/tendon/bursa disorder NOS
		802.4	Fx malar/maxillary, closed
		830.0	Dislocation jaw, closed
		848.1	Sprain of jaw
		905.0	Late effect, skull/face fracture
		905.2	Late effect, arm fracture
		905.4	Late effect, leg fracture
		905.5	Late effect NEC
		905.6	Late effect of dislocation
		905.7	Late effect of sprain/strain
		905.8	Late effect of tendon injury
		959.0	Face and neck injury NOS
		959.3	Elbow/forearm/wrist injury NOS

CPT CODE	SERVICE	ICD-9-CM
20605* (Cont'd.)		959.7 Lower leg injury NOS

REIMBURSEMENT INFORMATION

General

- ♦ See notes on page 286.
- ♦ Starred procedure.

Medicare

- ♦ Follow–up Days — 0
- ♦ Assistant Surgeon — not paid
- ♦ Supply Charges — not allowed
- ♦ Outpatient Limit — applies
- ♦ Minor Procedure Rules
- ♦ Fragments — 10160, 64450

CPT CODE	SERVICE
20610*	Arthrocentesis, aspiration and/or injection; major joint or bursa (eg, shoulder, hip, knee joint, subacromial bursa)

CPT NOTES

- ♦ For injection procedure for arthrography, see anatomical area.

ICD-9-CM

274.0	Gouty arthropathy
275.4	Disorders of calcium metabolism
711.0	Pyogenic arthritis
712.10	Dicalc phosphate cryst, unspecified
712.11	Dicalc phosphate cryst, shoulder
712.15	Dicalc phosphate cryst, pelv/thigh
712.19	Dicalc phosphate cryst, mult sites
712.20	Pyrophosphate cryst, unspecified
712.21	Pyrophosphate cryst, shoulder
712.25	Pyrophosphate cryst, pelvis/thigh
712.29	Pyrophosphate cryst, multiple sites
714.0	Rheumatoid arthritis
715.11	Loc prim osteoarthritis, shoulder
715.15	Loc prim osteoarthritis, pelv/thigh
715.16	Loc prim osteoarthritis, lower leg
715.18	Loc prim osteoarthritis NEC
715.21	Loc 2nd osteoarthritis, shoulder
715.25	Loc 2nd osteoarthritis, pelv/thigh
715.26	Loc 2nd osteoarthritis, lower leg
715.28	Loc 2nd osteoarthritis NEC
715.31	Loc osteoarthritis NOS, shoulder
715.35	Loc osteoarthritis NOS, pelv/thigh
715.36	Loc osteoarthritis NOS, lower leg
715.38	Loc osteoarthritis NOS, site NEC
718.01	Articular cartilage dis, shoulder
718.05	Articular cartilage dis, pelv/thigh
718.08	Articular cartilage dis, joint NEC
718.09	Articular cartilage dis, mult joint
718.11	Loose body in joint, shoulder
718.15	Loose body in joint, pelvis/thigh
718.17	Loose body in joint, ankle/foot
718.18	Loose body in joint, joint NEC
718.19	Loose body in joint, mult joints
718.21	Pathologic dislocation, shoulder
718.25	Pathologic dislocation, pelv/thigh
718.26	Pathologic dislocation, lower leg
718.27	Pathologic dislocation, ankle/foot
718.28	Pathologic dislocation, joint NEC
718.29	Pathologic dislocation, mult joints
718.31	Recurrent dislocation, shoulder
718.35	Recurrent dislocation, pelvis/thigh
718.36	Recurrent dislocation, lower leg
718.38	Recurrent dislocation, joint NEC
718.39	Recurrent dislocation, mult joints
719.01	Joint effusion, shoulder
719.05	Joint effusion, pelvis/thigh
719.06	Joint effusion, lower leg
719.51	Joint stiffness NEC, shoulder
719.55	Joint stiffness NEC, pelvis/thigh
719.56	Joint stiffness NEC, lower leg
726.0	Adhesive capsulitis of shoulder
726.10	Rotator cuff syndrome NOS
726.11	Calcifying tendinitis of shoulder
726.12	Bicipital tenosynovitis
726.19	Rotator cuff disorder NEC
726.2	Shoulder region disorder NEC

CPT CODE	SERVICE	ICD–9–CM	
20610* (Cont'd.)		726.5	Enthesopathy of hip
		726.6x	Enthesopathy of knee
		727.00	Synovitis NOS
		727.2	Occupational bursitis
		727.3	Bursitis NOS
		727.4x	Ganglion/cyst synovium/tendon/bursa
		727.50	Rupture of synovium NOS
		727.51	Popliteal synovial cyst
		727.59	Rupture of synovium NEC
		727.9	Synovium/tendon/bursa disorder NOS
		905.3	Late effect, femur neck fracture
		905.5	Late effect NEC
		905.6	Late effect of dislocation
		905.7	Late effect of sprain/strain
		905.8	Late effect of tendon injury
		959.2	Shoulder/upper arm injury NOS
		959.6	Hip/thigh injury NOS
		959.7	Lower leg injury NOS
		959.8	Injury, multiple sites, site NEC
		959.9	Injury, site NOS

REIMBURSEMENT INFORMATION

General

- ♦ See notes on page 286.
- ♦ Starred procedure.

Medicare

- ♦ Follow–up Days — 0
- ♦ Assistant Surgeon — not paid
- ♦ Supply Charges — not allowed
- ♦ Outpatient Limit — applies
- ♦ Minor Procedure Rules
- ♦ Fragments — 10160

CPT CODE	SERVICE
20615	Aspiration and injection for treatment of bone cyst

CPT NOTES

- For injection procedure for arthrography, see anatomical area.

ICD-9-CM

252.0	Hyperparathyroidism
526.0	Developmental odontogenic cysts
526.1	Fissural cysts of jaw
526.2	Jaw cysts NEC
526.89	Jaw disease NEC
733.20	Cyst of bone NOS
733.21	Solitary bone cyst
733.22	Aneurysmal bone cyst
733.29	Bone cyst NEC
756.54	Polyostotic fibrous bone dysplasia

REIMBURSEMENT INFORMATION

General

- See notes on page 286.

Medicare

- Follow-up Days — 10
- Assistant Surgeon — not paid
- Supply Charges — not allowed
- Outpatient Limit — applies
- Minor Procedure Rules

CPT CODE	SERVICE	ICD-9-CM	
20650*	Insertion of wire or pin with application of skeletal traction, including removal (separate procedure)	722.4	Cervical disc degeneration
		754.30	Congenital hip dislocation, unilat
		754.31	Congenital hip dislocation, bilat
		754.32	Congenital hip sublux, unilateral
		754.33	Congenital hip sublux, bilateral
		754.35	Congenital hip dislocation w/sublux
		754.40	Congenital genu recurvatum
		754.41	Congenital knee dislocation
		754.42	Congenital bowing of femur
		754.43	Congenital bowing of tibia/fibula
		802.30	Mandible Fx NOS, open
		802.31	Fx condylar proc mandible, open
		802.32	Subcondylar Fx, mandible, open
		802.33	Fx coronoid proc, mandible, open
		802.34	Fx ramus NOS, open
		802.35	Fx angle of jaw, open
		802.36	Fx symphysis mandible body, open
		802.37	Fx alveolar border mandible, open
		802.38	Fx mandible body NEC, open
		802.39	Multiple Fx mandible, open
		802.4	Fx malar/maxillary, closed
		802.5	Fx malar/maxillary, open
		802.9	Fx facial bone NEC, open
		808.0	Fracture acetabulum-closed
		808.1	Fracture acetabulum-open
		808.2	Fracture of pubis-closed
		808.3	Fracture of pubis-open
		808.41	Fracture of ilium-closed
		808.42	Fracture of ischium-closed
		808.43	Mult pelv Fx-closed w/pelv disrupt
		808.49	Pelvic fracture NEC, closed
		808.51	Fracture of ilium-open
		808.52	Fracture of ischium-open
		808.53	Mult pelvic Fx-open w/pelv disrupt
		808.59	Pelvic fracture NEC, open
		809.0	Fracture of trunk bone, closed
		809.1	Fracture of trunk bone, open
		810.x	Fracture of clavicle
		811.x	Fracture of scapula
		812.x	Fracture of humerus
		813.0x	Fracture of radius/ulna, upper end
		813.1x	Fracture of radius/ulna, lower end
		813.2x	Fracture of radius and ulna shaft
		813.3x	Fracture of radius and ulna shaft
		813.4x	Fracture of radius/ulna, lower end
		813.5x	Fracture of radius/ulna, lower end
		819.0	Fx arms with rib/sternum, closed
		819.1	Fx arms with rib/sternum, open
		820.x	Fracture of neck of femur
		821.x	Femur fracture NOS
		823.x	Fracture of tibia and fibula
		827.0	Fx lower limb NEC, closed
		827.1	Fx lower limb NEC, open
		828.0	Fx legs with arm/rib, closed
		828.1	FX legs with arm/rib, open

CPT NOTES

- ◆ For injection procedure for arthrography, see anatomical area.

CPT CODE	SERVICE	ICD–9–CM
20650* ((Cont'd.)		

REIMBURSEMENT INFORMATION

General

- ♦ See notes on page 286.
- ♦ Starred procedure.
- ♦ Separate procedure rules apply.

Medicare

- ♦ Follow–up Days — 10
- ♦ Assistant Surgeon — paid
- ♦ Supply Charges — not allowed
- ♦ Outpatient Limit — does not apply
- ♦ Minor Procedure Rules

CPT CODE	SERVICE	ICD–9–CM
20660	Application of cranial tongs, caliper, or stereotactic frame, including removal (separate procedure) **CPT NOTES** ◆ For injection procedure for arthrography, see anatomical area.	806.01 C1-C4 Fx-closed, compl cord lesion 806.03 C1-C4 Fx-closed, cen cord syndrome 806.06 C5-C7 Fx-closed, compl cord lesion 806.08 C5-C7 Fx-closed, cen cord syndrome 806.09 C5-C7 Fx-closed, cord injury NEC 806.11 C1-C4 Fx-open, compl cord lesion 806.13 C1-C4 Fx-open, cen cord syndrome 806.16 C5-C7 Fx-open, compl cord lesion 806.18 C5-C7 Fx-open, cen cord syndrome 806.19 C5-C7 Fx-open, cord injury NEC **REIMBURSEMENT INFORMATION** General ◆ See notes on page 286. ◆ Separate procedure rules apply. Medicare ◆ Follow–up Days — 0 ◆ Assistant Surgeon — not paid ◆ Supply Charges — not allowed ◆ Outpatient Limit — does not apply ◆ Minor Procedure Rules
20661	Application of halo, including removal; cranial **CPT NOTES** ◆ For injection procedure for arthrography, see anatomical area.	806.01 C1-C4 Fx-closed, compl cord lesion 806.03 C1-C4 Fx-closed, cen cord syndrome 806.06 C5-C7 Fx-closed, compl cord lesion 806.08 C5-C7 Fx-closed, cen cord syndrome 806.09 C5-C7 Fx-closed, cord injury NEC 806.11 C1-C4 Fx-open, compl cord lesion 806.13 C1-C4 Fx-open, cen cord syndrome 806.16 C5-C7 Fx-open, compl cord lesion 806.18 C5-C7 Fx-open, cen cord syndrome 806.19 C5-C7 Fx-open, cord injury NEC **REIMBURSEMENT INFORMATION** General ◆ See notes on page 286. Medicare ◆ Follow–up Days — 90 ◆ Assistant Surgeon — not paid ◆ Supply Charges — not allowed ◆ Outpatient Limit — does not apply ◆ Major Procedure Rules

CPT CODE **SERVICE**

20665* Removal of tongs or halo applied by another physician

CPT NOTES

- For injection procedure for arthrography, see anatomical area.

ICD–9–CM

806.01	C1-C4 Fx-closed, compl cord lesion
806.03	C1-C4 Fx-closed, cen cord syndrome
806.06	C5-C7 Fx-closed, compl cord lesion
806.08	C5-C7 Fx-closed, cen cord syndrome
806.09	C5-C7 Fx-closed, cord injury NEC
806.11	C1-C4 Fx-open, compl cord lesion
806.13	C1-C4 Fx-open, cen cord syndrome
806.16	C5-C7 Fx-open, compl cord lesion
806.18	C5-C7 Fx-open, cen cord syndrome
806.19	C5-C7 Fx-open, cord injury NEC
806.60	Fx sacrum-closed, cord injury NOS
806.61	Fx sacrum-closed, cauda equina les
806.62	Fx sacrum-closed, cauda injury NEC
806.69	Fx sacrum-closed, cord injury NEC
806.70	Fx sacrum-open, cord injury NOS
806.71	Fx sacrum-open, cauda equina lesion
806.72	Fx sacrum-open, cauda injury NEC
806.79	Fx sacrum-open, cord injury NEC
808.0	Fracture acetabulum-closed
808.1	Fracture acetabulum-open
808.2	Fracture of pubis-closed
808.3	Fracture of pubis-open
808.41	Fracture of ilium-closed
808.42	Fracture of ischium-closed
808.43	Mult pelv Fx-closed w/pelv disrupt
808.49	Pelvic fracture NEC, closed
808.51	Fracture of ilium-open
808.52	Fracture of ischium-open
808.53	Mult pelvic Fx-open w/pelv disrupt
808.59	Pelvic fracture NEC, open

REIMBURSEMENT INFORMATION

General

- See notes on page 286.
- Starred procedure.

Medicare

- Follow–up Days — 10
- Assistant Surgeon — not paid
- Supply Charges — not allowed
- Outpatient Limit — does not apply
- Minor Procedure Rules

CPT CODE	SERVICE
20670*	Removal of implant; superficial, (eg, buried wire, pin or rod) (separate procedure)

CPT NOTES

- ♦ For injection procedure for arthrography, see anatomical area.

ICD–9–CM

143.1	M-Neoplasm, Lower gum
802.20	Mandible Fx NOS, closed
802.21	Fx condylar proc mandible, closed
802.39	Multiple Fx mandible, open
802.4	Fx malar/maxillary, closed
802.5	Fx malar/maxillary, open
808.x	Fracture of pelvis
809.0	Fracture of trunk bone, closed
809.1	Fracture of trunk bone, open
810.0x	Clavicle fracture, closed
810.1x	Clavicle fracture, open
811.x	Fracture of scapula
812.x	Fracture of humerus
813.0x	Fracture of radius/ulna, upper end
813.1x	Fracture of radius/ulna, lower end
813.2x	Fracture of radius and ulna shaft
813.3x	Fracture of radius and ulna shaft
813.4x	Fracture of radius/ulna, lower end
813.5x	Fracture of radius/ulna, lower end
819.0	Fx arms with rib/sternum, closed
819.1	Fx arms with rib/sternum, open
820.x	Fracture of neck of femur
821.x	Femur fracture NOS
823.x	Fracture of tibia and fibula
827.0	Fx lower limb NEC, closed
827.1	Fx lower limb NEC, open
828.0	Fx legs with arm/rib, closed
828.1	FX legs with arm/rib, open
996.59	Malfunction other device/graft
996.60	Reaction, unspecified device/graft
996.70	Complication, unspec device/graft
V54.0	Removal of internal fixation device
V54.8	Orthopedic aftercare NEC

REIMBURSEMENT INFORMATION

General

- ♦ See notes on page 286.
- ♦ Starred procedure.
- ♦ Separate procedure rules apply.

Medicare

- ♦ Follow–up Days — 10
- ♦ Assistant Surgeon — not paid
- ♦ Supply Charges — not allowed
- ♦ Outpatient Limit — does not apply
- ♦ Minor Procedure Rules

CPT CODE **SERVICE**

20680 Removal of implant; deep, (eg, buried wire, pin, screw, metal band, nail, rod or plate)

CPT NOTES

- For injection procedure for arthrography, see anatomical area.

ICD–9–CM

143.1	M-Neoplasm, Lower gum
170.1	M-Neoplasm, Mandible
524.0x	Major anomaly of jaw size
524.1x	Jaw/cranial base relation anomaly
524.6x	Temporomandibular joint disorder
524.8	Dentofacial anomaly NEC
525.2	Atrophy, edentulous alveolar ridge
526.4	Inflammation of jaw
802.1	Nasal bone Fx, open
802.36	Fx symphysis mandible body, open
802.39	Multiple Fx mandible, open
802.4	Fx malar/maxillary, closed
802.5	Fx malar/maxillary, open
802.6	Fx orbital floor, closed
802.7	Fx orbital floor, open
802.8	Fx facial bone NEC, closed
802.9	Fx facial bone NEC, open
808.x	Fracture of pelvis
809.0	Fracture of trunk bone, closed
809.1	Fracture of trunk bone, open
810.0x	Clavicle fracture, closed
810.1x	Clavicle fracture, open
811.x	Fracture of scapula
812.x	Fracture of humerus
813.0x	Fracture of radius/ulna, upper end
813.1x	Fracture of radius/ulna, lower end
813.2x	Fracture of radius and ulna shaft
813.3x	Fracture of radius and ulna shaft
813.4x	Fracture of radius/ulna, lower end
813.5x	Fracture of radius/ulna, lower end
819.0	Fx arms with rib/sternum, closed
819.1	Fx arms with rib/sternum, open
820.x	Fracture of neck of femur
821.x	Femur fracture NOS
823.x	Fracture of tibia and fibula
827.0	Fx lower limb NEC, closed
827.1	Fx lower limb NEC, open
828.0	Fx legs with arm/rib, closed
828.1	FX legs with arm/rib, open
935.0	Foreign body in mouth
996.59	Malfunction other device/graft
996.60	Reaction, unspecified device/graft
996.70	Complication, unspec device/graft

REIMBURSEMENT INFORMATION

General

- See notes on page 286.

Medicare

- Follow–up Days — 90
- Assistant Surgeon — by report
- Supply Charges — not allowed
- Outpatient Limit — does not apply
- Major Procedure Rules
- Fragments — 11040, 11041, 11042

CPT CODE	SERVICE
20690	Application of a uniplane (pins or wires in one plane), unilateral, external fixation system

CPT NOTES

- For injection procedure for arthrography, see anatomical area.
- List in addition to code for treatment of the fracture or joint injury unless listed as part of basic procedure.

ICD–9–CM

144.9	M-Neoplasm, Floor of mouth NOS
170.1	M-Neoplasm, Mandible
524.8	Dentofacial anomaly NEC
802.2	Fracture, Mandible, closed
802.3	Fracture, Mandible, open
802.4	Fx malar/maxillary, closed
802.5	Fx malar/maxillary, open
808.x	Fracture of pelvis
809.0	Fracture of trunk bone, closed
809.1	Fracture of trunk bone, open
810.0x	Clavicle fracture, closed
810.1x	Clavicle fracture, open
811.x	Fracture of scapula
812.x	Fracture of humerus
813.0x	Fracture of radius/ulna, upper end
813.1x	Fracture of radius/ulna, lower end
813.2x	Fracture of radius and ulna shaft
813.3x	Fracture of radius and ulna shaft
813.4x	Fracture of radius/ulna, lower end
813.5x	Fracture of radius/ulna, lower end
819.0	Fx arms with rib/sternum, closed
819.1	Fx arms with rib/sternum, open
820.x	Fracture of neck of femur
821.x	Femur fracture NOS
823.x	Fracture of tibia and fibula
827.0	Fx lower limb NEC, closed
827.1	Fx lower limb NEC, open
828.0	Fx legs with arm/rib, closed
828.1	FX legs with arm/rib, open

REIMBURSEMENT INFORMATION

General

- See notes on page 286.

Medicare

- Follow–up Days — none; falls within global period of another procedure
- Assistant Surgeon — not paid
- Supply Charges — not allowed
- Outpatient Limit — does not apply

CPT CODE	SERVICE
20692	Application of a multiplane (pins or wires in more than one plane), unilateral, external fixation system (eg, Ilizarov, Monticelli type)

CPT NOTES

- ♦ For injection procedure for arthrography, see anatomical area.
- ♦ List in addition to code for treatment of the fracture or joint injury unless listed as part of basic procedure.

ICD–9–CM

144.9	M-Neoplasm, Floor of mouth NOS
170.1	M-Neoplasm, Mandible
524.8	Dentofacial anomaly NEC
526.4	Inflammation of jaw
802.2	Fracture, Mandible, closed
802.3	Fracture, Mandible, open
802.4	Fx malar/maxillary, closed
802.5	Fx malar/maxillary, open
808.x	Fracture of pelvis
809.0	Fracture of trunk bone, closed
809.1	Fracture of trunk bone, open
810.0x	Clavicle fracture, closed
810.1x	Clavicle fracture, open
811.x	Fracture of scapula
812.x	Fracture of humerus
813.0x	Fracture of radius/ulna, upper end
813.1x	Fracture of radius/ulna, lower end
813.2x	Fracture of radius and ulna shaft
813.3x	Fracture of radius and ulna shaft
813.4x	Fracture of radius/ulna, lower end
813.5x	Fracture of radius/ulna, lower end
819.0	Fx arms with rib/sternum, closed
819.1	Fx arms with rib/sternum, open
820.x	Fracture of neck of femur
821.x	Femur fracture NOS
823.x	Fracture of tibia and fibula
827.0	Fx lower limb NEC, closed
827.1	Fx lower limb NEC, open
828.0	Fx legs with arm/rib, closed
828.1	FX legs with arm/rib, open

REIMBURSEMENT INFORMATION

General

- ♦ See notes on page 286.

Medicare

- ♦ Follow–up Days — none; falls within global period of another procedure
- ♦ Assistant Surgeon — paid
- ♦ Supply Charges — not allowed
- ♦ Outpatient Limit — does not apply

CPT CODE **SERVICE**

20693 Adjustment or revision of external fixation system requiring anesthesia (eg, new pin(s) or wire(s) and/or new ring(s) or bar(s))

CPT NOTES

- For injection procedure for arthrography, see anatomical area.

ICD–9–CM

144.9	M-Neoplasm, Floor of mouth NOS
170.1	M-Neoplasm, Mandible
524.8	Dentofacial anomaly NEC
802.2	Fracture, Mandible, closed
802.3	Fracture, Mandible, open
802.4	Fx malar/maxillary, closed
802.5	Fx malar/maxillary, open
808.x	Fracture of pelvis
809.0	Fracture of trunk bone, closed
809.1	Fracture of trunk bone, open
810.0x	Clavicle fracture, closed
810.1x	Clavicle fracture, open
811.x	Fracture of scapula
812.x	Fracture of humerus
813.0x	Fracture of radius/ulna, upper end
813.1x	Fracture of radius/ulna, lower end
813.2x	Fracture of radius and ulna shaft
813.3x	Fracture of radius and ulna shaft
813.4x	Fracture of radius/ulna, lower end
813.5x	Fracture of radius/ulna, lower end
819.0	Fx arms with rib/sternum, closed
819.1	Fx arms with rib/sternum, open
820.x	Fracture of neck of femur
821.x	Femur fracture NOS
823.x	Fracture of tibia and fibula
827.0	Fx lower limb NEC, closed
827.1	Fx lower limb NEC, open
828.0	Fx legs with arm/rib, closed
828.1	FX legs with arm/rib, open

REIMBURSEMENT INFORMATION

General

- See notes on page 286.

Medicare

- Follow–up Days — 90
- Assistant Surgeon — not paid
- Supply Charges — not allowed
- Outpatient Limit — does not apply
- Major Procedure Rules

CPT CODE	SERVICE
20694	Removal, under anesthesia, of external fixation system

CPT NOTES

- For injection procedure for arthrography, see anatomical area.

ICD–9–CM

144.9	M-Neoplasm, Floor of mouth NOS
170.1	M-Neoplasm, Mandible
524.0x	Major anomaly of jaw size
524.1x	Jaw/cranial base relation anomaly
524.2	Dental arch relationship anomaly
524.8	Dentofacial anomaly NEC
524.9	Dentofacial anomaly NOS
526.4	Inflammation of jaw
802.2	Fracture, Mandible, closed
802.3	Fracture, Mandible, open
802.4	Fx malar/maxillary, closed
802.5	Fx malar/maxillary, open
808.x	Fracture of pelvis
809.0	Fracture of trunk bone, closed
809.1	Fracture of trunk bone, open
810.0x	Clavicle fracture, closed
810.1x	Clavicle fracture, open
811.x	Fracture of scapula
812.x	Fracture of humerus
813.0x	Fracture of radius/ulna, upper end
813.1x	Fracture of radius/ulna, lower end
813.2x	Fracture of radius and ulna shaft
813.3x	Fracture of radius and ulna shaft
813.4x	Fracture of radius/ulna, lower end
813.5x	Fracture of radius/ulna, lower end
819.0	Fx arms with rib/sternum, closed
819.1	Fx arms with rib/sternum, open
820.x	Fracture of neck of femur
821.x	Femur fracture NOS
823.x	Fracture of tibia and fibula
827.0	Fx lower limb NEC, closed
827.1	Fx lower limb NEC, open
828.0	Fx legs with arm/rib, closed
828.1	FX legs with arm/rib, open

REIMBURSEMENT INFORMATION

General

- See notes on page 286.

Medicare

- Follow–up Days — 90
- Assistant Surgeon — not paid
- Supply Charges — not allowed
- Outpatient Limit — does not apply
- Major Procedure Rules

CPT CODE	SERVICE	ICD-9-CM
20802	Replantation, arm (includes surgical neck of humerus through elbow joint); complete amputation	887.2 Amputation above elbow, unilateral 887.3 Amputation above elbow, unil, compl 887.6 Amputation of arm, bilateral 887.7 Amputation of arm, bilateral, compl
20804	Replantation, arm (includes surgical neck of humerus through elbow joint); incomplete amputation (devascularized extremity with soft tissue pedicle)	

REIMBURSEMENT INFORMATION

General

- See notes on page 286.

Medicare

- Follow-up Days — 90
- Assistant Surgeon — paid
- Supply Charges — not allowed
- Outpatient Limit — does not apply
- Major Procedure Rules

CPT CODE	SERVICE	ICD-9-CM
20805	Replantation, forearm (includes radius and ulna to radial carpal joint); complete amputation	887.0 Amputation below elbow, unilateral 887.1 Amputation below elbow, unil, compl 887.6 Amputation of arm, bilateral 887.7 Amputation of arm, bilateral, compl
20806	Replantation, forearm (includes radius and ulna to radial carpal joint); incomplete amputation (devascularized extremity with soft tissue pedicle)	

REIMBURSEMENT INFORMATION

General

- See notes on page 286.

Medicare

- Follow-up Days — 90
- Assistant Surgeon — paid
- Supply Charges — not allowed
- Outpatient Limit — does not apply
- Major Procedure Rules

CPT CODE	SERVICE	ICD-9-CM
20808	Replantation, hand (includes hand through metacarpophalangeal joints); complete amputation	887.0 Amputation below elbow, unilateral 887.1 Amputation below elbow, unil, compl 887.6 Amputation of arm, bilateral 887.7 Amputation of arm, bilateral, compl
20812	Replantation, hand (includes hand through metacarpophalangeal joints); incomplete amputation (devascularized extremity with soft tissue pedicle)	

REIMBURSEMENT INFORMATION

General

- See notes on page 286.

Medicare

- Follow-up Days — 90
- Assistant Surgeon — paid
- Supply Charges — not allowed
- Outpatient Limit — does not apply
- Major Procedure Rules

CPT CODE	SERVICE	ICD-9-CM
20816	Replantation, digit, excluding thumb (includes metacarpophalangeal joint to insertion of flexor sublimis tendon); complete amputation	886.0 Traumatic finger amputation 886.1 Traumatic finger amputation, compl **REIMBURSEMENT INFORMATION** General ◆ See notes on page 286. Medicare ◆ Follow-up Days — 90 ◆ Assistant Surgeon — paid ◆ Supply Charges — not allowed ◆ Outpatient Limit — does not apply ◆ Major Procedure Rules
20820	Replantation, digit, excluding thumb (includes metacarpophalangeal joint to insertion of flexor sublimis tendon); incomplete amputation (devascularized extremity with soft tissue pedicle)	
20822	Replantation, digit, excluding thumb (includes distal tip to sublimis tendon insertion); complete amputation	886.0 Traumatic finger amputation 886.1 Traumatic finger amputation, compl **REIMBURSEMENT INFORMATION** General ◆ See notes on page 286. Medicare ◆ Follow-up Days — 90 ◆ Assistant Surgeon — paid ◆ Supply Charges — not allowed ◆ Outpatient Limit — does not apply ◆ Major Procedure Rules
20823	Replantation, digit, excluding thumb (includes distal tip to sublimis tendon insertion); incomplete amputation (devascularized extremity with soft tissue pedicle)	
20824	Replantation, thumb (includes carpometacarpal joint to MP joint); complete amputation	885.0 Traumatic thumb amputation 885.1 Traumatic thumb amputation, compl **REIMBURSEMENT INFORMATION** General ◆ See notes on page 286. Medicare ◆ Follow-up Days — 90 ◆ Assistant Surgeon — paid ◆ Supply Charges — not allowed ◆ Outpatient Limit — does not apply ◆ Major Procedure Rules
20826	Replantation, thumb (includes carpometacarpal joint to MP joint); incomplete amputation (devascularized extremity with soft tissue pedicle)	

CPT CODE	SERVICE	ICD-9-CM
20827	Replantation, thumb (includes distal tip to MP joint); complete amputation	885.0 Traumatic thumb amputation 885.1 Traumatic thumb amputation, compl
20828	Replantation, thumb (includes distal tip to MP joint); incomplete amputation (devascularized extremity with soft tissue pedicle)	**REIMBURSEMENT INFORMATION** General ◆ See notes on page 286. Medicare ◆ Follow-up Days — 90 ◆ Assistant Surgeon — paid ◆ Supply Charges — not allowed ◆ Outpatient Limit — does not apply ◆ Major Procedure Rules
20832	Replantation, leg; complete amputation	897.0 Amputation below knee, unilateral 897.1 Amputate below knee, unilat, compl 897.2 Amputation above knee, unilateral 897.3 Amputate above knee, unilat, compl 897.6 Amputation of leg, bilateral 897.7 Amputation of leg, bilateral, compl
20834	Replantation, leg; incomplete amputation (devascularized extremity with soft tissue pedicle)	**REIMBURSEMENT INFORMATION** General ◆ See notes on page 286. Medicare ◆ Follow-up Days — 90 ◆ Assistant Surgeon — paid ◆ Supply Charges — not allowed ◆ Outpatient Limit — does not apply ◆ Major Procedure Rules
20838	Replantation, foot; complete amputation	896.x Traumatic amputation of foot **REIMBURSEMENT INFORMATION** General ◆ See notes on page 286. Medicare ◆ Follow-up Days — 90 ◆ Assistant Surgeon — paid ◆ Supply Charges — not allowed ◆ Outpatient Limit — does not apply ◆ Major Procedure Rules

CPT CODE	SERVICE
20840	Replantation, foot; incomplete amputation (devascularized extremity with soft tissue pedicle)

ICD–9–CM

896.0	Amputation of foot, unilateral
896.1	Amputation of foot, unilat, compl
896.2	Amputation of foot, bilateral
896.3	Amputation of foot, bilat, compl

REIMBURSEMENT INFORMATION

General

- See notes on page 286.

Medicare

- Follow–up Days — 90
- Assistant Surgeon — paid
- Supply Charges — not allowed
- Outpatient Limit — does not apply
- Major Procedure Rules

CPT CODE	SERVICE	ICD–9–CM	
20900	Bone graft, any donor area; minor or small (eg, dowel or button)	143.1	M-Neoplasm, Lower gum
		144.9	M-Neoplasm, Floor of mouth NOS
		170.0	M-Neoplasm, Skull/Face bone
		170.1	M-Neoplasm, Mandible
		170.5	M-Neoplasm, Wrist/Hand bones
		170.8	M-Neoplasm, Short bones, lower limb
		213.0	B-Neoplasm, Skull/Face bone
		213.1	B-Neoplasm, Lower jaw bone
		213.5	B-Neoplasm, Wrist/Hand bones
		213.8	B-Neoplasm, Short bones, lower limb
		376.40	Deformity of orbit NOS
		376.44	Craniofacial orbit deformity
		376.46	Enlargement of orbit
		376.47	Orbit deformity d/t trauma/surgery
		376.50	Enophthalmos NOS
		376.51	Enophthalmos d/t orbit atrophy
		376.52	Enophthalmos d/t trauma/surgery
		522.8	Radicular cyst
		523.4	Chronic periodontitis
		524.0x	Major anomaly of jaw size
		524.1x	Jaw/cranial base relation anomaly
		524.2	Dental arch relationship anomaly
		524.8	Dentofacial anomaly NEC
		524.9	Dentofacial anomaly NOS
		525.2	Atrophy, edentulous alveolar ridge
		526.0	Developmental odontogenic cysts
		526.1	Fissural cysts of jaw
		526.2	Jaw cysts NEC
		526.4	Inflammation of jaw
		526.89	Jaw disease NEC
		733.20	Cyst of bone NOS
		733.81	Malunion of fracture
		733.82	Nonunion of fracture
		738.12	Zygomatic hypoplasia
		754.0	Congen skull/face/jaw deformity
		755.21	Transverse arm deficiency
		755.29	Longitudinal defic, hand phalanges
		755.31	Transverse leg deficiency
		756.0	Anomaly of skull/face bones
		802.1	Nasal bone Fx, open
		802.2x	Fracture, Mandible, closed
		802.3x	Fracture, Mandible, open
		802.4	Fx malar/maxillary, closed
		802.5	Fx malar/maxillary, open
		802.6	Fx orbital floor, closed
		802.7	Fx orbital floor, open
		802.8	Fx facial bone NEC, closed
		802.9	Fx facial bone NEC, open
		815.x	Fracture of metacarpal bone(s)
		816.x	Fracture of phalanges of hand
		817.0	Multiple Fx hand, closed
		817.1	Multiple Fx hand, open
		822.0	Fracture of patella, closed
		822.1	Fracture of patella, open
		824.x	Fracture of ankle
		825.x	Tarsal/metatarsal fracture

CPT NOTES

- Codes for obtaining autogenous bone, cartilage, tendon, fascia lata grafts, or other tissues, through separate incisions are to be used only when graft is not already listed as part of basic procedure.

CPT CODE	SERVICE	ICD-9-CM
20900 (Cont'd.)		

826.0 Fx phalanx, foot, closed
826.1 Fx phalanx, foot, open
905.0 Late effect, skull/face fracture
905.2 Late effect, arm fracture
905.4 Late effect, leg fracture
905.5 Late effect NEC
905.9 Late effect of traumatic amputation

REIMBURSEMENT INFORMATION

General

- See notes on page 286.

Medicare

- Follow-up Days — 90
- Assistant Surgeon — paid
- Supply Charges — not allowed
- Outpatient Limit — does not apply
- Major Procedure Rules

CPT CODE	SERVICE
20902	Bone graft, any donor area; major or large

CPT NOTES

- Codes for obtaining autogenous bone, cartilage, tendon, fascia lata grafts, or other tissues, through separate incisions are to be used only when graft is not already listed as part of basic procedure.

ICD-9-CM	
143.1	M-Neoplasm, Lower gum
144.9	M-Neoplasm, Floor of mouth NOS
170.2	M-Neoplasm, Vertebrae
170.3	M-Neoplasm, Ribs/Sternum/Clavicle
170.4	M-Neoplasm, Long arm bones
170.5	M-Neoplasm, Wrist/Hand bones
170.6	M-Neoplasm, Pelvic girdle
170.7	M-Neoplasm, Long bones, lower limb
170.8	M-Neoplasm, Short bones, lower limb
213.2	B-Neoplasm, Vertebrae
213.3	B-Neoplasm, Ribs/Sternum/Clavicle
213.4	B-Neoplasm, Long bones, arm
213.5	B-Neoplasm, Wrist/Hand bones
213.6	B-Neoplasm, Pelvic girdle
213.7	B-Neoplasm, Long bones, lower limb
213.8	B-Neoplasm, Short bones, lower limb
376.40	Deformity of orbit NOS
376.44	Craniofacial orbit deformity
376.46	Enlargement of orbit
376.47	Orbit deformity d/t trauma/surgery
376.50	Enophthalmos NOS
376.51	Enophthalmos d/t orbit atrophy
376.52	Enophthalmos d/t trauma/surgery
522.8	Radicular cyst
523.4	Chronic periodontitis
524.0x	Major anomaly of jaw size
524.1x	Jaw/cranial base relation anomaly
524.2	Dental arch relationship anomaly
524.8	Dentofacial anomaly NEC
524.9	Dentofacial anomaly NOS
525.2	Atrophy, edentulous alveolar ridge
526.0	Developmental odontogenic cysts
526.1	Fissural cysts of jaw
526.2	Jaw cysts NEC
526.4	Inflammation of jaw
526.89	Jaw disease NEC
733.20	Cyst of bone NOS
733.81	Malunion of fracture
733.82	Nonunion of fracture
738.12	Zygomatic hypoplasia
754.0	Congen skull/face/jaw deformity
754.21	Congenital postural deformity
755.31	Transverse leg deficiency
756.0	Anomaly of skull/face bones
802.1	Nasal bone Fx, open
802.3x	Fracture, Mandible, open
802.5	Fx malar/maxillary, open
802.7	Fx orbital floor, open
802.9	Fx facial bone NEC, open
808.x	Fracture of pelvis
809.0	Fracture of trunk bone, closed
809.1	Fracture of trunk bone, open
810.00	Fx clavicle NOS, closed
810.01	Fx clavicle, sternum end, closed
810.02	Fx clavicle shaft, closed

CPT CODE	SERVICE	ICD-9-CM	
20902 (Cont'd.)		810.03	Fx clavicle, acromial end, closed
		810.10	Fx clavicle NOS, open
		810.11	Fx clavicle, sternum end, open
		810.12	Fx clavicle shaft, open
		810.13	Fx clavicle, acromial end, open
		811.x	Fracture of scapula
		812.x	Fracture of humerus
		813.0x	Fracture of radius/ulna, upper end
		813.1x	Fracture of radius/ulna, lower end
		813.2x	Fracture of radius and ulna shaft
		813.3x	Fracture of radius and ulna shaft
		813.4x	Fracture of radius/ulna, lower end
		813.5x	Fracture of radius/ulna, lower end
		819.0	Fx arms with rib/sternum, closed
		819.1	Fx arms with rib/sternum, open
		820.x	Fracture of neck of femur
		821.x	Femur fracture NOS
		823.x	Fracture of tibia and fibula
		827.0	Fx lower limb NEC, closed
		827.1	Fx lower limb NEC, open
		828.0	Fx legs with arm/rib, closed
		828.1	FX legs with arm/rib, open
		905.1	Late effect, spinal/trunk fracture
		905.2	Late effect, arm fracture
		905.3	Late effect, femur neck fracture
		905.4	Late effect, leg fracture
		905.5	Late effect NEC
		905.9	Late effect of traumatic amputation

REIMBURSEMENT INFORMATION

General

- See notes on page 286.

Medicare

- Follow–up Days — 90
- Assistant Surgeon — paid
- Supply Charges — not allowed
- Outpatient Limit — does not apply
- Major Procedure Rules

CPT CODE	SERVICE	ICD-9-CM

20910 Cartilage graft; costochondral

CPT NOTES

- Codes for obtaining autogenous bone, cartilage, tendon, fascia lata grafts, or other tissues, through separate incisions are to be used only when graft is not already listed as part of basic procedure.
- For ear cartilage, see 21235.

524.04	Mandibular hypoplasia
524.06	Microgenia
524.2	Dental arch relationship anomaly
524.4	Malocclusion NOS
524.60	TMJ disorders NOS
524.61	TMJ adhesions/ankylosis
526.89	Jaw disease NEC
754.0	Congen skull/face/jaw deformity
756.0	Anomaly of skull/face bones

REIMBURSEMENT INFORMATION

General

- See notes on page 286.

Medicare

- Follow-up Days — 90
- Assistant Surgeon — paid
- Supply Charges — not allowed
- Outpatient Limit — does not apply
- Major Procedure Rules

20912 Cartilage graft; nasal septum

CPT NOTES

- Codes for obtaining autogenous bone, cartilage, tendon, fascia lata grafts, or other tissues, through separate incisions are to be used only when graft is not already listed as part of basic procedure.
- For ear cartilage, see 21235.

170.0	M-Neoplasm, Skull/Face bone
213.0	B-Neoplasm, Skull/Face bone
374.1x	Ectropion
374.2x	Lagophthalmos
374.41	Eyelid retraction or lag
738.1	Acquired head deformity NEC
748.1	Congenital nose anomaly NEC
802.0	Nasal bone Fx, closed
802.1	Nasal bone Fx, open
802.6	Fx orbital floor, closed
802.7	Fx orbital floor, open
802.8	Fx facial bone NEC, closed
870.1	Full-thickness laceration eyelid
870.2	Eyelid laceration inv lacrimal pas
905.0	Late effect, skull/face fracture
906.0	Late effect, open wound head/trunk

REIMBURSEMENT INFORMATION

General

- See notes on page 286.

Medicare

- Follow-up Days — 90
- Assistant Surgeon — not paid
- Supply Charges — not allowed
- Outpatient Limit — does not apply
- Major Procedure Rules

CPT CODE	SERVICE
20924	Tendon graft, from a distance (eg, palmaris, toe extensor, plantaris)

CPT NOTES

- Codes for obtaining autogenous bone, cartilage, tendon, fascia lata grafts, or other tissues, through separate incisions are to be used only when graft is not already listed as part of basic procedure.

ICD–9–CM

374.1x	Ectropion
727.63	Rupture, hand/wrist extensor tendon
727.64	Rupture, hand/wrist flexor tendons
727.69	Nontraumatic tendon rupture NEC
727.81	Contracture of tendon
881.2	Elbow/forearm/wrist, tendon wound
882.2	Open wound of hand, w/tendon
883.2	Open wound of finger w/tendon
884.2	Open wound of arm NOS w/tendon
891.2	Open wound knee/leg/ankle w/tendon
892.2	Open wound of foot w/tendon
893.2	Open wound of toe w/tendon
894.2	Open wound of leg NEC w/tendon
905.8	Late effect of tendon injury
905.9	Late effect of traumatic amputation
927.11	Crushing injury, elbow
927.2x	Crushing injury, wrist and hand
927.3	Crushing injury, finger
928.11	Crushing injury, knee
928.20	Crushing injury, foot

REIMBURSEMENT INFORMATION

General

- See notes on page 286.

Medicare

- Follow–up Days — 90
- Assistant Surgeon — paid
- Supply Charges — not allowed
- Outpatient Limit — does not apply
- Major Procedure Rules

CPT CODE	SERVICE
20926	Tissue grafts, other (eg, paratenon, fat, dermis, etc)

CPT NOTES

- Codes for obtaining autogenous bone, cartilage, tendon, fascia lata grafts, or other tissues, through separate incisions are to be used only when graft is not already listed as part of basic procedure.

ICD–9–CM

524.6	Temporomandibular joint disorder
525.2	Atrophy, edentulous alveolar ridge
709.2	Scar/fibrosis of skin
830.1	Dislocation jaw, open
881.2	Elbow/forearm/wrist, tendon wound
882.2	Open wound of hand, w/tendon
883.2	Open wound of finger w/tendon
884.2	Open wound of arm NOS w/tendon
891.2	Open wound knee/leg/ankle w/tendon
892.2	Open wound of foot w/tendon
893.2	Open wound of toe w/tendon
894.2	Open wound of leg NEC w/tendon
927.11	Crushing injury, elbow
927.2x	Crushing injury, wrist and hand
927.3	Crushing injury, finger
928.11	Crushing injury, knee
928.20	Crushing injury, foot
928.3	Crushing injury, toe

REIMBURSEMENT INFORMATION

General

- See notes on page 286.

Medicare

- Follow–up Days — 90
- Assistant Surgeon — not paid
- Supply Charges — not allowed
- Outpatient Limit — does not apply
- Major Procedure Rules

CPT CODE	SERVICE
20950	Monitoring of interstitial fluid pressure (includes insertion of device eg, wick catheter technique, needle manometer technique) in detection of muscle compartment syndrome

ICD–9–CM

927.00	Crushing injury, shoulder region
927.1x	Crushing injury, elbow and forearm
927.2x	Crushing injury, wrist and hand
927.3	Crushing injury, finger
928.0x	Crushing injury, hip and thigh
928.1x	Crushing injury, knee, lower leg
928.20	Crushing injury, foot
928.8	Multiple crushing injuries, leg
958.8	Early complications of trauma NEC
959.1	Trunk injury NOS
959.2	Shoulder/upper arm injury NOS
959.3	Elbow/forearm/wrist injury NOS
959.4	Hand injury NOS
959.5	Finger injury NOS
959.6	Hip/thigh injury NOS
959.7	Lower leg injury NOS

REIMBURSEMENT INFORMATION

General

- See notes on page 286.

Medicare

- Follow–up Days — 0
- Assistant Surgeon — not paid
- Supply Charges — not allowed
- Outpatient Limit — does not apply
- Minor Procedure Rules

CPT CODE	SERVICE	ICD-9-CM
20972	Free osteocutaneous flap with microvascular anastomosis; metatarsal	524.9 Dentofacial anomaly NOS 754.0 Congen skull/face/jaw deformity 755.21 Transverse arm deficiency 755.28 Longitudinal deficiency, hand 755.31 Transverse leg deficiency 756.0 Anomaly of skull/face bones 885.1 Traumatic thumb amputation, compl 896.x Traumatic amputation of foot

REIMBURSEMENT INFORMATION

General

- See notes on page 286.

Medicare

- Follow–up Days — 90
- Assistant Surgeon — paid
- Supply Charges — not allowed
- Outpatient Limit — does not apply
- Major Procedure Rules

CPT CODE	SERVICE	ICD-9-CM
20973	Free osteocutaneous flap with microvascular anastomosis; great toe with web space	885.0 Traumatic thumb amputation 885.1 Traumatic thumb amputation, compl

REIMBURSEMENT INFORMATION

General

- See notes on page 286.

Medicare

- Follow–up Days — 90
- Assistant Surgeon — paid
- Supply Charges — not allowed
- Outpatient Limit — does not apply
- Major Procedure Rules

CPT CODE	SERVICE	ICD-9-CM

20974 Electrical stimulation to aid bone healing; noninvasive (nonoperative)

20975 Electrical stimulation to aid bone healing; invasive

CPT NOTES

- ♦ Use in addition to code for appropriate bony procedure, when applicable.

733.82 Nonunion of fracture

REIMBURSEMENT INFORMATION

General

- ♦ See notes on page 286.

Medicare

- ♦ Follow–up Days — none; falls within global period of another procedure
- ♦ Assistant Surgeon
- ♦ 90974 — not paid
  20975 — paid
- ♦ Supply Charges
  20974 — allowed
  20975 — not allowed
- ♦ Outpatient Limit — applies

21010 Arthrotomy, temporomandibular joint

CPT NOTES

- ♦ For drainage of superficial abscess and hematoma, see 20000.
- ♦ For removal of embedded foreign body from dentoalveolar structure, see 41805, 41806.

524.60	TMJ disorders NOS
524.61	TMJ adhesions/ankylosis
524.62	TMJ arthralgia
524.63	TMJ articular disc disorder
524.69	TMJ disorders NEC
526.4	Inflammation of jaw
830.0	Dislocation jaw, closed
830.1	Dislocation jaw, open
848.1	Sprain of jaw
905.6	Late effect of dislocation

REIMBURSEMENT INFORMATION

General

- ♦ See notes on page 286.

Medicare

- ♦ Follow–up Days — 90
- ♦ Assistant Surgeon — by report
- ♦ Supply Charges — not allowed
- ♦ Outpatient Limit — does not apply
- ♦ Major Procedure Rules

CPT CODE	SERVICE
21015	Radical resection of tumor (eg, malignant neoplasm), soft tissue of face or scalp

CPT NOTES

- For biopsy, see 20220, 20240.

ICD-9-CM

160.0	M-Neoplasm, Nasal cavities
160.2	M-Neoplasm, Maxillary sinus
160.3	M-Neoplasm, Ethmoidal sinus
160.4	M-Neoplasm, Frontal sinus
160.5	M-Neoplasm, Sphenoidal sinus
161.0	M-Neoplasm, Glottis
161.1	M-Neoplasm, Supraglottis
161.2	M-Neoplasm, Subglottis
161.3	M-Neoplasm, Laryngeal cartilages
161.8	M-Neoplasm, Larynx NEC
161.9	M-Neoplasm, Larynx NOS
162.0	M-Neoplasm, Trachea
171.0	M-Neoplasm, Soft tissue, head
172.0	Malignant melanoma, Lip
172.1	Malignant melanoma, eyelid/canthus
172.2	Malignant melanoma, Ear
172.3	Malignant melanoma, Face NEC/NOS
173.0	M-Neoplasm, Skin of lip
173.1	M-Neoplasm, Skin of eyelid/canthus
173.2	M-Neoplasm, Skin of ear
173.3	M-Neoplasm, Skin of face NEC
176.0	Kaposi's sarcoma, skin
176.1	Kaposi's sarcoma, soft tissue
195.0	M-Neoplasm, Head/face/neck
232.3	CA in situ, Skin of face NEC

REIMBURSEMENT INFORMATION

General

- See notes on page 286.

Medicare

- Follow-up Days — 90
- Assistant Surgeon — not paid
- Supply Charges — not allowed
- Outpatient Limit — does not apply
- Major Procedure Rules

CPT CODE **SERVICE**

21025 Excision of bone (eg, for osteomyelitis or bone abscess); mandible

CPT NOTES

- For biopsy, see 20220, 20240.

ICD-9-CM

350.2	Atypical face pain
524.0x	Major anomaly of jaw size
524.1x	Jaw/cranial base relation anomaly
524.6	Temporomandibular joint disorder
526.3	Jaw, central giant cell granuloma
526.4	Inflammation of jaw
526.81	Exostosis of jaw
526.89	Jaw disease NEC
528.3	Cellulitis/abscess of mouth
730.08	Acute osteomyelitis NEC
730.18	Chronic osteomyelitis NEC
730.28	Osteomyelitis NOS, other site
802.2	Fracture, Mandible, closed
802.3	Fracture, Mandible, open
905.0	Late effect, skull/face fracture
908.6	Late effect, trauma complications
909.2	Late effect of radiation
909.3	Late effect of surg/med complic

REIMBURSEMENT INFORMATION

General

- See notes on page 286.

Medicare

- Follow-up Days — 90
- Assistant Surgeon — not paid
- Supply Charges — not allowed
- Outpatient Limit — does not apply
- Major Procedure Rules

CPT CODE	SERVICE	ICD-9-CM

21026 Excision of bone (eg, for osteomyelitis or bone abscess); facial bone(s)

CPT NOTES

- For biopsy, see 20220, 20240.

350.2	Atypical face pain
376.42	Exostosis of orbit
526.4	Inflammation of jaw
726.91	Exostosis, site NOS
730.18	Chronic osteomyelitis NEC
756.4	Chondrodystrophy
905.0	Late effect, skull/face fracture
908.6	Late effect, trauma complications
909.2	Late effect of radiation
909.3	Late effect of surg/med complic
996.4	Malfunction, int orthoped dev/graft

REIMBURSEMENT INFORMATION

General

- See notes on page 286.

Medicare

- Follow-up Days — 90
- Assistant Surgeon — not paid
- Supply Charges — not allowed
- Outpatient Limit — does not apply
- Major Procedure Rules

21029 Removal by contouring of benign tumor of facial bone (eg, fibrous dysplasia)

CPT NOTES

- For biopsy, see 20220, 20240.

213.0	B-Neoplasm, Skull/Face bone
526.89	Jaw disease NEC
526.9	Jaw disease NOS
733.29	Bone cyst NEC
756.54	Polyostotic fibrous bone dysplasia

REIMBURSEMENT INFORMATION

General

- See notes on page 286.

Medicare

- Follow-up Days — 90
- Assistant Surgeon — not paid
- Supply Charges — not allowed
- Outpatient Limit — applies
- Major Procedure Rules

CPT CODE	SERVICE	ICD-9-CM	
21030	Excision of benign tumor or cyst or facial bone other than mandible	210.4	B-Neoplasm, Mouth NEC/NOS
		213.0	B-Neoplasm, Skull/Face bone
		238.0	UB-Neoplasm, Bone
		239.2	Bone/Skin neoplasm NOS
		522.7	Periapical abscess w/sinus
		522.8	Radicular cyst
		523.8	Periodontal disease NEC
		524.3	Tooth position anomaly
		526.0	Developmental odontogenic cysts
		526.1	Fissural cysts of jaw
		526.2	Jaw cysts NEC
		526.3	Jaw, central giant cell granuloma
		526.81	Exostosis of jaw
		733.2x	Cyst of bone

CPT NOTES

- For biopsy, see 20220, 20240.

REIMBURSEMENT INFORMATION

General

- See notes on page 286.

Medicare

- Follow-up Days — 90
- Assistant Surgeon — not paid
- Supply Charges — not allowed
- Outpatient Limit — applies
- Major Procedure Rules

CPT CODE	SERVICE	ICD-9-CM	
21031	Excision of torus mandibularis	525.8	Dental disorder NEC
		526.4	Inflammation of jaw
		526.81	Exostosis of jaw
		996.59	Malfunction other device/graft

CPT NOTES

- For biopsy, see 20220, 20240.

REIMBURSEMENT INFORMATION

General

- See notes on page 286.

Medicare

- Follow-up Days — 90
- Assistant Surgeon — not paid
- Supply Charges — not allowed
- Outpatient Limit — applies
- Major Procedure Rules

CPT CODE	SERVICE	ICD-9-CM
21032	Excision of maxillary torus palatinus	525.8 Dental disorder NEC 526.81 Exostosis of jaw 996.59 Malfunction other device/graft

CPT NOTES

- For biopsy, see 20220, 20240.

REIMBURSEMENT INFORMATION

General

- See notes on page 286.

Medicare

- Follow-up Days — 90
- Assistant Surgeon — not paid
- Supply Charges — not allowed
- Outpatient Limit — applies
- Major Procedure Rules

21034	Excision of malignant tumor of facial bone other than mandible	170.0 M-Neoplasm, Skull/Face bone 195.0 M-Neoplasm, Head/face/neck 198.5 M2-Neoplasm, Bone and bone marrow 199.0 M-Neoplasm, Disseminated 199.1 M-Neoplasm NOS 203.0 Multiple myeloma

CPT NOTES

- For biopsy, see 20220, 20240.

REIMBURSEMENT INFORMATION

General

- See notes on page 286.

Medicare

- Follow-up Days — 90
- Assistant Surgeon — not paid
- Supply Charges — not allowed
- Outpatient Limit — does not apply
- Major Procedure Rules

CPT CODE	SERVICE	ICD-9-CM	
21040	Excision of benign cyst or tumor of mandible; simple	145.6	M-Neoplasm, Retromolar area
21041	Excision of benign cyst or tumor of mandible; complex	210.4	B-Neoplasm, Mouth NEC/NOS
		213.1	B-Neoplasm, Lower jaw bone
		228.0	Hemangioma
		235.1	UB-Neoplasm, Oral cavity/pharynx
		238.0	UB-Neoplasm, Bone
		239.2	Bone/Skin neoplasm NOS
		520.6	Tooth eruption disturbances
		522.8	Radicular cyst
		523.8	Periodontal disease NEC
		526.0	Developmental odontogenic cysts
		526.1	Fissural cysts of jaw
		526.2	Jaw cysts NEC
		526.3	Jaw, central giant cell granuloma
		526.81	Exostosis of jaw
		526.89	Jaw disease NEC
		528.9	Oral soft tissue disease NEC
		756.54	Polyostotic fibrous bone dysplasia

CPT NOTES

- For biopsy, see 20220, 20240.

REIMBURSEMENT INFORMATION

General

- See notes on page 286.

Medicare

- Follow–up Days — 90
- Assistant Surgeon — not paid
- Supply Charges — not allowed
- Outpatient Limit — does not apply
- Major Procedure Rules

CPT CODE	SERVICE	ICD-9-CM	
21044	Excision of malignant tumor of mandible	170.1	M-Neoplasm, Mandible
21045	Excision of malignant tumor of mandible; radical resection	195.0	M-Neoplasm, Head/face/neck
		198.5	M2-Neoplasm, Bone and bone marrow
		199.0	M-Neoplasm, Disseminated
		199.1	M-Neoplasm NOS
		203.0	Multiple myeloma

CPT NOTES

- For biopsy, see 20220, 20240.
- For bone graft, see 21215.

REIMBURSEMENT INFORMATION

General

- See notes on page 286.

Medicare

- Follow–up Days — 90
- Assistant Surgeon — paid
- Supply Charges — not allowed
- Outpatient Limit — does not apply
- Major Procedure Rules

CPT CODE	SERVICE	ICD-9-CM

21050 Condylectomy, temporomandibular joint (separate procedure)

CPT NOTES

- For biopsy, see 20220, 20240.

170.0	M-Neoplasm, Skull/Face bone
170.1	M-Neoplasm, Mandible
524.6	Temporomandibular joint disorder
526.89	Jaw disease NEC
714.0	Rheumatoid arthritis
802.21	Fx condylar proc mandible, closed
802.31	Fx condylar proc mandible, open
905.0	Late effect, skull/face fracture
905.6	Late effect of dislocation

REIMBURSEMENT INFORMATION

General

- See notes on page 286.
- Separate procedure rules apply.

Medicare

- Follow-up Days — 90
- Assistant Surgeon — by report
- Supply Charges — not allowed
- Outpatient Limit — does not apply
- Major Procedure Rules

21060 Meniscectomy, partial or complete, temporomandibular joint (separate procedure)

CPT NOTES

- For biopsy, see 20220, 20240.

524.61	TMJ adhesions/ankylosis
524.62	TMJ arthralgia
524.63	TMJ articular disc disorder
524.69	TMJ disorders NEC
830.0	Dislocation jaw, closed
830.1	Dislocation jaw, open
848.1	Sprain of jaw
905.0	Late effect, skull/face fracture
905.6	Late effect of dislocation

REIMBURSEMENT INFORMATION

General

- See notes on page 286.
- Separate procedure rules apply.

Medicare

- Follow-up Days — 90
- Assistant Surgeon — not paid
- Supply Charges — not allowed
- Outpatient Limit — does not apply
- Major Procedure Rules

CPT CODE	SERVICE
21070	Coronoidectomy (separate procedure)

CPT NOTES

- For biopsy, see 20220, 20240.

ICD-9-CM

524.0x	Major anomaly of jaw size
524.1x	Jaw/cranial base relation anomaly
524.2	Dental arch relationship anomaly
524.5	Dentofacial functional abnormality
524.6	Temporomandibular joint disorder
524.8	Dentofacial anomaly NEC
524.9	Dentofacial anomaly NOS
526.89	Jaw disease NEC
733.99	Bone/Cartilage disorder NEC
802.23	Fx coronoid proc, mandible, closed
802.33	Fx coronoid proc, mandible, open

REIMBURSEMENT INFORMATION

General

- See notes on page 286.
- Separate procedure rules apply.

Medicare

- Follow-up Days — 90
- Assistant Surgeon — by report
- Supply Charges — not allowed
- Outpatient Limit — does not apply
- Major Procedure Rules

CPT CODE	SERVICE
21079	Impression and custom preparation; interim obturator prosthesis

CPT NOTES

- For application or removal of caliper or tongs, see 20660, 20665.
- Describes professional services for the rehabilitation of patients with oral, facial or other anatomical deficiencies by means of prostheses such as an artificial eye, ear, or nose or intraoral obturator to close a cleft. Code should only be used when the physician actually designs and prepares the prosthesis (i.e., not prepared by an outside laboratory.)

ICD–9–CM

143.0	M-Neoplasm, Upper gum
160.2	M-Neoplasm, Maxillary sinus
526.0	Developmental odontogenic cysts
526.1	Fissural cysts of jaw
526.2	Jaw cysts NEC
526.3	Jaw, central giant cell granuloma
526.89	Jaw disease NEC
526.9	Jaw disease NOS
749.0x	Cleft palate
754.0	Congen skull/face/jaw deformity
756.0	Anomaly of skull/face bones
784.49	Voice disturbance NEC
873.65	Open wound of palate
873.75	Open wound of palate, complicated
906.0	Late effect, open wound head/trunk
909.2	Late effect of radiation
909.3	Late effect of surg/med complic

REIMBURSEMENT INFORMATION

General

- See notes on page 286.

Medicare

- Follow–up Days — 90
- Assistant Surgeon — not paid
- Supply Charges — not allowed
- Outpatient Limit — applies
- Major Surgery Rules Apply

CPT CODE	SERVICE
21080	Impression and custom preparation; definitive obturator prosthesis

CPT NOTES

- For application or removal of caliper or tongs, see 20660, 20665.
- Describes professional services for the rehabilitation of patients with oral, facial or other anatomical deficiencies by means of prostheses such as an artificial eye, ear, or nose or intraoral obturator to close a cleft. Code should only be used when the physician actually designs and prepares the prosthesis (i.e., not prepared by an outside laboratory.)

ICD–9–CM

143.0	M-Neoplasm, Upper gum
144.1	M-Neoplasm, Lateral floor of mouth
145.2	M-Neoplasm, Hard palate
145.3	M-Neoplasm, Soft palate
160.2	M-Neoplasm, Maxillary sinus
526.0	Developmental odontogenic cysts
526.1	Fissural cysts of jaw
526.2	Jaw cysts NEC
526.3	Jaw, central giant cell granuloma
526.89	Jaw disease NEC
526.9	Jaw disease NOS
749.0x	Cleft palate
754.0	Congen skull/face/jaw deformity
756.0	Anomaly of skull/face bones
784.49	Voice disturbance NEC
873.65	Open wound of palate
873.75	Open wound of palate, complicated
906.0	Late effect, open wound head/trunk
909.2	Late effect of radiation
909.3	Late effect of surg/med complic

REIMBURSEMENT INFORMATION

General

- See notes on page 286.

Medicare

- Follow–up Days — 90
- Assistant Surgeon — not paid
- Supply Charges — not allowed
- Outpatient Limit — applies
- Major Surgery Rules Apply

CPT CODE	SERVICE	ICD-9-CM

21081 Impression and custom preparation; mandibular resection prosthesis

CPT NOTES

- For application or removal of caliper or tongs, see 20660, 20665.
- Describes professional services for the rehabilitation of patients with oral, facial or other anatomical deficiencies by means of prostheses such as an artificial eye, ear, or nose or intraoral obturator to close a cleft. Code should only be used when the physician actually designs and prepares the prosthesis (i.e., not prepared by an outside laboratory.)

141.0	M-Neoplasm, Tongue base
195.0	M-Neoplasm, Head/face/neck
526.0	Developmental odontogenic cysts
526.2	Jaw cysts NEC
526.3	Jaw, central giant cell granuloma
526.4	Inflammation of jaw
906.0	Late effect, open wound head/trunk
908.6	Late effect, trauma complications
909.2	Late effect of radiation
909.3	Late effect of surg/med complic

REIMBURSEMENT INFORMATION

General

- See notes on page 286.

Medicare

- Follow–up Days — 90
- Assistant Surgeon — not paid
- Supply Charges — not allowed
- Outpatient Limit — applies
- Major Surgery Rules Apply

21082 Impression and custom preparation; palatal augmentation prosthesis

CPT NOTES

- For application or removal of caliper or tongs, see 20660, 20665.
- Describes professional services for the rehabilitation of patients with oral, facial or other anatomical deficiencies by means of prostheses such as an artificial eye, ear, or nose or intraoral obturator to close a cleft. Code should only be used when the physician actually designs and prepares the prosthesis (i.e., not prepared by an outside laboratory.)

141.0	M-Neoplasm, Tongue base
145.2	M-Neoplasm, Hard palate
145.3	M-Neoplasm, Soft palate
145.4	M-Neoplasm, Uvula
145.5	M-Neoplasm, Palate NOS
145.8	M-Neoplasm, Mouth NEC
210.4	B-Neoplasm, Mouth NEC/NOS
230.0	CA in situ, Oral cavity/pharynx
235.1	UB-Neoplasm, Oral cavity/pharynx
239.0	Digestive neoplasm NOS
749.0x	Cleft palate
749.2x	Cleft palate w/cleft lip
784.49	Voice disturbance NEC

REIMBURSEMENT INFORMATION

General

- See notes on page 286.

Medicare

- Follow–up Days — 90
- Assistant Surgeon — by report
- Supply Charges — not allowed
- Outpatient Limit — applies
- Major Surgery Rules Apply

CPT CODE	SERVICE	ICD-9-CM

21083 Impression and custom preparation; palatal lift prosthesis

CPT NOTES

- ♦ For application or removal of caliper or tongs, see 20660, 20665.
- ♦ Describes professional services for the rehabilitation of patients with oral, facial or other anatomical deficiencies by means of prostheses such as an artificial eye, ear, or nose or intraoral obturator to close a cleft. Code should only be used when the physician actually designs and prepares the prosthesis (i.e., not prepared by an outside laboratory.)

145.2	M-Neoplasm, Hard palate
145.3	M-Neoplasm, Soft palate
145.4	M-Neoplasm, Uvula
145.5	M-Neoplasm, Palate NOS
145.8	M-Neoplasm, Mouth NEC
210.4	B-Neoplasm, Mouth NEC/NOS
230.0	CA in situ, Oral cavity/pharynx
235.1	UB-Neoplasm, Oral cavity/pharynx
239.0	Digestive neoplasm NOS
749.0x	Cleft palate
749.2x	Cleft palate w/cleft lip
784.49	Voice disturbance NEC

REIMBURSEMENT INFORMATION

General

- ♦ See notes on page 286.

Medicare

- ♦ Follow–up Days — 90
- ♦ Assistant Surgeon — by report
- ♦ Supply Charges — not allowed
- ♦ Outpatient Limit — applies
- ♦ Major Surgery Rules Apply

21110* Application of interdental fixation device for conditions other than fracture or dislocation, includes removal

CPT NOTES

- ♦ For application or removal of caliper or tongs, see 20660, 20665.
- ♦ For removal of interdental fixation by another physician, see 20670-20680.

145.3	M-Neoplasm, Soft palate
170.0	M-Neoplasm, Skull/Face bone
170.1	M-Neoplasm, Mandible
213.1	B-Neoplasm, Lower jaw bone
524.6	Temporomandibular joint disorder
525.2	Atrophy, edentulous alveolar ridge
784.0	Headache

REIMBURSEMENT INFORMATION

General

- ♦ See notes on page 286.
- ♦ Starred procedure.

Medicare

- ♦ Follow–up Days — 90
- ♦ Assistant Surgeon — not paid
- ♦ Supply Charges — not allowed
- ♦ Outpatient Limit — does not apply
- ♦ Major Surgery Rules Apply

CPT CODE	SERVICE	ICD–9–CM
21116	Injection procedure for temporomandibular joint arthrography	524.6 Temporomandibular joint disorder 524.60 TMJ disorders NOS 524.61 TMJ adhesions/ankylosis 524.62 TMJ arthralgia 524.63 TMJ articular disc disorder 524.69 TMJ disorders NEC 714.0 Rheumatoid arthritis 728.85 Spasm of muscle 784.0 Headache 830.0 Dislocation jaw, closed 830.1 Dislocation jaw, open 848.1 Sprain of jaw

CPT NOTES

- For application or removal of caliper or tongs, see 20660, 20665.
- For radiological supervision and interpretation, see 70332.

REIMBURSEMENT INFORMATION

General

- See notes on page 286.

Medicare

- Follow–up Days — 0
- Assistant Surgeon — not paid
- Supply Charges — not allowed
- Outpatient Limit — does not apply
- Minor Surgery Rules Apply

CPT CODE	SERVICE	ICD–9–CM
21120	Genioplasty; augmentation (autograft, allograft, prosthetic material)	524.0x Major anomaly of jaw size 524.1x Jaw/cranial base relation anomaly 524.2 Dental arch relationship anomaly 524.8 Dentofacial anomaly NEC 524.9 Dentofacial anomaly NOS 526.89 Jaw disease NEC 754.0 Congen skull/face/jaw deformity 756.4 Chondrodystrophy 905.0 Late effect, skull/face fracture
21121	Genioplasty; sliding osteotomy, single piece	
21122	Genioplasty; sliding osteotomies, two or more osteotomies (eg, wedge excision or bone wedge reversal for asymmetrical chin)	
21123	Genioplasty; sliding, augmentation with interpositional bone grafts (includes obtaining autografts)	

CPT NOTES

- For cranioplasty, see 21179, 21180 and 62116, 62120, 62140-62147.

REIMBURSEMENT INFORMATION

General

- See notes on page 286.

Medicare

- Follow–up Days — 90
- Assistant Surgeon — paid
- Supply Charges — not allowed
- Outpatient Limit — does not apply
- Major Surgery Rules Apply

CPT CODE	SERVICE
21125	Augmentation, mandibular body or angle; prosthetic material
21127	Augmentation, mandibular body or angle; with bone graft, onlay or interpositional (includes obtaining autograft)

CPT NOTES

- For cranioplasty, see 21179, 21180 and 62116, 62120, 62140-62147.

ICD–9–CM

170.1	M-Neoplasm, Mandible
522.8	Radicular cyst
523.4	Chronic periodontitis
524.0x	Major anomaly of jaw size
524.1x	Jaw/cranial base relation anomaly
524.2	Dental arch relationship anomaly
524.8	Dentofacial anomaly NEC
524.9	Dentofacial anomaly NOS
525.2	Atrophy, edentulous alveolar ridge
526.0	Developmental odontogenic cysts
526.1	Fissural cysts of jaw
526.2	Jaw cysts NEC
526.4	Inflammation of jaw
526.89	Jaw disease NEC
733.20	Cyst of bone NOS
733.81	Malunion of fracture
733.82	Nonunion of fracture
738.19	Acquired head deformity NEC
754.0	Congen skull/face/jaw deformity
802.30	Mandible Fx NOS, open
802.31	Fx condylar proc mandible, open
802.32	Subcondylar Fx, mandible, open
802.34	Fx ramus NOS, open
802.35	Fx angle of jaw, open
802.36	Fx symphysis mandible body, open
802.37	Fx alveolar border mandible, open
802.38	Fx mandible body NEC, open
802.39	Multiple Fx mandible, open
905.0	Late effect, skull/face fracture
906.0	Late effect, open wound head/trunk
909.3	Late effect of surg/med complic

REIMBURSEMENT INFORMATION

General

- See notes on page 286.

Medicare

- Follow–up Days — 90
- Assistant Surgeon — paid
- Supply Charges — not allowed
- Outpatient Limit — does not apply
- Major Surgery Rules Apply

CPT CODE	SERVICE
21137	Reduction forehead; contouring only
21138	Reduction forehead; contouring and application of prosthetic material or bone graft (includes obtaining autograft)
21139	Reduction forehead; contouring and setback of anterior frontal sinus wall

CPT NOTES

- For cranioplasty, see 21179, 21180 and 62116, 62120, 62140-62147.

ICD-9-CM

733.3	Hypertosis of skull
733.81	Malunion of fracture
733.99	Bone/Cartilage disorder NEC
738.1	Acquired head deformity NEC
754.0	Congen skull/face/jaw deformity
756.0	Anomaly of skull/face bones

REIMBURSEMENT INFORMATION

General

- See notes on page 286.

Medicare

- Follow–up Days — 90
- Assistant Surgeon — paid
- Supply Charges — not allowed
- Outpatient Limit — does not apply
- Major Surgery Rules Apply

21144	Reconstruction midface, LeFort I; intrusion, single piece (eg, for Long Face Syndrome)
21145	Reconstruction midface, LeFort I; single piece, any direction, requiring bone grafts (includes obtaining autografts)
21146	Reconstruction midface, LeFort I; two pieces, any direction, requiring bone grafts (includes obtaining autografts) (eg, ungrafted unilateral alveolar cleft)
21147	Reconstruction midface, LeFort I; three or more pieces, any direction, requiring bone grafts (includes obtaining autografts) (eg, ungrafted bilateral alveolar cleft or multiple osteotomies)

CPT NOTES

- For cranioplasty, see 21179, 21180 and 62116, 62120, 62140-62147.

524.0x	Major anomaly of jaw size
524.1x	Jaw/cranial base relation anomaly
524.2	Dental arch relationship anomaly
524.5	Dentofacial functional abnormality
524.8	Dentofacial anomaly NEC
524.9	Dentofacial anomaly NOS
526.89	Jaw disease NEC
733.81	Malunion of fracture
738.1	Acquired head deformity NEC
749.0x	Cleft palate
749.2x	Cleft palate w/cleft lip
754.0	Congen skull/face/jaw deformity
905.0	Late effect, skull/face fracture
V13.6	Hx of congenital malformation

REIMBURSEMENT INFORMATION

General

- See notes on page 286.

Medicare

- Follow–up Days — 90
- Assistant Surgeon — paid
- Supply Charges — not allowed
- Outpatient Limit — does not apply
- Major Surgery Rules Apply

CPT CODE	SERVICE	ICD-9-CM
21150	Reconstruction midface, LeFort II; anterior intrusion (eg, Treacher-Collins Syndrome)	524.0x Major anomaly of jaw size
21151	Reconstruction midface, LeFort II; any direction, requiring bone grafts (includes obtaining autografts)	524.1x Jaw/cranial base relation anomaly

CPT NOTES

- For cranioplasty, see 21179, 21180 and 62116, 62120, 62140-62147.

ICD-9-CM

- 524.0x Major anomaly of jaw size
- 524.1x Jaw/cranial base relation anomaly
- 524.2 Dental arch relationship anomaly
- 524.8 Dentofacial anomaly NEC
- 524.9 Dentofacial anomaly NOS
- 526.89 Jaw disease NEC
- 733.81 Malunion of fracture
- 754.0 Congen skull/face/jaw deformity
- 756.0 Anomaly of skull/face bones
- 905.0 Late effect, skull/face fracture
- V13.6 Hx of congenital malformation

REIMBURSEMENT INFORMATION

General

- See notes on page 286.

Medicare

- Follow–up Days — 90
- Assistant Surgeon — paid
- Supply Charges — not allowed
- Outpatient Limit — does not apply
- Major Surgery Rules Apply

21154 Reconstruction midface, LeFort III (extracranial), any type, requiring bone grafts (includes obtaining autografts); without LeFort I

21155 Reconstruction midface, LeFort III (extracranial), any type, requiring bone grafts (includes obtaining autografts); with LeFort I

CPT NOTES

- For cranioplasty, see 21179, 21180 and 62116, 62120, 62140-62147.

ICD-9-CM

- 524.0x Major anomaly of jaw size
- 524.1x Jaw/cranial base relation anomaly
- 524.2 Dental arch relationship anomaly
- 524.8 Dentofacial anomaly NEC
- 524.9 Dentofacial anomaly NOS
- 526.89 Jaw disease NEC
- 733.81 Malunion of fracture
- 754.0 Congen skull/face/jaw deformity
- 756.0 Anomaly of skull/face bones
- 905.0 Late effect, skull/face fracture
- V13.6 Hx of congenital malformation

REIMBURSEMENT INFORMATION

General

- See notes on page 286.

Medicare

- Follow–up Days — 90
- Assistant Surgeon — paid
- Supply Charges — not allowed
- Outpatient Limit — does not apply
- Major Surgery Rules Apply

CPT CODE	SERVICE
21159	Reconstruction midface, LeFort III (extra and intracranial) with forehead advancement (eg, mono bloc), requiring bone grafts (includes obtaining autografts); without LeFort I
21160	Reconstruction midface, LeFort III (extra and intracranial) with forehead advancement (eg, mono bloc), requiring bone grafts (includes obtaining autografts); with LeFort I

CPT NOTES

- For cranioplasty, see 21179, 21180 and 62116, 62120, 62140-62147.

ICD–9–CM

374.22	Mechanical lagophthalmos
376.30	Exophthalmos NOS
376.40	Deformity of orbit NOS
376.43	Orbit deformity d/t bone disease
376.44	Craniofacial orbit deformity
376.45	Atrophy of orbit
376.46	Enlargement of orbit
376.47	Orbit deformity d/t trauma/surgery
524.0x	Major anomaly of jaw size
524.1x	Jaw/cranial base relation anomaly
524.2	Dental arch relationship anomaly
524.8	Dentofacial anomaly NEC
524.9	Dentofacial anomaly NOS
526.89	Jaw disease NEC
733.81	Malunion of fracture
754.0	Congen skull/face/jaw deformity
756.0	Anomaly of skull/face bones
905.0	Late effect, skull/face fracture
V13.6	Hx of congenital malformation

REIMBURSEMENT INFORMATION

General

- See notes on page 286.

Medicare

- Follow–up Days — 90
- Assistant Surgeon — paid
- Supply Charges — not allowed
- Outpatient Limit — does not apply
- Major Surgery Rules Apply

CPT CODE	SERVICE
21172	Reconstruction superior-lateral orbital rim and lower forehead, advancement or alteration, with or without grafts (includes obtaining autografts)

CPT NOTES

- For cranioplasty, see 21179, 21180 and 62116, 62120, 62140-62147.
- For frontal or parietal craniotomy performed for craniosynostosis, see 61556.

ICD–9–CM

376.43	Orbit deformity d/t bone disease
376.44	Craniofacial orbit deformity
376.45	Atrophy of orbit
376.46	Enlargement of orbit
376.47	Orbit deformity d/t trauma/surgery
376.50	Enophthalmos NOS
376.51	Enophthalmos d/t orbit atrophy
376.52	Enophthalmos d/t trauma/surgery
733.81	Malunion of fracture
754.0	Congen skull/face/jaw deformity
756.0	Anomaly of skull/face bones
905.0	Late effect, skull/face fracture
V13.6	Hx of congenital malformation

REIMBURSEMENT INFORMATION

General

- See notes on page 286.

Medicare

- Follow–up Days — 90
- Assistant Surgeon — paid
- Supply Charges — not allowed
- Outpatient Limit — does not apply
- Major Surgery Rules Apply

CPT CODE	SERVICE	ICD-9-CM	
21175	Reconstruction, bifrontal, superior-lateral orbital rims and lower forehead, advancement or alteration (eg, plagiocephaly, trigonocephaly, brachycephaly), with or without grafts (includes obtaining autografts)	733.81	Malunion of fracture
		738.1	Acquired head deformity NEC
		754.0	Congen skull/face/jaw deformity
		756.0	Anomaly of skull/face bones
		905.0	Late effect, skull/face fracture
		V13.6	Hx of congenital malformation

CPT NOTES

- For cranioplasty, see 21179, 21180 and 62116, 62120, 62140-62147.
- For bifrontal craniotomy performed for craniosynostosis, see 61557.

REIMBURSEMENT INFORMATION

General

- See notes on page 286.

Medicare

- Follow–up Days — 90
- Assistant Surgeon — paid
- Supply Charges — not allowed
- Outpatient Limit — does not apply
- Major Surgery Rules Apply

CPT CODE	SERVICE	ICD-9-CM	
21179	Reconstruction, entire or majority of forehead and/or supraorbital rims; with grafts (allograft or prosthetic material)	733.81	Malunion of fracture
		754.0	Congen skull/face/jaw deformity
		756.0	Anomaly of skull/face bones
21180	Reconstruction, entire or majority of forehead and/or supraorbital rims; with autograft (includes obtaining grafts)	905.0	Late effect, skull/face fracture
		V13.6	Hx of congenital malformation

CPT NOTES

- For cranioplasty, see 21179, 21180 and 62116, 62120, 62140-62147.
- For extensive craniectomy for multiple suture craniosynostosis, use only 61558 or 61559.

REIMBURSEMENT INFORMATION

General

- See notes on page 286.

Medicare

- Follow–up Days — 90
- Assistant Surgeon — paid
- Supply Charges — not allowed
- Outpatient Limit — does not apply
- Major Surgery Rules Apply

CPT CODE	SERVICE	ICD-9-CM

21181 Removal by contouring of benign tumor of cranial bones (eg, fibrous dysplasia), extracranial

213.0 B-Neoplasm, Skull/Face bone
733.29 Bone cyst NEC
756.54 Polyostotic fibrous bone dysplasia

CPT NOTES

- For cranioplasty, see 21179, 21180 and 62116, 62120, 62140-62147.

REIMBURSEMENT INFORMATION

General

- See notes on page 286.

Medicare

- Follow-up Days — 90
- Assistant Surgeon — by report
- Supply Charges — not allowed
- Outpatient Limit — does not apply
- Major Surgery Rules Apply

21182 Reconstruction of orbital walls, rims, forehead, nasoethmoid complex following intra- and extracranial excision of benign tumor of cranial bone (eg, fibrous dysplasia), with multiple autografts (includes obtaining grafts); total area of bone grafting less than 40 sq cm

190.1 M-Neoplasm, Orbit
213.0 B-Neoplasm, Skull/Face bone
376.40 Deformity of orbit NOS
376.46 Enlargement of orbit
376.47 Orbit deformity d/t trauma/surgery
733.29 Bone cyst NEC
733.3 Hyperostosis of skull
738.1 Acquired head deformity NEC
756.54 Polyostotic fibrous bone dysplasia

CPT NOTES

- For cranioplasty, see 21179, 21180 and 62116, 62120, 62140-62147.
- For excision of benign tumor of cranial bones, see 61563, 61564.

REIMBURSEMENT INFORMATION

General

- See notes on page 286.

Medicare

- Follow-up Days — 90
- Assistant Surgeon — paid
- Supply Charges — not allowed
- Outpatient Limit — does not apply
- Major Surgery Rules Apply

CPT CODE	SERVICE	ICD–9–CM
21183	Reconstruction of orbital walls, rims, forehead, nasoethmoid complex following intra- and extracranial excision of benign tumor of cranial bone (eg, fibrous dysplasia), with multiple autografts (includes obtaining grafts); total area of bone grafting greater than 40 sq cm but less than 80 sq cm	376.40 Deformity of orbit NOS 376.46 Enlargement of orbit 376.47 Orbit deformity d/t trauma/surgery 733.29 Bone cyst NEC 733.3 Hyperostosis of skull 738.1 Acquired head deformity NEC 756.54 Polyostotic fibrous bone dysplasia
21184	Reconstruction of orbital walls, rims, forehead, nasoethmoid complex following intra- and extracranial excision of benign tumor of cranial bone (eg, fibrous dysplasia), with multiple autografts (includes obtaining grafts); total area of bone grafting greater than 80 sq cm	

CPT NOTES

- For cranioplasty, see 21179, 21180 and 62116, 62120, 62140-62147.
- For excision of benign tumor of cranial bones, see 61563, 61564.

REIMBURSEMENT INFORMATION

General

- See notes on page 286.

Medicare

- Follow–up Days — 90
- Assistant Surgeon — paid
- Supply Charges — not allowed
- Outpatient Limit — does not apply
- Major Surgery Rules Apply

CPT CODE	SERVICE	ICD–9–CM
21188	Reconstruction midface, osteotomies (other than LeFort type) and bone grafts (includes obtaining autografts)	524.0x Major anomaly of jaw size 524.1x Jaw/cranial base relation anomaly 524.2 Dental arch relationship anomaly 524.8 Dentofacial anomaly NEC 524.9 Dentofacial anomaly NOS 526.89 Jaw disease NEC 733.81 Malunion of fracture 738.1 Acquired head deformity NEC 754.0 Congen skull/face/jaw deformity 756.0 Anomaly of skull/face bones 905.0 Late effect, skull/face fracture

CPT NOTES

- For cranioplasty, see 21179, 21180 and 62116, 62120, 62140-62147.

REIMBURSEMENT INFORMATION

General

- See notes on page 286.

Medicare

- Follow–up Days — 90
- Assistant Surgeon — paid
- Supply Charges — not allowed
- Outpatient Limit — does not apply
- Major Surgery Rules Apply

CPT CODE	SERVICE
21193	Reconstruction of mandibular ramus, horizontal, vertical, "C" or "L" osteotomy; without bone graft
21194	Reconstruction of mandibular ramus, horizontal, vertical, "C" or "L" osteotomy; with bone graft (includes obtaining graft)

CPT NOTES

- For cranioplasty, see 21179, 21180 and 62116, 62120, 62140-62147.

ICD–9–CM

524.0x	Major anomaly of jaw size
524.1x	Jaw/cranial base relation anomaly
524.2	Dental arch relationship anomaly
524.8	Dentofacial anomaly NEC
524.9	Dentofacial anomaly NOS
526.89	Jaw disease NEC
733.81	Malunion of fracture
738.19	Acquired head deformity NEC
749.0x	Cleft palate
749.2x	Cleft palate w/cleft lip
754.0	Congen skull/face/jaw deformity
756.0	Anomaly of skull/face bones
780.53	Hypersomnia w/sleep apnea
780.57	Sleep apnea NOS
905.0	Late effect, skull/face fracture
V13.6	Hx of congenital malformation

REIMBURSEMENT INFORMATION

General

- See notes on page 286.

Medicare

- Follow–up Days — 90
- Assistant Surgeon — paid
- Supply Charges — not allowed
- Outpatient Limit — does not apply
- Major Surgery Rules Apply

CPT CODE	SERVICE
▲ 21195	Reconstruction of mandibular ramus and/or body, sagittal split; without internal rigid fixation
▲ 21196	Reconstruction of mandibular ramus and/or body, sagittal split; with internal rigid fixation

CPT NOTES

- For cranioplasty, see 21179, 21180 and 62116, 62120, 62140-62147.

ICD–9–CM

524.0x	Major anomaly of jaw size
524.1x	Jaw/cranial base relation anomaly
524.2	Dental arch relationship anomaly
524.8	Dentofacial anomaly NEC
524.9	Dentofacial anomaly NOS
526.89	Jaw disease NEC
733.81	Malunion of fracture
738.19	Acquired head deformity NEC
749.0x	Cleft palate
749.2x	Cleft palate w/cleft lip
754.0	Congen skull/face/jaw deformity
756.0	Anomaly of skull/face bones
780.53	Hypersomnia w/sleep apnea
780.57	Sleep apnea NOS
905.0	Late effect, skull/face fracture
V13.6	Hx of congenital malformation

REIMBURSEMENT INFORMATION

General

- See notes on page 286.
- Description changed in 1995 CPT.

Medicare

- Follow–up Days — 90
- Assistant Surgeon — paid
- Supply Charges — not allowed
- Outpatient Limit — does not apply
- Major Surgery Rules Apply

CPT CODE	SERVICE
21198	Osteotomy, mandible, segmental

CPT NOTES

- ♦ For cranioplasty, see 21179, 21180 and 62116, 62120, 62140-62147.

ICD–9–CM

524.0x	Major anomaly of jaw size
524.1x	Jaw/cranial base relation anomaly
524.2	Dental arch relationship anomaly
524.8	Dentofacial anomaly NEC
524.9	Dentofacial anomaly NOS
526.89	Jaw disease NEC
733.81	Malunion of fracture
738.19	Acquired head deformity NEC
749.0x	Cleft palate
749.2x	Cleft palate w/cleft lip
754.0	Congen skull/face/jaw deformity
756.0	Anomaly of skull/face bones
780.53	Hypersomnia w/sleep apnea
780.57	Sleep apnea NOS
905.0	Late effect, skull/face fracture
V13.6	Hx of congenital malformation

REIMBURSEMENT INFORMATION

General

- ♦ See notes on page 286.

Medicare

- ♦ Follow–up Days — 90
- ♦ Assistant Surgeon — paid
- ♦ Supply Charges — not allowed
- ♦ Outpatient Limit — does not apply
- ♦ Major Surgery Rules Apply

CPT CODE	SERVICE	ICD–9–CM	
21206	Osteotomy, maxilla, segmental (eg Wassmund or Schuchard)	213.0	B-Neoplasm, Skull/Face bone
		524.0x	Major anomaly of jaw size
		524.1x	Jaw/cranial base relation anomaly
		524.2	Dental arch relationship anomaly
		524.3	Tooth position anomaly
		524.8	Dentofacial anomaly NEC
		524.9	Dentofacial anomaly NOS
		526.89	Jaw disease NEC
		733.81	Malunion of fracture
		738.1	Acquired head deformity NEC
		749.0x	Cleft palate
		749.2x	Cleft palate w/cleft lip
		754.0	Congen skull/face/jaw deformity
		905.0	Late effect, skull/face fracture

CPT NOTES

- For cranioplasty, see 21179, 21180 and 62116, 62120, 62140-62147.

REIMBURSEMENT INFORMATION

General

- See notes on page 286.

Medicare

- Follow–up Days — 90
- Assistant Surgeon — paid
- Supply Charges — not allowed
- Outpatient Limit — does not apply
- Major Surgery Rules Apply

CPT CODE	SERVICE	ICD–9–CM	
21208	Osteoplasty, facial bones; augmentation (autograft, allograft, or prosthetic implant)	144.9	M-Neoplasm, Floor of mouth NOS
		524.0x	Major anomaly of jaw size
		524.1x	Jaw/cranial base relation anomaly
		524.2	Dental arch relationship anomaly
		524.8	Dentofacial anomaly NEC
		524.9	Dentofacial anomaly NOS
		526.89	Jaw disease NEC
		733.81	Malunion of fracture
		738.12	Zygomatic hypoplasia
		749.0x	Cleft palate
		749.2x	Cleft palate w/cleft lip
		754.0	Congen skull/face/jaw deformity
		905.0	Late effect, skull/face fracture
		V50.1	Plastic surgery NEC

CPT NOTES

- For cranioplasty, see 21179, 21180 and 62116, 62120, 62140-62147.

REIMBURSEMENT INFORMATION

General

- See notes on page 286.

Medicare

- Follow–up Days — 90
- Assistant Surgeon — not paid
- Supply Charges — not allowed
- Outpatient Limit — does not apply
- Major Surgery Rules Apply

CPT CODE	SERVICE
21209	Osteoplasty, facial bones; reduction

CPT NOTES

- For cranioplasty, see 21179, 21180 and 62116, 62120, 62140-62147.

ICD–9–CM

524.0x	Major anomaly of jaw size
524.1x	Jaw/cranial base relation anomaly
524.6	Temporomandibular joint disorder
524.8	Dentofacial anomaly NEC
524.9	Dentofacial anomaly NOS
526.89	Jaw disease NEC
726.91	Exostosis, site NOS
731.0	Osteitis deformans NOS
733.81	Malunion of fracture
738.0	Acquired nose deformity
738.10	Acquired head deformity NOS
738.11	Zygomatic hyperplasia
738.19	Acquired head deformity NEC
754.0	Congen skull/face/jaw deformity
905.0	Late effect, skull/face fracture
V50.1	Plastic surgery NEC

REIMBURSEMENT INFORMATION

General

- See notes on page 286.

Medicare

- Follow–up Days — 90
- Assistant Surgeon — paid
- Supply Charges — not allowed
- Outpatient Limit — does not apply
- Major Surgery Rules Apply

CPT CODE	SERVICE
21210	Graft, bone; nasal, maxillary or malar areas (includes obtaining graft)

CPT NOTES

- For cranioplasty, see 21179, 21180 and 62116, 62120, 62140-62147.
- For cleft palate repair, see 42200-42225.

ICD–9–CM

522.8	Radicular cyst
523.4	Chronic periodontitis
524.0x	Major anomaly of jaw size
524.1x	Jaw/cranial base relation anomaly
524.2	Dental arch relationship anomaly
524.8	Dentofacial anomaly NEC
524.9	Dentofacial anomaly NOS
525.2	Atrophy, edentulous alveolar ridge
526.0	Developmental odontogenic cysts
526.1	Fissural cysts of jaw
526.2	Jaw cysts NEC
526.89	Jaw disease NEC
733.20	Cyst of bone NOS
733.81	Malunion of fracture
733.82	Nonunion of fracture
738.0	Acquired nose deformity
738.10	Acquired head deformity NOS
738.11	Zygomatic hyperplasia
738.19	Acquired head deformity NEC
754.0	Congen skull/face/jaw deformity
802.1	Nasal bone Fx, open
802.30	Mandible Fx NOS, open
802.31	Fx condylar proc mandible, open
802.32	Subcondylar Fx, mandible, open
802.34	Fx ramus NOS, open
802.35	Fx angle of jaw, open
802.36	Fx symphysis mandible body, open
802.37	Fx alveolar border mandible, open
802.38	Fx mandible body NEC, open
802.39	Multiple Fx mandible, open
802.5	Fx malar/maxillary, open
802.7	Fx orbital floor, open
802.9	Fx facial bone NEC, open
905.0	Late effect, skull/face fracture
909.3	Late effect of surg/med complic
V50.1	Plastic surgery NEC

REIMBURSEMENT INFORMATION

General

- See notes on page 286.

Medicare

- Follow–up Days — 90
- Assistant Surgeon — not paid
- Supply Charges — not allowed
- Outpatient Limit — does not apply
- Major Surgery Rules Apply

CPT CODE **SERVICE**

21215 Graft, bone; mandible (includes obtaining graft)

CPT NOTES

- For cranioplasty, see 21179, 21180 and 62116, 62120, 62140-62147.

ICD–9–CM

143.1	M-Neoplasm, Lower gum
144.9	M-Neoplasm, Floor of mouth NOS
213.1	B-Neoplasm, Lower jaw bone
522.8	Radicular cyst
523.4	Chronic periodontitis
524.0x	Major anomaly of jaw size
524.1x	Jaw/cranial base relation anomaly
524.2	Dental arch relationship anomaly
524.8	Dentofacial anomaly NEC
524.9	Dentofacial anomaly NOS
525.2	Atrophy, edentulous alveolar ridge
526.0	Developmental odontogenic cysts
526.1	Fissural cysts of jaw
526.2	Jaw cysts NEC
526.4	Inflammation of jaw
526.89	Jaw disease NEC
733.20	Cyst of bone NOS
733.22	Aneurysmal bone cyst
733.81	Malunion of fracture
733.82	Nonunion of fracture
802.2	Fracture, Mandible, closed
802.30	Mandible Fx NOS, open
802.31	Fx condylar proc mandible, open
802.32	Subcondylar Fx, mandible, open
802.34	Fx ramus NOS, open
802.35	Fx angle of jaw, open
802.36	Fx symphysis mandible body, open
802.37	Fx alveolar border mandible, open
802.38	Fx mandible body NEC, open
802.39	Multiple Fx mandible, open
802.9	Fx facial bone NEC, open
905.0	Late effect, skull/face fracture

REIMBURSEMENT INFORMATION

General

- See notes on page 286.

Medicare

- Follow–up Days — 90
- Assistant Surgeon — paid
- Supply Charges — not allowed
- Outpatient Limit — does not apply
- Major Surgery Rules Apply

CPT CODE	SERVICE	ICD–9–CM

21230 Graft; rib cartilage, autogenous, to face, chin, nose or ear (includes obtaining graft)

CPT NOTES

- For cranioplasty, see 21179, 21180 and 62116, 62120, 62140-62147.

374.11	Senile ectropion
380.32	Acquired deformity auricle/pinna
380.89	External ear disorder NEC
524.0x	Major anomaly of jaw size
524.1x	Jaw/cranial base relation anomaly
524.6	Temporomandibular joint disorder
524.61	TMJ adhesions/ankylosis
524.62	TMJ arthralgia
524.8	Dentofacial anomaly NEC
524.9	Dentofacial anomaly NOS
738.0	Acquired nose deformity
738.1	Acquired head deformity NEC
738.6	Acquired pelvic deformity
744.01	Congenital absence of external ear
754.0	Congen skull/face/jaw deformity
905.0	Late effect, skull/face fracture
906.5	Late effect of head/neck burn

REIMBURSEMENT INFORMATION

General

- See notes on page 286.

Medicare

- Follow–up Days — 90
- Assistant Surgeon — by report
- Supply Charges — not allowed
- Outpatient Limit — does not apply
- Major Surgery Rules Apply

21235 Graft; ear cartilage, autograft, to nose or ear (includes obtaining graft)

CPT NOTES

- For cranioplasty, see 21179, 21180 and 62116, 62120, 62140-62147.

380.32	Acquired deformity auricle/pinna
380.89	External ear disorder NEC
478.1	Nasal and sinus disease NEC
738.0	Acquired nose deformity
748.1	Congenital nose anomaly NEC
906.0	Late effect, open wound head/trunk
906.5	Late effect of head/neck burn
V10.83	Hx of skin malignancy NEC

REIMBURSEMENT INFORMATION

General

- See notes on page 286.

Medicare

- Follow–up Days — 90
- Assistant Surgeon — not paid
- Supply Charges — not allowed
- Outpatient Limit — does not apply
- Major Surgery Rules Apply

CPT CODE	SERVICE	ICD-9-CM
21240	Arthroplasty, temporomandibular joint, with or without autograft (includes obtaining graft)	524.6x Temporomandibular joint disorder 714.0 Rheumatoid arthritis 714.3x Juvenile chronic polyarthritis 714.4 Chronic postrheumatic arthritis 733.81 Malunion of fracture 830.0 Dislocation jaw, closed 830.1 Dislocation jaw, open 905.0 Late effect, skull/face fracture 905.6 Late effect of dislocation 996.67 Reaction, internal ortho device NEC 996.77 Complication, int joint prosthesis

CPT NOTES

- For cranioplasty, see 21179, 21180 and 62116, 62120, 62140-62147.

REIMBURSEMENT INFORMATION

General

- See notes on page 286.

Medicare

- Follow-up Days — 90
- Assistant Surgeon — paid
- Supply Charges — not allowed
- Outpatient Limit — does not apply
- Major Surgery Rules Apply

CPT CODE	SERVICE	ICD-9-CM
21242	Arthroplasty, temporomandibular joint, with allograft	524.6x Temporomandibular joint disorder 714.3x Juvenile chronic polyarthritis 714.4 Chronic postrheumatic arthritis 733.81 Malunion of fracture 905.0 Late effect, skull/face fracture 905.6 Late effect of dislocation 996.67 Reaction, internal ortho device NEC 996.77 Complication, int joint prosthesis

CPT NOTES

- For cranioplasty, see 21179, 21180 and 62116, 62120, 62140-62147.

REIMBURSEMENT INFORMATION

General

- See notes on page 286.

Medicare

- Follow-up Days — 90
- Assistant Surgeon — paid
- Supply Charges — not allowed
- Outpatient Limit — does not apply
- Major Surgery Rules Apply

CPT CODE	SERVICE
21243	Arthroplasty, temporomandibular joint, with prosthetic joint replacement

CPT NOTES

- For cranioplasty, see 21179, 21180 and 62116, 62120, 62140-62147.

ICD–9–CM

524.6x	Temporomandibular joint disorder
714.0	Rheumatoid arthritis
714.3x	Juvenile chronic polyarthritis
714.4	Chronic postrheumatic arthritis
733.81	Malunion of fracture
905.0	Late effect, skull/face fracture
905.6	Late effect of dislocation
996.67	Reaction, internal ortho device NEC
996.77	Complication, int joint prosthesis

REIMBURSEMENT INFORMATION

General

- See notes on page 286.

Medicare

- Follow–up Days — 90
- Assistant Surgeon — paid
- Supply Charges — not allowed
- Outpatient Limit — does not apply
- Major Surgery Rules Apply

CPT CODE	SERVICE
21244	Reconstruction of mandible, extraoral, with transosteal bone plate (eg, mandibular staple bone plate)

CPT NOTES

- For cranioplasty, see 21179, 21180 and 62116, 62120, 62140-62147.

ICD–9–CM

210.4	B-Neoplasm, Mouth NEC/NOS
524.0x	Major anomaly of jaw size
524.8	Dentofacial anomaly NEC
524.9	Dentofacial anomaly NOS
525.0	Tooth exfoliation, systemic cause
525.1	Tooth loss, acquired
525.2	Atrophy, edentulous alveolar ridge
525.8	Dental disorder NEC
525.9	Dental disorder NOS
526.4	Inflammation of jaw
526.89	Jaw disease NEC
526.9	Jaw disease NOS
733.81	Malunion of fracture
733.82	Nonunion of fracture
802.3x	Fracture, Mandible, open
905.0	Late effect, skull/face fracture
996.4	Malfunction, int orthoped dev/graft
996.60	Reaction, unspecified device/graft
V10.01	Hx of tongue malignancy
V10.02	Hx of oral/pharynx malignancy NEC
V51.	Aftercare w/plastic surgery

REIMBURSEMENT INFORMATION

General

- See notes on page 286.

Medicare

- Follow–up Days — 90
- Assistant Surgeon — paid
- Supply Charges — not allowed
- Outpatient Limit — does not apply
- Major Surgery Rules Apply

CPT CODE	SERVICE
21245	Reconstruction of mandible or maxilla, subperiosteal implant; partial

CPT NOTES

- For cranioplasty, see 21179, 21180 and 62116, 62120, 62140-62147.

ICD–9–CM

524.0x	Major anomaly of jaw size
524.8	Dentofacial anomaly NEC
524.9	Dentofacial anomaly NOS
525.0	Tooth exfoliation, systemic cause
525.1	Tooth loss, acquired
525.2	Atrophy, edentulous alveolar ridge
525.8	Dental disorder NEC
525.9	Dental disorder NOS
526.4	Inflammation of jaw
526.89	Jaw disease NEC
526.9	Jaw disease NOS
754.0	Congen skull/face/jaw deformity
905.0	Late effect, skull/face fracture
996.4	Malfunction, int orthoped dev/graft
996.60	Reaction, unspecified device/graft
V10.01	Hx of tongue malignancy
V10.02	Hx of oral/pharynx malignancy NEC
V51.	Aftercare w/plastic surgery

REIMBURSEMENT INFORMATION

General

- See notes on page 286.

Medicare

- Follow–up Days — 90
- Assistant Surgeon — paid
- Supply Charges — not allowed
- Outpatient Limit — does not apply
- Major Surgery Rules Apply

CPT CODE	SERVICE
21246	Reconstruction of mandible or maxilla, subperiosteal implant; complete
21247	Reconstruction of mandibular condyle with bone and cartilage autografts (includes obtaining grafts) (eg, for hemifacial microsomia)

CPT NOTES

- For cranioplasty, see 21179, 21180 and 62116, 62120, 62140-62147.

ICD–9–CM

524.0x	Major anomaly of jaw size
524.8	Dentofacial anomaly NEC
524.9	Dentofacial anomaly NOS
525.0	Tooth exfoliation, systemic cause
525.1	Tooth loss, acquired
525.2	Atrophy, edentulous alveolar ridge
525.8	Dental disorder NEC
525.9	Dental disorder NOS
526.4	Inflammation of jaw
526.89	Jaw disease NEC
526.9	Jaw disease NOS
754.0	Congen skull/face/jaw deformity
996.4	Malfunction, int orthoped dev/graft
996.60	Reaction, unspecified device/graft
V10.01	Hx of tongue malignancy
V10.02	Hx of oral/pharynx malignancy NEC
V51.	Aftercare w/plastic surgery

REIMBURSEMENT INFORMATION

General

- See notes on page 286.

Medicare

- Follow–up Days — 90
- Assistant Surgeon — paid
- Supply Charges — not allowed
- Outpatient Limit — does not apply
- Major Surgery Rules Apply

CPT CODE	SERVICE
21248	Reconstruction of mandible or maxilla, endosteal implant (eg, blade, cylinder); partial

CPT NOTES

- For cranioplasty, see 21179, 21180 and 62116, 62120, 62140-62147.

ICD–9–CM

170.0	M-Neoplasm, Skull/Face bone
170.1	M-Neoplasm, Mandible
524.0x	Major anomaly of jaw size
524.3	Tooth position anomaly
524.8	Dentofacial anomaly NEC
524.9	Dentofacial anomaly NOS
525.0	Tooth exfoliation, systemic cause
525.1	Tooth loss, acquired
525.2	Atrophy, edentulous alveolar ridge
525.8	Dental disorder NEC
525.9	Dental disorder NOS
526.4	Inflammation of jaw
526.9	Jaw disease NOS
733.81	Malunion of fracture
754.0	Congen skull/face/jaw deformity
905.0	Late effect, skull/face fracture
996.4	Malfunction, int orthoped dev/graft
996.52	Other tissue graft malfunction
996.59	Malfunction other device/graft
996.60	Reaction, unspecified device/graft
996.70	Complication, unspec device/graft
V10.01	Hx of tongue malignancy
V10.02	Hx of oral/pharynx malignancy NEC
V51.	Aftercare w/plastic surgery

REIMBURSEMENT INFORMATION

General

- See notes on page 286.

Medicare

- Follow–up Days — 90
- Assistant Surgeon — not paid
- Supply Charges — not allowed
- Outpatient Limit — does not apply
- Major Surgery Rules Apply

CPT CODE	SERVICE
21249	Reconstruction of mandible or maxilla, endosteal implant (eg, blade, cylinder); complete

CPT NOTES

- For cranioplasty, see 21179, 21180 and 62116, 62120, 62140-62147.

ICD–9–CM

145.3	M-Neoplasm, Soft palate
524.0x	Major anomaly of jaw size
524.8	Dentofacial anomaly NEC
524.9	Dentofacial anomaly NOS
525.0	Tooth exfoliation, systemic cause
525.1	Tooth loss, acquired
525.2	Atrophy, edentulous alveolar ridge
525.8	Dental disorder NEC
525.9	Dental disorder NOS
526.4	Inflammation of jaw
526.9	Jaw disease NOS
905.0	Late effect, skull/face fracture
906.0	Late effect, open wound head/trunk
996.4	Malfunction, int orthoped dev/graft
996.52	Other tissue graft malfunction
996.59	Malfunction other device/graft
996.60	Reaction, unspecified device/graft
996.70	Complication, unspec device/graft
V10.01	Hx of tongue malignancy
V10.02	Hx of oral/pharynx malignancy NEC
V51.	Aftercare w/plastic surgery

REIMBURSEMENT INFORMATION

General

- See notes on page 286.

Medicare

- Follow–up Days — 90
- Assistant Surgeon — not paid
- Supply Charges — not allowed
- Outpatient Limit — does not apply
- Major Surgery Rules Apply

CPT CODE	SERVICE
21255	Reconstruction of zygomatic arch and glenoid fossa with bone and cartilage (includes obtaining autografts)

CPT NOTES

- For cranioplasty, see 21179, 21180 and 62116, 62120, 62140-62147.

ICD–9–CM

170.0	M-Neoplasm, Skull/Face bone
349.89	Nervous system disorder NEC
524.0x	Major anomaly of jaw size
524.1	Jaw/cranial base relation anomaly
524.10	Jaw/cranial relation anomaly NOS
524.11	Maxillary asymmetry
524.12	Jaw asymmetry NEC
524.19	Jaw/cranial relation anomaly NEC
524.2	Dental arch relationship anomaly
524.8	Dentofacial anomaly NEC
524.9	Dentofacial anomaly NOS
526.89	Jaw disease NEC
733.81	Malunion of fracture
754.0	Congen skull/face/jaw deformity
905.0	Late effect, skull/face fracture
906.0	Late effect, open wound head/trunk
996.4	Malfunction, int orthoped dev/graft
996.5	Complication, prosthetic device
996.6	Infection due to prosthetic device

REIMBURSEMENT INFORMATION

General

- See notes on page 286.

Medicare

- Follow–up Days — 90
- Assistant Surgeon — paid
- Supply Charges — not allowed
- Outpatient Limit — does not apply
- Major Surgery Rules Apply

CPT CODE	SERVICE
21256	Reconstruction of orbit with osteotomies (extracranial) and with bone grafts (includes obtaining autografts) (eg, microophthalmia)

CPT NOTES

- For cranioplasty, see 21179, 21180 and 62116, 62120, 62140-62147.

ICD–9–CM

212.0	B-Neoplasm, Nasal cavity/sinus
213.0	B-Neoplasm, Skull/Face bone
376.43	Orbit deformity d/t bone disease
376.46	Enlargement of orbit
376.47	Orbit deformity d/t trauma/surgery
376.51	Enophthalmos d/t orbit atrophy
376.52	Enophthalmos d/t trauma/surgery
524.0x	Major anomaly of jaw size
524.1	Jaw/cranial base relation anomaly
524.10	Jaw/cranial relation anomaly NOS
524.11	Maxillary asymmetry
524.12	Jaw asymmetry NEC
524.19	Jaw/cranial relation anomaly NEC
524.2	Dental arch relationship anomaly
524.8	Dentofacial anomaly NEC
524.9	Dentofacial anomaly NOS
526.89	Jaw disease NEC
733.29	Bone cyst NEC
743.06	Cryptophthalmos
743.10	Microphthalmos NOS
754.0	Congen skull/face/jaw deformity
756.0	Anomaly of skull/face bones
756.54	Polyostotic fibrous bone dysplasia
905.0	Late effect, skull/face fracture

REIMBURSEMENT INFORMATION

General

- See notes on page 286.

Medicare

- Follow–up Days — 90
- Assistant Surgeon — paid
- Supply Charges — not allowed
- Outpatient Limit — does not apply
- Major Surgery Rules Apply

CPT CODE	SERVICE	ICD–9–CM
21260	Periorbital osteotomies for orbital hypertelorism, with bone grafts; extracranial approach	
21261	Periorbital osteotomies for orbital hypertelorism, with bone grafts; combined intra- and extracranial approach	
21263	Periorbital osteotomies for orbital hypertelorism, with bone grafts; with forehead advancement	

376.41 Hypertelorism of orbit
376.44 Craniofacial orbit deformity
376.47 Orbit deformity d/t trauma/surgery
756.0 Anomaly of skull/face bones

CPT NOTES

- For cranioplasty, see 21179, 21180 and 62116, 62120, 62140-62147.

REIMBURSEMENT INFORMATION

General

- See notes on page 286.

Medicare

- Follow–up Days — 90
- Assistant Surgeon — paid
- Supply Charges — not allowed
- Outpatient Limit — does not apply
- Major Surgery Rules Apply

21267 Orbital repositioning, periorbital osteotomies, unilateral, with bone grafts; extracranial approach

242.0 Thyrotoxicosis
376.21 Thyrotoxic exophthalmos
376.22 Exophthalmic ophthalmoplegia
376.40 Deformity of orbit NOS
376.41 Hypertelorism of orbit
376.43 Orbit deformity d/t bone disease
376.44 Craniofacial orbit deformity
376.46 Enlargement of orbit
376.47 Orbit deformity d/t trauma/surgery
733.81 Malunion of fracture
756.0 Anomaly of skull/face bones

CPT NOTES

- For cranioplasty, see 21179, 21180 and 62116, 62120, 62140-62147.

REIMBURSEMENT INFORMATION

General

- See notes on page 286.

Medicare

- Follow–up Days — 90
- Assistant Surgeon — paid
- Supply Charges — not allowed
- Outpatient Limit — does not apply
- Major Surgery Rules Apply

CPT CODE	SERVICE	ICD-9-CM

21268 Orbital repositioning, periorbital osteotomies, unilateral, with bone grafts; combined intra- and extracranial approach

CPT NOTES

- For cranioplasty, see 21179, 21180 and 62116, 62120, 62140-62147.

376.40	Deformity of orbit NOS
376.41	Hypertelorism of orbit
376.43	Orbit deformity d/t bone disease
376.44	Craniofacial orbit deformity
376.46	Enlargement of orbit
376.47	Orbit deformity d/t trauma/surgery
733.81	Malunion of fracture
756.0	Anomaly of skull/face bones
905.0	Late effect, skull/face fracture

REIMBURSEMENT INFORMATION

General

- See notes on page 286.

Medicare

- Follow-up Days — 90
- Assistant Surgeon — paid
- Supply Charges — not allowed
- Outpatient Limit — does not apply
- Major Surgery Rules Apply

21270 Malar augmentation, prosthetic material

CPT NOTES

- For cranioplasty, see 21179, 21180 and 62116, 62120, 62140-62147.
- For malar augmentation with bone graft, see 21210.

349.89	Nervous system disorder NEC
376.47	Orbit deformity d/t trauma/surgery
524.8	Dentofacial anomaly NEC
524.9	Dentofacial anomaly NOS
733.81	Malunion of fracture
733.91	Arrest of bone growth
754.0	Congen skull/face/jaw deformity
905.0	Late effect, skull/face fracture
V50.1	Plastic surgery NEC

REIMBURSEMENT INFORMATION

General

- See notes on page 286.

Medicare

- Follow-up Days — 90
- Assistant Surgeon — paid
- Supply Charges — not allowed
- Outpatient Limit — does not apply
- Major Surgery Rules Apply

CPT CODE	SERVICE	ICD-9-CM
21275	Secondary revision of orbitocraniofacial reconstruction	376.40 Deformity of orbit NOS 376.41 Hypertelorism of orbit 376.43 Orbit deformity d/t bone disease 376.44 Craniofacial orbit deformity 376.46 Enlargement of orbit 376.47 Orbit deformity d/t trauma/surgery 733.81 Malunion of fracture 756.0 Anomaly of skull/face bones 905.0 Late effect, skull/face fracture

CPT NOTES

- For cranioplasty, see 21179, 21180 and 62116, 62120, 62140-62147.

REIMBURSEMENT INFORMATION

General

- See notes on page 286.

Medicare

- Follow-up Days — 90
- Assistant Surgeon — paid
- Supply Charges — not allowed
- Outpatient Limit — does not apply
- Major Surgery Rules Apply

CPT CODE	SERVICE	ICD-9-CM
21345	Closed treatment of nasomaxillary complex fracture (LeFort II type), with interdental wire fixation or fixation of denture or splint	802.0 Nasal bone Fx, closed 802.1 Nasal bone Fx, open 802.4 Fx malar/maxillary, closed 802.5 Fx malar/maxillary, open

REIMBURSEMENT INFORMATION

General

- See notes on page 286.

Medicare

- Follow-up Days — 90
- Assistant Surgeon — by report
- Supply Charges — not allowed
- Outpatient Limit — does not apply
- Major Surgery Rules Apply

CPT CODE	SERVICE	ICD-9-CM
21346	Open treatment of nasomaxillary complex fracture (LeFort II type); with wiring and/or local fixation	802.0 Nasal bone Fx, closed 802.1 Nasal bone Fx, open 802.4 Fx malar/maxillary, closed 802.5 Fx malar/maxillary, open
21347	Open treatment of nasomaxillary complex fracture (LeFort II type); requiring multiple open approaches	

REIMBURSEMENT INFORMATION

General

- ♦ See notes on page 286.

Medicare

- ♦ Follow-up Days — 90
- ♦ Assistant Surgeon — paid
- ♦ Supply Charges — not allowed
- ♦ Outpatient Limit — does not apply
- ♦ Major Surgery Rules Apply

21355* Percutaneous treatment of fracture of malar area, including zygomatic arch and malar tripod, with manipulation

802.4 Fx malar/maxillary, closed
802.5 Fx malar/maxillary, open

REIMBURSEMENT INFORMATION

General

- ♦ See notes on page 286.
- ♦ Starred procedure.

Medicare

- ♦ Follow-up Days — 10
- ♦ Assistant Surgeon — by report
- ♦ Supply Charges — not allowed
- ♦ Outpatient Limit — does not apply
- ♦ Minor Surgery Rules Apply

21360 Open treatment of depressed malar fracture, including zygomatic arch and malar tripod

802.4 Fx malar/maxillary, closed
802.5 Fx malar/maxillary, open

REIMBURSEMENT INFORMATION

General

- ♦ See notes on page 286.

Medicare

- ♦ Follow-up Days — 90
- ♦ Assistant Surgeon — paid
- ♦ Supply Charges — not allowed
- ♦ Outpatient Limit — does not apply
- ♦ Major Surgery Rules Apply

CPT CODE	SERVICE	ICD–9–CM
21365	Open treatment of complicated, (eg, comminuted or involving cranial nerve foramina) fracture(s) of malar area, including zygomatic arch and malar tripod; with internal fixation and multiple surgical approaches	802.4 Fx malar/maxillary, closed 802.5 Fx malar/maxillary, open 802.6 Fx orbital floor, closed 802.7 Fx orbital floor, open

REIMBURSEMENT INFORMATION

General

- ◆ See notes on page 286.

Medicare

- ◆ Follow–up Days — 90
- ◆ Assistant Surgeon — paid
- ◆ Supply Charges — not allowed
- ◆ Outpatient Limit — does not apply
- ◆ Major Surgery Rules Apply

CPT CODE	SERVICE	ICD–9–CM
21385	Open treatment of orbital floor "blowout" fracture; transantral approach (Caldwell-Luc type operation)	802.6 Fx orbital floor, closed 802.7 Fx orbital floor, open 802.8 Fx facial bone NEC, closed 802.9 Fx facial bone NEC, open
21386	Open treatment of orbital floor "blowout" fracture; periorbital approach	
21387	Open treatment of orbital floor "blowout" fracture; combined approach	
21390	Open treatment of orbital floor "blowout" fracture; periorbital approach, with alloplastic or other implant	
21395	Open treatment of orbital floor "blowout" fracture; periorbital approach with bone graft (includes obtaining graft)	

REIMBURSEMENT INFORMATION

General

- ◆ See notes on page 286.

Medicare

- ◆ Follow–up Days — 90
- ◆ Assistant Surgeon — paid
- ◆ Supply Charges — not allowed
- ◆ Outpatient Limit — does not apply
- ◆ Major Surgery Rules Apply

CPT CODE	SERVICE	ICD-9-CM
21400	Closed treatment of fracture of orbit, except "blowout"; without manipulation	801.00 Closed skull base fracture 801.06 Closed skull base Fx, coma NOS 801.16 Closed skull base Fx, coma NOS 801.26 Closed skull base Fx, coma NOS 801.50 Open skull base Fracture 801.56 Open skull base Fx, coma NOS 801.66 Open skull base Fx, coma NOS 801.76 Open skull base Fx, coma NOS 802.8 Fx facial bone NEC, closed
21401	Closed treatment of fracture of orbit, except "blowout"; with manipulation	

REIMBURSEMENT INFORMATION

General

- See notes on page 286.

Medicare

- Follow-up Days — 90
- Assistant Surgeon — not paid
- Supply Charges — not allowed
- Outpatient Limit — does not apply
- Major Surgery Rules Apply

CPT CODE	SERVICE	ICD-9-CM
21406	Open treatment of fracture of orbit, except "blowout"; without implant	801.00 Closed skull base fracture 801.06 Closed skull base Fx, coma NOS 801.16 Closed skull base Fx, coma NOS 801.26 Closed skull base Fx, coma NOS 801.50 Open skull base Fracture 801.56 Open skull base Fx, coma NOS 801.66 Open skull base Fx, coma NOS 801.76 Open skull base Fx, coma NOS 802.8 Fx facial bone NEC, closed 802.9 Fx facial bone NEC, open
21407	Open treatment of fracture of orbit, except "blowout"; with implant	

REIMBURSEMENT INFORMATION

General

- See notes on page 286.

Medicare

- Follow-up Days — 90
- Assistant Surgeon — paid
- Supply Charges — not allowed
- Outpatient Limit — does not apply
- Major Surgery Rules Apply

CPT CODE	SERVICE	ICD–9–CM
21421	Closed treatment of palatal or maxillary fracture (LeFort I type), with interdental wire fixation or fixation of denture or splint	802.4 Fx malar/maxillary, closed 802.5 Fx malar/maxillary, open 802.8 Fx facial bone NEC, closed 802.9 Fx facial bone NEC, open **REIMBURSEMENT INFORMATION** General ◆ See notes on page 286. Medicare ◆ Follow–up Days — 90 ◆ Assistant Surgeon — not paid ◆ Supply Charges — not allowed ◆ Outpatient Limit — does not apply ◆ Major Surgery Rules Apply
21422	Open treatment of palatal or maxillary fractures (LeFort I type);	802.4 Fx malar/maxillary, closed 802.5 Fx malar/maxillary, open 802.8 Fx facial bone NEC, closed 802.9 Fx facial bone NEC, open **REIMBURSEMENT INFORMATION** General ◆ See notes on page 286. Medicare ◆ Follow–up Days — 90 ◆ Assistant Surgeon — paid ◆ Supply Charges — not allowed ◆ Outpatient Limit — does not apply ◆ Major Surgery Rules Apply
21431	Closed treatment of craniofacial separation (Lefort III type) using interdental wire fixation of denture or splint	802.4 Fx malar/maxillary, closed 802.5 Fx malar/maxillary, open 802.8 Fx facial bone NEC, closed 802.9 Fx facial bone NEC, open **REIMBURSEMENT INFORMATION** General ◆ See notes on page 286. Medicare ◆ Follow–up Days — 90 ◆ Assistant Surgeon — paid ◆ Supply Charges — not allowed ◆ Outpatient Limit — does not apply ◆ Major Surgery Rules Apply

CPT CODE	SERVICE	ICD–9–CM

21432 Open treatment of craniofacial separation (LeFort III type); with wiring and/or internal fixation

CPT NOTES

- ♦ For removal of internal or external fixation device, see 20670.

802.4	Fx malar/maxillary, closed
802.5	Fx malar/maxillary, open
802.8	Fx facial bone NEC, closed
802.9	Fx facial bone NEC, open

REIMBURSEMENT INFORMATION

General

- ♦ See notes on page 286.

Medicare

- ♦ Follow–up Days — 90
- ♦ Assistant Surgeon — paid
- ♦ Supply Charges — not allowed
- ♦ Outpatient Limit — does not apply
- ♦ Major Surgery Rules Apply

21433 Open treatment of craniofacial separation (LeFort III type); complicated (eg, comminuted or involving cranial nerve foramina), multiple surgical approaches

CPT NOTES

- ♦ For removal of internal or external fixation device, see 20670.

802.0	Nasal bone Fx, closed
802.1	Nasal bone Fx, open
802.4	Fx malar/maxillary, closed
802.5	Fx malar/maxillary, open
802.8	Fx facial bone NEC, closed
802.9	Fx facial bone NEC, open
959.0	Face and neck injury NOS

REIMBURSEMENT INFORMATION

General

- ♦ See notes on page 286.

Medicare

- ♦ Follow–up Days — 90
- ♦ Assistant Surgeon — paid
- ♦ Supply Charges — not allowed
- ♦ Outpatient Limit — does not apply
- ♦ Major Surgery Rules Apply

CPT CODE	SERVICE	ICD-9-CM
21435	Open treatment of craniofacial separation (LeFort III type); complicated, utilizing internal and/or external fixation techniques (eg, head cap, halo device, and/or intermaxillary fixation)	802.0 Nasal bone Fx, closed 802.1 Nasal bone Fx, open 802.4 Fx malar/maxillary, closed 802.5 Fx malar/maxillary, open 802.8 Fx facial bone NEC, closed 802.9 Fx facial bone NEC, open

CPT NOTES

- For removal of interna or externall fixation device, see 20670.

REIMBURSEMENT INFORMATION

General

- See notes on page 286.

Medicare

- Follow–up Days — 90
- Assistant Surgeon — paid
- Supply Charges — not allowed
- Outpatient Limit — does not apply
- Major Surgery Rules Apply

CPT CODE	SERVICE	ICD-9-CM
21440	Closed treatment of mandibular or maxillary alveolar ridge fracture (separate procedure)	802.22 Subcondylar Fx, mandible, closed 802.27 Fx alveolar border mandible, closed 802.29 Multiple Fx mandible, closed 802.37 Fx alveolar border mandible, open 802.39 Multiple Fx mandible, open

REIMBURSEMENT INFORMATION

General

- See notes on page 286.
- Separate procedure rules apply.

Medicare

- Follow–up Days — 90
- Assistant Surgeon — not paid
- Supply Charges — not allowed
- Outpatient Limit — does not apply
- Major Surgery Rules Apply

CPT CODE	SERVICE	ICD–9–CM
21445	Open treatment of mandibular or maxillary alveolar ridge fracture (separate procedure)	802.27 Fx alveolar border mandible, closed 802.29 Multiple Fx mandible, closed 802.37 Fx alveolar border mandible, open 802.39 Multiple Fx mandible, open

REIMBURSEMENT INFORMATION

General

- ♦ See notes on page 286.
- ♦ Separate procedure rules apply.

Medicare

- ♦ Follow–up Days — 90
- ♦ Assistant Surgeon — paid
- ♦ Supply Charges — not allowed
- ♦ Outpatient Limit — does not apply
- ♦ Major Surgery Rules Apply

CPT CODE	SERVICE	ICD–9–CM
21450	Closed treatment of mandibular fracture; without manipulation	802.20 Mandible Fx NOS, closed 802.21 Fx condylar proc mandible, closed 802.22 Subcondylar Fx, mandible, closed 802.23 Fx coronoid proc, mandible, closed 802.24 Fx ramus NOS, closed 802.25 Fx angle of jaw, closed 802.26 Fx symphysis mandible body, closed 802.27 Fx alveolar border mandible, closed 802.28 Fx mandible body NEC, closed 802.29 Multiple Fx mandible, closed 802.30 Mandible Fx NOS, open 802.31 Fx condylar proc mandible, open 802.32 Subcondylar Fx, mandible, open 802.33 Fx coronoid proc, mandible, open 802.34 Fx ramus NOS, open 802.35 Fx angle of jaw, open 802.36 Fx symphysis mandible body, open 802.37 Fx alveolar border mandible, open 802.38 Fx mandible body NEC, open 802.39 Multiple Fx mandible, open

REIMBURSEMENT INFORMATION

General

- ♦ See notes on page 286.

Medicare

- ♦ Follow–up Days — 90
- ♦ Assistant Surgeon — not paid
- ♦ Supply Charges — not allowed
- ♦ Outpatient Limit — does not apply
- ♦ Major Surgery Rules Apply

CPT CODE	SERVICE
21451	Closed treatment of mandibular fracture; with manipulation

ICD–9–CM

733.82	Nonunion of fracture
802.20	Mandible Fx NOS, closed
802.21	Fx condylar proc mandible, closed
802.22	Subcondylar Fx, mandible, closed
802.23	Fx coronoid proc, mandible, closed
802.24	Fx ramus NOS, closed
802.25	Fx angle of jaw, closed
802.26	Fx symphysis mandible body, closed
802.27	Fx alveolar border mandible, closed
802.28	Fx mandible body NEC, closed
802.29	Multiple Fx mandible, closed
802.30	Mandible Fx NOS, open
802.31	Fx condylar proc mandible, open
802.32	Subcondylar Fx, mandible, open
802.33	Fx coronoid proc, mandible, open
802.34	Fx ramus NOS, open
802.35	Fx angle of jaw, open
802.36	Fx symphysis mandible body, open
802.37	Fx alveolar border mandible, open
802.38	Fx mandible body NEC, open
802.39	Multiple Fx mandible, open

REIMBURSEMENT INFORMATION

General

- See notes on page 286.

Medicare

- Follow–up Days — 90
- Assistant Surgeon — not paid
- Supply Charges — not allowed
- Outpatient Limit — does not apply
- Major Surgery Rules Apply

CPT CODE	SERVICE
21452	Percutaneous treatment of mandibular fracture, with external fixation

ICD–9–CM

733.82	Nonunion of fracture
802.20	Mandible Fx NOS, closed
802.21	Fx condylar proc mandible, closed
802.22	Subcondylar Fx, mandible, closed
802.23	Fx coronoid proc, mandible, closed
802.24	Fx ramus NOS, closed
802.25	Fx angle of jaw, closed
802.26	Fx symphysis mandible body, closed
802.27	Fx alveolar border mandible, closed
802.28	Fx mandible body NEC, closed
802.29	Multiple Fx mandible, closed
802.30	Mandible Fx NOS, open
802.31	Fx condylar proc mandible, open
802.32	Subcondylar Fx, mandible, open
802.33	Fx coronoid proc, mandible, open
802.34	Fx ramus NOS, open
802.35	Fx angle of jaw, open
802.36	Fx symphysis mandible body, open
802.37	Fx alveolar border mandible, open
802.38	Fx mandible body NEC, open
802.39	Multiple Fx mandible, open

REIMBURSEMENT INFORMATION

General

- See notes on page 286.

Medicare

- Follow–up Days — 90
- Assistant Surgeon — paid
- Supply Charges — not allowed
- Outpatient Limit — does not apply
- Major Surgery Rules Apply

CPT CODE	SERVICE	ICD-9-CM	
21453	Closed treatment of mandibular fracture with interdental fixation	733.82	Nonunion of fracture
		802.2	Fracture, Mandible, closed
		802.20	Mandible Fx NOS, closed
		802.21	Fx condylar proc mandible, closed
		802.22	Subcondylar Fx, mandible, closed
		802.23	Fx coronoid proc, mandible, closed
		802.24	Fx ramus NOS, closed
		802.25	Fx angle of jaw, closed
		802.26	Fx symphysis mandible body, closed
		802.27	Fx alveolar border mandible, closed
		802.28	Fx mandible body NEC, closed
		802.29	Multiple Fx mandible, closed
		802.30	Mandible Fx NOS, open
		802.31	Fx condylar proc mandible, open
		802.32	Subcondylar Fx, mandible, open
		802.33	Fx coronoid proc, mandible, open
		802.34	Fx ramus NOS, open
		802.35	Fx angle of jaw, open
		802.36	Fx symphysis mandible body, open
		802.37	Fx alveolar border mandible, open
		802.38	Fx mandible body NEC, open
		802.39	Multiple Fx mandible, open

REIMBURSEMENT INFORMATION

General

- See notes on page 286.

Medicare

- Follow-up Days — 90
- Assistant Surgeon — paid
- Supply Charges — not allowed
- Outpatient Limit — does not apply
- Major Surgery Rules Apply

CPT CODE	SERVICE
21454	Open treatment of mandibular fracture with external fixation

ICD–9–CM

733.82	Nonunion of fracture
802.20	Mandible Fx NOS, closed
802.21	Fx condylar proc mandible, closed
802.22	Subcondylar Fx, mandible, closed
802.23	Fx coronoid proc, mandible, closed
802.24	Fx ramus NOS, closed
802.25	Fx angle of jaw, closed
802.26	Fx symphysis mandible body, closed
802.27	Fx alveolar border mandible, closed
802.28	Fx mandible body NEC, closed
802.29	Multiple Fx mandible, closed
802.30	Mandible Fx NOS, open
802.31	Fx condylar proc mandible, open
802.32	Subcondylar Fx, mandible, open
802.34	Fx ramus NOS, open
802.35	Fx angle of jaw, open
802.36	Fx symphysis mandible body, open
802.37	Fx alveolar border mandible, open
802.38	Fx mandible body NEC, open
802.39	Multiple Fx mandible, open

REIMBURSEMENT INFORMATION

General

- See notes on page 286.

Medicare

- Follow–up Days — 90
- Assistant Surgeon — paid
- Supply Charges — not allowed
- Outpatient Limit — does not apply
- Major Surgery Rules Apply

CPT CODE	SERVICE	ICD–9–CM	
21461	Open treatment of mandibular fracture; without interdental fixation	733.82	Nonunion of fracture
		802.20	Mandible Fx NOS, closed
		802.21	Fx condylar proc mandible, closed
		802.22	Subcondylar Fx, mandible, closed
		802.23	Fx coronoid proc, mandible, closed
		802.24	Fx ramus NOS, closed
		802.25	Fx angle of jaw, closed
		802.26	Fx symphysis mandible body, closed
		802.27	Fx alveolar border mandible, closed
		802.28	Fx mandible body NEC, closed
		802.29	Multiple Fx mandible, closed
		802.30	Mandible Fx NOS, open
		802.31	Fx condylar proc mandible, open
		802.32	Subcondylar Fx, mandible, open
		802.33	Fx coronoid proc, mandible, open
		802.34	Fx ramus NOS, open
		802.35	Fx angle of jaw, open
		802.36	Fx symphysis mandible body, open
		802.37	Fx alveolar border mandible, open
		802.38	Fx mandible body NEC, open
		802.39	Multiple Fx mandible, open

REIMBURSEMENT INFORMATION

General

- See notes on page 286.

Medicare

- Follow–up Days — 90
- Assistant Surgeon — paid
- Supply Charges — not allowed
- Outpatient Limit — does not apply
- Major Surgery Rules Apply

CPT CODE	SERVICE
21462	Open treatment of mandibular fracture; with interdental fixation

ICD–9–CM

802.20	Mandible Fx NOS, closed
802.21	Fx condylar proc mandible, closed
802.22	Subcondylar Fx, mandible, closed
802.23	Fx coronoid proc, mandible, closed
802.24	Fx ramus NOS, closed
802.25	Fx angle of jaw, closed
802.26	Fx symphysis mandible body, closed
802.27	Fx alveolar border mandible, closed
802.28	Fx mandible body NEC, closed
802.29	Multiple Fx mandible, closed
802.30	Mandible Fx NOS, open
802.31	Fx condylar proc mandible, open
802.32	Subcondylar Fx, mandible, open
802.33	Fx coronoid proc, mandible, open
802.34	Fx ramus NOS, open
802.35	Fx angle of jaw, open
802.36	Fx symphysis mandible body, open
802.37	Fx alveolar border mandible, open
802.38	Fx mandible body NEC, open
802.39	Multiple Fx mandible, open

REIMBURSEMENT INFORMATION

General

- See notes on page 286.

Medicare

- Follow–up Days — 90
- Assistant Surgeon — paid
- Supply Charges — not allowed
- Outpatient Limit — does not apply
- Major Surgery Rules Apply

CPT CODE	SERVICE	ICD–9–CM
21465	Open treatment of mandibular condylar fracture	802.21 Fx condylar proc mandible, closed 802.22 Subcondylar Fx, mandible, closed 802.31 Fx condylar proc mandible, open 802.32 Subcondylar Fx, mandible, open

REIMBURSEMENT INFORMATION

General

- ◆ See notes on page 286.

Medicare

- ◆ Follow–up Days — 90
- ◆ Assistant Surgeon — paid
- ◆ Supply Charges — not allowed
- ◆ Outpatient Limit — does not apply
- ◆ Major Surgery Rules Apply

CPT CODE	SERVICE	ICD–9–CM
21470	Open treatment of complicated mandibular fracture by multiple surgical approaches including internal fixation, interdental fixation, and/or wiring of dentures or splints	733.81 Malunion of fracture 802.20 Mandible Fx NOS, closed 802.21 Fx condylar proc mandible, closed 802.22 Subcondylar Fx, mandible, closed 802.23 Fx coronoid proc, mandible, closed 802.24 Fx ramus NOS, closed 802.25 Fx angle of jaw, closed 802.26 Fx symphysis mandible body, closed 802.27 Fx alveolar border mandible, closed 802.28 Fx mandible body NEC, closed 802.29 Multiple Fx mandible, closed 802.30 Mandible Fx NOS, open 802.31 Fx condylar proc mandible, open 802.32 Subcondylar Fx, mandible, open 802.33 Fx coronoid proc, mandible, open 802.34 Fx ramus NOS, open 802.35 Fx angle of jaw, open 802.36 Fx symphysis mandible body, open 802.37 Fx alveolar border mandible, open 802.38 Fx mandible body NEC, open 802.39 Multiple Fx mandible, open

REIMBURSEMENT INFORMATION

General

- ◆ See notes on page 286.

Medicare

- ◆ Follow–up Days — 90
- ◆ Assistant Surgeon — paid
- ◆ Supply Charges — not allowed
- ◆ Outpatient Limit — does not apply
- ◆ Major Surgery Rules Apply

CPT CODE SERVICE	ICD-9-CM
21480 Closed treatment of temporomandibular dislocation; initial or subsequent	830.0 Dislocation jaw, closed 830.1 Dislocation jaw, open 848.1 Sprain of jaw **REIMBURSEMENT INFORMATION** General ♦ See notes on page 286. Medicare ♦ Follow-up Days — 0 ♦ Assistant Surgeon — not paid ♦ Supply Charges — not allowed ♦ Outpatient Limit — does not apply ♦ Minor Surgery Rules Apply
21485 Closed treatment of temporomandibular dislocation; complicated (eg, recurrent requiring intermaxillary fixation or splinting), initial or subsequent	728.85 Spasm of muscle 830.0 Dislocation jaw, closed 830.1 Dislocation jaw, open 848.1 Sprain of jaw 905.6 Late effect of dislocation **REIMBURSEMENT INFORMATION** General ♦ See notes on page 286. Medicare ♦ Follow-up Days — 90 ♦ Assistant Surgeon — not paid ♦ Supply Charges — not allowed ♦ Outpatient Limit — does not apply ♦ Major Surgery Rules Apply
21490 Open treatment of temporomandibular dislocation **CPT NOTES** ♦ For interdental wire fixation, see 21462.	830.0 Dislocation jaw, closed 830.1 Dislocation jaw, open **REIMBURSEMENT INFORMATION** General ♦ See notes on page 286. Medicare ♦ Follow-up Days — 90 ♦ Assistant Surgeon — not paid ♦ Supply Charges — not allowed ♦ Outpatient Limit — does not apply ♦ Major Surgery Rules Apply

CPT CODE **SERVICE** | **ICD–9–CM**

21497 Interdental wiring, for condition other than fracture

170.0	M-Neoplasm, Skull/Face bone
170.1	M-Neoplasm, Mandible
213.0	B-Neoplasm, Skull/Face bone
213.1	B-Neoplasm, Lower jaw bone
239.2	Bone/Skin neoplasm NOS
524.6	Temporomandibular joint disorder
526.0	Developmental odontogenic cysts
526.1	Fissural cysts of jaw
526.2	Jaw cysts NEC
526.3	Jaw, central giant cell granuloma
526.89	Jaw disease NEC
526.9	Jaw disease NOS
733.82	Nonunion of fracture

REIMBURSEMENT INFORMATION

General

- See notes on page 286.

Medicare

- Follow–up Days — 90
- Assistant Surgeon — by report
- Supply Charges — not allowed
- Outpatient Limit — does not apply
- Major Surgery Rules Apply

21501 Incision and drainage, deep abscess or hematoma, soft tissues of neck or thorax

CPT NOTES

- For cervical spine and back, see 21920 et seq.
- For injection of fracture site or trigger point, see 20550.
- For incision and drainage of abscess or hematoma, superficial, see 10060, 10140.

682.1	Cellulitis of neck
682.2	Cellulitis of trunk
728.0	Infective myositis
728.89	Muscle/ligament disorder NEC
906.3	Late effect of contusion
906.4	Late effect of crushing
909.3	Late effect of surg/med complic
920.	Contusion face/scalp/neck
922.1	Contusion of chest wall
925.	Crushing injury, face/scalp/neck
926.19	Crushing injury, trunk NEC
998.1	Hemorrhage complicating a procedure
998.5	Postoperative infection

REIMBURSEMENT INFORMATION

General

- See notes on page 286.

Medicare

- Follow–up Days — 90
- Assistant Surgeon — not paid
- Supply Charges — not allowed
- Outpatient Limit — does not apply
- Major Surgery Rules Apply

CPT CODE	SERVICE
21502	Incision and drainage, deep abscess or hematoma, soft tissues of neck or thorax; with partial rib ostectomy

CPT NOTES

- For cervical spine and back, see 21920 et seq.
- For injection of fracture site or trigger point, see 20550.
- For incision and drainage of abscess or hematoma, superficial, see 10060, 10140.

ICD–9–CM

682.1	Cellulitis of neck
682.2	Cellulitis of trunk
728.0	Infective myositis
728.89	Muscle/ligament disorder NEC
730.08	Acute osteomyelitis NEC
730.18	Chronic osteomyelitis NEC
757.2	Dermatoglyphic anomaly
906.3	Late effect of contusion
906.4	Late effect of crushing
909.3	Late effect of surg/med complic
920.	Contusion face/scalp/neck
922.1	Contusion of chest wall
925.	Crushing injury, face/scalp/neck
926.19	Crushing injury, trunk NEC
998.1	Hemorrhage complicating a procedure

REIMBURSEMENT INFORMATION

General

- See notes on page 286.

Medicare

- Follow–up Days — 90
- Assistant Surgeon — paid
- Supply Charges — not allowed
- Outpatient Limit — does not apply
- Major Surgery Rules Apply

CPT CODE	SERVICE
21550	Biopsy, soft tissue of neck or thorax

CPT NOTES

- For cervical spine and back, see 21920 et seq.
- For injection of fracture site or trigger point, see 20550.
- For bone biopsy, see 20220-20251.
- For needle biopsy of soft tissue, see 20206.

ICD–9–CM

171.0	M-Neoplasm, Soft tissue, head
171.4	M-Neoplasm, Soft tissue, thorax
171.8	M-Neoplasm, Soft tissue NEC
195.0	M-Neoplasm, Head/face/neck
195.1	M-Neoplasm, Thorax
196.0	M-Neoplasm, Lymph head/neck/face
196.1	M-Neoplasm, Lymph intrathoracic
200.01	Reticulosarcoma, head/neck/face
200.11	Lymphosarcoma, head/neck/face
200.21	Burkitt's tumor, head/neck face
215.0	B-Neoplasm, Soft tissue, head
215.4	B-Neoplasm, Soft tissue, thorax
229.0	B-Neoplasm, Lymph nodes
229.8	Benign neoplasm NEC
229.9	Benign neoplasm NOS
238.1	UB-Neoplasm, Soft tissue
239.2	Bone/Skin neoplasm NOS
241.0	Nontoxic uninodular goiter
706.2	Sebaceous cyst
709.4	Foreign body granuloma, skin
728.82	Foreign body granuloma of muscle
729.6	Old foreign body in soft tissue
744.41	Branchial cleft sinus/fistula
744.42	Branchial cleft cyst
784.2	Swelling in head/neck

REIMBURSEMENT INFORMATION

General

- See notes on page 286.

Medicare

- Follow–up Days — 10
- Assistant Surgeon — not paid
- Supply Charges — not allowed
- Outpatient Limit — does not apply
- Minor Surgery Rules Apply

CPT CODE	SERVICE
21555	Excision tumor, soft tissue of neck or thorax; subcutaneous

CPT NOTES

- ♦ For cervical spine and back, see 21920 et seq.
- ♦ For injection of fracture site or trigger point, see 20550.
- ♦ For bone biopsy, see 20220-20251.

ICD–9–CM

171.0	M-Neoplasm, Soft tissue, head
171.4	M-Neoplasm, Soft tissue, thorax
171.8	M-Neoplasm, Soft tissue NEC
195.0	M-Neoplasm, Head/face/neck
195.1	M-Neoplasm, Thorax
196.0	M-Neoplasm, Lymph head/neck/face
196.1	M-Neoplasm, Lymph intrathoracic
200.01	Reticulosarcoma, head/neck/face
200.11	Lymphosarcoma, head/neck/face
200.21	Burkitt's tumor, head/neck face
214.1	Lipoma, Skin NEC
215.0	B-Neoplasm, Soft tissue, head
215.4	B-Neoplasm, Soft tissue, thorax
229.0	B-Neoplasm, Lymph nodes
229.8	Benign neoplasm NEC
229.9	Benign neoplasm NOS
238.1	UB-Neoplasm, Soft tissue
239.2	Bone/Skin neoplasm NOS
706.2	Sebaceous cyst
709.4	Foreign body granuloma, skin
728.82	Foreign body granuloma of muscle
729.6	Old foreign body in soft tissue
744.41	Branchial cleft sinus/fistula
744.42	Branchial cleft cyst
784.2	Swelling in head/neck

REIMBURSEMENT INFORMATION

General

- ♦ See notes on page 286.

Medicare

- ♦ Follow–up Days — 90
- ♦ Assistant Surgeon — not paid
- ♦ Supply Charges — not allowed
- ♦ Outpatient Limit — does not apply
- ♦ Major Surgery Rules Apply

CPT CODE	SERVICE
21556	Excision tumor, soft tissue of neck or thorax; deep, subfascial, intramuscular

CPT NOTES

- For cervical spine and back, see 21920 et seq.
- For injection of fracture site or trigger point, see 20550.
- For bone biopsy, see 20220-20251.

ICD–9–CM

171.0	M-Neoplasm, Soft tissue, head
171.4	M-Neoplasm, Soft tissue, thorax
171.8	M-Neoplasm, Soft tissue NEC
195.0	M-Neoplasm, Head/face/neck
195.1	M-Neoplasm, Thorax
196.0	M-Neoplasm, Lymph head/neck/face
196.1	M-Neoplasm, Lymph intrathoracic
200.01	Reticulosarcoma, head/neck/face
200.11	Lymphosarcoma, head/neck/face
200.12	Lymphosarcoma, intrathoracic
200.21	Burkitt's tumor, head/neck face
214.1	Lipoma, Skin NEC
214.2	Lipoma, Intrathoracic
215.0	B-Neoplasm, Soft tissue, head
215.4	B-Neoplasm, Soft tissue, thorax
229.0	B-Neoplasm, Lymph nodes
229.8	Benign neoplasm NEC
229.9	Benign neoplasm NOS
238.1	UB-Neoplasm, Soft tissue
239.2	Bone/Skin neoplasm NOS
706.2	Sebaceous cyst
709.4	Foreign body granuloma, skin
728.82	Foreign body granuloma of muscle
729.6	Old foreign body in soft tissue
744.41	Branchial cleft sinus/fistula
744.42	Branchial cleft cyst
784.2	Swelling in head/neck

REIMBURSEMENT INFORMATION

General

- See notes on page 286.

Medicare

- Follow–up Days — 90
- Assistant Surgeon — not paid
- Supply Charges — not allowed
- Outpatient Limit — does not apply
- Major Surgery Rules Apply

CPT CODE	SERVICE

21557 Radical resection of tumor (eg, malignant neoplasm), soft tissue of neck or thorax

CPT NOTES

- For cervical spine and back, see 21920 et seq.
- For injection of fracture site or trigger point, see 20550.
- For bone biopsy, see 20220-20251.

ICD–9–CM

171.4	M-Neoplasm, Soft tissue, thorax
171.8	M-Neoplasm, Soft tissue NEC
195.0	M-Neoplasm, Head/face/neck
195.1	M-Neoplasm, Thorax
200.11	Lymphosarcoma, head/neck/face
200.12	Lymphosarcoma, intrathoracic
238.1	UB-Neoplasm, Soft tissue
239.2	Bone/Skin neoplasm NOS

REIMBURSEMENT INFORMATION

General

- See notes on page 286.

Medicare

- Follow–up Days — 90
- Assistant Surgeon — paid
- Supply Charges — not allowed
- Outpatient Limit — does not apply
- Major Surgery Rules Apply

21600 Excision of rib, partial

CPT NOTES

- For cervical spine and back, see 21920 et seq.
- For injection of fracture site or trigger point, see 20550.
- For bone biopsy, see 20220-20251.
- For radical resection of chest wall and rib cage for tumor, see 19260.
- For radical debridement of chest wall and rib case for injury, see 11040-11044.

170.3	M-Neoplasm, Ribs/Sternum/Clavicle
196.1	M-Neoplasm, Lymph intrathoracic
198.5	M2-Neoplasm, Bone and bone marrow
213.3	B-Neoplasm, Ribs/Sternum/Clavicle
238.0	UB-Neoplasm, Bone
239.2	Bone/Skin neoplasm NOS
733.99	Bone/Cartilage disorder NEC
756.2	Cervical rib

REIMBURSEMENT INFORMATION

General

- See notes on page 286.

Medicare

- Follow–up Days — 90
- Assistant Surgeon — paid
- Supply Charges — not allowed
- Outpatient Limit — does not apply
- Major Surgery Rules Apply

CPT CODE	SERVICE	ICD–9–CM

▲ **21615** Excision first and/or cervical rib

CPT NOTES

- For cervical spine and back, see 21920 et seq.
- For injection of fracture site or trigger point, see 20550.
- For bone biopsy, see 20220-20251.

ICD–9–CM

353.0	Brachial plexus lesions
733.99	Bone/Cartilage disorder NEC
756.2	Cervical rib

REIMBURSEMENT INFORMATION

General

- See notes on page 286.
- Description changed in 1995 CPT.

Medicare

- Follow–up Days — 90
- Assistant Surgeon — paid
- Supply Charges — not allowed
- Outpatient Limit — does not apply
- Major Surgery Rules Apply

▲ **21616** Excision first and/or cervical rib; with sympathectomy

CPT NOTES

- For cervical spine and back, see 21920 et seq.
- For injection of fracture site or trigger point, see 20550.
- For bone biopsy, see 20220-20251.

ICD–9–CM

353.0	Brachial plexus lesions

REIMBURSEMENT INFORMATION

General

- See notes on page 286.
- Description changed in 1995 CPT.

Medicare

- Follow–up Days — 90
- Assistant Surgeon — paid
- Supply Charges — not allowed
- Outpatient Limit — does not apply
- Major Surgery Rules Apply

CPT CODE	SERVICE	ICD–9–CM

21620 Ostectomy of sternum, partial

CPT NOTES

- ♦ For cervical spine and back, see 21920 et seq.
- ♦ For injection of fracture site or trigger point, see 20550.
- ♦ For bone biopsy, see 20220-20251.

170.3	M-Neoplasm, Ribs/Sternum/Clavicle
198.5	M2-Neoplasm, Bone and bone marrow
213.3	B-Neoplasm, Ribs/Sternum/Clavicle
238.0	UB-Neoplasm, Bone
239.2	Bone/Skin neoplasm NOS
730.08	Acute osteomyelitis NEC
730.18	Chronic osteomyelitis NEC
875.1	Open wound of chest, complicated
998.3	Postop wound disruption
998.5	Postoperative infection

REIMBURSEMENT INFORMATION

General

- ♦ See notes on page 286.

Medicare

- ♦ Follow–up Days — 90
- ♦ Assistant Surgeon — paid
- ♦ Supply Charges — not allowed
- ♦ Outpatient Limit — does not apply
- ♦ Major Surgery Rules Apply

21627 Sternal debridement

CPT NOTES

- ♦ For cervical spine and back, see 21920 et seq.
- ♦ For injection of fracture site or trigger point, see 20550.
- ♦ For bone biopsy, see 20220-20251.
- ♦ For debridement and closure, see 21750.

170.3	M-Neoplasm, Ribs/Sternum/Clavicle
198.5	M2-Neoplasm, Bone and bone marrow
213.3	B-Neoplasm, Ribs/Sternum/Clavicle
238.0	UB-Neoplasm, Bone
239.2	Bone/Skin neoplasm NOS
730.08	Acute osteomyelitis NEC
730.18	Chronic osteomyelitis NEC
875.1	Open wound of chest, complicated
998.3	Postop wound disruption
998.5	Postoperative infection

REIMBURSEMENT INFORMATION

General

- ♦ See notes on page 286.

Medicare

- ♦ Follow–up Days — 90
- ♦ Assistant Surgeon — paid
- ♦ Supply Charges — not allowed
- ♦ Outpatient Limit — does not apply
- ♦ Major Surgery Rules Apply

CPT CODE	SERVICE	ICD-9-CM
▲ **21630**	Radical resection of sternum	170.3 M-Neoplasm, Ribs/Sternum/Clavicle 198.5 M2-Neoplasm, Bone and bone marrow 213.3 B-Neoplasm, Ribs/Sternum/Clavicle 238.0 UB-Neoplasm, Bone 239.2 Bone/Skin neoplasm NOS 730.28 Osteomyelitis NOS, other site 998.5 Postoperative infection

CPT NOTES

- ♦ For cervical spine and back, see 21920 et seq.
- ♦ For injection of fracture site or trigger point, see 20550.
- ♦ For bone biopsy, see 20220-20251.

REIMBURSEMENT INFORMATION

General

- ♦ See notes on page 286.
- ♦ Description change in 1995 CPT.

Medicare

- ♦ Follow–up Days — 90
- ♦ Assistant Surgeon — paid
- ♦ Supply Charges — not allowed
- ♦ Outpatient Limit — does not apply
- ♦ Major Surgery Rules Apply

21632	Radical resection of sternum; with mediastinal lymphadenectomy	170.3 M-Neoplasm, Ribs/Sternum/Clavicle 196.1 M-Neoplasm, Lymph intrathoracic 198.5 M2-Neoplasm, Bone and bone marrow 213.3 B-Neoplasm, Ribs/Sternum/Clavicle 238.0 UB-Neoplasm, Bone 239.2 Bone/Skin neoplasm NOS 998.5 Postoperative infection

CPT NOTES

- ♦ For cervical spine and back, see 21920 et seq.
- ♦ For injection of fracture site or trigger point, see 20550.
- ♦ For bone biopsy, see 20220-20251.

REIMBURSEMENT INFORMATION

General

- ♦ See notes on page 286.

Medicare

- ♦ Follow–up Days — 90
- ♦ Assistant Surgeon — paid
- ♦ Supply Charges — not allowed
- ♦ Outpatient Limit — does not apply
- ♦ Major Surgery Rules Apply

CPT CODE	SERVICE	ICD–9–CM

21700 Division of scalenus anticus; without resection of cervical rib

21705 Division of scalenus anticus; with resection of cervical rib

CPT NOTES

- ♦ For cervical spine and back, see 21920 et seq.
- ♦ For injection of fracture site or trigger point, see 20550.
- ♦ For superficial wound, see Integumentary System section under Repair-Simple.

353.0 Brachial plexus lesions

REIMBURSEMENT INFORMATION

General

- ♦ See notes on page 286.

Medicare

- ♦ Follow–up Days — 90
- ♦ Assistant Surgeon — paid
- ♦ Supply Charges — not allowed
- ♦ Outpatient Limit — does not apply
- ♦ Major Surgery Rules Apply

21720 Division of sternocleidomastoid for torticollis, open operation; without cast application

21725 Division of sternocleidomastoid for torticollis, open operation; with cast application

CPT NOTES

- ♦ For cervical spine and back, see 21920 et seq.
- ♦ For injection of fracture site or trigger point, see 20550.
- ♦ For superficial wound, see Integumentary System section under Repair-Simple.
- ♦ For transection of spinal accessory and cervical nerves, see 63191, 64722.

723.5 Torticollis NOS
754.1 Congen sternomastoid torticollis

REIMBURSEMENT INFORMATION

General

- ♦ See notes on page 286.

Medicare

- ♦ Follow–up Days — 90
- ♦ Assistant Surgeon — paid
- ♦ Supply Charges — not allowed
- ♦ Outpatient Limit — does not apply
- ♦ Major Surgery Rules Apply

21740 Reconstructive repair of pectus excavatum or carinatum

CPT NOTES

- ♦ For cervical spine and back, see 21920 et seq.
- ♦ For injection of fracture site or trigger point, see 20550.
- ♦ For superficial wound, see Integumentary System section under Repair-Simple.

738.3 Acquired chest/rib deformity
754.81 Pectus excavatum
754.82 Pectus carinatum

REIMBURSEMENT INFORMATION

General

- ♦ See notes on page 286.

Medicare

- ♦ Follow–up Days — 90
- ♦ Assistant Surgeon — paid
- ♦ Supply Charges — not allowed
- ♦ Outpatient Limit — does not apply
- ♦ Major Surgery Rules Apply

CPT CODE	SERVICE	ICD-9-CM

21750 Closure of sternotomy separation with or without debridement (separate procedure)

CPT NOTES

- For cervical spine and back, see 21920 et seq.
- For injection of fracture site or trigger point, see 20550.
- For superficial wound, see Integumentary System section under Repair-Simple.

170.3	M-Neoplasm, Ribs/Sternum/Clavicle
198.5	M2-Neoplasm, Bone and bone marrow
213.3	B-Neoplasm, Ribs/Sternum/Clavicle
238.0	UB-Neoplasm, Bone
239.2	Bone/Skin neoplasm NOS
998.3	Postop wound disruption

REIMBURSEMENT INFORMATION

General

- See notes on page 286.
- Separate procedure rules apply.

Medicare

- Follow-up Days — 90
- Assistant Surgeon — paid
- Supply Charges — not allowed
- Outpatient Limit — does not apply
- Major Surgery Rules Apply

21800 Closed treatment of rib fracture, uncomplicated, each

CPT NOTES

- For cervical spine and back, see 21920 et seq.
- For injection of fracture site or trigger point, see 20550.

807.00	Fracture, rib NOS, closed
807.01	Fracture, one rib, closed
807.02	Fracture, two ribs, closed
807.03	Fracture, three ribs, closed
807.04	Fracture, four ribs, closed
807.05	Fracture, five ribs, closed
807.06	Fracture, six ribs, closed
807.07	Fracture, seven ribs, closed
807.08	Fracture, eight/more ribs, closed
807.09	Fracture, multiple ribs, closed

REIMBURSEMENT INFORMATION

General

- See notes on page 286.

Medicare

- Follow-up Days — 90
- Assistant Surgeon — not paid
- Supply Charges — not allowed
- Outpatient Limit — does not apply
- Major Surgery Rules Apply

CPT CODE	SERVICE	ICD-9-CM

21805 Open treatment of rib fracture without fixation, each

CPT NOTES

- For cervical spine and back, see 21920 et seq.
- For injection of fracture site or trigger point, see 20550.

ICD-9-CM

807.10 Fracture, rib NOS, open
807.11 Fracture, one rib, open
807.12 Fracture, two ribs, open
807.13 Fracture, three ribs, open
807.14 Fracture, four ribs, open
807.15 Fracture, five ribs, open
807.16 Fracture, six ribs, open
807.17 Fracture, seven ribs, open
807.18 Fracture, eight/more ribs, open
807.19 Fracture, multiple ribs, open

REIMBURSEMENT INFORMATION

General

- See notes on page 286.

Medicare

- Follow-up Days — 90
- Assistant Surgeon — by report
- Supply Charges — not allowed
- Outpatient Limit — does not apply
- Major Surgery Rules Apply

21810 Treatment of rib fracture requiring external fixation ("flail chest")

CPT NOTES

- For cervical spine and back, see 21920 et seq.
- For injection of fracture site or trigger point, see 20550.

ICD-9-CM

807.4 Flail chest

REIMBURSEMENT INFORMATION

General

- See notes on page 286.

Medicare

- Follow-up Days — 90
- Assistant Surgeon — paid
- Supply Charges — not allowed
- Outpatient Limit — does not apply
- Major Surgery Rules Apply

CPT CODE SERVICE	ICD–9–CM
21820 Closed treatment of sternum fracture **CPT NOTES** ◆ For cervical spine and back, see 21920 et seq. ◆ For injection of fracture site or trigger point, see 20550.	807.2 Fracture of sternum, closed 807.3 Fracture of sternum, open **REIMBURSEMENT INFORMATION** General ◆ See notes on page 286. Medicare ◆ Follow–up Days — 90 ◆ Assistant Surgeon — not paid ◆ Supply Charges — not allowed ◆ Outpatient Limit — does not apply ◆ Major Surgery Rules Apply
21825 Open treatment of sternum fracture with or without skeletal fixation **CPT NOTES** ◆ For cervical spine and back, see 21920 et seq. ◆ For injection of fracture site or trigger point, see 20550. ◆ For sternoclavicular dislocation, see 23520-23532.	807.2 Fracture of sternum, closed 807.3 Fracture of sternum, open **REIMBURSEMENT INFORMATION** General ◆ See notes on page 286. Medicare ◆ Follow–up Days — 90 ◆ Assistant Surgeon — paid ◆ Supply Charges — not allowed ◆ Outpatient Limit — does not apply ◆ Major Surgery Rules Apply
21920 Biopsy, soft tissue of back or flank; superficial **CPT NOTES** ◆ For needle biopsy of soft tissue, use 20206.	171.7 M-Neoplasm, Trunk NOS 171.8 M-Neoplasm, Soft tissue NEC 195.8 M-Neoplasm, site NEC 215.7 B-Neoplasm, Trunk NOS 238.1 UB-Neoplasm, Soft tissue 239.2 Bone/Skin neoplasm NOS 690. Erythematosquamous dermatosis 706.2 Sebaceous cyst **REIMBURSEMENT INFORMATION** General ◆ See notes on page 286. Medicare ◆ Follow–up Days — 10 ◆ Assistant Surgeon — not paid ◆ Supply Charges — not allowed ◆ Outpatient Limit — does not apply ◆ Minor Surgery Rules Apply

CPT CODE	SERVICE	ICD–9–CM
21925	Biopsy, soft tissue of back or flank; deep	171.7 M-Neoplasm, Trunk NOS 171.8 M-Neoplasm, Soft tissue NEC 171.9 M-Neoplasm, Soft tissue NOS 195.8 M-Neoplasm, site NEC 214.1 Lipoma, Skin NEC 215.7 B-Neoplasm, Trunk NOS 238.1 UB-Neoplasm, Soft tissue 238.2 UB-Neoplasm, Skin 239.2 Bone/Skin neoplasm NOS 690. Erythematosquamous dermatosis 706.2 Sebaceous cyst 709.3 Degenerative skin disorders 709.4 Foreign body granuloma, skin

CPT NOTES

- For needle biopsy of soft tissue, use 20206.

REIMBURSEMENT INFORMATION

General

- See notes on page 286.

Medicare

- Follow–up Days — 90
- Assistant Surgeon — not paid
- Supply Charges — not allowed
- Outpatient Limit — does not apply
- Major Surgery Rules Apply

CPT CODE	SERVICE	ICD–9–CM
21930	Excision, tumor, soft tissue of back or flank	171.7 M-Neoplasm, Trunk NOS 171.8 M-Neoplasm, Soft tissue NEC 171.9 M-Neoplasm, Soft tissue NOS 195.8 M-Neoplasm, site NEC 214.1 Lipoma, Skin NEC 215.7 B-Neoplasm, Trunk NOS 238.1 UB-Neoplasm, Soft tissue 238.2 UB-Neoplasm, Skin 239.2 Bone/Skin neoplasm NOS 709.3 Degenerative skin disorders 709.4 Foreign body granuloma, skin

REIMBURSEMENT INFORMATION

General

- See notes on page 286.

Medicare

- Follow–up Days — 10
- Assistant Surgeon — not paid
- Supply Charges — not allowed
- Outpatient Limit — does not apply
- Minor Surgery Rules Apply

CPT CODE	SERVICE	ICD-9-CM	
21935	Radical resection of tumor (eg, malignant neoplasm), soft tissue of back or flank	171.7	M-Neoplasm, Trunk NOS
		171.8	M-Neoplasm, Soft tissue NEC
		171.9	M-Neoplasm, Soft tissue NOS
		195.8	M-Neoplasm, site NEC
		214.1	Lipoma, Skin NEC
		238.1	UB-Neoplasm, Soft tissue
		238.2	UB-Neoplasm, Skin
		239.2	Bone/Skin neoplasm NOS
		709.3	Degenerative skin disorders
		709.4	Foreign body granuloma, skin

REIMBURSEMENT INFORMATION

General

- ♦ See notes on page 286.

Medicare

- ♦ Follow–up Days — 10
- ♦ Assistant Surgeon — paid
- ♦ Supply Charges — not allowed
- ♦ Outpatient Limit — does not apply
- ♦ Minor Surgery Rules Apply

22100 Partial resection of vertebral component, spinous processes; cervical

22101 Partial resection of vertebral component, spinous processes; thoracic

22102 Partial resection of vertebral component, spinous processes; lumbar

707.0	Decubitus ulcer
721.5	Kissing spine
876.1	Open wound of back, complicated

CPT NOTES

- ♦ For injection procedure for myelography, use 62284.
- ♦ For injection procedure for diskography, see 62290, 62291.
- ♦ For injection procedure, chemonucleolysis, single or multiple levels, use 62292.
- ♦ For injection procedure for facet joints, see 64442, 64443, 64622, 64623.
- ♦ For needle or trocar biopsy, see 20220-20225.
- ♦ For bone biopsy, see 20220-20251.

REIMBURSEMENT INFORMATION

General

- ♦ See notes on page 286.

Medicare

- ♦ Follow–up Days — 90
- ♦ Assistant Surgeon — paid
- ♦ Supply Charges — not allowed
- ♦ Outpatient Limit — does not apply
- ♦ Major Surgery Rules Apply

CPT CODE	SERVICE	ICD–9–CM
22900	Excision, abdominal wall tumor, subfascial (eg, desmoid)	171.5 M-Neoplasm, Soft tissue, abdomen 198.89 M2-Neoplasm NEC 215.5 B-Neoplasm, Soft tissue, abdomen 238.1 UB-Neoplasm, Soft tissue 239.2 Bone/Skin neoplasm NOS **REIMBURSEMENT INFORMATION** General ♦ See notes on page 286. Medicare ♦ Follow–up Days — 90 ♦ Assistant Surgeon — paid ♦ Supply Charges — not allowed ♦ Outpatient Limit — does not apply ♦ Major Surgery Rules Apply
23030	Incision and drainage, shoulder area; deep abscess or hematoma	682.3 Cellulitis of arm 711.01 Pyogenic arthritis, shoulder 711.91 Infect arthritis NOS, shoulder 726.1x Rotator cuff syndrome of shoulder 726.2 Shoulder region disorder NEC 727.2 Occupational bursitis 727.3 Bursitis NOS 727.4x Ganglion/cyst synovium/tendon/bursa 727.89 Synovium/tendon/bursa disorder NEC 728.0 Infective myositis 729.4 Fasciitis NOS 730.01 Acute osteomyelitis, shoulder 730.11 Chronic osteomyelitis, shoulder 906.3 Late effect of contusion 906.4 Late effect of crushing 909.3 Late effect of surg/med complic 923.0x Contusion, shoulder and upper arm 927.0x Crushing injury, shoulder/upper arm **REIMBURSEMENT INFORMATION** General ♦ See notes on page 286. Medicare ♦ Follow–up Days — 10 ♦ Assistant Surgeon — not paid ♦ Supply Charges — not allowed ♦ Outpatient Limit — does not apply ♦ Minor Surgery Rules Apply

CPT CODE	SERVICE
23031	Incision and drainage, shoulder area; infected bursa

ICD–9–CM

682.3	Cellulitis of arm
711.01	Pyogenic arthritis, shoulder
711.91	Infect arthritis NOS, shoulder
726.1x	Rotator cuff syndrome of shoulder
726.2	Shoulder region disorder NEC
727.2	Occupational bursitis
727.3	Bursitis NOS
727.4x	Ganglion/cyst synovium/tendon/bursa
727.89	Synovium/tendon/bursa disorder NEC
906.3	Late effect of contusion
906.4	Late effect of crushing
909.3	Late effect of surg/med complic
923.0x	Contusion, shoulder and upper arm
927.0x	Crushing injury, shoulder/upper arm

REIMBURSEMENT INFORMATION

General

- See notes on page 286.

Medicare

- Follow–up Days — 10
- Assistant Surgeon — not paid
- Supply Charges — not allowed
- Outpatient Limit — applies
- Minor Surgery Rules Apply

CPT CODE	SERVICE	ICD-9-CM
23035	Incision, deep, with opening of cortex (eg, for osteomyelitis or bone abscess), shoulder area	730.01 Acute osteomyelitis, shoulder 730.11 Chronic osteomyelitis, shoulder 730.21 Osteomyelitis NOS, shoulder 730.91 Bone infection NOS, shoulder

REIMBURSEMENT INFORMATION

General

- ♦ See notes on page 286.

Medicare

- ♦ Follow–up Days — 90
- ♦ Assistant Surgeon — paid
- ♦ Supply Charges — not allowed
- ♦ Outpatient Limit — does not apply
- ♦ Minor Surgery Rules Apply

CPT CODE	SERVICE	ICD-9-CM
23065	Biopsy, soft tissue of shoulder area; superficial	171.2 M-Neoplasm, Soft tissue, arm 198.89 M2-Neoplasm NEC 215.2 B-Neoplasm, Soft tissue, arm 238.1 UB-Neoplasm, Soft tissue 239.2 Bone/Skin neoplasm NOS

CPT NOTES

- ♦ For needle biopsy of soft tissue, use 20206.

REIMBURSEMENT INFORMATION

General

- ♦ See notes on page 286.

Medicare

- ♦ Follow–up Days — 10
- ♦ Assistant Surgeon — not paid
- ♦ Supply Charges — not allowed
- ♦ Outpatient Limit — applies
- ♦ Minor Surgery Rules Apply

CPT CODE	SERVICE	ICD–9–CM
23066	Biopsy, soft tissue of shoulder area; deep	171.2 M-Neoplasm, Soft tissue, arm 198.89 M2-Neoplasm NEC 215.2 B-Neoplasm, Soft tissue, arm 238.1 UB-Neoplasm, Soft tissue 239.2 Bone/Skin neoplasm NOS 728.82 Foreign body granuloma of muscle

CPT NOTES

- For needle biopsy of soft tissue, use 20206.

REIMBURSEMENT INFORMATION

General

- See notes on page 286.

Medicare

- Follow–up Days — 90
- Assistant Surgeon — not paid
- Supply Charges — not allowed
- Outpatient Limit — does not apply
- Major Surgery Rules Apply

CPT CODE	SERVICE	ICD–9–CM
23075	Excision, tumor, shoulder area; subcutaneous	171.2 M-Neoplasm, Soft tissue, arm 198.89 M2-Neoplasm NEC 215.2 B-Neoplasm, Soft tissue, arm 238.1 UB-Neoplasm, Soft tissue 239.2 Bone/Skin neoplasm NOS 709.4 Foreign body granuloma, skin 729.6 Old foreign body in soft tissue

REIMBURSEMENT INFORMATION

General

- See notes on page 286.

Medicare

- Follow–up Days — 10
- Assistant Surgeon — not paid
- Supply Charges — not allowed
- Outpatient Limit — does not apply
- Minor Surgery Rules Apply

CPT CODE	SERVICE	ICD-9-CM
23077	Radical resection of tumor (eg, malignant neoplasm), soft tissue of shoulder area	171.2 M-Neoplasm, Soft tissue, arm 198.89 M2-Neoplasm NEC 215.2 B-Neoplasm, Soft tissue, arm 238.1 UB-Neoplasm, Soft tissue 239.2 Bone/Skin neoplasm NOS

REIMBURSEMENT INFORMATION

General

- See notes on page 286.

Medicare

- Follow–up Days — 90
- Assistant Surgeon — paid
- Supply Charges — not allowed
- Outpatient Limit — does not apply
- Major Surgery Rules Apply

CPT CODE	SERVICE	ICD-9-CM
23120	Claviculectomy; partial	170.3 M-Neoplasm, Ribs/Sternum/Clavicle 198.5 M2-Neoplasm, Bone and bone marrow 213.3 B-Neoplasm, Ribs/Sternum/Clavicle 715.11 Loc prim osteoarthritis, shoulder 715.21 Loc 2nd osteoarthritis, shoulder 715.31 Loc osteoarthritis NOS, shoulder 730.01 Acute osteomyelitis, shoulder 730.11 Chronic osteomyelitis, shoulder 730.21 Osteomyelitis NOS, shoulder 733.82 Nonunion of fracture 840.0 Sprain acromioclavicular
23125	Claviculectomy; total	

REIMBURSEMENT INFORMATION

General

- See notes on page 286.

Medicare

- Follow–up Days — 90
- Assistant Surgeon — paid
- Supply Charges — not allowed
- Outpatient Limit — does not apply
- Major Surgery Rules Apply

CPT CODE	SERVICE	ICD–9–CM	
23140	Excision or curettage of bone cyst or benign tumor of clavicle or scapula	213.3	B-Neoplasm, Ribs/Sternum/Clavicle
23145	Excision or curettage of bone cyst or benign tumor of clavicle or scapula; with autograft (includes obtaining graft)	213.4	B-Neoplasm, Long bones, arm
		731.0	Osteitis deformans NOS
		733.20	Cyst of bone NOS
		733.21	Solitary bone cyst
		733.22	Aneurysmal bone cyst
		733.29	Bone cyst NEC
		733.40	Aseptic necrosis of bone NOS
		733.49	Aseptic necrosis of bone NEC

REIMBURSEMENT INFORMATION

General

- See notes on page 286.

Medicare

- Follow–up Days — 90
- Assistant Surgeon — not paid
- Supply Charges — not allowed
- Outpatient Limit — does not apply
- Major Surgery Rules Apply

CPT CODE	SERVICE	ICD–9–CM	
23170	Sequestrectomy (eg, for osteomyelitis or bone abscess), clavicle	730.01	Acute osteomyelitis, shoulder
		730.11	Chronic osteomyelitis, shoulder
		730.21	Osteomyelitis NOS, shoulder
		730.31	Periostitis, shoulder
		731.0	Osteitis deformans NOS
		733.20	Cyst of bone NOS
		733.21	Solitary bone cyst
		733.22	Aneurysmal bone cyst
		733.29	Bone cyst NEC
		733.40	Aseptic necrosis of bone NOS
		733.49	Aseptic necrosis of bone NEC

REIMBURSEMENT INFORMATION

General

- See notes on page 286.

Medicare

- Follow–up Days — 90
- Assistant Surgeon — paid
- Supply Charges — not allowed
- Outpatient Limit — does not apply
- Major Surgery Rules Apply

CPT CODE	SERVICE	ICD-9-CM
23172	Sequestrectomy (eg, for osteomyelitis or bone abscess), scapula	730.01 Acute osteomyelitis, shoulder 730.11 Chronic osteomyelitis, shoulder 730.21 Osteomyelitis NOS, shoulder 730.31 Periostitis, shoulder 731.0 Osteitis deformans NOS 733.20 Cyst of bone NOS 733.21 Solitary bone cyst 733.22 Aneurysmal bone cyst 733.29 Bone cyst NEC 733.40 Aseptic necrosis of bone NOS **REIMBURSEMENT INFORMATION** General ♦ See notes on page 286. Medicare ♦ Follow-up Days — 90 ♦ Assistant Surgeon — paid ♦ Supply Charges — not allowed ♦ Outpatient Limit — does not apply ♦ Major Surgery Rules Apply
23174	Sequestrectomy (eg, for osteomyelitis or bone abscess), humeral head to surgical neck	730.02 Acute osteomyelitis, upper arm 730.12 Chronic osteomyelitis, upper arm 730.21 Osteomyelitis NOS, shoulder 730.22 Osteomyelitis NOS, upper arm 730.31 Periostitis, shoulder 730.32 Periostitis, upper arm 731.0 Osteitis deformans NOS 733.20 Cyst of bone NOS 733.21 Solitary bone cyst 733.22 Aneurysmal bone cyst 733.29 Bone cyst NEC 733.41 Aseptic necrosis, head of humerus 733.49 Aseptic necrosis of bone NEC **REIMBURSEMENT INFORMATION** General ♦ See notes on page 286. Medicare ♦ Follow-up Days — 90 ♦ Assistant Surgeon — paid ♦ Supply Charges — not allowed ♦ Outpatient Limit — does not apply ♦ Major Surgery Rules Apply

CPT CODE	SERVICE	ICD-9-CM
23180	Partial excision, (craterization, saucerization, or diaphysectomy) of bone (eg, for osteomyelitis), clavicle	730.01 Acute osteomyelitis, shoulder 730.11 Chronic osteomyelitis, shoulder 730.21 Osteomyelitis NOS, shoulder 730.31 Periostitis, shoulder 731.0 Osteitis deformans NOS 733.20 Cyst of bone NOS 733.21 Solitary bone cyst 733.22 Aneurysmal bone cyst 733.29 Bone cyst NEC 733.49 Aseptic necrosis of bone NEC

REIMBURSEMENT INFORMATION

General

- ◆ See notes on page 286.

Medicare

- ◆ Follow-up Days — 90
- ◆ Assistant Surgeon — paid
- ◆ Supply Charges — not allowed
- ◆ Outpatient Limit — does not apply
- ◆ Major Surgery Rules Apply

CPT CODE	SERVICE	ICD-9-CM
23182	Partial excision, (craterization, saucerization, or diaphysectomy) of bone (eg, for osteomyelitis), scapula	730.01 Acute osteomyelitis, shoulder 730.11 Chronic osteomyelitis, shoulder 730.21 Osteomyelitis NOS, shoulder 730.31 Periostitis, shoulder 731.0 Osteitis deformans NOS 733.20 Cyst of bone NOS 733.21 Solitary bone cyst 733.22 Aneurysmal bone cyst 733.29 Bone cyst NEC

REIMBURSEMENT INFORMATION

General

- ◆ See notes on page 286.

Medicare

- ◆ Follow-up Days — 90
- ◆ Assistant Surgeon — paid
- ◆ Supply Charges — not allowed
- ◆ Outpatient Limit — does not apply
- ◆ Major Surgery Rules Apply

CPT CODE	SERVICE	ICD–9–CM
23184	Partial excision, (craterization, saucerization, or diaphysectomy) of bone (eg, for osteomyelitis), proximal humerus	730.01 Acute osteomyelitis, shoulder 730.02 Acute osteomyelitis, upper arm 730.11 Chronic osteomyelitis, shoulder 730.12 Chronic osteomyelitis, upper arm 730.21 Osteomyelitis NOS, shoulder 730.22 Osteomyelitis NOS, upper arm 730.31 Periostitis, shoulder 730.32 Periostitis, upper arm 731.0 Osteitis deformans NOS 733.20 Cyst of bone NOS 733.21 Solitary bone cyst 733.22 Aneurysmal bone cyst 733.29 Bone cyst NEC 733.41 Aseptic necrosis, head of humerus 733.49 Aseptic necrosis of bone NEC

REIMBURSEMENT INFORMATION

General

- See notes on page 286.

Medicare

- Follow–up Days — 90
- Assistant Surgeon — paid
- Supply Charges — not allowed
- Outpatient Limit — does not apply
- Major Surgery Rules Apply

CPT CODE	SERVICE	ICD–9–CM
23330	Removal of foreign body, shoulder; subcutaneous	709.4 Foreign body granuloma, skin 912.6 Foreign body, shoulder/arm 912.7 Foreign body, should/arm, infected

CPT NOTES

- For arthrocentesis or needling of bursa, see 20610.
- For K-wire or pin insertion or removal, see 20650, 20670, 20680.

REIMBURSEMENT INFORMATION

General

- See notes on page 286.

Medicare

- Follow–up Days — 10
- Assistant Surgeon — not paid
- Supply Charges — not allowed
- Outpatient Limit — does not apply
- Minor Surgery Rules Apply

CPT CODE	SERVICE
23331	Removal of foreign body, shoulder; deep (eg, Neer prosthesis removal)

CPT NOTES

- For arthrocentesis or needling of bursa, see 20610.
- For K-wire or pin insertion or removal, see 20650, 20670, 20680.

ICD–9–CM

728.82	Foreign body granuloma of muscle
733.82	Nonunion of fracture
733.99	Bone/Cartilage disorder NEC
880.10	Open wound of shoulder, complicated
996.66	Reaction, internal joint prosthesis
996.67	Reaction, internal ortho device NEC
996.77	Complication, int joint prosthesis
998.7	Postop foreign subst acute reaction

REIMBURSEMENT INFORMATION

General

- See notes on page 286.

Medicare

- Follow–up Days — 90
- Assistant Surgeon — not paid
- Supply Charges — not allowed
- Outpatient Limit — does not apply
- Major Surgery Rules Apply

CPT CODE	SERVICE
23930	Incision and drainage, upper arm or elbow area; deep abscess or hematoma

CPT NOTES

- For incision and drainage procedures, superficial, see 10040-10160.

ICD–9–CM

682.3	Cellulitis of arm
711.02	Pyogenic arthritis, upper arm
711.92	Infect arthritis NOS, upper arm
726.30	Elbow enthesopathy NOS
726.31	Medial epicondylitis
726.32	Lateral epicondylitis
726.33	Olecranon bursitis
726.39	Elbow enthesopathy NEC
727.2	Occupational bursitis
727.3	Bursitis NOS
727.4x	Ganglion/cyst synovium/tendon/bursa
727.89	Synovium/tendon/bursa disorder NEC
906.3	Late effect of contusion
906.4	Late effect of crushing
909.3	Late effect of surg/med complic
923.03	Contusion of upper arm
923.09	Contusion of shoulder & arm
923.11	Contusion of elbow
927.03	Crushing injury, upper arm
927.09	Crushing injury, shoulder & arm
927.11	Crushing injury, elbow
996.66	Reaction, internal joint prosthesis
996.77	Complication, int joint prosthesis
998.1	Hemorrhage complicating a procedure

REIMBURSEMENT INFORMATION

General

- See notes on page 286.

Medicare

- Follow–up Days — 10
- Assistant Surgeon — not paid
- Supply Charges — not allowed
- Outpatient Limit — does not apply
- Minor Surgery Rules Apply

CPT CODE	SERVICE
23931	Incision and drainage, upper arm or elbow area; infected bursa

CPT NOTES

- For incision and drainage procedures, superficial, see 10040-10160.

ICD–9–CM

682.3	Cellulitis of arm
711.02	Pyogenic arthritis, upper arm
711.92	Infect arthritis NOS, upper arm
726.30	Elbow enthesopathy NOS
726.31	Medial epicondylitis
726.32	Lateral epicondylitis
726.33	Olecranon bursitis
726.39	Elbow enthesopathy NEC
727.2	Occupational bursitis
727.3	Bursitis NOS
727.4x	Ganglion/cyst synovium/tendon/bursa
727.89	Synovium/tendon/bursa disorder NEC
906.1	Late effect, open wound extremity
906.3	Late effect of contusion
906.4	Late effect of crushing
909.3	Late effect of surg/med complic
923.03	Contusion of upper arm
923.09	Contusion of shoulder & arm
923.11	Contusion of elbow
927.03	Crushing injury, upper arm
927.09	Crushing injury, shoulder & arm
927.11	Crushing injury, elbow
998.5	Postoperative infection

REIMBURSEMENT INFORMATION

General

- See notes on page 286.

Medicare

- Follow–up Days — 10
- Assistant Surgeon — not paid
- Supply Charges — not allowed
- Outpatient Limit — does not apply
- Minor Surgery Rules Apply

CPT CODE	SERVICE
23935	Incision, deep, with opening of bone cortex (eg, for osteomyelitis or bone abscess), humerus or elbow

CPT NOTES

- ♦ For incision and drainage procedures, superficial, see 10040-10160.

ICD–9–CM

730.02	Acute osteomyelitis, upper arm
730.12	Chronic osteomyelitis, upper arm
730.22	Osteomyelitis NOS, upper arm
730.92	Bone infection NOS, upper arm

REIMBURSEMENT INFORMATION

General

- ♦ See notes on page 286.

Medicare

- ♦ Follow–up Days — 90
- ♦ Assistant Surgeon — not paid
- ♦ Supply Charges — not allowed
- ♦ Outpatient Limit — does not apply
- ♦ Major Surgery Rules Apply

CPT CODE	SERVICE
24000	Arthrotomy, elbow, for infection, with exploration, drainage or removal of foreign body

CPT NOTES

- For incision and drainage procedures, superficial, see 10040-10160.

ICD–9–CM

711.02	Pyogenic arthritis, upper arm
711.92	Infect arthritis NOS, upper arm
714.0	Rheumatoid arthritis
715.12	Loc prim osteoarthritis, upper arm
715.22	Loc 2nd osteoarthritis, upper arm
715.32	Loc osteoarthritis NOS, upper arm
716.12	Traumatic arthropathy, upper arm
718.12	Loose body in joint, upper arm
719.02	Joint effusion, upper arm
719.22	Villonodular synovitis, upper arm
729.6	Old foreign body in soft tissue
730.02	Acute osteomyelitis, upper arm
730.12	Chronic osteomyelitis, upper arm
730.22	Osteomyelitis NOS, upper arm
732.3	Juvenile osteochondrosis, arm
733.99	Bone/Cartilage disorder NEC
881.11	Open wound of elbow, complicated
913.7	Foreign body, forearm, infected
923.03	Contusion of upper arm
996.66	Reaction, internal joint prosthesis
996.77	Complication, int joint prosthesis
998.4	Foreign body left during procedure
998.5	Postoperative infection

REIMBURSEMENT INFORMATION

General

- See notes on page 286.

Medicare

- Follow–up Days — 90
- Assistant Surgeon — paid
- Supply Charges — not allowed
- Outpatient Limit — does not apply
- Major Surgery Rules Apply

CPT CODE	SERVICE
24006	Arthrotomy of the elbow, with capsular excision for capsular release (separate procedure)

CPT NOTES

- For incision and drainage procedures, superficial, see 10040-10160.

ICD–9–CM

711.02	Pyogenic arthritis, upper arm
711.92	Infect arthritis NOS, upper arm
714.0	Rheumatoid arthritis
715.12	Loc prim osteoarthritis, upper arm
715.22	Loc 2nd osteoarthritis, upper arm
715.32	Loc osteoarthritis NOS, upper arm
716.12	Traumatic arthropathy, upper arm
718.12	Loose body in joint, upper arm
718.42	Contracture of joint, upper arm
719.02	Joint effusion, upper arm
719.22	Villonodular synovitis, upper arm
719.42	Pain in joint, upper arm
719.52	Joint stiffness NEC, upper arm
726.30	Elbow enthesopathy NOS
729.6	Old foreign body in soft tissue
730.02	Acute osteomyelitis, upper arm
730.12	Chronic osteomyelitis, upper arm
730.22	Osteomyelitis NOS, upper arm
732.3	Juvenile osteochondrosis, arm

REIMBURSEMENT INFORMATION

General

- See notes on page 286.
- Separate procedure rules apply.

Medicare

- Follow–up Days — 90
- Assistant Surgeon — paid
- Supply Charges — not allowed
- Outpatient Limit — does not apply
- Major Surgery Rules Apply

CPT CODE	SERVICE	ICD-9-CM
24065	Biopsy, soft tissue of upper arm or elbow area; superficial	171.2 M-Neoplasm, Soft tissue, arm 215.2 B-Neoplasm, Soft tissue, arm 228.1 Lymphangioma, any site 238.1 UB-Neoplasm, Soft tissue 239.2 Bone/Skin neoplasm NOS 706.2 Sebaceous cyst

CPT NOTES

- For needle biopsy of soft tissue, use 20206.

REIMBURSEMENT INFORMATION

General

- See notes on page 286.

Medicare

- Follow-up Days — 10
- Assistant Surgeon — not paid
- Supply Charges — not allowed
- Outpatient Limit — does not apply
- Minor Surgery Rules Apply

CPT CODE	SERVICE	ICD-9-CM
24066	Biopsy, soft tissue of upper arm or elbow area; deep	171.2 M-Neoplasm, Soft tissue, arm 195.4 M-Neoplasm, Upper limb 215.2 B-Neoplasm, Soft tissue, abdomen 228.1 Lymphangioma, any site 238.1 UB-Neoplasm, Soft tissue 239.2 Bone/Skin neoplasm NOS

CPT NOTES

- For needle biopsy of soft tissue, use 20206.

REIMBURSEMENT INFORMATION

General

- See notes on page 286.

Medicare

- Follow-up Days — 90
- Assistant Surgeon — not paid
- Supply Charges — not allowed
- Outpatient Limit — does not apply
- Major Surgery Rules Apply

CPT CODE	SERVICE	ICD-9-CM
24075	Excision, tumor, upper arm or elbow area; subcutaneous	171.2 M-Neoplasm, Soft tissue, arm 195.4 M-Neoplasm, Upper limb 215.2 B-Neoplasm, Soft tissue, arm 238.1 UB-Neoplasm, Soft tissue 239.2 Bone/Skin neoplasm NOS 709.2 Scar/fibrosis of skin

REIMBURSEMENT INFORMATION

General

- ♦ See notes on page 286.

Medicare

- ♦ Follow-up Days — 90
- ♦ Assistant Surgeon — not paid
- ♦ Supply Charges — not allowed
- ♦ Outpatient Limit — does not apply
- ♦ Major Surgery Rules Apply

CPT CODE	SERVICE	ICD-9-CM
24076	Excision, tumor, upper arm or elbow area; deep, subfascial or intramuscular	171.2 M-Neoplasm, Soft tissue, arm 195.4 M-Neoplasm, Upper limb 215.2 B-Neoplasm, Soft tissue, arm 238.1 UB-Neoplasm, Soft tissue 239.2 Bone/Skin neoplasm NOS 728.82 Foreign body granuloma of muscle

REIMBURSEMENT INFORMATION

General

- ♦ See notes on page 286.

Medicare

- ♦ Follow-up Days — 90
- ♦ Assistant Surgeon — not paid
- ♦ Supply Charges — not allowed
- ♦ Outpatient Limit — does not apply
- ♦ Major Surgery Rules Apply

CPT CODE	SERVICE	ICD–9–CM	
24077	Radical resection of tumor (eg, malignant neoplasm), soft tissue of upper arm or elbow area	171.2	M-Neoplasm, Soft tissue, arm
		238.1	UB-Neoplasm, Soft tissue
		239.2	Bone/Skin neoplasm NOS

REIMBURSEMENT INFORMATION

General

- See notes on page 286.

Medicare

- Follow–up Days — 90
- Assistant Surgeon — paid
- Supply Charges — not allowed
- Outpatient Limit — does not apply
- Major Surgery Rules Apply

CPT CODE	SERVICE
▲ **24100**	Arthrotomy, elbow; with synovial biopsy only

ICD–9–CM

015.5	Tuberculosis, Limb bones
095.7	Syphilis of tendon/bursa/synovium
098.51	Gonococcal synovitis
171.2	M-Neoplasm, Soft tissue, arm
238.1	UB-Neoplasm, Soft tissue
239.2	Bone/Skin neoplasm NOS
274.0	Gouty arthropathy
275.4	Disorders of calcium metabolism
277.5	Mucopolysaccharidosis
710.1	Systemic sclerosis
711.92	Infect arthritis NOS, upper arm
714.0	Rheumatoid arthritis
714.30	Juvenile rheumatoid arthritis NOS
714.31	Juvenile acute rheumatoid arthritis
714.32	Pauciarticular juv rheum arthritis
714.33	Monoarticular juv rheum arthritis
714.4	Chronic postrheumatic arthritis
715.12	Loc prim osteoarthritis, upper arm
715.22	Loc 2nd osteoarthritis, upper arm
715.32	Loc osteoarthritis NOS, upper arm
716.12	Traumatic arthropathy, upper arm
718.12	Loose body in joint, upper arm
719.02	Joint effusion, upper arm
719.22	Villonodular synovitis, upper arm
727.00	Synovitis NOS
727.01	Synovitis in other diseases
729.6	Old foreign body in soft tissue
732.3	Juvenile osteochondrosis, arm

REIMBURSEMENT INFORMATION

General

- See notes on page 286.
- Description changed in 1995 CPT.

Medicare

- Follow–up Days — 90
- Assistant Surgeon — paid
- Supply Charges — not allowed
- Outpatient Limit — does not apply
- Major Surgery Rules Apply

CPT CODE	SERVICE
24101	Arthrotomy, elbow; with joint exploration, with or without biopsy, with or without removal of loose or foreign body

ICD–9–CM

171.2	M-Neoplasm, Soft tissue, arm
238.1	UB-Neoplasm, Soft tissue
239.2	Bone/Skin neoplasm NOS
277.5	Mucopolysaccharidosis
710.1	Systemic sclerosis
711.92	Infect arthritis NOS, upper arm
714.0	Rheumatoid arthritis
714.30	Juvenile rheumatoid arthritis NOS
714.31	Juvenile acute rheumatoid arthritis
714.32	Pauciarticular juv rheum arthritis
714.33	Monoarticular juv rheum arthritis
714.4	Chronic postrheumatic arthritis
715.12	Loc prim osteoarthritis, upper arm
715.22	Loc 2nd osteoarthritis, upper arm
715.32	Loc osteoarthritis NOS, upper arm
716.12	Traumatic arthropathy, upper arm
718.12	Loose body in joint, upper arm
719.02	Joint effusion, upper arm
719.22	Villonodular synovitis, upper arm
729.6	Old foreign body in soft tissue
732.3	Juvenile osteochondrosis, arm

REIMBURSEMENT INFORMATION

General

- See notes on page 286.

Medicare

- Follow–up Days — 90
- Assistant Surgeon — paid
- Supply Charges — not allowed
- Outpatient Limit — does not apply
- Major Surgery Rules Apply

CPT CODE	SERVICE
▲ **24102**	Arthrotomy, elbow; with synovectomy

ICD–9–CM

015.5	Tuberculosis, Limb bones
095.7	Syphilis of tendon/bursa/synovium
098.51	Gonococcal synovitis
171.2	M-Neoplasm, Soft tissue, arm
238.1	UB-Neoplasm, Soft tissue
239.2	Bone/Skin neoplasm NOS
274.0	Gouty arthropathy
275.4	Disorders of calcium metabolism
277.5	Mucopolysaccharidosis
710.1	Systemic sclerosis
711.92	Infect arthritis NOS, upper arm
714.0	Rheumatoid arthritis
714.30	Juvenile rheumatoid arthritis NOS
714.31	Juvenile acute rheumatoid arthritis
714.32	Pauciarticular juv rheum arthritis
714.33	Monoarticular juv rheum arthritis
714.4	Chronic postrheumatic arthritis
715.12	Loc prim osteoarthritis, upper arm
715.22	Loc 2nd osteoarthritis, upper arm
715.32	Loc osteoarthritis NOS, upper arm
716.12	Traumatic arthropathy, upper arm
718.12	Loose body in joint, upper arm
719.02	Joint effusion, upper arm
719.22	Villonodular synovitis, upper arm
727.00	Synovitis NOS
727.01	Synovitis in other diseases
729.6	Old foreign body in soft tissue
732.3	Juvenile osteochondrosis, arm

REIMBURSEMENT INFORMATION

General

- See notes on page 286.
- Description changed in 1995 CPT.

Medicare

- Follow–up Days — 90
- Assistant Surgeon — paid
- Supply Charges — not allowed
- Outpatient Limit — does not apply
- Major Surgery Rules Apply

CPT CODE	SERVICE	ICD-9-CM	
24105	Excision, olecranon bursa	726.33	Olecranon bursitis
		727.2	Occupational bursitis
		727.3	Bursitis NOS

REIMBURSEMENT INFORMATION

General

- See notes on page 286.

Medicare

- Follow–up Days — 90
- Assistant Surgeon — not paid
- Supply Charges — not allowed
- Outpatient Limit — does not apply
- Major Surgery Rules Apply

CPT CODE	SERVICE	ICD-9-CM	
24120	Excision or curettage of bone cyst or benign tumor of head or neck of radius or olecranon process	213.4	B-Neoplasm, Long bones, arm
24125	Excision or curettage of bone cyst or benign tumor of head or neck of radius or olecranon process; with autograft (includes obtaining graft)	733.20	Cyst of bone NOS
24126	Excision or curettage of bone cyst or benign tumor of head or neck of radius or olecranon process; with allograft	733.21	Solitary bone cyst
		733.22	Aneurysmal bone cyst
		733.29	Bone cyst NEC
		733.49	Aseptic necrosis of bone NEC

REIMBURSEMENT INFORMATION

General

- See notes on page 286.

Medicare

- Follow–up Days — 90
- Assistant Surgeon — not paid
- Supply Charges — not allowed
- Outpatient Limit — does not apply
- Major Surgery Rules Apply

CPT CODE	SERVICE
24130	Excision, radial head

CPT NOTES

- For replacement with implant, see 24366.

ICD–9–CM

213.4	B-Neoplasm, Long bones, arm
714.0	Rheumatoid arthritis
714.30	Juvenile rheumatoid arthritis NOS
714.31	Juvenile acute rheumatoid arthritis
714.32	Pauciarticular juv rheum arthritis
714.33	Monoarticular juv rheum arthritis
714.4	Chronic postrheumatic arthritis
715.92	Osteoarthrosis NOS, upper arm
716.12	Traumatic arthropathy, upper arm
730.12	Chronic osteomyelitis, upper arm
730.22	Osteomyelitis NOS, upper arm
730.32	Periostitis, upper arm
733.81	Malunion of fracture
733.82	Nonunion of fracture
813.05	Fx radius head, closed
813.15	Fx radius head, open
832.0x	Elbow dislocation, closed
832.1x	Elbow dislocation, open
905.2	Late effect, arm fracture
906.4	Late effect of crushing

REIMBURSEMENT INFORMATION

General

- See notes on page 286.

Medicare

- Follow–up Days — 90
- Assistant Surgeon — paid
- Supply Charges — not allowed
- Outpatient Limit — does not apply
- Major Surgery Rules Apply

CPT CODE	SERVICE	ICD–9–CM	
24134	Sequestrectomy (eg, for osteomyelitis or bone abscess), shaft or distal humerus	730.02	Acute osteomyelitis, upper arm
		730.12	Chronic osteomyelitis, upper arm
		730.22	Osteomyelitis NOS, upper arm
		730.32	Periostitis, upper arm
		731.0	Osteitis deformans NOS
		733.20	Cyst of bone NOS
		733.21	Solitary bone cyst
		733.22	Aneurysmal bone cyst
		733.29	Bone cyst NEC
		733.49	Aseptic necrosis of bone NEC

REIMBURSEMENT INFORMATION

General

- ◆ See notes on page 286.

Medicare

- ◆ Follow–up Days — 90
- ◆ Assistant Surgeon — paid
- ◆ Supply Charges — not allowed
- ◆ Outpatient Limit — does not apply
- ◆ Major Surgery Rules Apply

CPT CODE	SERVICE	ICD–9–CM	
24136	Sequestrectomy (eg, for osteomyelitis or bone abscess), radial head or neck	730.03	Acute osteomyelitis, forearm
		730.13	Chronic osteomyelitis, forearm
		730.23	Osteomyelitis NOS, forearm
		730.33	Periostitis, forearm
		731.0	Osteitis deformans NOS
		733.49	Aseptic necrosis of bone NEC

REIMBURSEMENT INFORMATION

General

- ◆ See notes on page 286.

Medicare

- ◆ Follow–up Days — 90
- ◆ Assistant Surgeon — paid
- ◆ Supply Charges — not allowed
- ◆ Outpatient Limit — does not apply
- ◆ Major Surgery Rules Apply

CPT CODE	SERVICE	ICD-9-CM
24138	Sequestrectomy (eg, for osteomyelitis or bone abscess), olecranon process	730.13 Chronic osteomyelitis, forearm 730.23 Osteomyelitis NOS, forearm 730.33 Periostitis, forearm 731.0 Osteitis deformans NOS 733.49 Aseptic necrosis of bone NEC

REIMBURSEMENT INFORMATION

General

- See notes on page 286.

Medicare

- Follow-up Days — 90
- Assistant Surgeon — paid
- Supply Charges — not allowed
- Outpatient Limit — does not apply
- Major Surgery Rules Apply

CPT CODE	SERVICE	ICD-9-CM
24140	Partial excision (craterization, saucerization or diaphysectomy) of bone (eg, for osteomyelitis), humerus	730.02 Acute osteomyelitis, upper arm 730.12 Chronic osteomyelitis, upper arm 730.22 Osteomyelitis NOS, upper arm 730.32 Periostitis, upper arm 733.21 Solitary bone cyst

REIMBURSEMENT INFORMATION

General

- See notes on page 286.

Medicare

- Follow-up Days — 90
- Assistant Surgeon — paid
- Supply Charges — not allowed
- Outpatient Limit — does not apply
- Major Surgery Rules Apply

CPT CODE	SERVICE	ICD–9–CM
24145	Partial excision (craterization, saucerization or diaphysectomy), of bone (eg, for osteomyelitis), radial head or neck	730.03 Acute osteomyelitis, forearm 730.13 Chronic osteomyelitis, forearm 730.23 Osteomyelitis NOS, forearm 730.33 Periostitis, forearm 733.21 Solitary bone cyst 754.89 Nonteratogenic anomaly NEC

REIMBURSEMENT INFORMATION

General

- See notes on page 286.

Medicare

- Follow–up Days — 90
- Assistant Surgeon — paid
- Supply Charges — not allowed
- Outpatient Limit — does not apply
- Major Surgery Rules Apply

CPT CODE	SERVICE	ICD–9–CM
24147	Partial excision (craterization, saucerization or diaphysectomy), of bone (eg, for osteomyelitis), olecranon process	730.03 Acute osteomyelitis, forearm 730.13 Chronic osteomyelitis, forearm 730.23 Osteomyelitis NOS, forearm 730.33 Periostitis, forearm 731.0 Osteitis deformans NOS 733.21 Solitary bone cyst 733.22 Aneurysmal bone cyst 733.29 Bone cyst NEC 733.49 Aseptic necrosis of bone NEC

REIMBURSEMENT INFORMATION

General

- See notes on page 286.

Medicare

- Follow–up Days — 90
- Assistant Surgeon — paid
- Supply Charges — not allowed
- Outpatient Limit — does not apply
- Major Surgery Rules Apply

CPT CODE	SERVICE	ICD-9-CM
24150	Radical resection for tumor, shaft or distal humerus	170.4 M-Neoplasm, Long arm bones 198.5 M2-Neoplasm, Bone and bone marrow 238.0 UB-Neoplasm, Bone 239.2 Bone/Skin neoplasm NOS
24151	Radical resection for tumor, shaft or distal humerus; with autograft (includes obtaining graft)	

REIMBURSEMENT INFORMATION

General

- ♦ See notes on page 286.

Medicare

- ♦ Follow–up Days — 90
- ♦ Assistant Surgeon — paid
- ♦ Supply Charges — not allowed
- ♦ Outpatient Limit — does not apply
- ♦ Major Surgery Rules Apply

CPT CODE	SERVICE	ICD-9-CM
24152	Radical resection for tumor, radial head or neck	170.4 M-Neoplasm, Long arm bones 195.4 M-Neoplasm, Upper limb 198.5 M2-Neoplasm, Bone and bone marrow 199.0 M-Neoplasm, Disseminated 238.0 UB-Neoplasm, Bone 239.2 Bone/Skin neoplasm NOS
24153	Radical resection for tumor, radial head or neck; with autograft (includes obtaining graft)	

REIMBURSEMENT INFORMATION

General

- ♦ See notes on page 286.

Medicare

- ♦ Follow–up Days — 90
- ♦ Assistant Surgeon — paid
- ♦ Supply Charges — not allowed
- ♦ Outpatient Limit — does not apply
- ♦ Major Surgery Rules Apply

CPT CODE	SERVICE	ICD-9-CM	
24155	Resection of elbow joint (arthrectomy)	170.4	M-Neoplasm, Long arm bones
		198.5	M2-Neoplasm, Bone and bone marrow
		238.0	UB-Neoplasm, Bone
		239.2	Bone/Skin neoplasm NOS
		711.02	Pyogenic arthritis, upper arm
		711.92	Infect arthritis NOS, upper arm
		714.0	Rheumatoid arthritis
		714.30	Juvenile rheumatoid arthritis NOS
		714.31	Juvenile acute rheumatoid arthritis
		714.32	Pauciarticular juv rheum arthritis
		714.33	Monoarticular juv rheum arthritis
		714.4	Chronic postrheumatic arthritis
		715.12	Loc prim osteoarthritis, upper arm
		715.22	Loc 2nd osteoarthritis, upper arm
		715.32	Loc osteoarthritis NOS, upper arm
		716.12	Traumatic arthropathy, upper arm
		718.52	Ankylosis of joint, upper arm
		719.22	Villonodular synovitis, upper arm
		730.12	Chronic osteomyelitis, upper arm
		731.0	Osteitis deformans NOS
		732.3	Juvenile osteochondrosis, arm
		733.49	Aseptic necrosis of bone NEC
		905.2	Late effect, arm fracture
		906.4	Late effect of crushing
		996.66	Reaction, internal joint prosthesis
		996.77	Complication, int joint prosthesis

REIMBURSEMENT INFORMATION

General

- See notes on page 286.

Medicare

- Follow-up Days — 90
- Assistant Surgeon — paid
- Supply Charges — not allowed
- Outpatient Limit — does not apply
- Major Surgery Rules Apply

CPT CODE	SERVICE	ICD–9–CM

24200 Removal of foreign body, upper arm or elbow area; subcutaneous

CPT NOTES

- For K-wire or pin insertion or removal, see 20650, 20670, 20680.
- For arthrocentesis or needling of bursa or joint, see 20605.

709.4	Foreign body granuloma, skin
729.6	Old foreign body in soft tissue
912.6	Foreign body, shoulder/arm
912.7	Foreign body, should/arm, infected
913.6	Foreign body, forearm
913.7	Foreign body, forearm, infected
998.4	Foreign body left during procedure

REIMBURSEMENT INFORMATION

General

- See notes on page 286.

Medicare

- Follow–up Days — 10
- Assistant Surgeon — not paid
- Supply Charges — not allowed
- Outpatient Limit — applies
- Minor Surgery Rules Apply

24201 Removal of foreign body, upper arm or elbow area; deep

CPT NOTES

- For K-wire or pin insertion or removal, see 20650, 20670, 20680.
- For arthrocentesis or needling of bursa or joint, see 20605.

728.82	Foreign body granuloma of muscle
729.6	Old foreign body in soft tissue
733.99	Bone/Cartilage disorder NEC
880.13	Open wound of upper arm, complic
881.11	Open wound of elbow, complicated
996.66	Reaction, internal joint prosthesis
996.77	Complication, int joint prosthesis
998.4	Foreign body left during procedure
998.7	Postop foreign subst acute reaction

REIMBURSEMENT INFORMATION

General

- See notes on page 286.

Medicare

- Follow–up Days — 90
- Assistant Surgeon — not paid
- Supply Charges — not allowed
- Outpatient Limit — does not apply
- Major Surgery Rules Apply

CPT CODE	SERVICE	ICD–9–CM	
24301	Muscle or tendon transfer, any type, upper arm or elbow, single	045.0x	Acute paralytic poliomyelitis
		045.1x	Acute paralytic poliomyelitis
		045.9x	Acute poliomyelitis NOS
		343.x	Infantile cerebral palsy
		344.0	Quadriplegia NOS
		436.	Acute CVA, ill-defined
		728.83	Nontraumatic muscle rupture
		840.x	Upper arm/shoulder sprain/strain
		841.x	Elbow/forearm sprain and strain
		880.23	Open wound upper arm w/tendon
		881.21	Open wound of elbow w/tendon
		905.8	Late effect of tendon injury
		907.4	Late effect, nerve injury shld/arm
		953.0	Cervical root injury
		955.x	Injury to peripheral nerve(s)
		959.2	Shoulder/upper arm injury NOS
		959.3	Elbow/forearm/wrist injury NOS

REIMBURSEMENT INFORMATION

General

- See notes on page 286.

Medicare

- Follow–up Days — 90
- Assistant Surgeon — paid
- Supply Charges — not allowed
- Outpatient Limit — does not apply
- Major Surgery Rules Apply

CPT CODE	SERVICE
24305	Tendon lengthening, upper arm or elbow, single, each

ICD–9–CM

045.0x	Acute paralytic poliomyelitis
045.1x	Acute paralytic poliomyelitis
045.9x	Acute poliomyelitis NOS
343.x	Infantile cerebral palsy
436.	Acute CVA, ill-defined
728.81	Interstitial myositis
728.85	Spasm of muscle
840.x	Upper arm/shoulder sprain/strain
841.x	Elbow/forearm sprain and strain
880.23	Open wound upper arm w/tendon
881.21	Open wound of elbow w/tendon
953.0	Cervical root injury
955.x	Injury to peripheral nerve(s)
959.2	Shoulder/upper arm injury NOS
959.3	Elbow/forearm/wrist injury NOS

REIMBURSEMENT INFORMATION

General

- See notes on page 286.

Medicare

- Follow–up Days — 90
- Assistant Surgeon — paid
- Supply Charges — not allowed
- Outpatient Limit — does not apply
- Major Surgery Rules Apply

CPT CODE	SERVICE
24310	Tenotomy, open elbow to shoulder, single, each

ICD–9–CM

045.0x	Acute paralytic poliomyelitis
045.1x	Acute paralytic poliomyelitis
045.9x	Acute poliomyelitis NOS
343.x	Infantile cerebral palsy
436.	Acute CVA, ill-defined
728.85	Spasm of muscle
840.x	Upper arm/shoulder sprain/strain
841.x	Elbow/forearm sprain and strain
880.23	Open wound upper arm w/tendon
881.21	Open wound of elbow w/tendon
953.0	Cervical root injury
955.x	Injury to peripheral nerve(s)
959.2	Shoulder/upper arm injury NOS
959.3	Elbow/forearm/wrist injury NOS

REIMBURSEMENT INFORMATION

General

- See notes on page 286.

Medicare

- Follow–up Days — 90
- Assistant Surgeon — paid
- Supply Charges — not allowed
- Outpatient Limit — does not apply
- Major Surgery Rules Apply

CPT CODE	SERVICE	ICD-9-CM
24320	Tenoplasty, with muscle transfer, with or without free graft, elbow to shoulder, single (Seddon-Brookes type procedure)	045.0x Acute paralytic poliomyelitis 045.1x Acute paralytic poliomyelitis 045.9x Acute poliomyelitis NOS 343.x Infantile cerebral palsy 436. Acute CVA, ill-defined 840.x Upper arm/shoulder sprain/strain 841.x Elbow/forearm sprain and strain 880.23 Open wound upper arm w/tendon 881.21 Open wound of elbow w/tendon 953.0 Cervical root injury 955.x Injury to peripheral nerve(s) 959.2 Shoulder/upper arm injury NOS 959.3 Elbow/forearm/wrist injury NOS **REIMBURSEMENT INFORMATION** General ♦ See notes on page 286. Medicare ♦ Follow-up Days — 90 ♦ Assistant Surgeon — paid ♦ Supply Charges — not allowed ♦ Outpatient Limit — does not apply ♦ Major Surgery Rules Apply
24330 **24331**	Flexor-plasty, elbow, (eg, Steindler type advancement) Flexor-plasty, elbow, (eg, Steindler type advancement); with extensor advancement	045.0x Acute paralytic poliomyelitis 045.1x Acute paralytic poliomyelitis 045.9x Acute poliomyelitis NOS 343.x Infantile cerebral palsy 436. Acute CVA, ill-defined 841.x Elbow/forearm sprain and strain 881.21 Open wound of elbow w/tendon 907.4 Late effect, nerve injury shld/arm 953.0 Cervical root injury 955.x Injury to peripheral nerve(s) 959.3 Elbow/forearm/wrist injury NOS **REIMBURSEMENT INFORMATION** General ♦ See notes on page 286. Medicare ♦ Follow-up Days — 90 ♦ Assistant Surgeon — paid ♦ Supply Charges — not allowed ♦ Outpatient Limit — does not apply ♦ Major Surgery Rules Apply

CPT CODE	SERVICE	ICD–9–CM
▲ **24340**	Tenodesis of biceps tendon at elbow (separate procedure)	138. Late effects of acute polio 727.62 Biceps tendon rupture 881.01 Open wound of elbow 881.11 Open wound of elbow, complicated 881.21 Open wound of elbow w/tendon

REIMBURSEMENT INFORMATION

General

- ♦ See notes on page 286.
- ♦ Description changed in 1995 CPT.
- ♦ Separate procedure rules apply.

Medicare

- ♦ Follow–up Days — 90
- ♦ Assistant Surgeon — paid
- ♦ Supply Charges — not allowed
- ♦ Outpatient Limit — does not apply
- ♦ Major Surgery Rules Apply

CPT CODE	SERVICE	ICD–9–CM
24342	Reinsertion or repair of ruptured or lacerated biceps or triceps tendon, distal, with or without tendon graft	727.62 Biceps tendon rupture 881.01 Open wound of elbow 881.11 Open wound of elbow, complicated 881.21 Open wound of elbow w/tendon

REIMBURSEMENT INFORMATION

General

- ♦ See notes on page 286.

Medicare

- ♦ Follow–up Days — 90
- ♦ Assistant Surgeon — paid
- ♦ Supply Charges — not allowed
- ♦ Outpatient Limit — does not apply
- ♦ Major Surgery Rules Apply

CPT CODE	SERVICE
24350	Fasciotomy, lateral or medial (eg, "tennis elbow" or epicondylitis)
24351	Fasciotomy, lateral or medial (eg, "tennis elbow" or epicondylitis); with extensor origin detachment
24352	Fasciotomy, lateral or medial (eg, "tennis elbow" or epicondylitis); with annular ligament resection
24354	Fasciotomy, lateral or medial (eg, "tennis elbow" or epicondylitis); with stripping
24356	Fasciotomy, lateral or medial (eg, "tennis elbow" or epicondylitis); with partial ostectomy

ICD-9-CM

718.42	Contracture of joint, upper arm
726.31	Medial epicondylitis
726.32	Lateral epicondylitis
958.8	Early complications of trauma NEC

REIMBURSEMENT INFORMATION

General

- See notes on page 286.

Medicare

- Follow-up Days — 90
- Assistant Surgeon — paid
- Supply Charges — not allowed
- Outpatient Limit — does not apply
- Major Surgery Rules Apply

CPT CODE	SERVICE
24360	Arthroplasty, elbow; with membrane
24361	Arthroplasty, elbow; with distal humeral prosthetic replacement
24362	Arthroplasty, elbow; with implant and fascia lata ligament reconstruction
24363	Arthroplasty, elbow; with distal humerus and proximal ulnar prosthetic replacement ("total elbow")

ICD–9–CM

213.4	B-Neoplasm, Long bones, arm
711.02	Pyogenic arthritis, upper arm
711.92	Infect arthritis NOS, upper arm
714.0	Rheumatoid arthritis
714.30	Juvenile rheumatoid arthritis NOS
714.31	Juvenile acute rheumatoid arthritis
714.32	Pauciarticular juv rheum arthritis
714.33	Monoarticular juv rheum arthritis
714.4	Chronic postrheumatic arthritis
715.12	Loc prim osteoarthritis, upper arm
715.22	Loc 2nd osteoarthritis, upper arm
715.32	Loc osteoarthritis NOS, upper arm
716.12	Traumatic arthropathy, upper arm
718.02	Articular cartilage dis, upper arm
718.03	Articular cartilage dis, forearm
718.52	Ankylosis of joint, upper arm
718.53	Ankylosis of joint, forearm
719.22	Villonodular synovitis, upper arm
731.0	Osteitis deformans NOS
732.3	Juvenile osteochondrosis, arm
733.49	Aseptic necrosis of bone NEC

REIMBURSEMENT INFORMATION

General

- See notes on page 286.

Medicare

- Follow–up Days — 90
- Assistant Surgeon
  24360–24361, 24363 — paid
  24362 — not paid
- Supply Charges — not allowed
- Outpatient Limit — does not apply
- Major Surgery Rules Apply

CPT CODE	SERVICE	ICD-9-CM	
24495	Decompression fasciotomy, forearm, with brachial artery exploration	442.0	Upper extremity artery aneurysm
		443.1	Thromboangiitis obliterans
		444.21	Upper extremity embolism
		446.5	Giant cell arteritis
		447.0	Acquired arteriovenous fistula
		447.1	Stricture of artery
		453.1	Thrombophlebitis migrans
		812.41	Supracondylar Fx humerus, closed
		812.42	Fx humerus, lateral condyle, closed
		812.43	Fx humerus, medial condyle, closed
		812.44	Fx humerus, condyle NOS, closed
		812.49	Fx lower humerus NEC, closed
		812.51	Supracondylar Fx humerus, open
		812.52	Fx humerus, lateral condyle, open
		812.53	Fx humerus, medial condyle, open
		812.54	Fx humerus, condyle NOS, open
		812.59	Fx lower humerus NEC, open
		813.0x	Fracture of radius/ulna, upper end
		813.1x	Fracture of radius/ulna, lower end
		813.2x	Fracture of radius and ulna shaft
		813.3x	Fracture of radius and ulna shaft
		813.4x	Fracture of radius/ulna, lower end
		813.5x	Fracture of radius/ulna, lower end
		832.0x	Elbow dislocation, closed
		832.1x	Elbow dislocation, open
		881.00	Open wound of forearm
		881.01	Open wound of elbow
		881.10	Open wound of forearm, complicated
		881.11	Open wound of elbow, complicated
		881.20	Open wound of forearm w/tendon
		881.21	Open wound of elbow w/tendon
		908.3	Late effect, inj peripheral vessel
		923.1x	Contusion, elbow and forearm
		927.1x	Crushing injury, elbow and forearm
		958.8	Early complications of trauma NEC
		996.91	Complication, reattached forearm
		996.94	Complication, reattached arm NEC

REIMBURSEMENT INFORMATION

General

- See notes on page 286.

Medicare

- Follow–up Days — 90
- Assistant Surgeon — not paid
- Supply Charges — not allowed
- Outpatient Limit — does not apply
- Major Surgery Rules Apply

CPT CODE	SERVICE	ICD-9-CM
24500	Closed treatment of humeral shaft fracture; without manipulation	812.21 Fx humerus shaft, closed 812.31 Fx humerus shaft, open
24505	Closed treatment of humeral shaft fracture; with manipulation, with or without skeletal traction	**REIMBURSEMENT INFORMATION** General ◆ See notes on page 286. Medicare ◆ Follow-up Days — 90 ◆ Assistant Surgeon — not paid ◆ Supply Charges — not allowed ◆ Outpatient Limit — does not apply ◆ Major Surgery Rules Apply
24515	Open treatment of humeral shaft fracture with plate/screws, with or without cerclage	812.21 Fx humerus shaft, closed 812.31 Fx humerus shaft, open **REIMBURSEMENT INFORMATION** General ◆ See notes on page 286. Medicare ◆ Follow-up Days — 90 ◆ Assistant Surgeon — paid ◆ Supply Charges — not allowed ◆ Outpatient Limit — does not apply
24516	Open treatment of humeral shaft fracture, with insertion of intramedullary implant, with or without cerclage and/or locking screws	812.21 Fx humerus shaft, closed 812.31 Fx humerus shaft, open **REIMBURSEMENT INFORMATION** General ◆ See notes on page 286. Medicare ◆ Follow-up Days — 90 ◆ Assistant Surgeon — paid ◆ Supply Charges — not allowed ◆ Outpatient Limit — does not apply ◆ Major Surgery Rules Apply

CPT CODE	SERVICE	ICD–9–CM
24530	Closed treatment of supracondylar or transcondylar humeral fracture, with or without intercondylar extension; without manipulation	812.40 Fx lower humerus NOS, closed 812.41 Supracondylar Fx humerus, closed 812.50 Fx lower humerus NOS, open 812.51 Supracondylar Fx humerus, open 813.08 Fx upper end radius w/ulna, closed
24535	Closed treatment of supracondylar or transcondylar humeral fracture, with or without intercondylar extension; with manipulation, with or without skin or skeletal traction	

REIMBURSEMENT INFORMATION

General

- ♦ See notes on page 286.

Medicare

- ♦ Follow–up Days — 90
- ♦ Assistant Surgeon — not paid
- ♦ Supply Charges — not allowed
- ♦ Outpatient Limit — does not apply
- ♦ Major Surgery Rules Apply

CPT CODE	SERVICE	ICD–9–CM
24538	Percutaneous skeletal fixation of supracondylar or transcondylar humeral fracture, with or without intercondylar extension	812.40 Fx lower humerus NOS, closed 812.41 Supracondylar Fx humerus, closed 812.50 Fx lower humerus NOS, open 812.51 Supracondylar Fx humerus, open 813.08 Fx upper end radius w/ulna, closed 813.18 Fx upper end radius w/ulna, open

REIMBURSEMENT INFORMATION

General

- ♦ See notes on page 286.

Medicare

- ♦ Follow–up Days — 90
- ♦ Assistant Surgeon — paid
- ♦ Supply Charges — not allowed
- ♦ Outpatient Limit — does not apply
- ♦ Major Surgery Rules Apply

CPT CODE	SERVICE	ICD–9–CM
24545	Open treatment of humeral supracondylar or transcondylar fracture, with or without internal or external fixation; without intercondylar extension	812.40 Fx lower humerus NOS, closed 812.41 Supracondylar Fx humerus, closed 812.50 Fx lower humerus NOS, open 812.51 Supracondylar Fx humerus, open 813.08 Fx upper end radius w/ulna, closed 813.18 Fx upper end radius w/ulna, open

REIMBURSEMENT INFORMATION

General

- ♦ See notes on page 286.

Medicare

- ♦ Follow–up Days — 90
- ♦ Assistant Surgeon — paid
- ♦ Supply Charges — not allowed
- ♦ Outpatient Limit — does not apply
- ♦ Major Surgery Rules Apply

CPT CODE	SERVICE	ICD–9–CM
24546	Open treatment of humeral supracondylar or transcondylar fracture, with or without internal or external fixation; with intercondylar extension	812.40 Fx lower humerus NOS, closed 812.41 Supracondylar Fx humerus, closed 812.50 Fx lower humerus NOS, open 812.51 Supracondylar Fx humerus, open

REIMBURSEMENT INFORMATION

General

- ♦ See notes on page 286.

Medicare

- ♦ Follow–up Days — 90
- ♦ Assistant Surgeon — paid
- ♦ Supply Charges — not allowed
- ♦ Outpatient Limit — does not apply
- ♦ Major Surgery Rules Apply

CPT CODE	SERVICE	ICD-9-CM
24560	Closed treatment of humeral epicondylar fracture, medial or lateral; without manipulation	812.42 Fx humerus, lateral condyle, closed 812.43 Fx humerus, medial condyle, closed 812.52 Fx humerus, lateral condyle, open 812.53 Fx humerus, medial condyle, open 813.08 Fx upper end radius w/ulna, closed 813.18 Fx upper end radius w/ulna, open

REIMBURSEMENT INFORMATION

General

- ♦ See notes on page 286.

Medicare

- ♦ Follow-up Days — 90
- ♦ Assistant Surgeon — not paid
- ♦ Supply Charges — not allowed
- ♦ Outpatient Limit — does not apply
- ♦ Major Surgery Rules Apply

CPT CODE	SERVICE	ICD-9-CM
24586	Open treatment of periarticular fracture and/or dislocation of the elbow (fracture distal humerus and proximal ulna and/or proximal radius)	812.40 Fx lower humerus NOS, closed 812.50 Fx lower humerus NOS, open 813.08 Fx upper end radius w/ulna, closed 813.18 Fx upper end radius w/ulna, open 832.00 Dislocation elbow NOS, closed 832.01 Anterior disloc elbow, closed 832.02 Posterior disloc elbow, closed 832.03 Medial disloc elbow, closed 832.04 Lateral disloc elbow, closed 832.09 Dislocation elbow NEC, closed

CPT NOTES

- ♦ See also 24361.

REIMBURSEMENT INFORMATION

General

- ♦ See notes on page 286.

Medicare

- ♦ Follow-up Days — 90
- ♦ Assistant Surgeon — paid
- ♦ Supply Charges — not allowed
- ♦ Outpatient Limit — does not apply
- ♦ Major Surgery Rules Apply

CPT CODE	SERVICE	ICD-9-CM	
24587	Open treatment of periarticular fracture and/or dislocation of the elbow (fracture distal humerus and proximal ulna and/or proximal radius); with implant arthroplasty	812.40	Fx lower humerus NOS, closed
		812.50	Fx lower humerus NOS, open
		813.08	Fx upper end radius w/ulna, closed
		813.18	Fx upper end radius w/ulna, open

CPT NOTES

- See also 24361.

REIMBURSEMENT INFORMATION

General

- See notes on page 286.

Medicare

- Follow-up Days — 90
- Assistant Surgeon — paid
- Supply Charges — not allowed
- Outpatient Limit — does not apply
- Major Surgery Rules Apply

CPT CODE	SERVICE	ICD-9-CM	
24900	Amputation, arm through humerus; with primary closure	170.4	M-Neoplasm, Long arm bones
		198.5	M2-Neoplasm, Bone and bone marrow
		444.21	Upper extremity embolism
		682.3	Cellulitis of arm
		730.12	Chronic osteomyelitis, upper arm
		733.41	Aseptic necrosis, head of humerus
		785.4	Gangrene
		887.2	Amputation above elbow, unilateral
		887.3	Amputation above elbow, unil, compl
		906.4	Late effect of crushing
		906.6	Late effect of wrist/hand burn
		908.3	Late effect, inj peripheral vessel
		927.0x	Crushing injury, shoulder/upper arm
		927.11	Crushing injury, elbow
		958.8	Early complications of trauma NEC
		996.94	Complication, reattached arm NEC
		997.60	Late amputation stump complic NOS

REIMBURSEMENT INFORMATION

General

- See notes on page 286.

Medicare

- Follow-up Days — 90
- Assistant Surgeon — not paid
- Supply Charges — not allowed
- Outpatient Limit — does not apply
- Major Surgery Rules Apply

CPT CODE	SERVICE	ICD–9–CM	
24920	Amputation, arm through humerus; open, circular (guillotine)	170.4	M-Neoplasm, Long arm bones
		198.5	M2-Neoplasm, Bone and bone marrow
		444.21	Upper extremity embolism
		682.3	Cellulitis of arm
		730.12	Chronic osteomyelitis, upper arm
		733.41	Aseptic necrosis, head of humerus
		785.4	Gangrene
		887.2	Amputation above elbow, unilateral
		887.3	Amputation above elbow, unil, compl
		906.4	Late effect of crushing
		906.6	Late effect of wrist/hand burn
		908.3	Late effect, inj peripheral vessel
		927.0x	Crushing injury, shoulder/upper arm
		927.11	Crushing injury, elbow
		958.8	Early complications of trauma NEC
		996.94	Complication, reattached arm NEC
		997.60	Late amputation stump complic NOS
		997.62	Infection of amputated stump

REIMBURSEMENT INFORMATION

General

- See notes on page 286.

Medicare

- Follow–up Days — 90
- Assistant Surgeon — paid
- Supply Charges — not allowed
- Outpatient Limit — does not apply
- Major Surgery Rules Apply

CPT CODE	SERVICE
24925	Amputation, arm through humerus; secondary closure or scar revision
24930	Amputation, arm through humerus; reamputation

ICD–9–CM

170.4	M-Neoplasm, Long arm bones
198.5	M2-Neoplasm, Bone and bone marrow
444.21	Upper extremity embolism
682.3	Cellulitis of arm
730.12	Chronic osteomyelitis, upper arm
733.41	Aseptic necrosis, head of humerus
785.4	Gangrene
887.2	Amputation above elbow, unilateral
887.3	Amputation above elbow, unil, compl
906.4	Late effect of crushing
906.6	Late effect of wrist/hand burn
908.3	Late effect, inj peripheral vessel
927.0x	Crushing injury, shoulder/upper arm
927.11	Crushing injury, elbow
958.8	Early complications of trauma NEC
996.94	Complication, reattached arm NEC
997.60	Late amputation stump complic NOS
997.61	Neuroma of amputation stump
997.62	Infection of amputated stump
997.69	Late amputation stump complic NEC
V49.66	Above elbow amputation status

REIMBURSEMENT INFORMATION

General

- See notes on page 286.

Medicare

- Follow–up Days — 90
- Assistant Surgeon — paid
- Supply Charges — not allowed
- Outpatient Limit — does not apply
- Major Surgery Rules Apply

CPT CODE	SERVICE
24931	Amputation, arm through humerus; with implant

ICD–9–CM

170.4	M-Neoplasm, Long arm bones
198.5	M2-Neoplasm, Bone and bone marrow
444.21	Upper extremity embolism
682.3	Cellulitis of arm
730.12	Chronic osteomyelitis, upper arm
733.41	Aseptic necrosis, head of humerus
785.4	Gangrene
887.2	Amputation above elbow, unilateral
887.3	Amputation above elbow, unil, compl
906.4	Late effect of crushing
906.6	Late effect of wrist/hand burn
908.3	Late effect, inj peripheral vessel
927.0x	Crushing injury, shoulder/upper arm
927.11	Crushing injury, elbow
958.8	Early complications of trauma NEC
996.94	Complication, reattached arm NEC
997.60	Late amputation stump complic NOS
997.62	Infection of amputated stump
V53.0	Fit/adjust nervous system device

REIMBURSEMENT INFORMATION

General

- See notes on page 286.

Medicare

- Follow–up Days — 90
- Assistant Surgeon — paid
- Supply Charges — not allowed
- Outpatient Limit — does not apply
- Major Surgery Rules Apply

CPT CODE	SERVICE	ICD–9–CM
24935	Stump elongation, upper extremity	170.4 M-Neoplasm, Long arm bones 198.5 M2-Neoplasm, Bone and bone marrow 730.12 Chronic osteomyelitis, upper arm 733.41 Aseptic necrosis, head of humerus 785.4 Gangrene 887.2 Amputation above elbow, unilateral 887.3 Amputation above elbow, unil, compl 927.0x Crushing injury, shoulder/upper arm 927.11 Crushing injury, elbow V49.66 Above elbow amputation status

REIMBURSEMENT INFORMATION

General

- ◆ See notes on page 286.

Medicare

- ◆ Follow–up Days — 90
- ◆ Assistant Surgeon — by report
- ◆ Supply Charges — not allowed
- ◆ Outpatient Limit — does not apply
- ◆ Major Surgery Rules Apply

CPT CODE	SERVICE	ICD–9–CM
24940	Cineplasty, upper extremity, complete procedure	170.4 M-Neoplasm, Long arm bones 198.5 M2-Neoplasm, Bone and bone marrow 730.12 Chronic osteomyelitis, upper arm 733.41 Aseptic necrosis, head of humerus 785.4 Gangrene 887.2 Amputation above elbow, unilateral 887.3 Amputation above elbow, unil, compl 927.0x Crushing injury, shoulder/upper arm 927.11 Crushing injury, elbow

REIMBURSEMENT INFORMATION

General

- ◆ See notes on page 286.

Medicare

- ◆ Follow–up Days — 90
- ◆ Assistant Surgeon — paid
- ◆ Supply Charges — not allowed
- ◆ Outpatient Limit — does not apply
- ◆ Major Surgery Rules Apply

CPT CODE	SERVICE	ICD–9–CM

▲ **25000** Tendon sheath incision; at radial styloid (eg, for deQuervain's disease)

CPT NOTES

- For decompression median nerve or for carpal tunnel syndrome, see 64721.

ICD–9–CM

727.04	Radial styloid tenosynovitis
727.05	Tenosynovitis of hand/wrist NEC

REIMBURSEMENT INFORMATION

General

- See notes on page 286.
- Description changed in 1995 CPT.

Medicare

- Follow–up Days — 90
- Assistant Surgeon — not paid
- Supply Charges — not allowed
- Outpatient Limit — does not apply
- Major Surgery Rules Apply

25020 Decompression fasciotomy, forearm and/or wrist; flexor or extensor compartment

CPT NOTES

- For decompression fasciotomy with brachial artery exploration, see 24495.
- For incision and drainage procedures, superficial, see 10040-10160.
- For debridement, see also 11000-11044.

ICD–9–CM

813.4x	Fracture of radius/ulna, lower end
833.0x	Wrist dislocation, closed
833.1x	Wrist dislocation, open
881.00	Open wound of forearm
881.01	Open wound of elbow
881.10	Open wound of forearm, complicated
881.11	Open wound of elbow, complicated
881.20	Open wound of forearm w/tendon
881.21	Open wound of elbow w/tendon
905.2	Late effect, arm fracture
906.6	Late effect of wrist/hand burn
923.1x	Contusion, elbow and forearm
927.10	Crushing injury, forearm
927.21	Crushing injury, wrist
958.8	Early complications of trauma NEC
989.5	Toxic effect of venom
996.94	Complication, reattached arm NEC
998.1	Hemorrhage complicating a procedure
998.5	Postoperative infection

REIMBURSEMENT INFORMATION

General

- See notes on page 286.

Medicare

- Follow–up Days — 90
- Assistant Surgeon — not paid
- Supply Charges — not allowed
- Outpatient Limit — does not apply
- Major Surgery Rules Apply

CPT CODE	SERVICE
25023	Decompression fasciotomy, forearm and/or wrist; with debridement of nonviable muscle and/or nerve

CPT NOTES

- For decompression fasciotomy with brachial artery exploration, see 24495.
- For incision and drainage procedures, superficial, see 10040-10160.
- For debridement, see also 11000-11044.

ICD–9–CM

813.4x	Fracture of radius/ulna, lower end
833.0x	Wrist dislocation, closed
833.1x	Wrist dislocation, open
881.00	Open wound of forearm
881.01	Open wound of elbow
881.10	Open wound of forearm, complicated
881.11	Open wound of elbow, complicated
881.20	Open wound of forearm w/tendon
881.21	Open wound of elbow w/tendon
905.2	Late effect, arm fracture
906.6	Late effect of wrist/hand burn
923.1x	Contusion, elbow and forearm
927.10	Crushing injury, forearm
927.21	Crushing injury, wrist
958.6	Volkmann's ischemic contracture
958.8	Early complications of trauma NEC
989.5	Toxic effect of venom
996.94	Complication, reattached arm NEC
998.1	Hemorrhage complicating a procedure
998.5	Postoperative infection

REIMBURSEMENT INFORMATION

General

- See notes on page 286.

Medicare

- Follow–up Days — 90
- Assistant Surgeon — not paid
- Supply Charges — not allowed
- Outpatient Limit — does not apply
- Major Surgery Rules Apply

CPT CODE	SERVICE
25028	Incision and drainage, forearm and/or wrist; deep abscess or hematoma
25031	Incision and drainage, forearm and/or wrist; infected bursa

ICD–9–CM

682.3	Cellulitis of arm
682.4	Cellulitis of hand
711.03	Pyogenic arthritis, forearm
711.04	Pyogenic arthritis, hand
711.93	Infect arthritis NOS, forearm
711.94	Infect arthritis NOS, hand
726.4	Enthesopathy of wrist/carpus
727.2	Occupational bursitis
727.3	Bursitis NOS
727.4x	Ganglion/cyst synovium/tendon/bursa
727.89	Synovium/tendon/bursa disorder NEC
906.3	Late effect of contusion
906.4	Late effect of crushing
909.3	Late effect of surg/med complic
923.10	Contusion of forearm
923.21	Contusion of wrist
927.10	Crushing injury, forearm
927.21	Crushing injury, wrist
927.8	Multiple crushing injuries, arm
996.67	Reaction, internal ortho device NEC
997.62	Infection of amputated stump
998.5	Postoperative infection

REIMBURSEMENT INFORMATION

General

- See notes on page 286.

Medicare

- Follow–up Days — 90
- Assistant Surgeon
  25028 — not paid
  25031 — by report
- Supply Charges — not allowed
- Outpatient Limit — does not apply
- Major Surgery Rules Apply

CPT CODE	SERVICE	ICD–9–CM
25035	Incision, deep, with opening of bone cortex (eg, for osteomyelitis or bone abscess), forearm and/or wrist	730.03 Acute osteomyelitis, forearm 730.13 Chronic osteomyelitis, forearm 730.23 Osteomyelitis NOS, forearm 730.93 Bone infection NOS, forearm

REIMBURSEMENT INFORMATION

General

- ◆ See notes on page 286.

Medicare

- ◆ Follow–up Days — 90
- ◆ Assistant Surgeon — by report
- ◆ Supply Charges — not allowed
- ◆ Outpatient Limit — does not apply
- ◆ Major Surgery Rules Apply

CPT CODE	SERVICE	ICD–9–CM
▲ 25040	Arthrotomy, radiocarpal or midcarpal joint, with exploration, drainage, or removal of foreign body	711.03 Pyogenic arthritis, forearm 711.93 Infect arthritis NOS, forearm 714.0 Rheumatoid arthritis 715.13 Loc prim osteoarthritis, forearm 715.23 Loc 2nd osteoarthritis, forearm 715.33 Loc osteoarthritis NOS, forearm 716.13 Traumatic arthropathy, forearm 718.13 Loose body in joint, forearm 719.03 Joint effusion, forearm 719.23 Villonodular synovitis, forearm 727.02 Giant cell tumor of tendon sheath 727.05 Tenosynovitis of hand/wrist NEC 727.40 Synovial cyst NOS 729.6 Old foreign body in soft tissue 730.03 Acute osteomyelitis, forearm 730.13 Chronic osteomyelitis, forearm 730.23 Osteomyelitis NOS, forearm 732.3 Juvenile osteochondrosis, arm 881.12 Open wound of wrist, complicated 913.7 Foreign body, forearm, infected 996.66 Reaction, internal joint prosthesis 998.4 Foreign body left during procedure 998.5 Postoperative infection

REIMBURSEMENT INFORMATION

General

- ◆ See notes on page 286.
- ◆ Description changed in 1995 CPT.

Medicare

- ◆ Follow–up Days — 90
- ◆ Assistant Surgeon — not paid
- ◆ Supply Charges — not allowed
- ◆ Outpatient Limit — does not apply
- ◆ Major Surgery Rules Apply

CPT CODE	SERVICE	ICD-9-CM

25065 Biopsy, soft tissue of forearm and/or wrist; superficial

CPT NOTES

- For needle biopsy of soft tissue, use 20206.

170.5	M-Neoplasm, Wrist/Hand bones
171.2	M-Neoplasm, Soft tissue, arm
172.6	Malignant melanoma, Arm
195.4	M-Neoplasm, Upper limb
198.2	M2-Neoplasm, Skin
198.89	M2-Neoplasm NEC
199.0	M-Neoplasm, Disseminated
215.2	B-Neoplasm, Soft tissue, arm
238.1	UB-Neoplasm, Soft tissue
239.2	Bone/Skin neoplasm NOS
727.02	Giant cell tumor of tendon sheath
727.05	Tenosynovitis of hand/wrist NEC
727.40	Synovial cyst NOS

REIMBURSEMENT INFORMATION

General

- See notes on page 286.

Medicare

- Follow-up Days — 10
- Assistant Surgeon — not paid
- Supply Charges — not allowed
- Outpatient Limit — does not apply
- Minor Surgery Rules Apply

25066 Biopsy, soft tissue of forearm and/or wrist; deep

CPT NOTES

- For needle biopsy of soft tissue, use 20206.

170.5	M-Neoplasm, Wrist/Hand bones
171.2	M-Neoplasm, Soft tissue, arm
172.6	Malignant melanoma, Arm
195.4	M-Neoplasm, Upper limb
198.89	M2-Neoplasm NEC
199.0	M-Neoplasm, Disseminated
215.2	B-Neoplasm, Soft tissue, arm
238.1	UB-Neoplasm, Soft tissue
239.2	Bone/Skin neoplasm NOS
728.12	Traumatic myositis ossificans
728.13	Postop heterotopic calcification
728.2	Muscular disuse atrophy NEC
728.81	Interstitial myositis
728.89	Muscle/ligament disorder NEC

REIMBURSEMENT INFORMATION

General

- See notes on page 286.

Medicare

- Follow-up Days — 90
- Assistant Surgeon — not paid
- Supply Charges — not allowed
- Outpatient Limit — does not apply
- Major Surgery Rules Apply

CPT CODE	SERVICE	ICD-9-CM	
25075	Excision, tumor, forearm and/or wrist area; subcutaneous	171.2	M-Neoplasm, Soft tissue, arm
		172.6	Malignant melanoma, Arm
		195.4	M-Neoplasm, Upper limb
		198.2	M2-Neoplasm, Skin
		199.0	M-Neoplasm, Disseminated
		215.2	B-Neoplasm, Soft tissue, arm
		238.1	UB-Neoplasm, Soft tissue
		239.2	Bone/Skin neoplasm NOS

REIMBURSEMENT INFORMATION

General

- See notes on page 286.

Medicare

- Follow–up Days — 90
- Assistant Surgeon — not paid
- Supply Charges — not allowed
- Outpatient Limit — does not apply
- Major Surgery Rules Apply

CPT CODE	SERVICE	ICD-9-CM	
25076	Excision, tumor, forearm and/or wrist area; deep, subfascial or intramuscular	171.2	M-Neoplasm, Soft tissue, arm
		195.4	M-Neoplasm, Upper limb
		215.2	B-Neoplasm, Soft tissue, arm
		238.1	UB-Neoplasm, Soft tissue
		239.2	Bone/Skin neoplasm NOS

REIMBURSEMENT INFORMATION

General

- See notes on page 286.

Medicare

- Follow–up Days — 90
- Assistant Surgeon — not paid
- Supply Charges — not allowed
- Outpatient Limit — does not apply
- Major Surgery Rules Apply

CPT CODE	SERVICE	ICD–9–CM	
25077	Radical resection of tumor (eg, malignant neoplasm), soft tissue of forearm and/or wrist area	171.2	M-Neoplasm, Soft tissue, arm
		172.6	Malignant melanoma, Arm
		195.4	M-Neoplasm, Upper limb
		238.1	UB-Neoplasm, Soft tissue
		239.2	Bone/Skin neoplasm NOS

REIMBURSEMENT INFORMATION

General

- ♦ See notes on page 286.

Medicare

- ♦ Follow–up Days — 90
- ♦ Assistant Surgeon — not paid
- ♦ Supply Charges — not allowed
- ♦ Outpatient Limit — does not apply
- ♦ Major Surgery Rules Apply

CPT CODE	SERVICE	ICD–9–CM	
25085	Capsulotomy, wrist (eg, for contracture)	344.0	Quadriplegia NOS
		718.43	Contracture of joint, forearm
		718.53	Ankylosis of joint, forearm
		719.43	Pain in joint, forearm
		719.53	Joint stiffness NEC, forearm
		727.81	Contracture of tendon
		927.21	Crushing injury, wrist
		958.6	Volkmann's ischemic contracture

REIMBURSEMENT INFORMATION

General

- ♦ See notes on page 286.

Medicare

- ♦ Follow–up Days — 90
- ♦ Assistant Surgeon — paid
- ♦ Supply Charges — not allowed
- ♦ Outpatient Limit — does not apply
- ♦ Major Surgery Rules Apply

CPT CODE	SERVICE
▲ **25100**	Arthrotomy, wrist joint; with biopsy

ICD–9–CM

170.5	M-Neoplasm, Wrist/Hand bones
171.2	M-Neoplasm, Soft tissue, arm
198.89	M2-Neoplasm NEC
215.2	B-Neoplasm, Soft tissue, arm
238.1	UB-Neoplasm, Soft tissue
239.2	Bone/Skin neoplasm NOS
711.03	Pyogenic arthritis, forearm
711.93	Infect arthritis NOS, forearm
714.0	Rheumatoid arthritis
714.30	Juvenile rheumatoid arthritis NOS
714.31	Juvenile acute rheumatoid arthritis
714.32	Pauciarticular juv rheum arthritis
714.33	Monoarticular juv rheum arthritis
714.4	Chronic postrheumatic arthritis
715.13	Loc prim osteoarthritis, forearm
715.23	Loc 2nd osteoarthritis, forearm
715.33	Loc osteoarthritis NOS, forearm
716.13	Traumatic arthropathy, forearm
718.13	Loose body in joint, forearm
719.03	Joint effusion, forearm
719.23	Villonodular synovitis, forearm
727.00	Synovitis NOS
727.05	Tenosynovitis of hand/wrist NEC
727.40	Synovial cyst NOS
727.49	Bursal cyst NEC
729.6	Old foreign body in soft tissue
730.13	Chronic osteomyelitis, forearm
730.23	Osteomyelitis NOS, forearm
732.3	Juvenile osteochondrosis, arm
881.12	Open wound of wrist, complicated
913.7	Foreign body, forearm, infected
996.66	Reaction, internal joint prosthesis
998.4	Foreign body left during procedure
998.5	Postoperative infection

REIMBURSEMENT INFORMATION

General

- See notes on page 286.
- Description changed in 1995 CPT.

Medicare

- Follow–up Days — 90
- Assistant Surgeon — not paid
- Supply Charges — not allowed
- Outpatient Limit — does not apply
- Major Surgery Rules Apply

CPT CODE	SERVICE
25101	Arthrotomy, wrist joint; with joint exploration, with or without biopsy, with or without removal of loose or foreign body

ICD–9–CM

170.5	M-Neoplasm, Wrist/Hand bones
198.89	M2-Neoplasm NEC
215.2	B-Neoplasm, Soft tissue, arm
238.0	UB-Neoplasm, Bone
239.2	Bone/Skin neoplasm NOS
711.03	Pyogenic arthritis, forearm
711.93	Infect arthritis NOS, forearm
714.0	Rheumatoid arthritis
714.30	Juvenile rheumatoid arthritis NOS
714.31	Juvenile acute rheumatoid arthritis
714.32	Pauciarticular juv rheum arthritis
714.33	Monoarticular juv rheum arthritis
714.4	Chronic postrheumatic arthritis
715.13	Loc prim osteoarthritis, forearm
715.23	Loc 2nd osteoarthritis, forearm
715.33	Loc osteoarthritis NOS, forearm
716.13	Traumatic arthropathy, forearm
718.13	Loose body in joint, forearm
719.03	Joint effusion, forearm
719.23	Villonodular synovitis, forearm
729.6	Old foreign body in soft tissue
730.13	Chronic osteomyelitis, forearm
730.23	Osteomyelitis NOS, forearm
732.3	Juvenile osteochondrosis, arm
881.12	Open wound of wrist, complicated
913.7	Foreign body, forearm, infected
996.66	Reaction, internal joint prosthesis
998.4	Foreign body left during procedure
998.5	Postoperative infection

REIMBURSEMENT INFORMATION

General

- See notes on page 286.

Medicare

- Follow–up Days — 90
- Assistant Surgeon — not paid
- Supply Charges — not allowed
- Outpatient Limit — does not apply
- Major Surgery Rules Apply

CPT CODE	SERVICE
▲ **25105**	Arthrotomy, wrist joint; with synovectomy

ICD–9–CM

170.5	M-Neoplasm, Wrist/Hand bones
171.2	M-Neoplasm, Soft tissue, arm
198.89	M2-Neoplasm NEC
215.2	B-Neoplasm, Soft tissue, arm
238.1	UB-Neoplasm, Soft tissue
239.2	Bone/Skin neoplasm NOS
714.0	Rheumatoid arthritis
719.03	Joint effusion, forearm
719.23	Villonodular synovitis, forearm
727.00	Synovitis NOS
732.3	Juvenile osteochondrosis, arm
881.12	Open wound of wrist, complicated
913.7	Foreign body, forearm, infected
996.66	Reaction, internal joint prosthesis
998.5	Postoperative infection

REIMBURSEMENT INFORMATION

General

- See notes on page 286.
- Description changed in 1995 CPT.

Medicare

- Follow–up Days — 90
- Assistant Surgeon — paid
- Supply Charges — not allowed
- Outpatient Limit — does not apply
- Major Surgery Rules Apply

CPT CODE	SERVICE	ICD-9-CM
25107	Arthrotomy, distal radioulnar joint for repair of triangular cartilage complex	718.03 Articular cartilage dis, forearm 718.33 Recurrent dislocation, forearm 719.43 Pain in joint, forearm 833.01 Disloc distal radioulnar, closed 833.11 Disloc distal radioulnar, open 842.09 Sprain of wrist NEC

REIMBURSEMENT INFORMATION

General

- ♦ See notes on page 286.

Medicare

- ♦ Follow–up Days — 90
- ♦ Assistant Surgeon — paid
- ♦ Supply Charges — not allowed
- ♦ Outpatient Limit — does not apply
- ♦ Major Surgery Rules Apply

CPT CODE	SERVICE	ICD-9-CM
25110	Excision, lesion of tendon sheath, forearm and/or wrist	727.02 Giant cell tumor of tendon sheath 727.41 Ganglion of joint 727.42 Ganglion of tendon sheath 727.43 Ganglion NOS

REIMBURSEMENT INFORMATION

General

- ♦ See notes on page 286.

Medicare

- ♦ Follow–up Days — 90
- ♦ Assistant Surgeon — not paid
- ♦ Supply Charges — not allowed
- ♦ Outpatient Limit — does not apply
- ♦ Major Surgery Rules Apply

CPT CODE	SERVICE	ICD–9–CM
25111	Excision of ganglion, wrist (dorsal or volar); primary	727.41 Ganglion of joint 727.42 Ganglion of tendon sheath 727.43 Ganglion NOS
25112	Excision of ganglion, wrist (dorsal or volar); recurrent	

CPT NOTES

- For hand or finger, see 26160.

REIMBURSEMENT INFORMATION

General

- See notes on page 286.

Medicare

- Follow–up Days — 90
- Assistant Surgeon — not paid
- Supply Charges
  25111 — allowed
  25112 — not allowed
- Outpatient Limit — does not apply
- Major Surgery Rules Apply

CPT CODE	SERVICE	ICD–9–CM
25115	Radical excision of bursa, synovia of wrist, or forearm tendon sheaths (eg, tenosynovitis, fungus, Tbc, or other granulomas, rheumatoid arthritis); flexors	015.8 Tuberculosis, Joint 714.0 Rheumatoid arthritis 714.30 Juvenile rheumatoid arthritis NOS 714.31 Juvenile acute rheumatoid arthritis 714.32 Pauciarticular juv rheum arthritis 714.33 Monoarticular juv rheum arthritis 714.4 Chronic postrheumatic arthritis 719.23 Villonodular synovitis, forearm 727.00 Synovitis NOS 727.01 Synovitis in other diseases 727.05 Tenosynovitis of hand/wrist NEC 727.2 Occupational bursitis 727.89 Synovium/tendon/bursa disorder NEC
25116	Radical excision of bursa, synovia of wrist, or forearm tendon sheaths (eg, tenosynovitis, fungus, Tbc, or other granulomas, rheumatoid arthritis); extensors (with or without transposition of dorsal retinaculum)	

CPT NOTES

- For finger synovectomies, see 26145.

REIMBURSEMENT INFORMATION

General

- See notes on page 286.

Medicare

- Follow–up Days — 90
- Assistant Surgeon
  25115 — not paid
  25116 — paid
- Supply Charges — not allowed
- Outpatient Limit — does not apply
- Major Surgery Rules Apply

CPT CODE	SERVICE	ICD–9–CM	
25118	Synovectomy, extensor tendon sheath, wrist, single compartment	015.8	Tuberculosis, Joint
		170.5	M-Neoplasm, Wrist/Hand bones
		171.2	M-Neoplasm, Soft tissue, arm
		198.89	M2-Neoplasm NEC
		215.2	B-Neoplasm, Soft tissue, arm
		238.1	UB-Neoplasm, Soft tissue
		239.2	Bone/Skin neoplasm NOS
		711.03	Pyogenic arthritis, forearm
		711.93	Infect arthritis NOS, forearm
		714.0	Rheumatoid arthritis
		715.13	Loc prim osteoarthritis, forearm
		715.23	Loc 2nd osteoarthritis, forearm
		715.33	Loc osteoarthritis NOS, forearm
		716.13	Traumatic arthropathy, forearm
		718.13	Loose body in joint, forearm
		719.03	Joint effusion, forearm
		719.23	Villonodular synovitis, forearm
		727.00	Synovitis NOS
		727.01	Synovitis in other diseases
		727.05	Tenosynovitis of hand/wrist NEC
		727.2	Occupational bursitis
		729.6	Old foreign body in soft tissue
		730.03	Acute osteomyelitis, forearm
		730.13	Chronic osteomyelitis, forearm
		730.23	Osteomyelitis NOS, forearm
		732.3	Juvenile osteochondrosis, arm
		881.12	Open wound of wrist, complicated
		913.7	Foreign body, forearm, infected
		996.66	Reaction, internal joint prosthesis
		998.4	Foreign body left during procedure
		998.5	Postoperative infection

REIMBURSEMENT INFORMATION

General

- See notes on page 286.

Medicare

- Follow–up Days — 90
- Assistant Surgeon — not paid
- Supply Charges — not allowed
- Outpatient Limit — does not apply
- Major Surgery Rules Apply

CPT CODE	SERVICE
25119	Synovectomy, extensor tendon sheath, wrist, single compartment; with resection of distal ulna

ICD–9–CM

015.8	Tuberculosis, Joint
098.51	Gonococcal synovitis
098.7	Gonococcal infection of anus/rectum
170.5	M-Neoplasm, Wrist/Hand bones
171.2	M-Neoplasm, Soft tissue, arm
198.89	M2-Neoplasm NEC
215.2	B-Neoplasm, Soft tissue, arm
238.1	UB-Neoplasm, Soft tissue
239.2	Bone/Skin neoplasm NOS
274.0	Gouty arthropathy
711.03	Pyogenic arthritis, forearm
711.93	Infect arthritis NOS, forearm
714.0	Rheumatoid arthritis
714.30	Juvenile rheumatoid arthritis NOS
714.31	Juvenile acute rheumatoid arthritis
714.32	Pauciarticular juv rheum arthritis
714.33	Monoarticular juv rheum arthritis
714.4	Chronic postrheumatic arthritis
715.13	Loc prim osteoarthritis, forearm
715.23	Loc 2nd osteoarthritis, forearm
715.33	Loc osteoarthritis NOS, forearm
716.13	Traumatic arthropathy, forearm
718.13	Loose body in joint, forearm
719.03	Joint effusion, forearm
719.23	Villonodular synovitis, forearm
727.00	Synovitis NOS
727.01	Synovitis in other diseases
727.05	Tenosynovitis of hand/wrist NEC
727.2	Occupational bursitis
729.6	Old foreign body in soft tissue
730.03	Acute osteomyelitis, forearm
730.13	Chronic osteomyelitis, forearm
730.23	Osteomyelitis NOS, forearm
732.3	Juvenile osteochondrosis, arm
881.12	Open wound of wrist, complicated
913.7	Foreign body, forearm, infected
996.66	Reaction, internal joint prosthesis
998.4	Foreign body left during procedure
998.5	Postoperative infection

REIMBURSEMENT INFORMATION

General

- See notes on page 286.

Medicare

- Follow–up Days — 90
- Assistant Surgeon — paid
- Supply Charges — not allowed
- Outpatient Limit — does not apply
- Major Surgery Rules Apply

CPT CODE	SERVICE	ICD-9-CM
25120	Excision or curettage of bone cyst or benign tumor of radius or ulna (excluding head or neck of radius and olecranon process)	213.4 B-Neoplasm, Long bones, arm 726.4 Enthesopathy of wrist/carpus 726.91 Exostosis, site NOS 733.2x Cyst of bone 733.49 Aseptic necrosis of bone NEC
25125	Excision or curettage of bone cyst or benign tumor of radius or ulna (excluding head or neck of radius and olecranon process); with auto graft (includes obtaining graft)	
25126	Excision or curettage of bone cyst or benign tumor of radius or ulna (excluding head or neck of radius and olecranon process); with allograft	

CPT NOTES

- For head or neck of radius or olecranon process, see 24120-24126.

REIMBURSEMENT INFORMATION

General

- See notes on page 286.

Medicare

- Follow-up Days — 90
- Assistant Surgeon
  25120 — not paid
  25125 — by report
  25126 — paid
- Supply Charges — not allowed
- Outpatient Limit — does not apply
- Major Surgery Rules Apply

CPT CODE	SERVICE	ICD-9-CM
25130	Excision or curettage of bone cyst or benign tumor of carpal bones	213.5 B-Neoplasm, Wrist/Hand bones 726.4 Enthesopathy of wrist/carpus 727.41 Ganglion of joint 733.20 Cyst of bone NOS 733.21 Solitary bone cyst 733.22 Aneurysmal bone cyst 733.29 Bone cyst NEC
25135	Excision or curettage of bone cyst or benign tumor of carpal bones; with autograft (includes obtaining graft)	
25136	Excision or curettage of bone cyst or benign tumor of carpal bones; with allograft	

REIMBURSEMENT INFORMATION

General

- See notes on page 286.

Medicare

- Follow-up Days — 90
- Assistant Surgeon
  25130 — not paid
  25135–25136 — not paid
- Supply Charges — not allowed
- Outpatient Limit — does not apply
- Major Surgery Rules Apply

CPT CODE	SERVICE	ICD-9-CM
25145	Sequestrectomy (eg, for osteomyelitis or bone abscess), forearm and/or wrist	730.03 Acute osteomyelitis, forearm 730.13 Chronic osteomyelitis, forearm 730.23 Osteomyelitis NOS, forearm 730.33 Periostitis, forearm

REIMBURSEMENT INFORMATION

General

- ♦ See notes on page 286.

Medicare

- ♦ Follow-up Days — 90
- ♦ Assistant Surgeon — paid
- ♦ Supply Charges — not allowed
- ♦ Outpatient Limit — does not apply
- ♦ Major Surgery Rules Apply

CPT CODE	SERVICE	ICD-9-CM
25150	Partial excision (craterization, saucerization or diaphysectomy) of bone (eg, for osteomyelitis); ulna	730.03 Acute osteomyelitis, forearm 730.13 Chronic osteomyelitis, forearm 730.23 Osteomyelitis NOS, forearm 730.33 Periostitis, forearm 731.0 Osteitis deformans NOS 733.21 Solitary bone cyst 733.22 Aneurysmal bone cyst 733.29 Bone cyst NEC 733.49 Aseptic necrosis of bone NEC
25151	Partial excision (craterization, saucerization or diaphysectomy) of bone (eg, for osteomyelitis); radius	

CPT NOTES

- ♦ For head or neck of radius or olecranon process, see 24145, 24147.

REIMBURSEMENT INFORMATION

General

- ♦ See notes on page 286.

Medicare

- ♦ Follow-up Days — 90
- ♦ Assistant Surgeon — paid
- ♦ Supply Charges — not allowed
- ♦ Outpatient Limit — does not apply
- ♦ Major Surgery Rules Apply

CPT CODE	SERVICE
25170	Radical resection for tumor, radius or ulna

ICD–9–CM

170.4	M-Neoplasm, Long arm bones
195.4	M-Neoplasm, Upper limb
199.0	M-Neoplasm, Disseminated
238.0	UB-Neoplasm, Bone
239.2	Bone/Skin neoplasm NOS

REIMBURSEMENT INFORMATION

General

- See notes on page 286.

Medicare

- Follow–up Days — 90
- Assistant Surgeon — paid
- Supply Charges — not allowed
- Outpatient Limit — does not apply
- Major Surgery Rules Apply

CPT CODE	SERVICE
25210	Carpectomy; one bone

CPT NOTES

- For carpectomy with implant, see 25441-25445.

ICD–9–CM

170.5	M-Neoplasm, Wrist/Hand bones
213.5	B-Neoplasm, Wrist/Hand bones
238.0	UB-Neoplasm, Bone
239.2	Bone/Skin neoplasm NOS
714.0	Rheumatoid arthritis
714.30	Juvenile rheumatoid arthritis NOS
714.31	Juvenile acute rheumatoid arthritis
714.32	Pauciarticular juv rheum arthritis
714.33	Monoarticular juv rheum arthritis
714.4	Chronic postrheumatic arthritis
715.13	Loc prim osteoarthritis, forearm
715.23	Loc 2nd osteoarthritis, forearm
715.33	Loc osteoarthritis NOS, forearm
730.03	Acute osteomyelitis, forearm
730.13	Chronic osteomyelitis, forearm
730.23	Osteomyelitis NOS, forearm
730.33	Periostitis, forearm
731.0	Osteitis deformans NOS
732.8	Osteochondropathy NEC
733.21	Solitary bone cyst
733.22	Aneurysmal bone cyst
733.29	Bone cyst NEC
733.49	Aseptic necrosis of bone NEC
733.81	Malunion of fracture
755.56	Accessory carpal bones
905.2	Late effect, arm fracture
V13.6	Hx of congenital malformation

REIMBURSEMENT INFORMATION

General

- See notes on page 286.

Medicare

- Follow–up Days — 90
- Assistant Surgeon — paid
- Supply Charges — not allowed
- Outpatient Limit — does not apply
- Major Surgery Rules Apply

CPT CODE	SERVICE
25215	Carpectomy; all bones of proximal row

ICD–9–CM

170.5	M-Neoplasm, Wrist/Hand bones
213.5	B-Neoplasm, Wrist/Hand bones
238.0	UB-Neoplasm, Bone
239.2	Bone/Skin neoplasm NOS
714.0	Rheumatoid arthritis
714.30	Juvenile rheumatoid arthritis NOS
714.31	Juvenile acute rheumatoid arthritis
714.32	Pauciarticular juv rheum arthritis
714.33	Monoarticular juv rheum arthritis
714.4	Chronic postrheumatic arthritis
715.13	Loc prim osteoarthritis, forearm
715.23	Loc 2nd osteoarthritis, forearm
715.33	Loc osteoarthritis NOS, forearm
715.80	Osteoarthrosis mult site, site NOS
718.43	Contracture of joint, forearm
730.03	Acute osteomyelitis, forearm
730.13	Chronic osteomyelitis, forearm
730.23	Osteomyelitis NOS, forearm
730.33	Periostitis, forearm
731.0	Osteitis deformans NOS
732.8	Osteochondropathy NEC
733.21	Solitary bone cyst
733.22	Aneurysmal bone cyst
733.29	Bone cyst NEC
733.49	Aseptic necrosis of bone NEC
733.81	Malunion of fracture
755.56	Accessory carpal bones
905.2	Late effect, arm fracture
V13.6	Hx of congenital malformation

REIMBURSEMENT INFORMATION

General

- See notes on page 286.

Medicare

- Follow–up Days — 90
- Assistant Surgeon — paid
- Supply Charges — not allowed
- Outpatient Limit — does not apply
- Major Surgery Rules Apply

CPT CODE	SERVICE	ICD–9–CM	
25230	Radial styloidectomy (separate procedure)	170.4	M-Neoplasm, Long arm bones
		213.4	B-Neoplasm, Long bones, arm
		238.0	UB-Neoplasm, Bone
		239.2	Bone/Skin neoplasm NOS
		714.0	Rheumatoid arthritis
		715.13	Loc prim osteoarthritis, forearm
		716.12	Traumatic arthropathy, upper arm
		716.13	Traumatic arthropathy, forearm
		730.03	Acute osteomyelitis, forearm
		730.13	Chronic osteomyelitis, forearm
		730.23	Osteomyelitis NOS, forearm
		730.33	Periostitis, forearm
		731.0	Osteitis deformans NOS
		733.21	Solitary bone cyst
		733.22	Aneurysmal bone cyst
		733.29	Bone cyst NEC
		733.49	Aseptic necrosis of bone NEC
		733.81	Malunion of fracture
		733.82	Nonunion of fracture

REIMBURSEMENT INFORMATION

General

- See notes on page 286.
- Separate procedure rules apply.

Medicare

- Follow–up Days — 90
- Assistant Surgeon — paid
- Supply Charges — not allowed
- Outpatient Limit — does not apply
- Major Surgery Rules Apply

CPT CODE	SERVICE
▲ 25240	Excision distal ulna partial or complete, (eg, Darrach type or matched resection)

CPT NOTES

- For implant replacement, distal ulna, see 25442.
- For obtaining fascia for interposition, see 20920, 20922.

ICD–9–CM

170.5	M-Neoplasm, Wrist/Hand bones
213.5	B-Neoplasm, Wrist/Hand bones
238.0	UB-Neoplasm, Bone
239.2	Bone/Skin neoplasm NOS
714.0	Rheumatoid arthritis
714.30	Juvenile rheumatoid arthritis NOS
714.31	Juvenile acute rheumatoid arthritis
714.32	Pauciarticular juv rheum arthritis
714.33	Monoarticular juv rheum arthritis
715.13	Loc prim osteoarthritis, forearm
715.33	Loc osteoarthritis NOS, forearm
716.13	Traumatic arthropathy, forearm
716.14	Traumatic arthropathy, hand
718.03	Articular cartilage dis, forearm
719.43	Pain in joint, forearm
906.2	Late effect of superficial injury

REIMBURSEMENT INFORMATION

General

- See notes on page 286.
- Description changed in 1995 CPT.

Medicare

- Follow–up Days — 90
- Assistant Surgeon — paid
- Supply Charges — not allowed
- Outpatient Limit — does not apply
- Major Surgery Rules Apply

CPT CODE	SERVICE
25246	Injection procedure for wrist arthrography

CPT NOTES

- For K-wire, pin or rod insertion or removal, see 20650, 20670, 20680.
- For radiological supervision and interpretation, see 73115.
- For foreign body removal, superficial see 20520.

ICD–9–CM

714.0	Rheumatoid arthritis
715.13	Loc prim osteoarthritis, forearm
715.23	Loc 2nd osteoarthritis, forearm
715.33	Loc osteoarthritis NOS, forearm
716.13	Traumatic arthropathy, forearm
716.43	Transient arthropathy, forearm
718.03	Articular cartilage dis, forearm
718.13	Loose body in joint, forearm
718.23	Pathologic dislocation, forearm
718.33	Recurrent dislocation, forearm
718.43	Contracture of joint, forearm
718.53	Ankylosis of joint, forearm
718.83	Joint derangement NEC, forearm
719.23	Villonodular synovitis, forearm
719.43	Pain in joint, forearm
719.53	Joint stiffness NEC, forearm
719.83	Joint disorder NEC, forearm
727.00	Synovitis NOS
729.6	Old foreign body in soft tissue
842.0x	Wrist sprain/strain

REIMBURSEMENT INFORMATION

General

- See notes on page 286.

Medicare

- Follow–up Days — 0
- Assistant Surgeon — not paid
- Supply Charges — not allowed
- Outpatient Limit — does not apply
- Minor Surgery Rules Apply

CPT CODE	SERVICE
▲ **25248**	Exploration with removal of deep foreign body, forearm or wrist

CPT NOTES

- For K-wire, pin or rod insertion or removal, see 20650, 20670, 20680.

ICD–9–CM

728.82	Foreign body granuloma of muscle
729.6	Old foreign body in soft tissue
996.66	Reaction, internal joint prosthesis
996.77	Complication, int joint prosthesis
998.7	Postop foreign subst acute reaction

REIMBURSEMENT INFORMATION

General

- See notes on page 286.
- Description changed in 1995 CPT.

Medicare

- Follow–up Days — 90
- Assistant Surgeon — not paid
- Supply Charges — not allowed
- Outpatient Limit — does not apply
- Major Surgery Rules Apply

CPT CODE	SERVICE	ICD–9–CM
25250	Removal of wrist prosthesis; (separate procedure)	996.4 Malfunction, int orthoped dev/graft 996.66 Reaction, internal joint prosthesis 996.67 Reaction, internal ortho device NEC 996.77 Complication, int joint prosthesis 996.78 Complication, oth int ortho device 998.5 Postoperative infection
25251	Removal of wrist prosthesis; complicated, including "total wrist"	

CPT NOTES

- For K-wire, pin or rod insertion or removal, see 20650, 20670, 20680.

REIMBURSEMENT INFORMATION

General

- See notes on page 286.
- Separate procedure rules apply. (25250)

Medicare

- Follow–up Days — 90
- Assistant Surgeon — paid
- Supply Charges — not allowed
- Outpatient Limit — does not apply
- Major Surgery Rules Apply

CPT CODE	SERVICE	ICD–9–CM
25260	Repair, tendon or muscle, flexor, forearm and/or wrist; primary, single, each tendon or muscle	727.64 Rupture, hand/wrist flexor tendons 881.12 Open wound of wrist, complicated 881.22 Open wound of wrist w/tendon 927.10 Crushing injury, forearm 927.21 Crushing injury, wrist

REIMBURSEMENT INFORMATION

General

- See notes on page 286.

Medicare

- Follow–up Days — 90
- Assistant Surgeon — not paid
- Supply Charges — not allowed
- Outpatient Limit — does not apply
- Major Surgery Rules Apply

CPT CODE	SERVICE	ICD–9–CM
25263	Repair, tendon or muscle, flexor, forearm and/or wrist; secondary, single, each tendon or muscle	727.64 Rupture, hand/wrist flexor tendons 881.12 Open wound of wrist, complicated 881.22 Open wound of wrist w/tendon 905.8 Late effect of tendon injury 927.10 Crushing injury, forearm 927.21 Crushing injury, wrist
25265	Repair, tendon or muscle, flexor, forearm and/or wrist; secondary, with free graft (includes obtaining graft), each tendon or muscle	

REIMBURSEMENT INFORMATION

General

- ♦ See notes on page 286.

Medicare

- ♦ Follow–up Days — 90
- ♦ Assistant Surgeon — paid
- ♦ Supply Charges — not allowed
- ♦ Outpatient Limit — does not apply
- ♦ Major Surgery Rules Apply

CPT CODE	SERVICE	ICD–9–CM
25270	Repair, tendon or muscle, extensor, forearm and/or wrist; primary, single, each tendon or muscle	727.63 Rupture, hand/wrist extensor tendon 881.12 Open wound of wrist, complicated 881.22 Open wound of wrist w/tendon 905.8 Late effect of tendon injury 927.10 Crushing injury, forearm 927.21 Crushing injury, wrist
25272	Repair, tendon or muscle, extensor, forearm and/or wrist; secondary, single, each tendon or muscle	

REIMBURSEMENT INFORMATION

General

- ♦ See notes on page 286.

Medicare

- ♦ Follow–up Days — 90
- ♦ Assistant Surgeon
  25270 — not paid
  25272 — paid
- ♦ Supply Charges — not allowed
- ♦ Outpatient Limit — does not apply
- ♦ Major Surgery Rules Apply

CPT CODE	SERVICE	ICD–9–CM	
25274	Repair, tendon or muscle, extensor, secondary, with tendon graft (includes obtaining graft), forearm and/or wrist, each tendon or muscle	727.63	Rupture, hand/wrist extensor tendon
		881.12	Open wound of wrist, complicated
		881.22	Open wound of wrist w/tendon
		905.8	Late effect of tendon injury
		927.10	Crushing injury, forearm
		927.21	Crushing injury, wrist

REIMBURSEMENT INFORMATION

General

- ♦ See notes on page 286.

Medicare

- ♦ Follow–up Days — 90
- ♦ Assistant Surgeon — paid
- ♦ Supply Charges — not allowed
- ♦ Outpatient Limit — does not apply
- ♦ Major Surgery Rules Apply

CPT CODE	SERVICE	ICD–9–CM	
25280	Lengthening or shortening of flexor or extensor tendon, forearm and/or wrist, single, each tendon	138.	Late effects of acute polio
		343.x	Infantile cerebral palsy
		344.0	Quadriplegia NOS
		436.	Acute CVA, ill-defined
		718.43	Contracture of joint, forearm
		727.81	Contracture of tendon
		881.22	Open wound of wrist w/tendon
		905.8	Late effect of tendon injury
		906.6	Late effect of wrist/hand burn
		907.2	Late effect, spinal cord injury
		927.21	Crushing injury, wrist
		958.6	Volkmann's ischemic contracture
		996.91	Complication, reattached forearm
		996.92	Complication, reattached hand

REIMBURSEMENT INFORMATION

General

- ♦ See notes on page 286.

Medicare

- ♦ Follow–up Days — 90
- ♦ Assistant Surgeon — paid
- ♦ Supply Charges — not allowed
- ♦ Outpatient Limit — does not apply
- ♦ Major Surgery Rules Apply

CPT CODE	SERVICE	ICD–9–CM	
25290	Tenotomy, open flexor or extensor tendon, forearm and/or wrist, single, each tendon	138.	Late effects of acute polio
		343.x	Infantile cerebral palsy
		344.0	Quadriplegia NOS
		436.	Acute CVA, ill-defined
		718.43	Contracture of joint, forearm
		727.81	Contracture of tendon
		881.22	Open wound of wrist w/tendon
		905.8	Late effect of tendon injury
		906.6	Late effect of wrist/hand burn
		907.2	Late effect, spinal cord injury
		927.21	Crushing injury, wrist
		958.6	Volkmann's ischemic contracture
		996.91	Complication, reattached forearm
		996.92	Complication, reattached hand

REIMBURSEMENT INFORMATION

General

- See notes on page 286.

Medicare

- Follow–up Days — 90
- Assistant Surgeon — not paid
- Supply Charges — not allowed
- Outpatient Limit — does not apply
- Major Surgery Rules Apply

CPT CODE	SERVICE	ICD–9–CM	
25295	Tenolysis, flexor or extensor tendon, forearm and/or wrist, single, each tendon	138.	Late effects of acute polio
		343.x	Infantile cerebral palsy
		436.	Acute CVA, ill-defined
		727.81	Contracture of tendon
		881.22	Open wound of wrist w/tendon
		905.8	Late effect of tendon injury
		927.21	Crushing injury, wrist
		996.91	Complication, reattached forearm
		996.92	Complication, reattached hand

REIMBURSEMENT INFORMATION

General

- See notes on page 286.

Medicare

- Follow–up Days — 90
- Assistant Surgeon — not paid
- Supply Charges — not allowed
- Outpatient Limit — does not apply
- Major Surgery Rules Apply

CPT CODE	SERVICE
25300	Tenodesis at wrist; flexors of fingers
25301	Tenodesis at wrist; extensors of fingers

ICD–9–CM

138.	Late effects of acute polio
343.1	Congenital hemiplegia
343.2	Congenital quadriplegia
343.3	Congenital monoplegia
343.4	Infantile hemiplegia
343.8	Infantile cerebral palsy NEC
343.9	Infantile cerebral palsy NOS
344.0	Quadriplegia NOS
436.	Acute CVA, ill-defined
727.05	Tenosynovitis of hand/wrist NEC
727.64	Rupture, hand/wrist flexor tendons
881.22	Open wound of wrist w/tendon
927.21	Crushing injury, wrist

REIMBURSEMENT INFORMATION

General

- See notes on page 286.

Medicare

- Follow–up Days — 90
- Assistant Surgeon — paid
- Supply Charges — not allowed
- Outpatient Limit — does not apply
- Major Surgery Rules Apply

CPT CODE	SERVICE	ICD–9–CM
25310	Tendon transplantation or transfer, flexor or extensor, forearm and/or wrist, single; each tendon	138. Late effects of acute polio 344.0 Quadriplegia NOS 344.2 Diplegia of upper limbs 344.4 Monoplegia of upper limb 727.63 Rupture, hand/wrist extensor tendon 727.64 Rupture, hand/wrist flexor tendons 767.6 Brachial plexus injury at birth 881.22 Open wound of wrist w/tendon 905.8 Late effect of tendon injury 907.4 Late effect, nerve injury shld/arm 927.21 Crushing injury, wrist 955.1 Injury median nerve 955.2 Injury ulnar nerve 955.3 Injury radial nerve 955.4 Injury musculocutaneous nerve 955.7 Injury nerve shoulder/arm NEC 955.8 Injury multiple nerves shoulder/arm
25312	Tendon transplantation or transfer, flexor or extensor, forearm and/or wrist, single; with tendon graft(s) (includes obtaining graft), each tendon	

REIMBURSEMENT INFORMATION

General

- See notes on page 286.

Medicare

- Follow–up Days — 90
- Assistant Surgeon — paid
- Supply Charges — not allowed
- Outpatient Limit — does not apply
- Major Surgery Rules Apply

CPT CODE	SERVICE	ICD–9–CM
▲ **25315**	Flexor origin slide (eg, for cerebral palsy, Volkmann contracture), forearm and/or wrist	343.x Infantile cerebral palsy 958.6 Volkmann's ischemic contracture
▲ **25316**	Flexor origin slide (eg, for cerebral palsy, Volkmann contracture), forearm and/or wrist; with tendon(s) transfer	

REIMBURSEMENT INFORMATION

General

- See notes on page 286.
- Description changed in 1995 CPT.

Medicare

- Follow–up Days — 90
- Assistant Surgeon — paid
- Supply Charges — not allowed
- Outpatient Limit — does not apply
- Major Surgery Rules Apply

CPT CODE	SERVICE
▲ 25320	Capsulorrhaphy or reconstruction, wrist any method (eg, capsulodesis, ligament repair, tendon transfer or graft) (includes synovectomy, capsulotomy and open reduction) for carpal instability

ICD–9–CM

714.0	Rheumatoid arthritis
714.30	Juvenile rheumatoid arthritis NOS
714.31	Juvenile acute rheumatoid arthritis
714.32	Pauciarticular juv rheum arthritis
714.33	Monoarticular juv rheum arthritis
714.4	Chronic postrheumatic arthritis
715.13	Loc prim osteoarthritis, forearm
718.43	Contracture of joint, forearm
719.43	Pain in joint, forearm
728.4	Laxity of ligament
728.5	Hypermobility syndrome
736.03	Valgus deformity of wrist
736.04	Varus deformity of wrist
736.05	Wrist drop
881.22	Open wound of wrist w/tendon

REIMBURSEMENT INFORMATION

General

- See notes on page 286.
- Description changed in 1995 CPT.

Medicare

- Follow–up Days — 90
- Assistant Surgeon — paid
- Supply Charges — not allowed
- Outpatient Limit — does not apply
- Major Surgery Rules Apply

CPT CODE **SERVICE**

25330 Arthroplasty, wrist

CPT NOTES

- For obtaining fascia for interposition, see 20920, 20922.

ICD–9–CM

711.03	Pyogenic arthritis, forearm
711.93	Infect arthritis NOS, forearm
714.0	Rheumatoid arthritis
714.30	Juvenile rheumatoid arthritis NOS
714.31	Juvenile acute rheumatoid arthritis
714.32	Pauciarticular juv rheum arthritis
714.33	Monoarticular juv rheum arthritis
714.4	Chronic postrheumatic arthritis
715.13	Loc prim osteoarthritis, forearm
715.23	Loc 2nd osteoarthritis, forearm
715.33	Loc osteoarthritis NOS, forearm
716.13	Traumatic arthropathy, forearm
718.03	Articular cartilage dis, forearm
718.33	Recurrent dislocation, forearm
718.43	Contracture of joint, forearm
718.53	Ankylosis of joint, forearm
719.23	Villonodular synovitis, forearm
719.43	Pain in joint, forearm
719.83	Joint disorder NEC, forearm
730.13	Chronic osteomyelitis, forearm
731.0	Osteitis deformans NOS
732.3	Juvenile osteochondrosis, arm
732.6	Juvenile osteochondrosis NEC
732.7	Osteochondritis dissecans
733.49	Aseptic necrosis of bone NEC
842.0x	Wrist sprain/strain
842.11	Sprain carpometacarpal
905.2	Late effect, arm fracture
906.4	Late effect of crushing
927.21	Crushing injury, wrist

REIMBURSEMENT INFORMATION

General

- See notes on page 286.

Medicare

- Follow–up Days — 90
- Assistant Surgeon —- paid
- Supply Charges — not allowed
- Outpatient Limit — does not apply
- Major Surgery Rules Apply

CPT CODE	SERVICE
25331	Arthroplasty, wrist; with implant

CPT NOTES

- For obtaining fascia for interposition, see 20920, 20922.

ICD–9–CM

696.0	Psoriatic arthropathy
711.03	Pyogenic arthritis, forearm
711.93	Infect arthritis NOS, forearm
713.5	Arthropathy w/neurological disorder
713.8	Arthropathy w/other disorders NEC
714.0	Rheumatoid arthritis
714.30	Juvenile rheumatoid arthritis NOS
714.31	Juvenile acute rheumatoid arthritis
714.32	Pauciarticular juv rheum arthritis
714.33	Monoarticular juv rheum arthritis
714.4	Chronic postrheumatic arthritis
715.13	Loc prim osteoarthritis, forearm
715.23	Loc 2nd osteoarthritis, forearm
715.33	Loc osteoarthritis NOS, forearm
716.13	Traumatic arthropathy, forearm
718.03	Articular cartilage dis, forearm
718.33	Recurrent dislocation, forearm
718.43	Contracture of joint, forearm
718.53	Ankylosis of joint, forearm
719.23	Villonodular synovitis, forearm
719.43	Pain in joint, forearm
719.83	Joint disorder NEC, forearm
730.13	Chronic osteomyelitis, forearm
731.0	Osteitis deformans NOS
732.3	Juvenile osteochondrosis, arm
732.6	Juvenile osteochondrosis NEC
732.7	Osteochondritis dissecans
733.49	Aseptic necrosis of bone NEC
842.x	Wrist/hand sprain/strain
905.2	Late effect, arm fracture
906.4	Late effect of crushing
927.21	Crushing injury, wrist

REIMBURSEMENT INFORMATION

General

- See notes on page 286.

Medicare

- Follow–up Days — 90
- Assistant Surgeon — paid
- Supply Charges — not allowed
- Outpatient Limit — does not apply
- Major Surgery Rules Apply

CPT CODE	SERVICE
25332	Arthroplasty, wrist; pseudarthrosis type with internal fixation

CPT NOTES

- For obtaining fascia for interposition, see 20920, 20922.

ICD–9–CM

696.0	Psoriatic arthropathy
711.03	Pyogenic arthritis, forearm
711.93	Infect arthritis NOS, forearm
713.5	Arthropathy w/neurological disorder
714.0	Rheumatoid arthritis
714.30	Juvenile rheumatoid arthritis NOS
714.31	Juvenile acute rheumatoid arthritis
714.32	Pauciarticular juv rheum arthritis
714.33	Monoarticular juv rheum arthritis
714.4	Chronic postrheumatic arthritis
715.13	Loc prim osteoarthritis, forearm
715.23	Loc 2nd osteoarthritis, forearm
715.33	Loc osteoarthritis NOS, forearm
715.8	Arthropathy w/other disorders NEC
716.13	Traumatic arthropathy, forearm
718.03	Articular cartilage dis, forearm
718.33	Recurrent dislocation, forearm
718.43	Contracture of joint, forearm
718.53	Ankylosis of joint, forearm
719.23	Villonodular synovitis, forearm
719.43	Pain in joint, forearm
719.83	Joint disorder NEC, forearm
730.13	Chronic osteomyelitis, forearm
731.0	Osteitis deformans NOS
732.3	Juvenile osteochondrosis, arm
732.6	Juvenile osteochondrosis NEC
732.7	Osteochondritis dissecans
733.49	Aseptic necrosis of bone NEC
733.82	Nonunion of fracture
842.0x	Wrist sprain/strain
842.11	Sprain carpometacarpal
905.2	Late effect, arm fracture
906.4	Late effect of crushing
927.21	Crushing injury, wrist

REIMBURSEMENT INFORMATION

General

- See notes on page 286.

Medicare

- Follow–up Days — 90
- Assistant Surgeon — paid
- Supply Charges — not allowed
- Outpatient Limit — does not apply
- Major Surgery Rules Apply

CPT CODE	SERVICE	ICD–9–CM
25335	Centralization of wrist on ulna (eg, radial club hand)	728.4 Laxity of ligament 736.07 Club hand, acquired 754.89 Nonteratogenic anomaly NEC 755.26 Longitudinal deficiency, radius 842.09 Sprain of wrist NEC 905.2 Late effect, arm fracture

REIMBURSEMENT INFORMATION

General

- ♦ See notes on page 286.

Medicare

- ♦ Follow–up Days — 90
- ♦ Assistant Surgeon — paid
- ♦ Supply Charges — not allowed
- ♦ Outpatient Limit — does not apply
- ♦ Major Surgery Rules Apply

CPT CODE	SERVICE	ICD–9–CM
● 25337	Reconstruction for stabilization of unstable distal ulna or distal radioulnar joint, secondary by soft tissue stabilization (eg, tendon transfer, tendon graft or weave, or tenodesis) with or without open reduction of distal radioulnar joint	755.54 Madelung's deformity 842.0x Wrist sprain/strain 905.2 Late effect, arm fracture

CPT NOTES

- ♦ For harvesting of fascia lata graft, see 20920, 20922.

REIMBURSEMENT INFORMATION

General

- ♦ See notes on page 286.
- ♦ New procedure, 1995 CPT.

Medicare

- ♦ Follow–up Days — 90
- ♦ Assistant Surgeon — paid
- ♦ Supply Charges — not allowed
- ♦ Outpatient Limit — does not apply
- ♦ Major Surgery Rules Apply

CPT CODE	SERVICE	ICD-9-CM
25350	Osteotomy, radius; distal third	715.13 Loc prim osteoarthritis, forearm 716.13 Traumatic arthropathy, forearm 732.3 Juvenile osteochondrosis, arm 733.81 Malunion of fracture 733.82 Nonunion of fracture 755.27 Longitudinal deficiency, ulna 755.54 Madelung's deformity 756.4 Chondrodystrophy 756.5x Osteodystrophy 905.2 Late effect, arm fracture V13.6 Hx of congenital malformation
25355	Osteotomy, radius; middle or proximal third	

REIMBURSEMENT INFORMATION

General

- ♦ See notes on page 286.

Medicare

- ♦ Follow–up Days — 90
- ♦ Assistant Surgeon — paid
- ♦ Supply Charges — not allowed
- ♦ Outpatient Limit — does not apply
- ♦ Major Surgery Rules Apply

CPT CODE	SERVICE	ICD-9-CM
25360	Osteotomy; ulna	715.13 Loc prim osteoarthritis, forearm 716.13 Traumatic arthropathy, forearm 730.03 Acute osteomyelitis, forearm 730.13 Chronic osteomyelitis, forearm 731.0 Osteitis deformans NOS 732.3 Juvenile osteochondrosis, arm 733.81 Malunion of fracture 733.82 Nonunion of fracture 755.26 Longitudinal deficiency, radius 755.54 Madelung's deformity 756.4 Chondrodystrophy 756.5x Osteodystrophy 905.2 Late effect, arm fracture V13.6 Hx of congenital malformation
25365	Osteotomy; radius and ulna	

REIMBURSEMENT INFORMATION

General

- ♦ See notes on page 286.

Medicare

- ♦ Follow–up Days — 90
- ♦ Assistant Surgeon — paid
- ♦ Supply Charges — not allowed
- ♦ Outpatient Limit — does not apply
- ♦ Major Surgery Rules Apply

CPT CODE	SERVICE	ICD–9–CM	
25370	Multiple osteotomies, with realignment on intramedullary rod (Sofield type procedure); radius OR ulna	715.13	Loc prim osteoarthritis, forearm
25375	Multiple osteotomies, with realignment on intramedullary rod (Sofield type procedure); radius AND ulna	716.13	Traumatic arthropathy, forearm
		730.03	Acute osteomyelitis, forearm
		730.13	Chronic osteomyelitis, forearm
		731.0	Osteitis deformans NOS
		732.3	Juvenile osteochondrosis, arm
		733.81	Malunion of fracture
		733.82	Nonunion of fracture
		755.54	Madelung's deformity
		756.4	Chondrodystrophy
		756.5x	Osteodystrophy
		905.2	Late effect, arm fracture
		V13.6	Hx of congenital malformation

REIMBURSEMENT INFORMATION

General

- ◆ See notes on page 286.

Medicare

- ◆ Follow–up Days — 90
- ◆ Assistant Surgeon — paid
- ◆ Supply Charges — not allowed
- ◆ Outpatient Limit — does not apply
- ◆ Major Surgery Rules Apply

CPT CODE	SERVICE	ICD–9–CM	
25390	Osteoplasty, radius OR ulna; shortening	715.13	Loc prim osteoarthritis, forearm
25391	Osteoplasty, radius OR ulna; lengthening with autograft	716.13	Traumatic arthropathy, forearm
		718.03	Articular cartilage dis, forearm
		730.03	Acute osteomyelitis, forearm
		730.13	Chronic osteomyelitis, forearm
		731.0	Osteitis deformans NOS
		732.3	Juvenile osteochondrosis, arm
		733.81	Malunion of fracture
		733.82	Nonunion of fracture
		755.26	Longitudinal deficiency, radius
		755.27	Longitudinal deficiency, ulna

REIMBURSEMENT INFORMATION

General

- ◆ See notes on page 286.

Medicare

- ◆ Follow–up Days — 90
- ◆ Assistant Surgeon — paid
- ◆ Supply Charges — not allowed
- ◆ Outpatient Limit — does not apply
- ◆ Major Surgery Rules Apply

CPT CODE	SERVICE	ICD-9-CM
25392	Osteoplasty, radius AND ulna; shortening (excluding 64876)	715.13 Loc prim osteoarthritis, forearm 716.13 Traumatic arthropathy, forearm 730.03 Acute osteomyelitis, forearm 730.13 Chronic osteomyelitis, forearm 731.0 Osteitis deformans NOS 732.3 Juvenile osteochondrosis, arm 733.81 Malunion of fracture 733.82 Nonunion of fracture 756.4 Chondrodystrophy 756.5x Osteodystrophy 905.2 Late effect, arm fracture
25393	Osteoplasty, radius AND ulna; lengthening with autograft	

REIMBURSEMENT INFORMATION

General

- ♦ See notes on page 286.

Medicare

- ♦ Follow-up Days — 90
- ♦ Assistant Surgeon — paid
- ♦ Supply Charges — not allowed
- ♦ Outpatient Limit — does not apply
- ♦ Major Surgery Rules Apply

CPT CODE	SERVICE	ICD-9-CM
25400	Repair of nonunion or malunion, radius OR ulna; without graft (eg, compression technique)	733.81 Malunion of fracture 733.82 Nonunion of fracture 905.2 Late effect, arm fracture
25405	Repair of nonunion or malunion, radius OR ulna; with iliac or other autograft (includes obtaining graft)	

REIMBURSEMENT INFORMATION

General

- ♦ See notes on page 286.

Medicare

- ♦ Follow-up Days — 90
- ♦ Assistant Surgeon — paid
- ♦ Supply Charges — not allowed
- ♦ Outpatient Limit — does not apply
- ♦ Major Surgery Rules Apply

CPT CODE	SERVICE	ICD-9-CM	
25415	Repair of nonunion or malunion, radius AND ulna; without graft (eg, compression technique, etc)	733.81	Malunion of fracture
25420	Repair of nonunion or malunion, radius AND ulna; with iliac or other autograft (includes obtaining graft)	733.82	Nonunion of fracture
		905.2	Late effect, arm fracture

REIMBURSEMENT INFORMATION

General
- ♦ See notes on page 286.

Medicare
- ♦ Follow-up Days — 90
- ♦ Assistant Surgeon — paid
- ♦ Supply Charges — not allowed
- ♦ Outpatient Limit — does not apply
- ♦ Major Surgery Rules Apply

CPT CODE	SERVICE	ICD-9-CM	
25425	Repair of defect with autograft; radius OR ulna	733.81	Malunion of fracture
25426	Repair of defect with autograft; radius AND ulna	733.82	Nonunion of fracture
		905.2	Late effect, arm fracture

REIMBURSEMENT INFORMATION

General
- ♦ See notes on page 286.

Medicare
- ♦ Follow-up Days — 90
- ♦ Assistant Surgeon — paid
- ♦ Supply Charges — not allowed
- ♦ Outpatient Limit — does not apply
- ♦ Major Surgery Rules Apply

CPT CODE	SERVICE
25440	Repair of nonunion, scaphoid (navicular) bone, with or without radial styloidectomy (includes obtaining graft and necessary fixation)

ICD–9–CM

733.82	Nonunion of fracture
905.2	Late effect, arm fracture

REIMBURSEMENT INFORMATION

General

- See notes on page 286.

Medicare

- Follow–up Days — 90
- Assistant Surgeon — paid
- Supply Charges — not allowed
- Outpatient Limit — does not apply
- Major Surgery Rules Apply

CPT CODE	SERVICE
25441	Arthroplasty with prosthetic replacement; distal radius
25442	Arthroplasty with prosthetic replacement; distal ulna

ICD–9–CM

094.0	Tabes dorsalis
250.6	Diabetes w/neurologic manifestation
336.0	Syringomyelia
711.03	Pyogenic arthritis, forearm
711.93	Infect arthritis NOS, forearm
713.5	Arthropathy w/neurological disorder
714.0	Rheumatoid arthritis
714.30	Juvenile rheumatoid arthritis NOS
714.31	Juvenile acute rheumatoid arthritis
714.32	Pauciarticular juv rheum arthritis
714.33	Monoarticular juv rheum arthritis
714.4	Chronic postrheumatic arthritis
715.13	Loc prim osteoarthritis, forearm
715.23	Loc 2nd osteoarthritis, forearm
715.33	Loc osteoarthritis NOS, forearm
716.13	Traumatic arthropathy, forearm
718.03	Articular cartilage dis, forearm
718.53	Ankylosis of joint, forearm
719.23	Villonodular synovitis, forearm
730.13	Chronic osteomyelitis, forearm
731.0	Osteitis deformans NOS
732.3	Juvenile osteochondrosis, arm
733.49	Aseptic necrosis of bone NEC
733.81	Malunion of fracture
733.82	Nonunion of fracture
905.2	Late effect, arm fracture

REIMBURSEMENT INFORMATION

General

- See notes on page 286.

Medicare

- Follow–up Days — 90
- Assistant Surgeon — paid
- Supply Charges — not allowed
- Outpatient Limit — does not apply
- Major Surgery Rules Apply

CPT CODE	SERVICE
25443	Arthroplasty with prosthetic replacement; scaphoid (navicular)
25444	Arthroplasty with prosthetic replacement; lunate

ICD–9–CM

711.03	Pyogenic arthritis, forearm
711.93	Infect arthritis NOS, forearm
714.0	Rheumatoid arthritis
715.13	Loc prim osteoarthritis, forearm
715.23	Loc 2nd osteoarthritis, forearm
715.33	Loc osteoarthritis NOS, forearm
716.13	Traumatic arthropathy, forearm
719.23	Villonodular synovitis, forearm
730.13	Chronic osteomyelitis, forearm
731.0	Osteitis deformans NOS
732.3	Juvenile osteochondrosis, arm
733.49	Aseptic necrosis of bone NEC
733.82	Nonunion of fracture
905.2	Late effect, arm fracture

REIMBURSEMENT INFORMATION

General

- See notes on page 286.

Medicare

- Follow–up Days — 90
- Assistant Surgeon — paid
- Supply Charges — not allowed
- Outpatient Limit — does not apply
- Major Surgery Rules Apply

CPT CODE	SERVICE
25446	Arthroplasty with prosthetic replacement; distal radius and partial or entire carpus ("total wrist")

ICD–9–CM

711.03	Pyogenic arthritis, forearm
711.93	Infect arthritis NOS, forearm
714.0	Rheumatoid arthritis
714.30	Juvenile rheumatoid arthritis NOS
714.31	Juvenile acute rheumatoid arthritis
714.32	Pauciarticular juv rheum arthritis
714.33	Monoarticular juv rheum arthritis
714.4	Chronic postrheumatic arthritis
715.13	Loc prim osteoarthritis, forearm
715.23	Loc 2nd osteoarthritis, forearm
715.33	Loc osteoarthritis NOS, forearm
716.13	Traumatic arthropathy, forearm
719.23	Villonodular synovitis, forearm
730.13	Chronic osteomyelitis, forearm
731.0	Osteitis deformans NOS
732.3	Juvenile osteochondrosis, arm
733.49	Aseptic necrosis of bone NEC
733.82	Nonunion of fracture
905.2	Late effect, arm fracture

REIMBURSEMENT INFORMATION

General

- See notes on page 286.

Medicare

- Follow–up Days — 90
- Assistant Surgeon — paid
- Supply Charges — not allowed
- Outpatient Limit — does not apply
- Major Surgery Rules Apply

CPT CODE	SERVICE
25447	Interposition arthroplasty, intercarpal or carpometacarpal joints

ICD–9–CM

711.03	Pyogenic arthritis, forearm
711.93	Infect arthritis NOS, forearm
714.0	Rheumatoid arthritis
714.30	Juvenile rheumatoid arthritis NOS
714.31	Juvenile acute rheumatoid arthritis
714.32	Pauciarticular juv rheum arthritis
714.33	Monoarticular juv rheum arthritis
714.4	Chronic postrheumatic arthritis
715.13	Loc prim osteoarthritis, forearm
715.23	Loc 2nd osteoarthritis, forearm
715.33	Loc osteoarthritis NOS, forearm
716.13	Traumatic arthropathy, forearm
719.23	Villonodular synovitis, forearm
730.13	Chronic osteomyelitis, forearm
731.0	Osteitis deformans NOS
732.3	Juvenile osteochondrosis, arm
733.49	Aseptic necrosis of bone NEC
733.82	Nonunion of fracture
905.2	Late effect, arm fracture

REIMBURSEMENT INFORMATION

General

- See notes on page 286.

Medicare

- Follow–up Days — 90
- Assistant Surgeon — paid
- Supply Charges — not allowed
- Outpatient Limit — does not apply
- Major Surgery Rules Apply

CPT CODE	SERVICE
25449	Revision of arthroplasty, including removal of implant, wrist joint

ICD-9-CM

711.03	Pyogenic arthritis, forearm
711.93	Infect arthritis NOS, forearm
714.0	Rheumatoid arthritis
714.30	Juvenile rheumatoid arthritis NOS
714.31	Juvenile acute rheumatoid arthritis
714.32	Pauciarticular juv rheum arthritis
714.33	Monoarticular juv rheum arthritis
714.4	Chronic postrheumatic arthritis
715.13	Loc prim osteoarthritis, forearm
715.23	Loc 2nd osteoarthritis, forearm
715.33	Loc osteoarthritis NOS, forearm
716.13	Traumatic arthropathy, forearm
719.23	Villonodular synovitis, forearm
730.13	Chronic osteomyelitis, forearm
731.0	Osteitis deformans NOS
732.3	Juvenile osteochondrosis, arm
733.49	Aseptic necrosis of bone NEC
733.82	Nonunion of fracture
905.2	Late effect, arm fracture
914.4	Insect bite, hand
996.4	Malfunction, int orthoped dev/graft
996.66	Reaction, internal joint prosthesis
996.67	Reaction, internal ortho device NEC
996.77	Complication, int joint prosthesis

REIMBURSEMENT INFORMATION

General

- See notes on page 286.

Medicare

- Follow-up Days — 90
- Assistant Surgeon — paid
- Supply Charges — not allowed
- Outpatient Limit — does not apply
- Major Surgery Rules Apply

CPT CODE	SERVICE	ICD-9-CM
25450	Epiphyseal arrest by epiphysiodesis or stapling; distal radius OR ulna	733.91 Arrest of bone growth 733.99 Bone/Cartilage disorder NEC 755.54 Madelung's deformity V13.6 Hx of congenital malformation
25455	Epiphyseal arrest by epiphysiodesis or stapling; distal radius AND ulna	

REIMBURSEMENT INFORMATION

General

- ♦ See notes on page 286.

Medicare

- ♦ Follow-up Days — 90
- ♦ Assistant Surgeon — paid
- ♦ Supply Charges — not allowed
- ♦ Outpatient Limit — does not apply
- ♦ Major Surgery Rules Apply

CPT CODE	SERVICE	ICD-9-CM
25500	Closed treatment of radial shaft fracture; without manipulation	813.21 Fx radius shaft, closed 813.31 Fx radius shaft, open

REIMBURSEMENT INFORMATION

General

- ♦ See notes on page 286.

Medicare

- ♦ Follow-up Days — 90
- ♦ Assistant Surgeon — not paid
- ♦ Supply Charges — not allowed
- ♦ Outpatient Limit — applies
- ♦ Major Surgery Rules Apply

CPT CODE	SERVICE	ICD-9-CM
25505	Closed treatment of radial shaft fracture; with manipulation	813.21 Fx radius shaft, closed

REIMBURSEMENT INFORMATION

General

- ♦ See notes on page 286.

Medicare

- ♦ Follow-up Days — 90
- ♦ Assistant Surgeon — not paid
- ♦ Supply Charges — not allowed
- ♦ Outpatient Limit — does not apply
- ♦ Major Surgery Rules Apply

CPT CODE	SERVICE	ICD-9-CM
25515	Open treatment of radial shaft fracture, with or without internal or external fixation	813.21 Fx radius shaft, closed 813.31 Fx radius shaft, open **REIMBURSEMENT INFORMATION** General ◆ See notes on page 286. Medicare ◆ Follow-up Days — 90 ◆ Assistant Surgeon — paid ◆ Supply Charges — not allowed ◆ Outpatient Limit — does not apply ◆ Major Surgery Rules Apply
25520	Closed treatment of radial shaft fracture, with dislocation of distal radioulnar joint (Galeazzi fracture/dislocation)	813.21 Fx radius shaft, closed 813.31 Fx radius shaft, open **REIMBURSEMENT INFORMATION** General ◆ See notes on page 286. Medicare ◆ Follow-up Days — 90 ◆ Assistant Surgeon — paid ◆ Supply Charges — not allowed ◆ Outpatient Limit — does not apply ◆ Major Surgery Rules Apply
25525	Open treatment of radial shaft fracture, with internal and/or external fixation and closed treatment of dislocation of distal radioulnar joint (Galeazzi fracture/dislocation), with or without percutaneous skeletal fixation	813.21 Fx radius shaft, closed 813.31 Fx radius shaft, open **REIMBURSEMENT INFORMATION** General ◆ See notes on page 286. Medicare ◆ Follow-up Days — 90 ◆ Assistant Surgeon — paid ◆ Supply Charges — not allowed ◆ Outpatient Limit — does not apply ◆ Major Surgery Rules Apply

CPT CODE	SERVICE	ICD-9-CM
25526	Open treatment of radial shaft fracture, with internal and/or external fixation and open treatment, with or without internal or external fixation of distal radioulnar joint (Galeazzi fracture/dislocation), includes repair of triangular cartilage	813.21 Fx radius shaft, closed 813.31 Fx radius shaft, open **REIMBURSEMENT INFORMATION** General ♦ See notes on page 286. Medicare ♦ Follow-up Days — 90 ♦ Assistant Surgeon — paid ♦ Supply Charges — not allowed ♦ Outpatient Limit — does not apply ♦ Major Surgery Rules Apply
25530 **25535**	Closed treatment of ulnar shaft fracture; without manipulation Closed treatment of ulnar shaft fracture; with manipulation	813.22 Fx ulna shaft, closed 813.32 Fx ulna shaft, open **REIMBURSEMENT INFORMATION** General ♦ See notes on page 286. Medicare ♦ Follow-up Days — 90 ♦ Assistant Surgeon — not paid ♦ Supply Charges — not allowed ♦ Outpatient Limit 25530 — applies 25535 — does not apply ♦ Major Surgery Rules Apply
25545	Open treatment of ulnar shaft fracture, with or without internal or external fixation	813.22 Fx ulna shaft, closed 813.32 Fx ulna shaft, open **REIMBURSEMENT INFORMATION** General ♦ See notes on page 286. Medicare ♦ Follow-up Days — 90 ♦ Assistant Surgeon — paid ♦ Supply Charges — not allowed ♦ Outpatient Limit — does not apply ♦ Major Surgery Rules Apply

CPT CODE	SERVICE	ICD-9-CM
25560	Closed treatment of radial and ulnar shaft fractures; without manipulation	813.23 Fx shaft radius w/ulna, closed 813.33 Fx shaft radius w/ulna, open
25565	Closed treatment of radial and ulnar shaft fractures; with manipulation	**REIMBURSEMENT INFORMATION** General ◆ See notes on page 286. Medicare ◆ Follow-up Days — 90 ◆ Assistant Surgeon — not paid ◆ Supply Charges — not allowed ◆ Outpatient Limit — does not apply ◆ Major Surgery Rules Apply
25574	Open treatment of radial and ulnar shaft fractures, with internal or external fixation; of radius OR ulna	813.21 Fx radius shaft, closed 813.22 Fx ulna shaft, closed 813.31 Fx radius shaft, open 813.32 Fx ulna shaft, open **REIMBURSEMENT INFORMATION** General ◆ See notes on page 286. Medicare ◆ Follow-up Days — 90 ◆ Assistant Surgeon — paid ◆ Supply Charges — not allowed ◆ Outpatient Limit — does not apply ◆ Major Surgery Rules Apply
25575	Open treatment of radial and ulnar shaft fractures, with internal or external fixation; of radius AND ulna	813.23 Fx shaft radius w/ulna, closed 813.33 Fx shaft radius w/ulna, open **REIMBURSEMENT INFORMATION** General ◆ See notes on page 286. Medicare ◆ Follow-up Days — 90 ◆ Assistant Surgeon — paid ◆ Supply Charges — not allowed ◆ Outpatient Limit — does not apply ◆ Major Surgery Rules Apply

CPT CODE	SERVICE	ICD–9–CM
25600	Closed treatment of distal radial fracture (eg, Colles or Smith type) or epiphyseal separation, with or without fracture of ulnar styloid; without manipulation	813.40 Fx lower forearm NOS, closed 813.41 Colles' fracture, closed 813.42 Fx distal radius NEC, closed 813.43 Fx distal ulna, closed 813.44 Fx lower radius w/ulna, closed 813.50 Fx lower forearm NOS, open 813.51 Colles' fracture, open **REIMBURSEMENT INFORMATION** General ◆ See notes on page 286. Medicare ◆ Follow–up Days — 90 ◆ Assistant Surgeon — not paid ◆ Supply Charges — not allowed ◆ Outpatient Limit — applies ◆ Major Surgery Rules Apply ◆ Fragments — 29125
25605	Closed treatment of distal radial fracture (eg, Colles or Smith type) or epiphyseal separation, with or without fracture of ulnar styloid; with manipulation	813.40 Fx lower forearm NOS, closed 813.41 Colles' fracture, closed 813.42 Fx distal radius NEC, closed 813.43 Fx distal ulna, closed 813.44 Fx lower radius w/ulna, closed 813.50 Fx lower forearm NOS, open 813.51 Colles' fracture, open **REIMBURSEMENT INFORMATION** General ◆ See notes on page 286. Medicare ◆ Follow–up Days — 90 ◆ Assistant Surgeon — not paid ◆ Supply Charges — not allowed ◆ Outpatient Limit — does not apply ◆ Major Surgery Rules Apply ◆ Fragments — 25600, 29075, 29125

CPT CODE	SERVICE	ICD–9–CM
25611	Percutaneous skeletal fixation of distal radial fracture (eg, Colles or Smith type) or epiphyseal separation, with or without fracture of ulnar styloid, requiring manipulation, with or without external fixation	813.40 Fx lower forearm NOS, closed 813.41 Colles' fracture, closed 813.42 Fx distal radius NEC, closed 813.43 Fx distal ulna, closed 813.44 Fx lower radius w/ulna, closed 813.50 Fx lower forearm NOS, open 813.51 Colles' fracture, open **REIMBURSEMENT INFORMATION** General ◆ See notes on page 286. Medicare ◆ Follow–up Days — 90 ◆ Assistant Surgeon — not paid ◆ Supply Charges — not allowed ◆ Outpatient Limit — does not apply ◆ Major Surgery Rules Apply
25620	Open treatment of distal radial fracture (eg, Colles or Smith type) or epiphyseal separation, with or without fracture of ulnar styloid, with or without internal or external fixation	813.40 Fx lower forearm NOS, closed 813.41 Colles' fracture, closed 813.42 Fx distal radius NEC, closed 813.43 Fx distal ulna, closed 813.44 Fx lower radius w/ulna, closed 813.50 Fx lower forearm NOS, open 813.51 Colles' fracture, open **REIMBURSEMENT INFORMATION** General ◆ See notes on page 286. Medicare ◆ Follow–up Days — 90 ◆ Assistant Surgeon — paid ◆ Supply Charges — not allowed ◆ Outpatient Limit — does not apply ◆ Major Surgery Rules Apply

CPT CODE	SERVICE	ICD-9-CM
25622	Closed treatment of carpal scaphoid (navicular) fracture; without manipulation	814.01 Fx navicular, wrist, closed 814.11 Fx navicular, wrist, open
25624	Closed treatment of carpal scaphoid (navicular) fracture; with manipulation	

REIMBURSEMENT INFORMATION

General

- ♦ See notes on page 286.

Medicare

- ♦ Follow-up Days — 90
- ♦ Assistant Surgeon — not paid
- ♦ Supply Charges — not allowed
- ♦ Outpatient Limit — applies
- ♦ Major Surgery Rules Apply

CPT CODE	SERVICE	ICD-9-CM
25628	Open treatment of carpal scaphoid (navicular) fracture, with or without internal or external fixation	814.01 Fx navicular, wrist, closed 814.11 Fx navicular, wrist, open

REIMBURSEMENT INFORMATION

General

- ♦ See notes on page 286.

Medicare

- ♦ Follow-up Days — 90
- ♦ Assistant Surgeon — paid
- ♦ Supply Charges — not allowed
- ♦ Outpatient Limit — does not apply
- ♦ Major Surgery Rules Apply

CPT CODE	SERVICE	ICD–9–CM
25630	Closed treatment of carpal bone fracture (excluding carpal scaphoid (navicular)); without manipulation, each bone	814.00 Fx carpal bone NOS, closed 814.02 Fx lunate bone, wrist, closed 814.03 Fx triquetral bone, wrist, closed 814.04 Fx pisiform, closed 814.05 Fx trapezium bone, closed 814.06 Fx trapezoid bone, closed 814.07 Fx capitate bone, closed 814.08 Fx hamate bone, closed 814.09 Fx carpal bone NEC, closed 814.10 Fx carpal bone NOS, open 814.12 Fx lunate bone, wrist, open 814.13 Fx triquetral bone, wrist, open 814.14 Fx pisiform, open 814.15 Fx trapezium bone, open 814.16 Fx trapezoid bone, open 814.17 Fx capitate bone, open 814.18 Fx hamate bone, open 814.19 Fx carpal bone NEC, open
25635	Closed treatment of carpal bone fracture (excluding carpal scaphoid (navicular)); with manipulation, each bone	

REIMBURSEMENT INFORMATION

General

- See notes on page 286.

Medicare

- Follow–up Days — 90
- Assistant Surgeon — not paid
- Supply Charges — not allowed
- Outpatient Limit — applies
- Major Surgery Rules Apply

CPT CODE	SERVICE	ICD-9-CM	
25645	Open treatment of carpal bone fracture (excluding carpal scaphoid (navicular)), each bone	814.00	Fx carpal bone NOS, closed
		814.02	Fx lunate bone, wrist, closed
		814.03	Fx triquetral bone, wrist, closed
		814.04	Fx pisiform, closed
		814.05	Fx trapezium bone, closed
		814.06	Fx trapezoid bone, closed
		814.07	Fx capitate bone, closed
		814.08	Fx hamate bone, closed
		814.09	Fx carpal bone NEC, closed
		814.10	Fx carpal bone NOS, open
		814.12	Fx lunate bone, wrist, open
		814.13	Fx triquetral bone, wrist, open
		814.14	Fx pisiform, open
		814.15	Fx trapezium bone, open
		814.16	Fx trapezoid bone, open
		814.17	Fx capitate bone, open
		814.18	Fx hamate bone, open
		814.19	Fx carpal bone NEC, open

REIMBURSEMENT INFORMATION

General

- See notes on page 286.

Medicare

- Follow-up Days — 90
- Assistant Surgeon — paid
- Supply Charges — not allowed
- Outpatient Limit — does not apply
- Major Surgery Rules Apply

CPT CODE	SERVICE	ICD–9–CM
25650	Closed treatment of ulnar styloid fracture	813.43 Fx distal ulna, closed

REIMBURSEMENT INFORMATION

General

- See notes on page 286.

Medicare

- Follow–up Days — 90
- Assistant Surgeon — not paid
- Supply Charges — not allowed
- Outpatient Limit — applies
- Major Surgery Rules Apply

CPT CODE	SERVICE	ICD–9–CM
25660	Closed treatment of radiocarpal or intercarpal dislocation, one or more bones, with manipulation	833.02 Disloc radiocarpal, closed 833.03 Disloc midcarpal, closed 833.04 Disloc carpometacarpal, closed 833.05 Disloc metacarpal, closed 833.12 Disloc radiocarpal, open 833.13 Disloc midcarpal, open 833.14 Disloc carpometacarpal, open 833.15 Disloc metacarpal, open

REIMBURSEMENT INFORMATION

General

- See notes on page 286.

Medicare

- Follow–up Days — 90
- Assistant Surgeon — not paid
- Supply Charges — not allowed
- Outpatient Limit — does not apply
- Major Surgery Rules Apply

CPT CODE	SERVICE	ICD-9-CM
25670	Open treatment of radiocarpal or intercarpal dislocation, one or more bones	833.02 Disloc radiocarpal, closed 833.03 Disloc midcarpal, closed 833.04 Disloc carpometacarpal, closed 833.05 Disloc metacarpal, closed 833.12 Disloc radiocarpal, open 833.13 Disloc midcarpal, open 833.14 Disloc carpometacarpal, open 833.15 Disloc metacarpal, open **REIMBURSEMENT INFORMATION** General ♦ See notes on page 286. Medicare ♦ Follow–up Days — 90 ♦ Assistant Surgeon — paid ♦ Supply Charges — not allowed ♦ Outpatient Limit — does not apply ♦ Major Surgery Rules Apply
25675	Closed treatment of distal radioulnar dislocation with manipulation	833.01 Disloc distal radioulnar, closed **REIMBURSEMENT INFORMATION** General ♦ See notes on page 286. Medicare ♦ Follow–up Days — 90 ♦ Assistant Surgeon — by report ♦ Supply Charges — not allowed ♦ Outpatient Limit — does not apply ♦ Major Surgery Rules Apply
25676	Open treatment of distal radioulnar dislocation, acute or chronic	833.01 Disloc distal radioulnar, closed 833.11 Disloc distal radioulnar, open **REIMBURSEMENT INFORMATION** General ♦ See notes on page 286. Medicare ♦ Follow–up Days — 90 ♦ Assistant Surgeon — paid ♦ Supply Charges — not allowed ♦ Outpatient Limit — does not apply ♦ Major Surgery Rules Apply

CPT CODE	SERVICE	ICD-9-CM
25680	Closed treatment of trans-scaphoperilunar type of fracture dislocation, with manipulation	814.01 Fx navicular, wrist, closed 814.02 Fx lunate bone, wrist, closed 833.00 Dislocation wrist NOS, closed 833.03 Disloc midcarpal, closed

REIMBURSEMENT INFORMATION

General

- ♦ See notes on page 286.

Medicare

- ♦ Follow–up Days — 90
- ♦ Assistant Surgeon — by report
- ♦ Supply Charges — not allowed
- ♦ Outpatient Limit — does not apply
- ♦ Major Surgery Rules Apply

CPT CODE	SERVICE	ICD-9-CM
25685	Open treatment of trans-scaphoperilunar type of fracture dislocation	814.01 Fx navicular, wrist, closed 814.02 Fx lunate bone, wrist, closed 814.11 Fx navicular, wrist, open 814.12 Fx lunate bone, wrist, open 833.00 Dislocation wrist NOS, closed 833.03 Disloc midcarpal, closed 833.10 Dislocation wrist NOS, open 833.13 Disloc midcarpal, open

REIMBURSEMENT INFORMATION

General

- ♦ See notes on page 286.

Medicare

- ♦ Follow–up Days — 90
- ♦ Assistant Surgeon — paid
- ♦ Supply Charges — not allowed
- ♦ Outpatient Limit — does not apply
- ♦ Major Surgery Rules Apply

CPT CODE	SERVICE	ICD-9-CM
25690	Closed treatment of lunate dislocation, with manipulation	833.00 Dislocation wrist NOS, closed 833.03 Disloc midcarpal, closed 833.10 Dislocation wrist NOS, open

REIMBURSEMENT INFORMATION

General

- ♦ See notes on page 286.

Medicare

- ♦ Follow-up Days — 90
- ♦ Assistant Surgeon — by report
- ♦ Supply Charges — not allowed
- ♦ Outpatient Limit — does not apply
- ♦ Major Surgery Rules Apply

CPT CODE	SERVICE	ICD-9-CM
25695	Open treatment of lunate dislocation	833.00 Dislocation wrist NOS, closed 833.03 Disloc midcarpal, closed 833.10 Dislocation wrist NOS, open 833.13 Disloc midcarpal, open

REIMBURSEMENT INFORMATION

General

- ♦ See notes on page 286.

Medicare

- ♦ Follow-up Days — 90
- ♦ Assistant Surgeon — paid
- ♦ Supply Charges — not allowed
- ♦ Outpatient Limit — does not apply
- ♦ Major Surgery Rules Apply

CPT CODE	SERVICE
25800	Arthrodesis, wrist joint (including radiocarpal and/or ulnocarpal fusion); without bone graft
25805	Arthrodesis, wrist joint (including radiocarpal and/or ulnocarpal fusion); with sliding graft
25810	Arthrodesis, wrist joint (including radiocarpal and/or ulnocarpal fusion); with iliac or other autograft (includes obtaining graft)

ICD–9–CM

138.	Late effects of acute polio
711.03	Pyogenic arthritis, forearm
711.93	Infect arthritis NOS, forearm
714.0	Rheumatoid arthritis
714.3x	Juvenile chronic polyarthritis
714.4	Chronic postrheumatic arthritis
715.13	Loc prim osteoarthritis, forearm
715.23	Loc 2nd osteoarthritis, forearm
715.33	Loc osteoarthritis NOS, forearm
715.93	Osteoarthrosis NOS, forearm
716.03	Kaschin-Beck disease, forearm
716.13	Traumatic arthropathy, forearm
716.23	Allergic arthritis, forearm
716.33	Climacteric arthritis, forearm
716.43	Transient arthropathy, forearm
718.03	Articular cartilage dis, forearm
718.23	Pathologic dislocation, forearm
718.33	Recurrent dislocation, forearm
730.13	Chronic osteomyelitis, forearm
733.82	Nonunion of fracture
813.4x	Fracture of radius/ulna, lower end
813.5x	Fracture of radius/ulna, lower end
905.2	Late effect, arm fracture
906.4	Late effect of crushing
996.4	Malfunction, int orthoped dev/graft
996.66	Reaction, internal joint prosthesis
996.67	Reaction, internal ortho device NEC
996.77	Complication, int joint prosthesis

REIMBURSEMENT INFORMATION

General

- See notes on page 286.

Medicare

- Follow–up Days — 90
- Assistant Surgeon — paid
- Supply Charges — not allowed
- Outpatient Limit — does not apply
- Major Surgery Rules Apply

CPT CODE	SERVICE
25820	Intercarpal fusion; without bone graft
25825	Intercarpal fusion; with autograft (includes obtaining graft)

ICD–9–CM

711.03	Pyogenic arthritis, forearm
711.93	Infect arthritis NOS, forearm
714.0	Rheumatoid arthritis
714.3x	Juvenile chronic polyarthritis
714.4	Chronic postrheumatic arthritis
715.13	Loc prim osteoarthritis, forearm
715.23	Loc 2nd osteoarthritis, forearm
715.33	Loc osteoarthritis NOS, forearm
715.93	Osteoarthrosis NOS, forearm
716.03	Kaschin-Beck disease, forearm
716.13	Traumatic arthropathy, forearm
716.23	Allergic arthritis, forearm
716.33	Climacteric arthritis, forearm
716.43	Transient arthropathy, forearm
718.03	Articular cartilage dis, forearm
718.23	Pathologic dislocation, forearm
718.33	Recurrent dislocation, forearm
730.13	Chronic osteomyelitis, forearm
733.82	Nonunion of fracture
813.4x	Fracture of radius/ulna, lower end
813.5x	Fracture of radius/ulna, lower end
814.0x	Carpal fracture, closed
814.1x	Carpal fracture, open
833.0x	Wrist dislocation, closed
833.1x	Wrist dislocation, open
905.2	Late effect, arm fracture
905.6	Late effect of dislocation
906.4	Late effect of crushing
996.66	Reaction, internal joint prosthesis
996.67	Reaction, internal ortho device NEC

REIMBURSEMENT INFORMATION

General

- See notes on page 286.

Medicare

- Follow–up Days — 90
- Assistant Surgeon — paid
- Supply Charges — not allowed
- Outpatient Limit — does not apply
- Major Surgery Rules Apply

CPT CODE	SERVICE	ICD-9-CM
▲ 25830	Distal radioulnar joint arthrodesis and segmental resection of ulna (eg, Sauve-Kapandji procedure), with or without bone graft	714.0 Rheumatoid arthritis 716.93 Arthropathy NOS, forearm 728.4 Laxity of ligament 755.59 Upper limb anomaly NEC 756.83 Ehlers-Danlos syndrome 842.09 Sprain of wrist NEC

REIMBURSEMENT INFORMATION

General

- ♦ See notes on page 286.
- ♦ New procedure, 1995 CPT.

Medicare

- ♦ Follow–up Days — 90
- ♦ Assistant Surgeon — paid
- ♦ Supply Charges — not allowed
- ♦ Outpatient Limit — does not apply
- ♦ Major Surgery Rules Apply

CPT CODE	SERVICE	ICD-9-CM
25900	Amputation, forearm, through radius and ulna	170.4 M-Neoplasm, Long arm bones 198.5 M2-Neoplasm, Bone and bone marrow 238.0 UB-Neoplasm, Bone 239.2 Bone/Skin neoplasm NOS 682.3 Cellulitis of arm 682.4 Cellulitis of hand 728.0 Infective myositis 730.13 Chronic osteomyelitis, forearm 785.4 Gangrene 887.0 Amputation below elbow, unilateral 887.1 Amputation below elbow, unil, compl 927.10 Crushing injury, forearm
25905	Amputation, forearm, through radius and ulna; open, circular (guillotine)	

REIMBURSEMENT INFORMATION

General

- ♦ See notes on page 286.

Medicare

- ♦ Follow–up Days — 90
- ♦ Assistant Surgeon — paid
- ♦ Supply Charges — not allowed
- ♦ Outpatient Limit — does not apply
- ♦ Major Surgery Rules Apply

CPT CODE	SERVICE	ICD-9-CM	
25907	Amputation, forearm, through radius and ulna; secondary closure or scar revision	170.4	M-Neoplasm, Long arm bones
		198.5	M2-Neoplasm, Bone and bone marrow
		238.0	UB-Neoplasm, Bone
25909	Amputation, forearm, through radius and ulna; reamputation	239.2	Bone/Skin neoplasm NOS
		730.13	Chronic osteomyelitis, forearm
		733.49	Aseptic necrosis of bone NEC
		785.4	Gangrene
		887.0	Amputation below elbow, unilateral
		887.1	Amputation below elbow, unil, compl
		905.9	Late effect of traumatic amputation
		927.10	Crushing injury, forearm
		996.91	Complication, reattached forearm
		997.60	Late amputation stump complic NOS
		997.61	Neuroma of amputation stump
		997.62	Infection of amputated stump
		997.69	Late amputation stump complic NEC
		V58.41	Planned postoperative wound closure

REIMBURSEMENT INFORMATION

General

- ♦ See notes on page 286.

Medicare

- ♦ Follow–up Days — 90
- ♦ Assistant Surgeon — paid
- ♦ Supply Charges — not allowed
- ♦ Outpatient Limit — does not apply
- ♦ Major Surgery Rules Apply

CPT CODE	SERVICE	ICD-9-CM	
25915	Krukenberg procedure	369.00	Both eyes blind, WHO definition
		755.25	Longitudinal deficiency, radioulna
		887.6	Amputation of arm, bilateral
		887.7	Amputation of arm, bilateral, compl
		905.9	Late effect of traumatic amputation

REIMBURSEMENT INFORMATION

General

- ♦ See notes on page 286.

Medicare

- ♦ Follow–up Days — 90
- ♦ Assistant Surgeon — paid
- ♦ Supply Charges — not allowed
- ♦ Outpatient Limit — does not apply
- ♦ Major Surgery Rules Apply

CPT CODE	SERVICE
25920	Disarticulation through wrist

ICD–9–CM

170.5	M-Neoplasm, Wrist/Hand bones
198.5	M2-Neoplasm, Bone and bone marrow
238.0	UB-Neoplasm, Bone
239.2	Bone/Skin neoplasm NOS
443.0	Raynaud's syndrome
444.21	Upper extremity embolism
730.04	Acute osteomyelitis, hand
730.14	Chronic osteomyelitis, hand
733.49	Aseptic necrosis of bone NEC
785.4	Gangrene
887.0	Amputation below elbow, unilateral
887.1	Amputation below elbow, unil, compl
906.4	Late effect of crushing
927.2x	Crushing injury, wrist and hand

REIMBURSEMENT INFORMATION

General

- See notes on page 286.

Medicare

- Follow–up Days — 90
- Assistant Surgeon — paid
- Supply Charges — not allowed
- Outpatient Limit — does not apply
- Major Surgery Rules Apply

CPT CODE	SERVICE
25922	Disarticulation through wrist; secondary closure or scar revision
25924	Disarticulation through wrist; reamputation

ICD–9–CM

170.5	M-Neoplasm, Wrist/Hand bones
198.5	M2-Neoplasm, Bone and bone marrow
238.0	UB-Neoplasm, Bone
239.2	Bone/Skin neoplasm NOS
443.0	Raynaud's syndrome
444.21	Upper extremity embolism
730.04	Acute osteomyelitis, hand
730.14	Chronic osteomyelitis, hand
733.49	Aseptic necrosis of bone NEC
785.4	Gangrene
887.0	Amputation below elbow, unilateral
887.1	Amputation below elbow, unil, compl
906.4	Late effect of crushing
927.10	Crushing injury, forearm
927.2x	Crushing injury, wrist and hand
996.91	Complication, reattached forearm
997.60	Late amputation stump complic NOS
997.61	Neuroma of amputation stump
997.62	Infection of amputated stump
997.69	Late amputation stump complic NEC

REIMBURSEMENT INFORMATION

General

- ♦ See notes on page 286.

Medicare

- ♦ Follow–up Days — 90
- ♦ Assistant Surgeon — paid
- ♦ Supply Charges — not allowed
- ♦ Outpatient Limit — does not apply
- ♦ Major Surgery Rules Apply

CPT CODE	SERVICE	ICD–9–CM	
25927	Transmetacarpal amputation	170.5	M-Neoplasm, Wrist/Hand bones
		198.5	M2-Neoplasm, Bone and bone marrow
		238.0	UB-Neoplasm, Bone
		239.2	Bone/Skin neoplasm NOS
		733.49	Aseptic necrosis of bone NEC
		785.4	Gangrene
		882.1	Open wound of hand, complicated
		887.0	Amputation below elbow, unilateral
		887.1	Amputation below elbow, unil, compl
		906.4	Late effect of crushing
		927.10	Crushing injury, forearm

REIMBURSEMENT INFORMATION

General

- See notes on page 286.

Medicare

- Follow–up Days — 90
- Assistant Surgeon — not paid
- Supply Charges — not allowed
- Outpatient Limit — does not apply
- Major Surgery Rules Apply

CPT CODE	SERVICE
25929	Transmetacarpal amputation; secondary closure or scar revision
25931	Transmetacarpal amputation; reamputation

ICD–9–CM

170.5	M-Neoplasm, Wrist/Hand bones
198.5	M2-Neoplasm, Bone and bone marrow
238.0	UB-Neoplasm, Bone
239.2	Bone/Skin neoplasm NOS
730.13	Chronic osteomyelitis, forearm
733.49	Aseptic necrosis of bone NEC
785.4	Gangrene
887.0	Amputation below elbow, unilateral
887.1	Amputation below elbow, unil, compl
906.4	Late effect of crushing
927.10	Crushing injury, forearm
996.91	Complication, reattached forearm
997.60	Late amputation stump complic NOS
997.61	Neuroma of amputation stump
997.62	Infection of amputated stump
997.69	Late amputation stump complic NEC

REIMBURSEMENT INFORMATION

General

- See notes on page 286.

Medicare

- Follow–up Days — 90
- Assistant Surgeon — paid
- Supply Charges — not allowed
- Outpatient Limit — does not apply
- Major Surgery Rules Apply

CPT CODE	SERVICE	ICD–9–CM
26010*	Drainage of finger abscess; simple	681.0x Cellulitis and abscess, finger 906.1 Late effect, open wound extremity 909.3 Late effect of surg/med complic 923.3 Contusion of finger 927.3 Crushing injury, finger
26011*	Drainage of finger abscess; complicated (eg, felon, etc)	

REIMBURSEMENT INFORMATION

General

- ♦ See notes on page 286.
- ♦ Starred procedure.

Medicare

- ♦ Follow–up Days — 10
- ♦ Assistant Surgeon — not paid
- ♦ Supply Charges — not allowed
- ♦ Outpatient Limit — applies
- ♦ Minor Surgery Rules Apply

CPT CODE	SERVICE	ICD–9–CM
26020	Drainage of tendon sheath, one digit and/or palm	681.00 Cellulitis, finger NOS 726.4 Enthesopathy of wrist/carpus 727.2 Occupational bursitis 727.3 Bursitis NOS 727.4x Ganglion/cyst synovium/tendon/bursa 727.89 Synovium/tendon/bursa disorder NEC 906.1 Late effect, open wound extremity 906.3 Late effect of contusion 906.4 Late effect of crushing 909.3 Late effect of surg/med complic

REIMBURSEMENT INFORMATION

General

- ♦ See notes on page 286.

Medicare

- ♦ Follow–up Days — 90
- ♦ Assistant Surgeon — not paid
- ♦ Supply Charges — not allowed
- ♦ Outpatient Limit — does not apply
- ♦ Major Surgery Rules Apply

CPT CODE	SERVICE	ICD-9-CM	
26025	Drainage of palmar bursa; single, ulnar or radial	682.4	Cellulitis of hand
		711.04	Pyogenic arthritis, hand
26030	Drainage of palmar bursa; multiple or complicated	711.94	Infect arthritis NOS, hand
		726.4	Enthesopathy of wrist/carpus
		727.2	Occupational bursitis
		727.3	Bursitis NOS
		727.4x	Ganglion/cyst synovium/tendon/bursa
		727.89	Synovium/tendon/bursa disorder NEC
		906.1	Late effect, open wound extremity
		906.3	Late effect of contusion
		906.4	Late effect of crushing
		909.3	Late effect of surg/med complic
		923.20	Contusion of hand(s)
		927.20	Crushing injury, hand
		927.8	Multiple crushing injuries, arm

REIMBURSEMENT INFORMATION

General

- ♦ See notes on page 286.

Medicare

- ♦ Follow–up Days — 90
- ♦ Assistant Surgeon — not paid
- ♦ Supply Charges — not allowed
- ♦ Outpatient Limit — does not apply
- ♦ Major Surgery Rules Apply

CPT CODE	SERVICE	ICD-9-CM	
26034	Incision, deep, with opening of bone cortex (eg, for osteomyelitis or bone abscess), hand or finger	730.04	Acute osteomyelitis, hand
		730.14	Chronic osteomyelitis, hand
		730.94	Bone infection NOS, hand

REIMBURSEMENT INFORMATION

General

- ♦ See notes on page 286.

Medicare

- ♦ Follow–up Days — 90
- ♦ Assistant Surgeon — not paid
- ♦ Supply Charges — not allowed
- ♦ Outpatient Limit — does not apply
- ♦ Major Surgery Rules Apply

CPT CODE	SERVICE	ICD-9-CM
26035	Decompression fingers and/or hand, injection injury (eg, grease gun, etc)	727.89 Synovium/tendon/bursa disorder NEC 882.1 Open wound of hand, complicated 883.1 Open wound of finger, complicated

REIMBURSEMENT INFORMATION

General

- ♦ See notes on page 286.

Medicare

- ♦ Follow-up Days — 90
- ♦ Assistant Surgeon — not paid
- ♦ Supply Charges — not allowed
- ♦ Outpatient Limit — does not apply
- ♦ Major Surgery Rules Apply

26037 Decompressive fasciotomy, hand (excludes 26035)

CPT NOTES

- ♦ For injection injury, see 26035.

ICD-9-CM	
814.0x	Carpal fracture, closed
814.1x	Carpal fracture, open
815.0x	Metacarpal fracture, closed
815.1x	Metacarpal fracture, open
833.0x	Wrist dislocation, closed
833.1x	Wrist dislocation, open
882.x	Open wound of hand
927.20	Crushing injury, hand
958.5	Traumatic anuria
958.6	Volkmann's ischemic contracture
989.5	Toxic effect of venom
996.66	Reaction, internal joint prosthesis
996.77	Complication, int joint prosthesis
998.5	Postoperative infection

REIMBURSEMENT INFORMATION

General

- ♦ See notes on page 286.

Medicare

- ♦ Follow-up Days — 90
- ♦ Assistant Surgeon — not paid
- ♦ Supply Charges — not allowed
- ♦ Outpatient Limit — does not apply
- ♦ Major Surgery Rules Apply

CPT CODE	SERVICE	ICD-9-CM
26040	Fasciotomy, palmar, for Dupuytren's contracture; closed (subcutaneous)	728.6 Contracture of palmar fascia
26045	Fasciotomy, palmar, for Dupuytren's contracture; open, partial	

CPT NOTES

- For fasciectomy, see 26121-26125.

REIMBURSEMENT INFORMATION

General

- See notes on page 286.

Medicare

- Follow-up Days — 90
- Assistant Surgeon — not paid
- Supply Charges — not allowed
- Outpatient Limit — does not apply
- Major Surgery Rules Apply

CPT CODE	SERVICE	ICD-9-CM
▲ **26055**	Tendon sheath incision (eg, for trigger finger)	727.03 Trigger finger 756.89 Congenital soft tissue anomaly NEC

REIMBURSEMENT INFORMATION

General

- See notes on page 286.
- Description changed in 1995 CPT.

Medicare

- Follow-up Days — 90
- Assistant Surgeon — not paid
- Supply Charges — not allowed
- Outpatient Limit — does not apply
- Major Surgery Rules Apply
- Fragments — 29125

CPT CODE	SERVICE	ICD–9–CM	
26060	Tenotomy, subcutaneous, single, each digit	344.00	Quadriplegia NOS
		434.00	Cerebral thrombosis
		727.81	Contracture of tendon
		728.85	Spasm of muscle
		736.06	Claw hand
		736.07	Club hand, acquired
		736.20	Acquired finger deformity NOS
		736.29	Acquired finger deformity NEC

REIMBURSEMENT INFORMATION

General

- ♦ See notes on page 286.

Medicare

- ♦ Follow–up Days — 90
- ♦ Assistant Surgeon — not paid
- ♦ Supply Charges — not allowed
- ♦ Outpatient Limit — does not apply
- ♦ Major Surgery Rules Apply

CPT CODE	SERVICE
26070	Arthrotomy, for infection, with exploration, drainage or removal of foreign body; carpometacarpal joint
26075	Arthrotomy, for infection, with exploration, drainage or removal of foreign body; metacarpophalangeal joint
26080	Arthrotomy, for infection, with exploration, drainage or removal of foreign body; interphalangeal joint, each

ICD–9–CM

277.5	Mucopolysaccharidosis
711.04	Pyogenic arthritis, hand
711.94	Infect arthritis NOS, hand
712.14	Dicalc phosphate cryst, hand
714.0	Rheumatoid arthritis
714.30	Juvenile rheumatoid arthritis NOS
714.31	Juvenile acute rheumatoid arthritis
714.32	Pauciarticular juv rheum arthritis
714.33	Monoarticular juv rheum arthritis
714.4	Chronic postrheumatic arthritis
715.14	Loc prim osteoarthritis, hand
715.24	Loc 2nd osteoarthritis, hand
715.34	Loc osteoarthritis NOS, hand
716.14	Traumatic arthropathy, hand
718.14	Loose body in joint, hand
719.04	Joint effusion, hand
719.14	Hemarthrosis, hand
719.24	Villonodular synovitis, hand
727.00	Synovitis NOS
727.05	Tenosynovitis of hand/wrist NEC
729.6	Old foreign body in soft tissue
730.04	Acute osteomyelitis, hand
730.14	Chronic osteomyelitis, hand
730.24	Osteomyelitis NOS, hand
732.3	Juvenile osteochondrosis, arm
882.1	Open wound of hand, complicated
914.7	Foreign body, hand, infected
996.66	Reaction, internal joint prosthesis
998.4	Foreign body left during procedure
998.5	Postoperative infection

REIMBURSEMENT INFORMATION

General

- See notes on page 286.

Medicare

- Follow–up Days — 90
- Assistant Surgeon — not paid
- Supply Charges — not allowed
- Outpatient Limit — does not apply
- Major Surgery Rules Apply

CPT CODE	SERVICE
▲ **26100**	Arthrotomy with synovial biopsy; carpometacarpal joint

ICD–9–CM

170.5	M-Neoplasm, Wrist/Hand bones
171.2	M-Neoplasm, Soft tissue, arm
198.89	M2-Neoplasm NEC
215.2	B-Neoplasm, Soft tissue, arm
238.1	UB-Neoplasm, Soft tissue
239.2	Bone/Skin neoplasm NOS
277.5	Mucopolysaccharidosis
712.14	Dicalc phosphate cryst, hand
714.0	Rheumatoid arthritis
714.30	Juvenile rheumatoid arthritis NOS
714.31	Juvenile acute rheumatoid arthritis
714.32	Pauciarticular juv rheum arthritis
714.33	Monoarticular juv rheum arthritis
714.4	Chronic postrheumatic arthritis
719.04	Joint effusion, hand
719.14	Hemarthrosis, hand
719.24	Villonodular synovitis, hand
727.00	Synovitis NOS
727.05	Tenosynovitis of hand/wrist NEC
729.6	Old foreign body in soft tissue
732.3	Juvenile osteochondrosis, arm
914.7	Foreign body, hand, infected
996.66	Reaction, internal joint prosthesis
998.4	Foreign body left during procedure

REIMBURSEMENT INFORMATION

General

- See notes on page 286.
- Description changed in 1995 CPT.

Medicare

- Follow–up Days — 90
- Assistant Surgeon — not paid
- Supply Charges — not allowed
- Outpatient Limit — does not apply
- Major Surgery Rules Apply

CPT CODE	SERVICE	ICD–9–CM	
26105	Arthrotomy with synovial biopsy; metacarpophalangeal joint	170.5	M-Neoplasm, Wrist/Hand bones
		171.2	M-Neoplasm, Soft tissue, arm
		198.89	M2-Neoplasm NEC
		215.2	B-Neoplasm, Soft tissue, arm
		238.1	UB-Neoplasm, Soft tissue
		239.2	Bone/Skin neoplasm NOS
		277.5	Mucopolysaccharidosis
		712.14	Dicalc phosphate cryst, hand
		714.0	Rheumatoid arthritis
		714.30	Juvenile rheumatoid arthritis NOS
		714.31	Juvenile acute rheumatoid arthritis
		714.32	Pauciarticular juv rheum arthritis
		714.33	Monoarticular juv rheum arthritis
		714.4	Chronic postrheumatic arthritis
		719.04	Joint effusion, hand
		719.14	Hemarthrosis, hand
		719.24	Villonodular synovitis, hand
		727.00	Synovitis NOS
		727.05	Tenosynovitis of hand/wrist NEC
		727.4	Ganglion/cyst synovium/tendon/bursa
		729.6	Old foreign body in soft tissue
		732.3	Juvenile osteochondrosis, arm
		914.7	Foreign body, hand, infected
		996.66	Reaction, internal joint prosthesis
		998.4	Foreign body left during procedure

REIMBURSEMENT INFORMATION

General

- See notes on page 286.

Medicare

- Follow–up Days — 90
- Assistant Surgeon — by report
- Supply Charges — not allowed
- Outpatient Limit — does not apply
- Major Surgery Rules Apply

CPT CODE	SERVICE	ICD-9-CM
26110	Arthrotomy with synovial biopsy; interphalangeal joint, each	170.5 M-Neoplasm, Wrist/Hand bones 171.2 M-Neoplasm, Soft tissue, arm 198.89 M2-Neoplasm NEC 215.2 B-Neoplasm, Soft tissue, arm 238.1 UB-Neoplasm, Soft tissue 239.2 Bone/Skin neoplasm NOS 714.0 Rheumatoid arthritis 719.04 Joint effusion, hand 719.24 Villonodular synovitis, hand 729.6 Old foreign body in soft tissue 732.3 Juvenile osteochondrosis, arm 914.7 Foreign body, hand, infected 996.66 Reaction, internal joint prosthesis 998.4 Foreign body left during procedure **REIMBURSEMENT INFORMATION** General ◆ See notes on page 286. Medicare ◆ Follow-up Days — 90 ◆ Assistant Surgeon — not paid ◆ Supply Charges — not allowed ◆ Outpatient Limit — does not apply ◆ Major Surgery Rules Apply
26115 **26116**	Excision, tumor or vascular malformation, hand or finger; subcutaneous Excision, tumor or vascular malformation, hand or finger; deep, subfascial, intramuscular	170.5 M-Neoplasm, Wrist/Hand bones 171.2 M-Neoplasm, Soft tissue, arm 198.89 M2-Neoplasm NEC 214.1 Lipoma, Skin NEC 215.2 B-Neoplasm, Soft tissue, arm 228.01 Hemangioma, Skin 228.1 Lymphangioma, any site 238.1 UB-Neoplasm, Soft tissue 239.2 Bone/Skin neoplasm NOS 442.0 Upper extremity artery aneurysm 747.6 Peripheral vascular anomaly NEC **REIMBURSEMENT INFORMATION** General ◆ See notes on page 286. Medicare ◆ Follow-up Days — 90 ◆ Assistant Surgeon — not paid ◆ Supply Charges — not allowed ◆ Outpatient Limit — does not apply ◆ Major Surgery Rules Apply

CPT CODE	SERVICE	ICD–9–CM
26117	Radical resection of tumor (eg, malignant neoplasm), soft tissue of hand or finger	171.2 M-Neoplasm, Soft tissue, arm 198.89 M2-Neoplasm NEC

REIMBURSEMENT INFORMATION

General

- See notes on page 286.

Medicare

- Follow–up Days — 90
- Assistant Surgeon — not paid
- Supply Charges — not allowed
- Outpatient Limit — does not apply
- Major Surgery Rules Apply

26121 Fasciectomy, palmar only, with or without z-plasty, other local tissue rearrangement, or skin grafting (includes obtaining graft);

26123 Fasciectomy, palmar only, with or without z-plasty, other local tissue rearrangement, or skin grafting (includes obtaining graft); partial palmar excision with release of single digit including proximal interphalangeal joint

26125 Fasciectomy, palmar only, with or without z-plasty, other local tissue rearrangement, or skin grafting (includes obtaining graft); partial palmar excision with release of each additional digit, including proximal interphalangeal joint

CPT NOTES

- For fasciotomy, see 26040, 26045.

718.44 Contracture of joint, hand
728.6 Contracture of palmar fascia
958.8 Early complications of trauma NEC

REIMBURSEMENT INFORMATION

General

- See notes on page 286.

Medicare

- Follow–up Days
  26121–26123 — 90
  26125 — none; falls within global period of another procedure
- Assistant Surgeon — not paid
- Supply Charges — not allowed
- Outpatient Limit — does not apply
- Major Surgery Rules Apply

CPT CODE	SERVICE	ICD–9–CM	
26130	Synovectomy, carpometacarpal joint	170.5	M-Neoplasm, Wrist/Hand bones
		171.2	M-Neoplasm, Soft tissue, arm
		198.89	M2-Neoplasm NEC
		215.2	B-Neoplasm, Soft tissue, arm
		238.1	UB-Neoplasm, Soft tissue
		239.2	Bone/Skin neoplasm NOS
		711.04	Pyogenic arthritis, hand
		711.94	Infect arthritis NOS, hand
		714.0	Rheumatoid arthritis
		714.30	Juvenile rheumatoid arthritis NOS
		714.31	Juvenile acute rheumatoid arthritis
		714.32	Pauciarticular juv rheum arthritis
		714.33	Monoarticular juv rheum arthritis
		714.4	Chronic postrheumatic arthritis
		715.14	Loc prim osteoarthritis, hand
		715.24	Loc 2nd osteoarthritis, hand
		715.34	Loc osteoarthritis NOS, hand
		716.14	Traumatic arthropathy, hand
		718.14	Loose body in joint, hand
		719.04	Joint effusion, hand
		719.24	Villonodular synovitis, hand
		727.00	Synovitis NOS
		727.02	Giant cell tumor of tendon sheath
		727.03	Trigger finger
		727.04	Radial styloid tenosynovitis
		727.05	Tenosynovitis of hand/wrist NEC
		729.6	Old foreign body in soft tissue
		730.04	Acute osteomyelitis, hand
		730.14	Chronic osteomyelitis, hand
		730.24	Osteomyelitis NOS, hand
		732.3	Juvenile osteochondrosis, arm
		882.1	Open wound of hand, complicated
		914.7	Foreign body, hand, infected
		996.66	Reaction, internal joint prosthesis
		998.4	Foreign body left during procedure
		998.5	Postoperative infection

REIMBURSEMENT INFORMATION

General

- See notes on page 286.

Medicare

- Follow–up Days — 90
- Assistant Surgeon — not paid
- Supply Charges — not allowed
- Outpatient Limit — does not apply
- Major Surgery Rules Apply

CPT CODE	SERVICE	ICD-9-CM	
26140	Synovectomy, proximal interphalangeal joint, including extensor reconstruction, each interphalangeal joint	170.5	M-Neoplasm, Wrist/Hand bones
		171.2	M-Neoplasm, Soft tissue, arm
		198.89	M2-Neoplasm NEC
		215.2	B-Neoplasm, Soft tissue, arm
		238.1	UB-Neoplasm, Soft tissue
		239.2	Bone/Skin neoplasm NOS
		711.04	Pyogenic arthritis, hand
		711.94	Infect arthritis NOS, hand
		714.0	Rheumatoid arthritis
		714.30	Juvenile rheumatoid arthritis NOS
		714.31	Juvenile acute rheumatoid arthritis
		714.32	Pauciarticular juv rheum arthritis
		714.33	Monoarticular juv rheum arthritis
		714.4	Chronic postrheumatic arthritis
		715.14	Loc prim osteoarthritis, hand
		715.24	Loc 2nd osteoarthritis, hand
		715.34	Loc osteoarthritis NOS, hand
		716.14	Traumatic arthropathy, hand
		718.14	Loose body in joint, hand
		719.04	Joint effusion, hand
		719.24	Villonodular synovitis, hand
		727.00	Synovitis NOS
		727.02	Giant cell tumor of tendon sheath
		727.03	Trigger finger
		727.04	Radial styloid tenosynovitis
		727.05	Tenosynovitis of hand/wrist NEC
		729.6	Old foreign body in soft tissue
		730.04	Acute osteomyelitis, hand
		730.14	Chronic osteomyelitis, hand
		730.24	Osteomyelitis NOS, hand
		732.3	Juvenile osteochondrosis, arm
		883.1	Open wound of finger, complicated
		915.7	Foreign body, finger, infected
		996.66	Reaction, internal joint prosthesis
		998.4	Foreign body left during procedure
		998.5	Postoperative infection

REIMBURSEMENT INFORMATION

General

- See notes on page 286.

Medicare

- Follow–up Days — 90
- Assistant Surgeon — not paid
- Supply Charges — not allowed
- Outpatient Limit — does not apply
- Major Surgery Rules Apply

CPT CODE	SERVICE
26145	Synovectomy tendon sheath, radical (tenosynovectomy), flexor, palm or finger, single, each digit

CPT NOTES

- For tendon sheath synovectomies at wrist, see 25115, 15116.

ICD–9–CM

170.5	M-Neoplasm, Wrist/Hand bones
171.2	M-Neoplasm, Soft tissue, arm
198.89	M2-Neoplasm NEC
215.2	B-Neoplasm, Soft tissue, arm
238.1	UB-Neoplasm, Soft tissue
239.2	Bone/Skin neoplasm NOS
711.04	Pyogenic arthritis, hand
711.94	Infect arthritis NOS, hand
714.0	Rheumatoid arthritis
714.30	Juvenile rheumatoid arthritis NOS
714.31	Juvenile acute rheumatoid arthritis
714.32	Pauciarticular juv rheum arthritis
714.33	Monoarticular juv rheum arthritis
714.4	Chronic postrheumatic arthritis
715.14	Loc prim osteoarthritis, hand
715.24	Loc 2nd osteoarthritis, hand
715.34	Loc osteoarthritis NOS, hand
716.14	Traumatic arthropathy, hand
718.14	Loose body in joint, hand
719.04	Joint effusion, hand
719.24	Villonodular synovitis, hand
727.00	Synovitis NOS
727.02	Giant cell tumor of tendon sheath
727.03	Trigger finger
727.04	Radial styloid tenosynovitis
727.05	Tenosynovitis of hand/wrist NEC
729.6	Old foreign body in soft tissue
730.04	Acute osteomyelitis, hand
730.14	Chronic osteomyelitis, hand
730.24	Osteomyelitis NOS, hand
732.3	Juvenile osteochondrosis, arm
883.1	Open wound of finger, complicated
915.7	Foreign body, finger, infected
996.66	Reaction, internal joint prosthesis
998.4	Foreign body left during procedure
998.5	Postoperative infection

REIMBURSEMENT INFORMATION

General

- See notes on page 286.

Medicare

- Follow–up Days — 90
- Assistant Surgeon — not paid
- Supply Charges — not allowed
- Outpatient Limit — does not apply
- Major Surgery Rules Apply

CPT CODE	SERVICE	ICD–9–CM
26160	Excision of lesion of tendon sheath or capsule (eg, cyst, mucous cyst, or ganglion), hand or finger	719.24 Villonodular synovitis, hand 727.00 Synovitis NOS 727.02 Giant cell tumor of tendon sheath 727.4x Ganglion/cyst synovium/tendon/bursa

CPT NOTES

- For wrist ganglion, see 25111, 25112.
- For trigger digit, see 26055.

REIMBURSEMENT INFORMATION

General

- See notes on page 286.

Medicare

- Follow–up Days — 90
- Assistant Surgeon — not paid
- Supply Charges — not allowed
- Outpatient Limit — does not apply
- Major Surgery Rules Apply

CPT CODE	SERVICE	ICD–9–CM
26170	Excision of tendon, palm, flexor, single (separate procedure), each	682.4 Cellulitis of hand 714.0 Rheumatoid arthritis 727.81 Contracture of tendon 882.2 Open wound of hand, w/tendon 905.8 Late effect of tendon injury

REIMBURSEMENT INFORMATION

General

- See notes on page 286.
- Separate procedure rules apply.

Medicare

- Follow–up Days — 90
- Assistant Surgeon — not paid
- Supply Charges — not allowed
- Outpatient Limit — does not apply
- Major Surgery Rules Apply

CPT CODE	SERVICE	ICD–9–CM
26180	Excision of tendon, finger, flexor (separate procedure)	682.4 Cellulitis of hand 714.0 Rheumatoid arthritis 727.81 Contracture of tendon 882.2 Open wound of hand, w/tendon 905.8 Late effect of tendon injury

REIMBURSEMENT INFORMATION

General

- See notes on page 286.
- Separate procedure rules apply.

Medicare

- Follow–up Days — 90
- Assistant Surgeon — not paid
- Supply Charges — not allowed
- Outpatient Limit — does not apply
- Major Surgery Rules Apply

CPT CODE	SERVICE	ICD–9–CM
26200	Excision or curettage of bone cyst or benign tumor of metacarpal	213.5 B-Neoplasm, Wrist/Hand bones 733.20 Cyst of bone NOS 733.21 Solitary bone cyst 733.22 Aneurysmal bone cyst 733.29 Bone cyst NEC
26205	Excision or curettage of bone cyst or benign tumor of metacarpal; with autograft (includes obtaining graft)	

REIMBURSEMENT INFORMATION

General

- See notes on page 286.

Medicare

- Follow–up Days — 90
- Assistant Surgeon — not paid
- Supply Charges — not allowed
- Outpatient Limit — does not apply
- Major Surgery Rules Apply

CPT CODE	SERVICE	ICD-9-CM
26210	Excision or curettage of bone cyst or benign tumor of proximal, middle or distal phalanx of finger	213.5 B-Neoplasm, Wrist/Hand bones 733.20 Cyst of bone NOS 733.21 Solitary bone cyst 733.22 Aneurysmal bone cyst 733.29 Bone cyst NEC
26215	Excision or curettage of bone cyst or benign tumor of proximal, middle or distal phalanx of finger; with autograft (includes obtaining graft)	

REIMBURSEMENT INFORMATION

General

- See notes on page 286.

Medicare

- Follow–up Days — 90
- Assistant Surgeon
  26210 — not paid
  26215 — paid
- Supply Charges — not allowed
- Outpatient Limit — does not apply
- Major Surgery Rules Apply

CPT CODE	SERVICE	ICD-9-CM
26230	Partial excision (craterization, saucerization, or diaphysectomy) of bone (eg, for osteomyelitis); metacarpal	170.5 M-Neoplasm, Wrist/Hand bones 213.5 B-Neoplasm, Wrist/Hand bones 238.0 UB-Neoplasm, Bone 239.2 Bone/Skin neoplasm NOS 730.04 Acute osteomyelitis, hand 730.14 Chronic osteomyelitis, hand 730.24 Osteomyelitis NOS, hand
26235	Partial excision (craterization, saucerization, or diaphysectomy) of bone (eg, for osteomyelitis); proximal or middle phalanx of finger	
26236	Partial excision (craterization, saucerization, or diaphysectomy) of bone (eg, for osteomyelitis); distal phalanx of finger	

REIMBURSEMENT INFORMATION

General

- See notes on page 286.

Medicare

- Follow–up Days — 90
- Assistant Surgeon — not paid
- Supply Charges — not allowed
- Outpatient Limit — does not apply
- Major Surgery Rules Apply

CPT CODE	SERVICE	ICD–9–CM
26250	Radical resection (ostectomy) for tumor, metacarpal	170.5 M-Neoplasm, Wrist/Hand bones 198.5 M2-Neoplasm, Bone and bone marrow 238.0 UB-Neoplasm, Bone 239.2 Bone/Skin neoplasm NOS 730.14 Chronic osteomyelitis, hand **REIMBURSEMENT INFORMATION** General ◆ See notes on page 286. Medicare ◆ Follow–up Days — 90 ◆ Assistant Surgeon — by report ◆ Supply Charges — not allowed ◆ Outpatient Limit — does not apply ◆ Major Surgery Rules Apply
26255	Radical resection (ostectomy) for tumor, metacarpal; with autograft (includes obtaining graft)	170.5 M-Neoplasm, Wrist/Hand bones 198.5 M2-Neoplasm, Bone and bone marrow 238.0 UB-Neoplasm, Bone 239.2 Bone/Skin neoplasm NOS 730.14 Chronic osteomyelitis, hand **REIMBURSEMENT INFORMATION** General ◆ See notes on page 286. Medicare ◆ Follow–up Days — 90 ◆ Assistant Surgeon — paid ◆ Supply Charges — not allowed ◆ Outpatient Limit — does not apply ◆ Major Surgery Rules Apply

CPT CODE	SERVICE	ICD–9–CM
26260	Radical resection (ostectomy) for tumor, proximal or middle phalanx of finger	170.5 M-Neoplasm, Wrist/Hand bones 198.5 M2-Neoplasm, Bone and bone marrow 238.0 UB-Neoplasm, Bone 239.2 Bone/Skin neoplasm NOS 730.14 Chronic osteomyelitis, hand
26261	Radical resection (ostectomy) for tumor, proximal or middle phalanx of finger; with autograft (includes obtaining graft)	

REIMBURSEMENT INFORMATION

General

- ♦ See notes on page 286.

Medicare

- ♦ Follow–up Days — 90
- ♦ Assistant Surgeon — paid
- ♦ Supply Charges — not allowed
- ♦ Outpatient Limit — does not apply
- ♦ Major Surgery Rules Apply

CPT CODE	SERVICE	ICD–9–CM
26262	Radical resection (ostectomy) for tumor, distal phalanx of finger	170.5 M-Neoplasm, Wrist/Hand bones 198.5 M2-Neoplasm, Bone and bone marrow 238.0 UB-Neoplasm, Bone 239.2 Bone/Skin neoplasm NOS 730.14 Chronic osteomyelitis, hand

REIMBURSEMENT INFORMATION

General

- ♦ See notes on page 286.

Medicare

- ♦ Follow–up Days — 90
- ♦ Assistant Surgeon — paid
- ♦ Supply Charges — not allowed
- ♦ Outpatient Limit — does not apply
- ♦ Major Surgery Rules Apply

CPT CODE	SERVICE	ICD–9–CM

26320 Removal of implant from finger or hand

CPT NOTES

- For removal of foreign body in hand or finger, see 20520, 20525.

714.0	Rheumatoid arthritis
996.4	Malfunction, int orthoped dev/graft
996.66	Reaction, internal joint prosthesis
996.77	Complication, int joint prosthesis
996.78	Complication, oth int ortho device
V54.0	Removal of internal fixation device

REIMBURSEMENT INFORMATION

General

- See notes on page 286.

Medicare

- Follow–up Days — 90
- Assistant Surgeon — not paid
- Supply Charges — not allowed
- Outpatient Limit — does not apply
- Major Surgery Rules Apply

26350 Flexor tendon repair or advancement, single, not in "no man's land"; primary or secondary without free graft, each tendon

727.64	Rupture, hand/wrist flexor tendons
882.2	Open wound of hand, w/tendon
883.2	Open wound of finger w/tendon
927.20	Crushing injury, hand
927.3	Crushing injury, finger

REIMBURSEMENT INFORMATION

General

- See notes on page 286.

Medicare

- Follow–up Days — 90
- Assistant Surgeon — not paid
- Supply Charges — not allowed
- Outpatient Limit — does not apply
- Major Surgery Rules Apply

CPT CODE	SERVICE	ICD-9-CM
26352	Flexor tendon repair or advancement, single, not in "no man's land"; secondary with free graft (includes obtaining graft), each tendon	727.64 Rupture, hand/wrist flexor tendons 882.2 Open wound of hand, w/tendon 883.2 Open wound of finger w/tendon 927.20 Crushing injury, hand 927.3 Crushing injury, finger

REIMBURSEMENT INFORMATION

General

- ◆ See notes on page 286.

Medicare

- ◆ Follow-up Days — 90
- ◆ Assistant Surgeon — paid
- ◆ Supply Charges — not allowed
- ◆ Outpatient Limit — does not apply
- ◆ Major Surgery Rules Apply

CPT CODE	SERVICE	ICD-9-CM
26356	Flexor tendon repair or advancement, single, in "no man's land"; primary, each tendon	727.64 Rupture, hand/wrist flexor tendons 882.2 Open wound of hand, w/tendon 883.2 Open wound of finger w/tendon 927.20 Crushing injury, hand 927.3 Crushing injury, finger
26357	Flexor tendon repair or advancement, single, in "no man's land"; secondary, each tendon	
26358	Flexor tendon repair or advancement, single, in "no man's land"; secondary with free graft (includes obtaining graft), each tendon	

REIMBURSEMENT INFORMATION

General

- ◆ See notes on page 286.

Medicare

- ◆ Follow-up Days — 90
- ◆ Assistant Surgeon
  26356 — not paid
  26357–26358 — paid
- ◆ Supply Charges — not allowed
- ◆ Outpatient Limit — does not apply
- ◆ Major Surgery Rules Apply

CPT CODE	SERVICE	ICD-9-CM
26370	Profundus tendon repair or advancement, with intact sublimis; primary	727.64 Rupture, hand/wrist flexor tendons 882.2 Open wound of hand, w/tendon 883.2 Open wound of finger w/tendon 927.20 Crushing injury, hand 927.3 Crushing injury, finger
26372	Profundus tendon repair or advancement, with intact sublimis; secondary with free graft (includes obtaining graft)	
26373	Profundus tendon repair or advancement, with intact sublimis; secondary without free graft	

REIMBURSEMENT INFORMATION

General

- See notes on page 286.

Medicare

- Follow-up Days — 90
- Assistant Surgeon
  26370 — not paid
  26372–26373 — paid
- Supply Charges — not allowed
- Outpatient Limit — does not apply
- Major Surgery Rules Apply

CPT CODE	SERVICE	ICD-9-CM
26390	Flexor tendon excision, implantation of plastic tube or rod for delayed tendon graft, hand or finger	882.2 Open wound of hand, w/tendon 883.2 Open wound of finger w/tendon 905.8 Late effect of tendon injury

REIMBURSEMENT INFORMATION

General

- See notes on page 286.

Medicare

- Follow-up Days — 90
- Assistant Surgeon — paid
- Supply Charges — not allowed
- Outpatient Limit — does not apply
- Major Surgery Rules Apply

CPT CODE	SERVICE	ICD-9-CM
26392	Removal of tube or rod and insertion of flexor tendon graft (includes obtaining graft), hand or finger	905.8 Late effect of tendon injury V51. Aftercare w/plastic surgery

REIMBURSEMENT INFORMATION

General

- See notes on page 286.

Medicare

- Follow-up Days — 90
- Assistant Surgeon — paid
- Supply Charges — not allowed
- Outpatient Limit — does not apply
- Major Surgery Rules Apply

CPT CODE	SERVICE	ICD-9-CM
26410	Extensor tendon repair, dorsum of hand, single, primary or secondary; without free graft, each tendon	727.63 Rupture, hand/wrist extensor tendon 882.2 Open wound of hand, w/tendon 883.2 Open wound of finger w/tendon 905.8 Late effect of tendon injury 927.20 Crushing injury, hand 927.3 Crushing injury, finger
26412	Extensor tendon repair, dorsum of hand, single, primary or secondary; with free graft, (includes obtaining graft), each tendon	

REIMBURSEMENT INFORMATION

General

- See notes on page 286.

Medicare

- Follow-up Days — 90
- Assistant Surgeon
  26410 — not paid
  26412 — paid
- Supply Charges — not allowed
- Outpatient Limit — does not apply
- Major Surgery Rules Apply

CPT CODE	SERVICE	ICD-9-CM
26415	Extensor tendon excision, implantation of plastic tube or rod for delayed extensor tendon graft, hand or finger	882.2 Open wound of hand, w/tendon 883.2 Open wound of finger w/tendon 905.8 Late effect of tendon injury

REIMBURSEMENT INFORMATION

General

- See notes on page 286.

Medicare

- Follow-up Days — 90
- Assistant Surgeon — not paid
- Supply Charges — not allowed
- Outpatient Limit — does not apply
- Major Surgery Rules Apply

CPT CODE	SERVICE	ICD-9-CM
26416	Removal of tube or rod and insertion of extensor tendon graft (includes obtaining graft), hand or finger	905.8 Late effect of tendon injury V51. Aftercare w/plastic surgery

REIMBURSEMENT INFORMATION

General

- See notes on page 286.

Medicare

- Follow-up Days — 90
- Assistant Surgeon — paid
- Supply Charges — not allowed
- Outpatient Limit — does not apply
- Major Surgery Rules Apply

CPT CODE	SERVICE	ICD-9-CM
26418	Extensor tendon repair, dorsum of finger, single, primary or secondary, without free graft, each tendon	727.63 Rupture, hand/wrist extensor tendon 882.2 Open wound of hand, w/tendon 883.2 Open wound of finger w/tendon 905.8 Late effect of tendon injury 927.20 Crushing injury, hand 927.3 Crushing injury, finger
26420	Extensor tendon repair, dorsum of finger, single, primary or secondary, with free graft, (includes obtaining graft) each tendon	

REIMBURSEMENT INFORMATION

General

- See notes on page 286.

Medicare

- Follow-up Days — 90
- Assistant Surgeon
  26418 — not paid
  26420 — paid
- Supply Charges — not allowed
- Outpatient Limit — does not apply
- Major Surgery Rules Apply

CPT CODE	SERVICE	ICD-9-CM
26426	Extensor tendon repair, central slip repair, secondary (boutonniere deformity); using local tissues	714.0 Rheumatoid arthritis 736.21 Boutonniere deformity, finger 883.2 Open wound of finger w/tendon 905.8 Late effect of tendon injury 927.20 Crushing injury, hand 927.3 Crushing injury, finger
26428	Extensor tendon repair, central slip repair, secondary (boutonniere deformity); with free graft (includes obtaining graft)	

REIMBURSEMENT INFORMATION

General

- See notes on page 286.

Medicare

- Follow-up Days — 90
- Assistant Surgeon
  26426 — paid
- 26428 — paid
- Supply Charges — not allowed
- Outpatient Limit — does not apply
- Major Surgery Rules Apply

CPT CODE	SERVICE	ICD-9-CM
26432	Extensor tendon repair, distal insertion ("mallet finger"), closed, splinting with or without percutaneous pinning	736.1 Mallet finger 883.2 Open wound of finger w/tendon 905.2 Late effect, arm fracture 905.8 Late effect of tendon injury 906.4 Late effect of crushing 927.3 Crushing injury, finger

REIMBURSEMENT INFORMATION

General

- ♦ See notes on page 286.

Medicare

- ♦ Follow-up Days — 90
- ♦ Assistant Surgeon — not paid
- ♦ Supply Charges — not allowed
- ♦ Outpatient Limit — does not apply
- ♦ Major Surgery Rules Apply

CPT CODE	SERVICE	ICD-9-CM
26433	Extensor tendon repair, distal insertion ("mallet finger"), open, primary or secondary repair; without graft	736.1 Mallet finger 883.2 Open wound of finger w/tendon 905.2 Late effect, arm fracture 905.8 Late effect of tendon injury 906.4 Late effect of crushing 927.3 Crushing injury, finger
26434	Extensor tendon repair, distal insertion ("mallet finger"), open, primary or secondary repair; with free graft (includes obtaining graft)	

CPT NOTES

- ♦ For tenovaginotomy for trigger finger, see 26055.

REIMBURSEMENT INFORMATION

General

- ♦ See notes on page 286.

Medicare

- ♦ Follow-up Days — 90
- ♦ Assistant Surgeon
  26433— not paid
  26434 — paid
- ♦ Supply Charges — not allowed
- ♦ Outpatient Limit — does not apply
- ♦ Major Surgery Rules Apply

CPT CODE	SERVICE	ICD–9–CM
26437	Extensor tendon realignment, hand	714.0 Rheumatoid arthritis 714.30 Juvenile rheumatoid arthritis NOS 714.31 Juvenile acute rheumatoid arthritis 714.32 Pauciarticular juv rheum arthritis 714.33 Monoarticular juv rheum arthritis 714.4 Chronic postrheumatic arthritis

REIMBURSEMENT INFORMATION

General

- ◆ See notes on page 286.

Medicare

- ◆ Follow–up Days — 90
- ◆ Assistant Surgeon — not paid
- ◆ Supply Charges — not allowed
- ◆ Outpatient Limit — does not apply
- ◆ Major Surgery Rules Apply

CPT CODE	SERVICE	ICD–9–CM
26440	Tenolysis, simple, flexor tendon; palm OR finger, single, each tendon	736.29 Acquired finger deformity NEC 905.2 Late effect, arm fracture 905.5 Late effect NEC
26442	Tenolysis, simple, flexor tendon; palm AND finger, each tendon	905.6 Late effect of dislocation 905.8 Late effect of tendon injury 906.4 Late effect of crushing

REIMBURSEMENT INFORMATION

General

- ◆ See notes on page 286.

Medicare

- ◆ Follow–up Days — 90
- ◆ Assistant Surgeon — not paid
- ◆ Supply Charges — not allowed
- ◆ Outpatient Limit — does not apply
- ◆ Major Surgery Rules Apply

CPT CODE	SERVICE	ICD–9–CM
26445	Tenolysis, extensor tendon, dorsum of hand or finger, each tendon	736.29 Acquired finger deformity NEC 905.2 Late effect, arm fracture 905.5 Late effect NEC 905.6 Late effect of dislocation 905.8 Late effect of tendon injury 906.4 Late effect of crushing

REIMBURSEMENT INFORMATION

General

- ♦ See notes on page 286.

Medicare

- ♦ Follow–up Days — 90
- ♦ Assistant Surgeon — not paid
- ♦ Supply Charges — not allowed
- ♦ Outpatient Limit — does not apply
- ♦ Major Surgery Rules Apply

CPT CODE	SERVICE	ICD–9–CM
26449	Tenolysis, complex, extensor tendon, dorsum of hand or finger, including hand and forearm	736.29 Acquired finger deformity NEC 905.2 Late effect, arm fracture 905.5 Late effect NEC 905.6 Late effect of dislocation 905.8 Late effect of tendon injury 906.4 Late effect of crushing

REIMBURSEMENT INFORMATION

General

- ♦ See notes on page 286.

Medicare

- ♦ Follow–up Days — 90
- ♦ Assistant Surgeon — not paid
- ♦ Supply Charges — not allowed
- ♦ Outpatient Limit — does not apply
- ♦ Major Surgery Rules Apply

CPT CODE	SERVICE	ICD–9–CM
26450	Tenotomy, flexor, single, palm, open, each	344.00 Quadriplegia NOS 434.00 Cerebral thrombosis 719.54 Joint stiffness NEC, hand 727.00 Synovitis NOS 727.05 Tenosynovitis of hand/wrist NEC 727.09 Synovitis NEC 727.81 Contracture of tendon 728.85 Spasm of muscle 736.06 Claw hand 736.07 Club hand, acquired 736.20 Acquired finger deformity NOS 736.29 Acquired finger deformity NEC **REIMBURSEMENT INFORMATION** General ◆ See notes on page 286. Medicare ◆ Follow–up Days — 90 ◆ Assistant Surgeon — not paid ◆ Supply Charges — not allowed ◆ Outpatient Limit — does not apply ◆ Major Surgery Rules Apply
26455	Tenotomy, flexor, single, finger, open, each	344.00 Quadriplegia NOS 434.00 Cerebral thrombosis 719.54 Joint stiffness NEC, hand 727.00 Synovitis NOS 727.05 Tenosynovitis of hand/wrist NEC 727.09 Synovitis NEC 727.81 Contracture of tendon 736.06 Claw hand 736.07 Club hand, acquired 736.20 Acquired finger deformity NOS 736.29 Acquired finger deformity NEC **REIMBURSEMENT INFORMATION** General ◆ See notes on page 286. Medicare ◆ Follow–up Days — 90 ◆ Assistant Surgeon — not paid ◆ Supply Charges — not allowed ◆ Outpatient Limit — does not apply ◆ Major Surgery Rules Apply

CPT CODE	SERVICE	ICD–9–CM
26460	Tenotomy, extensor hand or finger, single, open, each	344.00 Quadriplegia NOS 434.00 Cerebral thrombosis 719.54 Joint stiffness NEC, hand 727.00 Synovitis NOS 727.04 Radial styloid tenosynovitis 727.05 Tenosynovitis of hand/wrist NEC 727.09 Synovitis NEC 727.81 Contracture of tendon 728.85 Spasm of muscle 736.06 Claw hand 736.07 Club hand, acquired 736.20 Acquired finger deformity NOS 736.29 Acquired finger deformity NEC

REIMBURSEMENT INFORMATION

General

- ♦ See notes on page 286.

Medicare

- ♦ Follow–up Days — 90
- ♦ Assistant Surgeon — by report
- ♦ Supply Charges — not allowed
- ♦ Outpatient Limit — does not apply
- ♦ Major Surgery Rules Apply

CPT CODE	SERVICE
26471	Tenodesis; for proximal interphalangeal joint stabilization
26474	Tenodesis; for distal joint stabilization

ICD–9–CM

138.	Late effects of acute polio
344.00	Quadriplegia NOS
727.04	Radial styloid tenosynovitis
727.05	Tenosynovitis of hand/wrist NEC
727.63	Rupture, hand/wrist extensor tendon
727.64	Rupture, hand/wrist flexor tendons
727.69	Nontraumatic tendon rupture NEC
736.21	Boutonniere deformity, finger
736.22	Swan-neck deformity, finger
736.29	Acquired finger deformity NEC
842.13	Sprain interphalangeal
883.2	Open wound of finger w/tendon
905.8	Late effect of tendon injury
907.4	Late effect, nerve injury shld/arm
927.20	Crushing injury, hand

REIMBURSEMENT INFORMATION

General

- See notes on page 286.

Medicare

- Follow–up Days — 90
- Assistant Surgeon
  26471 — not paid
  26474 — not paid
- Supply Charges — not allowed
- Outpatient Limit — does not apply
- Major Surgery Rules Apply

CPT CODE	SERVICE
26476	Tendon lengthening, extensor, hand or finger, single, each

ICD–9–CM

138.	Late effects of acute polio
343.x	Infantile cerebral palsy
716.14	Traumatic arthropathy, hand
736.06	Claw hand
736.07	Club hand, acquired
736.20	Acquired finger deformity NOS
736.21	Boutonniere deformity, finger
736.22	Swan-neck deformity, finger
816.00	Fx phalanx, hand NOS, closed
816.01	Fx mid/prox phalanx, hand, closed
816.02	Fx distal phalanx, hand, closed
816.10	Fx phalanx, hand NOS, open
816.11	Fx mid/prox phalanx, hand, open
816.12	Fx distal phalanx, hand, open
834.0x	Finger dislocation, closed
834.1x	Finger dislocation, open
883.2	Open wound of finger w/tendon
905.8	Late effect of tendon injury
927.3	Crushing injury, finger
955.6	Injury digital nerve

REIMBURSEMENT INFORMATION

General

- See notes on page 286.

Medicare

- Follow–up Days — 90
- Assistant Surgeon — paid
- Supply Charges — not allowed
- Outpatient Limit — does not apply
- Major Surgery Rules Apply

CPT CODE	SERVICE	ICD-9-CM	
26477	Tendon shortening, extensor, hand or finger, single, each	138.	Late effects of acute polio
		343.x	Infantile cerebral palsy
		716.14	Traumatic arthropathy, hand
		736.05	Wrist drop
		736.06	Claw hand
		736.1	Mallet finger
		736.20	Acquired finger deformity NOS
		736.21	Boutonniere deformity, finger
		736.22	Swan-neck deformity, finger
		834.00	Dislocation finger NOS, closed
		834.01	Disloc metacarpophalangeal, closed
		834.02	Disloc interphalangeal hand, closed
		834.10	Dislocation finger NOS, open
		834.11	Disloc metacarpophalangeal, open
		834.12	Disloc interphalangeal hand, open
		842.13	Sprain interphalangeal
		883.2	Open wound of finger w/tendon
		905.8	Late effect of tendon injury
		927.3	Crushing injury, finger

REIMBURSEMENT INFORMATION

General

- See notes on page 286.

Medicare

- Follow-up Days — 90
- Assistant Surgeon — paid
- Supply Charges — not allowed
- Outpatient Limit — does not apply
- Major Surgery Rules Apply

CPT CODE	SERVICE	ICD–9–CM
26478	Tendon lengthening, flexor, hand or finger, single, each	138. Late effects of acute polio 343.x Infantile cerebral palsy 344.00 Quadriplegia NOS 716.14 Traumatic arthropathy, hand 727.81 Contracture of tendon 736.05 Wrist drop 736.06 Claw hand 736.1 Mallet finger 736.20 Acquired finger deformity NOS 755.59 Upper limb anomaly NEC 834.0x Finger dislocation, closed 834.1x Finger dislocation, open 883.2 Open wound of finger w/tendon 905.8 Late effect of tendon injury 927.3 Crushing injury, finger 958.6 Volkmann's ischemic contracture **REIMBURSEMENT INFORMATION** General ◆ See notes on page 286. Medicare ◆ Follow–up Days — 90 ◆ Assistant Surgeon — not paid ◆ Supply Charges — not allowed ◆ Outpatient Limit — does not apply ◆ Major Surgery Rules Apply
26479	Tendon shortening, flexor, hand or finger, single, each	138. Late effects of acute polio 343.x Infantile cerebral palsy 716.14 Traumatic arthropathy, hand 834.0x Finger dislocation, closed 834.1x Finger dislocation, open 883.2 Open wound of finger w/tendon 905.8 Late effect of tendon injury 927.3 Crushing injury, finger **REIMBURSEMENT INFORMATION** General ◆ See notes on page 286. Medicare ◆ Follow–up Days — 90 ◆ Assistant Surgeon — paid ◆ Supply Charges — not allowed ◆ Outpatient Limit — does not apply ◆ Major Surgery Rules Apply

CPT CODE	SERVICE
26480	Tendon transfer or transplant, carpometacarpal area or dorsum of hand, single; without free graft, each
26483	Tendon transfer or transplant, carpometacarpal area or dorsum of hand, single; with free tendon graft (includes obtaining graft), each tendon

ICD–9–CM

138.	Late effects of acute polio
342.90	Hemiplegia NOS, side NEC
342.91	Hemiplegia NOS, dominant side
342.92	Hemiplegia NOS, nondominant side
343.x	Infantile cerebral palsy
344.00	Quadriplegia NOS
354.0	Carpal tunnel syndrome
354.1	Lesion of median nerve NEC
354.2	Ulnar nerve lesion
354.3	Radial nerve lesion
359.1	Hered prog muscular dystrophy
434.00	Cerebral thrombosis
716.14	Traumatic arthropathy, hand
842.11	Sprain carpometacarpal
882.2	Open wound of hand, w/tendon
906.1	Late effect, open wound extremity
907.2	Late effect, spinal cord injury
907.3	Late effect, nerve injury trunk NEC
907.4	Late effect, nerve injury shld/arm
927.20	Crushing injury, hand
955.1	Injury median nerve
955.2	Injury ulnar nerve
955.3	Injury radial nerve

REIMBURSEMENT INFORMATION

General

- See notes on page 286.

Medicare

- Follow–up Days — 90
- Assistant Surgeon — paid
- Supply Charges — not allowed
- Outpatient Limit — does not apply
- Major Surgery Rules Apply

CPT CODE	SERVICE
26485	Tendon transfer or transplant, palmar, single, each tendon; without free tendon graft
26489	Tendon transfer or transplant, palmar, single, each tendon; with free tendon graft (includes obtaining graft), each tendon

ICD–9–CM

138.	Late effects of acute polio
342.90	Hemiplegia NOS, side NEC
342.91	Hemiplegia NOS, dominant side
342.92	Hemiplegia NOS, nondominant side
343.x	Infantile cerebral palsy
344.00	Quadriplegia NOS
354.0	Carpal tunnel syndrome
354.1	Lesion of median nerve NEC
354.2	Ulnar nerve lesion
354.3	Radial nerve lesion
359.1	Hered prog muscular dystrophy
434.00	Cerebral thrombosis
716.14	Traumatic arthropathy, hand
842.11	Sprain carpometacarpal
882.2	Open wound of hand, w/tendon
906.1	Late effect, open wound extremity
907.2	Late effect, spinal cord injury
907.3	Late effect, nerve injury trunk NEC
907.4	Late effect, nerve injury shld/arm
927.20	Crushing injury, hand
955.1	Injury median nerve
955.2	Injury ulnar nerve
955.3	Injury radial nerve

REIMBURSEMENT INFORMATION

General

- See notes on page 286.

Medicare

- Follow–up Days — 90
- Assistant Surgeon
  26485 — paid
  26489 — not paid
- Supply Charges — not allowed
- Outpatient Limit — does not apply
- Major Surgery Rules Apply

CPT CODE	SERVICE	ICD–9–CM
26490	Opponensplasty; sublimis tendon transfer type	138. Late effects of acute polio 343.x Infantile cerebral palsy 354.0 Carpal tunnel syndrome 354.1 Lesion of median nerve NEC 354.2 Ulnar nerve lesion 716.14 Traumatic arthropathy, hand 842.11 Sprain carpometacarpal 882.2 Open wound of hand, w/tendon 907.4 Late effect, nerve injury shld/arm 927.20 Crushing injury, hand 955.1 Injury median nerve 955.2 Injury ulnar nerve 996.92 Complication, reattached hand
26492	Opponensplasty; tendon transfer with graft (includes obtaining graft)	
26494	Opponensplasty; hypothenar muscle transfer	
26496	Opponensplasty; other methods	

CPT NOTES

- ♦ For thumb fusion in opposition, see 26820.

REIMBURSEMENT INFORMATION

General

- ♦ See notes on page 286.

Medicare

- ♦ Follow–up Days — 90
- ♦ Assistant Surgeon
  26490–26494— paid
  26496 — not paid
- ♦ Supply Charges — not allowed
- ♦ Outpatient Limit — does not apply
- ♦ Major Surgery Rules Apply

CPT CODE	SERVICE	ICD–9–CM
26497	Tendon transfer to restore intrinsic function; ring and small finger	354.2 Ulnar nerve lesion 736.00 Forearm deformity NOS 736.09 Forearm deformity NEC 736.20 Acquired finger deformity NOS 883.2 Open wound of finger w/tendon 907.4 Late effect, nerve injury shld/arm 927.3 Crushing injury, finger 955.2 Injury ulnar nerve 996.92 Complication, reattached hand

REIMBURSEMENT INFORMATION

General

- ♦ See notes on page 286.

Medicare

- ♦ Follow–up Days — 90
- ♦ Assistant Surgeon — paid
- ♦ Supply Charges — not allowed
- ♦ Outpatient Limit — does not apply
- ♦ Major Surgery Rules Apply

CPT CODE	SERVICE	ICD-9-CM
26498	Tendon transfer to restore intrinsic function; all four fingers	354.0 Carpal tunnel syndrome 354.1 Lesion of median nerve NEC 354.2 Ulnar nerve lesion 736.00 Forearm deformity NOS 736.09 Forearm deformity NEC 736.20 Acquired finger deformity NOS 883.2 Open wound of finger w/tendon 907.4 Late effect, nerve injury shld/arm 927.3 Crushing injury, finger 955.1 Injury median nerve 955.2 Injury ulnar nerve 996.92 Complication, reattached hand

REIMBURSEMENT INFORMATION

General

- See notes on page 286.

Medicare

- Follow-up Days — 90
- Assistant Surgeon — paid
- Supply Charges — not allowed
- Outpatient Limit — does not apply
- Major Surgery Rules Apply

CPT CODE	SERVICE	ICD-9-CM
26499	Correction claw finger, other methods	736.06 Claw hand 736.20 Acquired finger deformity NOS 907.4 Late effect, nerve injury shld/arm 996.92 Complication, reattached hand

REIMBURSEMENT INFORMATION

General

- See notes on page 286.

Medicare

- Follow-up Days — 90
- Assistant Surgeon — paid
- Supply Charges — not allowed
- Outpatient Limit — does not apply
- Major Surgery Rules Apply

CPT CODE	SERVICE	ICD-9-CM
26500	Tendon pulley reconstruction, with local tissues (separate procedure)	883.2 Open wound of finger w/tendon 905.8 Late effect of tendon injury 906.1 Late effect, open wound extremity 906.4 Late effect of crushing 909.3 Late effect of surg/med complic 927.3 Crushing injury, finger
26502	Tendon pulley reconstruction; with tendon or fascial graft (includes obtaining graft) (separate procedure)	
26504	Tendon pulley reconstruction; with tendon prosthesis (separate procedure)	

REIMBURSEMENT INFORMATION

General

- ◆ See notes on page 286.
- ◆ Separate procedure rules apply.

Medicare

- ◆ Follow-up Days — 90
- ◆ Assistant Surgeon
  26500 — not paid
  26502–26504 — paid
- ◆ Supply Charges — not allowed
- ◆ Outpatient Limit — does not apply
- ◆ Major Surgery Rules Apply

CPT CODE	SERVICE	ICD-9-CM
26508	Thenar muscle release for thumb contracture	714.0 Rheumatoid arthritis 714.30 Juvenile rheumatoid arthritis NOS 714.31 Juvenile acute rheumatoid arthritis 714.32 Pauciarticular juv rheum arthritis 714.33 Monoarticular juv rheum arthritis 714.4 Chronic postrheumatic arthritis 715.14 Loc prim osteoarthritis, hand 718.44 Contracture of joint, hand 755.55 Acrocephalosyndactyly

REIMBURSEMENT INFORMATION

General

- ◆ See notes on page 286.

Medicare

- ◆ Follow-up Days — 90
- ◆ Assistant Surgeon — not paid
- ◆ Supply Charges — not allowed
- ◆ Outpatient Limit — does not apply
- ◆ Major Surgery Rules Apply

CPT CODE	SERVICE	ICD-9-CM	
26510	Cross intrinsic transfer	714.0	Rheumatoid arthritis
		714.30	Juvenile rheumatoid arthritis NOS
		714.31	Juvenile acute rheumatoid arthritis
		714.32	Pauciarticular juv rheum arthritis
		714.33	Monoarticular juv rheum arthritis
		714.4	Chronic postrheumatic arthritis
		736.09	Forearm deformity NEC

REIMBURSEMENT INFORMATION

General

- ♦ See notes on page 286.

Medicare

- ♦ Follow–up Days — 90
- ♦ Assistant Surgeon — paid
- ♦ Supply Charges — not allowed
- ♦ Outpatient Limit — does not apply
- ♦ Major Surgery Rules Apply

CPT CODE	SERVICE	ICD-9-CM	
26516	Capsulodesis for M-P joint stabilization; single digit	714.0	Rheumatoid arthritis
		714.30	Juvenile rheumatoid arthritis NOS
		714.31	Juvenile acute rheumatoid arthritis
		714.32	Pauciarticular juv rheum arthritis
		714.33	Monoarticular juv rheum arthritis
		714.4	Chronic postrheumatic arthritis
		728.4	Laxity of ligament
		728.5	Hypermobility syndrome
		736.00	Forearm deformity NOS
		736.06	Claw hand
		736.09	Forearm deformity NEC
		907.4	Late effect, nerve injury shld/arm
		955.1	Injury median nerve
		955.2	Injury ulnar nerve

REIMBURSEMENT INFORMATION

General

- ♦ See notes on page 286.

Medicare

- ♦ Follow–up Days — 90
- ♦ Assistant Surgeon — paid
- ♦ Supply Charges — not allowed
- ♦ Outpatient Limit — does not apply
- ♦ Major Surgery Rules Apply

CPT CODE	SERVICE	ICD-9-CM
26517	Capsulodesis for M-P joint stabilization; two digits	714.0 Rheumatoid arthritis 714.30 Juvenile rheumatoid arthritis NOS 714.31 Juvenile acute rheumatoid arthritis 714.32 Pauciarticular juv rheum arthritis 714.33 Monoarticular juv rheum arthritis 714.4 Chronic postrheumatic arthritis 715.14 Loc prim osteoarthritis, hand 728.4 Laxity of ligament 728.5 Hypermobility syndrome 736.00 Forearm deformity NOS 736.06 Claw hand 736.09 Forearm deformity NEC 907.4 Late effect, nerve injury shld/arm 955.1 Injury median nerve 955.2 Injury ulnar nerve **REIMBURSEMENT INFORMATION** General ◆ See notes on page 286. Medicare ◆ Follow–up Days — 90 ◆ Assistant Surgeon — paid ◆ Supply Charges — not allowed ◆ Outpatient Limit — does not apply ◆ Major Surgery Rules Apply
26518	Capsulodesis for M-P joint stabilization; three or four digits	
26520	Capsulectomy or capsulotomy for contracture; metacarpophalangeal joint, single, each	715.14 Loc prim osteoarthritis, hand 718.44 Contracture of joint, hand 718.54 Ankylosis of joint, hand 719.54 Joint stiffness NEC, hand 736.09 Forearm deformity NEC 736.29 Acquired finger deformity NEC 907.4 Late effect, nerve injury shld/arm 958.6 Volkmann's ischemic contracture **REIMBURSEMENT INFORMATION** General ◆ See notes on page 286. Medicare ◆ Follow–up Days — 90 ◆ Assistant Surgeon — not paid ◆ Supply Charges — not allowed ◆ Outpatient Limit — does not apply ◆ Major Surgery Rules Apply

CPT CODE	SERVICE
26525	Capsulectomy or capsulotomy for contracture; interphalangeal joint, single each

ICD–9–CM

709.2	Scar/fibrosis of skin
714.0	Rheumatoid arthritis
715.14	Loc prim osteoarthritis, hand
727.81	Contracture of tendon
728.6	Contracture of palmar fascia
736.20	Acquired finger deformity NOS
736.29	Acquired finger deformity NEC
905.8	Late effect of tendon injury
906.4	Late effect of crushing
907.4	Late effect, nerve injury shld/arm
958.6	Volkmann's ischemic contracture
996.93	Complication, reattached finger

REIMBURSEMENT INFORMATION

General

- ♦ See notes on page 286.

Medicare

- ♦ Follow–up Days — 90
- ♦ Assistant Surgeon — paid
- ♦ Supply Charges — not allowed
- ♦ Outpatient Limit — does not apply
- ♦ Major Surgery Rules Apply

CPT CODE	SERVICE
26530	Arthroplasty, metacarpophalangeal joint; single, each
26531	Arthroplasty, metacarpophalangeal joint; with prosthetic implant, single, each

ICD–9–CM

711.04	Pyogenic arthritis, hand
711.94	Infect arthritis NOS, hand
714.0	Rheumatoid arthritis
714.30	Juvenile rheumatoid arthritis NOS
714.31	Juvenile acute rheumatoid arthritis
714.32	Pauciarticular juv rheum arthritis
714.33	Monoarticular juv rheum arthritis
714.4	Chronic postrheumatic arthritis
715.14	Loc prim osteoarthritis, hand
715.24	Loc 2nd osteoarthritis, hand
715.34	Loc osteoarthritis NOS, hand
716.14	Traumatic arthropathy, hand
718.04	Articular cartilage dis, hand
718.54	Ankylosis of joint, hand
719.24	Villonodular synovitis, hand
729.5	Pain in limb
730.14	Chronic osteomyelitis, hand
731.0	Osteitis deformans NOS
732.3	Juvenile osteochondrosis, arm
733.49	Aseptic necrosis of bone NEC
733.82	Nonunion of fracture
905.2	Late effect, arm fracture
927.20	Crushing injury, hand
927.3	Crushing injury, finger

REIMBURSEMENT INFORMATION

General

- See notes on page 286.

Medicare

- Follow–up Days — 90
- Assistant Surgeon — paid
- Supply Charges — not allowed
- Outpatient Limit — does not apply
- Major Surgery Rules Apply

CPT CODE	SERVICE	ICD–9–CM	
26535	Arthroplasty, interphalangeal joint; single, each	711.04	Pyogenic arthritis, hand
		711.94	Infect arthritis NOS, hand
		714.0	Rheumatoid arthritis
		714.30	Juvenile rheumatoid arthritis NOS
		714.31	Juvenile acute rheumatoid arthritis
		714.32	Pauciarticular juv rheum arthritis
		714.33	Monoarticular juv rheum arthritis
		714.4	Chronic postrheumatic arthritis
		715.14	Loc prim osteoarthritis, hand
		715.24	Loc 2nd osteoarthritis, hand
		715.34	Loc osteoarthritis NOS, hand
		716.14	Traumatic arthropathy, hand
		718.04	Articular cartilage dis, hand
		718.54	Ankylosis of joint, hand
		719.24	Villonodular synovitis, hand
		729.5	Pain in limb
		730.14	Chronic osteomyelitis, hand
		731.0	Osteitis deformans NOS
		732.3	Juvenile osteochondrosis, arm
		733.49	Aseptic necrosis of bone NEC
		733.82	Nonunion of fracture
		905.2	Late effect, arm fracture
		906.4	Late effect of crushing
		927.20	Crushing injury, hand
		927.3	Crushing injury, finger

REIMBURSEMENT INFORMATION

General

- ♦ See notes on page 286.

Medicare

- ♦ Follow–up Days — 90
- ♦ Assistant Surgeon — not paid
- ♦ Supply Charges — not allowed
- ♦ Outpatient Limit — does not apply
- ♦ Major Surgery Rules Apply

CPT CODE	SERVICE	ICD–9–CM	
26536	Arthroplasty, interphalangeal joint; with prosthetic implant, single, each	711.04	Pyogenic arthritis, hand
		711.94	Infect arthritis NOS, hand
		714.0	Rheumatoid arthritis
		714.30	Juvenile rheumatoid arthritis NOS
		714.31	Juvenile acute rheumatoid arthritis
		714.32	Pauciarticular juv rheum arthritis
		714.33	Monoarticular juv rheum arthritis
		714.4	Chronic postrheumatic arthritis
		715.14	Loc prim osteoarthritis, hand
		715.24	Loc 2nd osteoarthritis, hand
		715.34	Loc osteoarthritis NOS, hand
		716.14	Traumatic arthropathy, hand
		718.05	Articular cartilage dis, pelv/thigh
		718.54	Ankylosis of joint, hand
		719.24	Villonodular synovitis, hand
		729.5	Pain in limb
		730.14	Chronic osteomyelitis, hand
		731.0	Osteitis deformans NOS
		732.3	Juvenile osteochondrosis, arm
		733.49	Aseptic necrosis of bone NEC
		733.82	Nonunion of fracture
		905.2	Late effect, arm fracture
		906.4	Late effect of crushing
		927.20	Crushing injury, hand
		927.3	Crushing injury, finger

REIMBURSEMENT INFORMATION

General

- See notes on page 286.

Medicare

- Follow–up Days — 90
- Assistant Surgeon — paid
- Supply Charges — not allowed
- Outpatient Limit — does not apply
- Major Surgery Rules Apply

CPT CODE	SERVICE	ICD–9–CM
26540	Primary repair of collateral ligament, metacarpophalangeal joint	718.24 Pathologic dislocation, hand 718.34 Recurrent dislocation, hand 728.4 Laxity of ligament 728.5 Hypermobility syndrome 736.22 Swan-neck deformity, finger 834.01 Disloc metacarpophalangeal, closed 834.11 Disloc metacarpophalangeal, open 842.12 Sprain metacarpophalangeal 883.2 Open wound of finger w/tendon
26541	Primary repair of collateral ligament, metacarpophalangeal joint; with tendon or fascial graft (includes obtaining graft)	
26542	Primary repair of collateral ligament, metacarpophalangeal joint; with local tissue (eg, adductor advancement)	

REIMBURSEMENT INFORMATION

General

- ♦ See notes on page 286.

Medicare

- ♦ Follow–up Days — 90
- ♦ Assistant Surgeon — paid
- ♦ Supply Charges — not allowed
- ♦ Outpatient Limit — does not apply
- ♦ Major Surgery Rules Apply

CPT CODE	SERVICE	ICD–9–CM
26545	Reconstruction, collateral ligament, interphalangeal joint, single, including graft, each joint	718.24 Pathologic dislocation, hand 718.34 Recurrent dislocation, hand 728.4 Laxity of ligament 728.5 Hypermobility syndrome 736.22 Swan-neck deformity, finger 834.01 Disloc metacarpophalangeal, closed 834.11 Disloc metacarpophalangeal, open 842.13 Sprain interphalangeal 883.2 Open wound of finger w/tendon

REIMBURSEMENT INFORMATION

General

- ♦ See notes on page 286.

Medicare

- ♦ Follow–up Days — 90
- ♦ Assistant Surgeon — paid
- ♦ Supply Charges — not allowed
- ♦ Outpatient Limit — does not apply
- ♦ Major Surgery Rules Apply

CPT CODE	SERVICE	ICD–9–CM
26548	Repair and reconstruction, finger volar plate, interphalangeal joint	718.24 Pathologic dislocation, hand 718.34 Recurrent dislocation, hand 728.4 Laxity of ligament 728.5 Hypermobility syndrome 736.22 Swan-neck deformity, finger 834.02 Disloc interphalangeal hand, closed 834.12 Disloc interphalangeal hand, open 842.13 Sprain interphalangeal 883.2 Open wound of finger w/tendon

REIMBURSEMENT INFORMATION

General

- ◆ See notes on page 286.

Medicare

- ◆ Follow–up Days — 90
- ◆ Assistant Surgeon — not paid
- ◆ Supply Charges — not allowed
- ◆ Outpatient Limit — does not apply
- ◆ Major Surgery Rules Apply

CPT CODE	SERVICE	ICD–9–CM
26550	Pollicization of a digit	170.5 M-Neoplasm, Wrist/Hand bones 198.5 M2-Neoplasm, Bone and bone marrow 238.0 UB-Neoplasm, Bone 239.2 Bone/Skin neoplasm NOS 730.13 Chronic osteomyelitis, forearm 733.49 Aseptic necrosis of bone NEC 754.89 Nonteratogenic anomaly NEC 755.29 Longitudinal defic, hand phalanges 785.4 Gangrene 885.x Traumatic amputation of thumb 886.x Traumatic finger amputation 905.9 Late effect of traumatic amputation 906.4 Late effect of crushing 906.6 Late effect of wrist/hand burn 927.3 Crushing injury, finger V13.6 Hx of congenital malformation

REIMBURSEMENT INFORMATION

General

- ◆ See notes on page 286.

Medicare

- ◆ Follow–up Days — 90
- ◆ Assistant Surgeon — paid
- ◆ Supply Charges — not allowed
- ◆ Outpatient Limit — does not apply
- ◆ Major Surgery Rules Apply

CPT CODE	SERVICE
26552	Reconstruction thumb with toe

ICD–9–CM

170.5	M-Neoplasm, Wrist/Hand bones
198.5	M2-Neoplasm, Bone and bone marrow
238.0	UB-Neoplasm, Bone
239.2	Bone/Skin neoplasm NOS
730.13	Chronic osteomyelitis, forearm
733.49	Aseptic necrosis of bone NEC
754.89	Nonteratogenic anomaly NEC
755.29	Longitudinal defic, hand phalanges
785.4	Gangrene
885.x	Traumatic amputation of thumb
886.x	Traumatic finger amputation
905.9	Late effect of traumatic amputation
906.4	Late effect of crushing
906.6	Late effect of wrist/hand burn
927.3	Crushing injury, finger

REIMBURSEMENT INFORMATION

General

- See notes on page 286.

Medicare

- Follow–up Days — 90
- Assistant Surgeon — paid
- Supply Charges — not allowed
- Outpatient Limit — does not apply
- Major Surgery Rules Apply

CPT CODE	SERVICE
26555	Positional change of other finger

ICD–9–CM

170.5	M-Neoplasm, Wrist/Hand bones
198.5	M2-Neoplasm, Bone and bone marrow
238.0	UB-Neoplasm, Bone
239.2	Bone/Skin neoplasm NOS
730.13	Chronic osteomyelitis, forearm
733.49	Aseptic necrosis of bone NEC
754.89	Nonteratogenic anomaly NEC
755.29	Longitudinal defic, hand phalanges
785.4	Gangrene
885.x	Traumatic amputation of thumb
886.x	Traumatic finger amputation
905.9	Late effect of traumatic amputation
906.4	Late effect of crushing
906.6	Late effect of wrist/hand burn
927.3	Crushing injury, finger

REIMBURSEMENT INFORMATION

General

- See notes on page 286.

Medicare

- Follow–up Days — 90
- Assistant Surgeon — paid
- Supply Charges — not allowed
- Outpatient Limit — does not apply
- Major Surgery Rules Apply

CPT CODE	SERVICE	ICD-9-CM
26557	Toe to finger transfer; first stage	170.5 M-Neoplasm, Wrist/Hand bones 198.5 M2-Neoplasm, Bone and bone marrow 238.0 UB-Neoplasm, Bone 239.2 Bone/Skin neoplasm NOS 730.13 Chronic osteomyelitis, forearm 733.49 Aseptic necrosis of bone NEC 754.89 Nonteratogenic anomaly NEC 755.29 Longitudinal defic, hand phalanges 785.4 Gangrene 885.x Traumatic amputation of thumb 886.x Traumatic finger amputation 905.9 Late effect of traumatic amputation 906.4 Late effect of crushing 906.6 Late effect of wrist/hand burn 927.3 Crushing injury, finger
26558	Toe to finger transfer; each delay	
26559	Toe to finger transfer; second stage	

REIMBURSEMENT INFORMATION

General

- See notes on page 286.

Medicare

- Follow-up Days — 90
- Assistant Surgeon
  26557 — by report
  26558–26559 — paid
- Supply Charges — not allowed
- Outpatient Limit — does not apply
- Major Surgery Rules Apply

CPT CODE	SERVICE	ICD-9-CM
26560	Repair of syndactyly (web finger) each web space; with skin flaps	755.10 Syndactyly, multiple/NOS 755.11 Syndactyly of fingers, no fusion 755.12 Syndactyly of fingers, w/fusion 755.55 Acrocephalosyndactyly
26561	Repair of syndactyly (web finger) each web space; with skin flaps and grafts	
26562	Repair of syndactyly (web finger) each web space; complex, involving bone, nails, etc	

REIMBURSEMENT INFORMATION

General

- See notes on page 286.

Medicare

- Follow-up Days — 90
- Assistant Surgeon — paid
- Supply Charges — not allowed
- Outpatient Limit — does not apply
- Major Surgery Rules Apply

CPT CODE	SERVICE	ICD–9–CM
26565	Osteotomy for correction of deformity; metacarpal	733.81 Malunion of fracture 733.82 Nonunion of fracture
26567	Osteotomy for correction of deformity; phalanx of finger	**REIMBURSEMENT INFORMATION** General ◆ See notes on page 286. Medicare ◆ Follow–up Days — 90 ◆ Assistant Surgeon — paid ◆ Supply Charges — not allowed ◆ Outpatient Limit — does not apply ◆ Major Surgery Rules Apply
26568	Osteoplasty for lengthening of metacarpal or phalanx	733.81 Malunion of fracture 733.82 Nonunion of fracture 736.00 Forearm deformity NOS 755.28 Longitudinal deficiency, hand 755.29 Longitudinal defic, hand phalanges 905.9 Late effect of traumatic amputation 998.5 Postoperative infection **REIMBURSEMENT INFORMATION** General ◆ See notes on page 286. Medicare ◆ Follow–up Days — 90 ◆ Assistant Surgeon — paid ◆ Supply Charges — not allowed ◆ Outpatient Limit — does not apply ◆ Major Surgery Rules Apply
26580	Repair cleft hand	755.58 Congenital cleft hand V13.6 Hx of congenital malformation **REIMBURSEMENT INFORMATION** General ◆ See notes on page 286. Medicare ◆ Follow–up Days — 90 ◆ Assistant Surgeon — paid ◆ Supply Charges — not allowed ◆ Outpatient Limit — does not apply ◆ Major Surgery Rules Apply

CPT CODE	SERVICE	ICD–9–CM
26585	Repair bifid digit	755.01 Polydactyly, fingers 755.02 Polydactyly, toes 755.59 Upper limb anomaly NEC 755.66 Anomalies of toes NEC V13.6 Hx of congenital malformation **REIMBURSEMENT INFORMATION** General ♦ See notes on page 286. Medicare ♦ Follow–up Days — 90 ♦ Assistant Surgeon — paid ♦ Supply Charges — not allowed ♦ Outpatient Limit — does not apply ♦ Major Surgery Rules Apply
26587	Reconstruction of supernumerary digit, soft tissue and bone **CPT NOTES** ♦ For excision of supernumerary digit, soft tissue only, use 11200.	755.00 Polydactyly NOS 755.01 Polydactyly, fingers 755.02 Polydactyly, toes **REIMBURSEMENT INFORMATION** General ♦ See notes on page 286. Medicare ♦ Follow–up Days — 90 ♦ Assistant Surgeon — paid ♦ Supply Charges — not allowed ♦ Outpatient Limit — does not apply ♦ Major Surgery Rules Apply
26590	Repair macrodactylia	755.57 Macrodactylia (fingers) 755.65 Macrodactylia of toes V13.6 Hx of congenital malformation **REIMBURSEMENT INFORMATION** General ♦ See notes on page 286. Medicare ♦ Follow–up Days — 90 ♦ Assistant Surgeon — paid ♦ Supply Charges — not allowed ♦ Outpatient Limit — does not apply ♦ Major Surgery Rules Apply

CPT CODE	SERVICE	ICD–9–CM

26591 Repair, intrinsic muscles of hand (specify)

CPT NOTES

- For mircrosurgical technique, use modifier "-20" or 09920.

728.83	Nontraumatic muscle rupture
736.09	Forearm deformity NEC
883.2	Open wound of finger w/tendon
927.3	Crushing injury, finger

REIMBURSEMENT INFORMATION

General

- See notes on page 286.

Medicare

- Follow–up Days — 90
- Assistant Surgeon — not paid
- Supply Charges — not allowed
- Outpatient Limit — does not apply
- Major Surgery Rules Apply

26593 Release, intrinsic muscles of hand (specify)

CPT NOTES

- For mircrosurgical technique, use modifier "-20" or 09920.

714.0	Rheumatoid arthritis
716.14	Traumatic arthropathy, hand
718.44	Contracture of joint, hand
719.54	Joint stiffness NEC, hand
728.85	Spasm of muscle
736.09	Forearm deformity NEC
907.4	Late effect, nerve injury shld/arm
955.1	Injury median nerve
955.2	Injury ulnar nerve
955.3	Injury radial nerve
955.4	Injury musculocutaneous nerve
955.5	Injury cutaneous sensory nerve/arm

REIMBURSEMENT INFORMATION

General

- See notes on page 286.

Medicare

- Follow–up Days — 90
- Assistant Surgeon — not paid
- Supply Charges — not allowed
- Outpatient Limit — does not apply
- Major Surgery Rules Apply

CPT CODE	SERVICE	ICD–9–CM
26596	Excision of constricting ring of finger, with multiple Z-plasties	754.89 Nonteratogenic anomaly NEC V13.6 Hx of congenital malformation

REIMBURSEMENT INFORMATION

General

- ♦ See notes on page 286.

Medicare

- ♦ Follow–up Days — 90
- ♦ Assistant Surgeon — paid
- ♦ Supply Charges — not allowed
- ♦ Outpatient Limit — does not apply
- ♦ Major Surgery Rules Apply

CPT CODE	SERVICE	ICD–9–CM
26597	Release of scar contracture, flexor or extensor, with skin grafts, rearrangement flaps, or Z-plasties, hand and/or finger	709.2 Scar/fibrosis of skin 728.89 Muscle/ligament disorder NEC 905.8 Late effect of tendon injury 906.1 Late effect, open wound extremity 906.4 Late effect of crushing 906.6 Late effect of wrist/hand burn 907.4 Late effect, nerve injury shld/arm 996.92 Complication, reattached hand 996.93 Complication, reattached finger

REIMBURSEMENT INFORMATION

General

- ♦ See notes on page 286.

Medicare

- ♦ Follow–up Days — 90
- ♦ Assistant Surgeon — paid
- ♦ Supply Charges — not allowed
- ♦ Outpatient Limit — does not apply
- ♦ Major Surgery Rules Apply

CPT CODE	SERVICE	ICD-9-CM
26600	Closed treatment of metacarpal fracture, single; without manipulation, each bone	815.00 Fx metacarpal bone NOS, closed 815.02 Fx metacarpal base NEC, closed 815.03 Fx metacarpal shaft, closed 815.04 Fx metacarpal neck, closed 815.09 Metacarpus Fx, mult sites, closed

REIMBURSEMENT INFORMATION

General

- ♦ See notes on page 286.

Medicare

- ♦ Follow-up Days — 90
- ♦ Assistant Surgeon — not paid
- ♦ Supply Charges — not allowed
- ♦ Outpatient Limit — applies
- ♦ Major Surgery Rules Apply

CPT CODE	SERVICE	ICD-9-CM
26605	Closed treatment of metacarpal fracture, single; with manipulation, each bone	815.00 Fx metacarpal bone NOS, closed 815.02 Fx metacarpal base NEC, closed 815.03 Fx metacarpal shaft, closed 815.04 Fx metacarpal neck, closed 815.09 Metacarpus Fx, mult sites, closed 815.10 Fx metacarpal bone NOS, open 815.12 Fx metacarpal base NEC, open 815.13 Fx metacarpal shaft, open 815.14 Fx metacarpal neck, open 815.19 Metacarpus Fx, multiple sites, open

REIMBURSEMENT INFORMATION

General

- ♦ See notes on page 286.

Medicare

- ♦ Follow-up Days — 90
- ♦ Assistant Surgeon — not paid
- ♦ Supply Charges — not allowed
- ♦ Outpatient Limit — does not apply
- ♦ Major Surgery Rules Apply

CPT CODE	SERVICE	ICD-9-CM
26607	Closed treatment of metacarpal fracture, single; with manipulation, with internal or external fixation, each bone	815.00 Fx metacarpal bone NOS, closed 815.02 Fx metacarpal base NEC, closed 815.03 Fx metacarpal shaft, closed 815.04 Fx metacarpal neck, closed 815.09 Metacarpus Fx, mult sites, closed 815.10 Fx metacarpal bone NOS, open 815.12 Fx metacarpal base NEC, open 815.13 Fx metacarpal shaft, open 815.14 Fx metacarpal neck, open 815.19 Metacarpus Fx, multiple sites, open **REIMBURSEMENT INFORMATION** General ♦ See notes on page 286. Medicare ♦ Follow-up Days — 90 ♦ Assistant Surgeon — not paid ♦ Supply Charges — not allowed ♦ Outpatient Limit — does not apply ♦ Major Surgery Rules Apply
26608	Percutaneous skeletal fixation of metacarpal fracture, each bone	815.00 Fx metacarpal bone NOS, closed 815.02 Fx metacarpal base NEC, closed 815.03 Fx metacarpal shaft, closed 815.04 Fx metacarpal neck, closed 815.09 Metacarpus Fx, mult sites, closed 815.10 Fx metacarpal bone NOS, open 815.12 Fx metacarpal base NEC, open 815.13 Fx metacarpal shaft, open 815.14 Fx metacarpal neck, open 815.19 Metacarpus Fx, multiple sites, open **REIMBURSEMENT INFORMATION** General ♦ See notes on page 286. Medicare ♦ Follow-up Days — 90 ♦ Assistant Surgeon — by report ♦ Supply Charges — not allowed ♦ Outpatient Limit — does not apply ♦ Major Surgery Rules Apply

CPT CODE	SERVICE	ICD–9–CM
26615	Open treatment of metacarpal fracture, single, with or without internal or external fixation, each bone	815.00 Fx metacarpal bone NOS, closed 815.02 Fx metacarpal base NEC, closed 815.03 Fx metacarpal shaft, closed 815.04 Fx metacarpal neck, closed 815.09 Metacarpus Fx, mult sites, closed 815.10 Fx metacarpal bone NOS, open 815.12 Fx metacarpal base NEC, open 815.13 Fx metacarpal shaft, open 815.14 Fx metacarpal neck, open 815.19 Metacarpus Fx, multiple sites, open **REIMBURSEMENT INFORMATION** General ◆ See notes on page 286. Medicare ◆ Follow–up Days — 90 ◆ Assistant Surgeon — not paid ◆ Supply Charges — not allowed ◆ Outpatient Limit — does not apply ◆ Major Surgery Rules Apply
26641	Closed treatment of carpometacarpal dislocation, thumb, with manipulation	718.44 Contracture of joint, hand 833.04 Disloc carpometacarpal, closed 833.14 Disloc carpometacarpal, open **REIMBURSEMENT INFORMATION** General ◆ See notes on page 286. Medicare ◆ Follow–up Days — 90 ◆ Assistant Surgeon — not paid ◆ Supply Charges — not allowed ◆ Outpatient Limit — does not apply ◆ Major Surgery Rules Apply

CPT CODE	SERVICE	ICD-9-CM
26645	Closed treatment of carpometacarpal fracture dislocation, thumb (Bennett fracture), with manipulation	815.01 Fx thumb base metacarpal, closed 815.11 Fx thumb base metacarpal, open **REIMBURSEMENT INFORMATION** General ◆ See notes on page 286. Medicare ◆ Follow-up Days — 90 ◆ Assistant Surgeon — not paid ◆ Supply Charges — not allowed ◆ Outpatient Limit — does not apply ◆ Major Surgery Rules Apply
26650	Percutaneous skeletal fixation of carpometacarpal fracture dislocation, thumb (Bennett fracture), with manipulation, with or without external fixation	815.01 Fx thumb base metacarpal, closed 815.11 Fx thumb base metacarpal, open **REIMBURSEMENT INFORMATION** General ◆ See notes on page 286. Medicare ◆ Follow-up Days — 90 ◆ Assistant Surgeon — paid ◆ Supply Charges — not allowed ◆ Outpatient Limit — does not apply ◆ Major Surgery Rules Apply
26665	Open treatment of carpometacarpal fracture dislocation, thumb (Bennett fracture), with or without internal or external fixation	815.01 Fx thumb base metacarpal, closed 815.11 Fx thumb base metacarpal, open **REIMBURSEMENT INFORMATION** General ◆ See notes on page 286. Medicare ◆ Follow-up Days — 90 ◆ Assistant Surgeon — paid ◆ Supply Charges — not allowed ◆ Outpatient Limit — does not apply ◆ Major Surgery Rules Apply

CPT CODE	SERVICE	ICD–9–CM
26670	Closed treatment of carpometacarpal dislocation, other than thumb (Bennett fracture), single, with manipulation; without anesthesia	718.44 Contracture of joint, hand 833.04 Disloc carpometacarpal, closed 833.14 Disloc carpometacarpal, open
26675	Closed treatment of carpometacarpal dislocation, other than thumb (Bennett fracture), single, with manipulation; requiring anesthesia	

REIMBURSEMENT INFORMATION

General

- ◆ See notes on page 286.

Medicare

- ◆ Follow–up Days — 90
- ◆ Assistant Surgeon — by report
- ◆ Supply Charges — not allowed
- ◆ Outpatient Limit — does not apply
- ◆ Major Surgery Rules Apply

CPT CODE	SERVICE	ICD–9–CM
26676	Percutaneous skeletal fixation of carpometacarpal dislocation, other than thumb (Bennett fracture), single, with manipulation	718.44 Contracture of joint, hand 833.04 Disloc carpometacarpal, closed 833.14 Disloc carpometacarpal, open

REIMBURSEMENT INFORMATION

General

- ◆ See notes on page 286.

Medicare

- ◆ Follow–up Days — 90
- ◆ Assistant Surgeon — paid
- ◆ Supply Charges — not allowed
- ◆ Outpatient Limit — does not apply
- ◆ Major Surgery Rules Apply

CPT CODE	SERVICE	ICD–9–CM
26685	Open treatment of carpometacarpal dislocation, other than thumb (Bennett fracture); single, with or without internal or external fixation	718.44 Contracture of joint, hand 833.04 Disloc carpometacarpal, closed 833.14 Disloc carpometacarpal, open
26686	Open treatment of carpometacarpal dislocation, other than thumb (Bennett fracture); complex, multiple or delayed reduction	

REIMBURSEMENT INFORMATION

General

- ◆ See notes on page 286.

Medicare

- ◆ Follow–up Days — 90
- ◆ Assistant Surgeon — paid
- ◆ Supply Charges — not allowed
- ◆ Outpatient Limit — does not apply
- ◆ Major Surgery Rules Apply

CPT CODE	SERVICE	ICD-9-CM
26700	Closed treatment of metacarpophalangeal dislocation, single, with manipulation; without anesthesia	718.44 Contracture of joint, hand 833.04 Disloc carpometacarpal, closed 833.14 Disloc carpometacarpal, open
26705	Closed treatment of metacarpophalangeal dislocation, single, with manipulation; requiring anesthesia	**REIMBURSEMENT INFORMATION** General ◆ See notes on page 286. Medicare ◆ Follow-up Days — 90 ◆ Assistant Surgeon — not paid ◆ Supply Charges — not allowed ◆ Outpatient Limit — does not apply ◆ Major Surgery Rules Apply
26706	Percutaneous skeletal fixation of metacarpophalangeal dislocation, single, with manipulation	718.44 Contracture of joint, hand 833.04 Disloc carpometacarpal, closed 833.14 Disloc carpometacarpal, open **REIMBURSEMENT INFORMATION** General ◆ See notes on page 286. Medicare ◆ Follow-up Days — 90 ◆ Assistant Surgeon — paid ◆ Supply Charges — not allowed ◆ Outpatient Limit — does not apply ◆ Major Surgery Rules Apply
26715	Open treatment of metacarpophalangeal dislocation, single, with or without internal or external fixation	718.44 Contracture of joint, hand 833.04 Disloc carpometacarpal, closed 833.14 Disloc carpometacarpal, open **REIMBURSEMENT INFORMATION** General ◆ See notes on page 286. Medicare ◆ Follow-up Days — 90 ◆ Assistant Surgeon — not paid ◆ Supply Charges — not allowed ◆ Outpatient Limit — does not apply ◆ Major Surgery Rules Apply

CPT CODE	SERVICE	ICD–9–CM
26720	Closed treatment of phalangeal shaft fracture, proximal or middle phalanx, finger or thumb; without manipulation, each	816.01 Fx mid/prox phalanx, hand, closed 816.11 Fx mid/prox phalanx, hand, open **REIMBURSEMENT INFORMATION** General ♦ See notes on page 286. Medicare ♦ Follow–up Days — 90 ♦ Assistant Surgeon — not paid ♦ Supply Charges — not allowed ♦ Outpatient Limit — applies ♦ Major Surgery Rules Apply
26725	Closed treatment of phalangeal shaft fracture, proximal or middle phalanx, finger or thumb; with manipulation, with or without skin or skeletal traction, each	816.01 Fx mid/prox phalanx, hand, closed 816.03 Fx mult phalanx, hand, closed 816.11 Fx mid/prox phalanx, hand, open 816.13 Fx mult phalanx, hand, open **REIMBURSEMENT INFORMATION** General ♦ See notes on page 286. Medicare ♦ Follow–up Days — 90 ♦ Assistant Surgeon — not paid ♦ Supply Charges — not allowed ♦ Outpatient Limit — applies ♦ Major Surgery Rules Apply
26727	Percutaneous skeletal fixation of unstable phalangeal shaft fracture, proximal or middle phalanx, finger or thumb, with manipulation, each	816.01 Fx mid/prox phalanx, hand, closed 816.03 Fx mult phalanx, hand, closed 816.11 Fx mid/prox phalanx, hand, open 816.13 Fx mult phalanx, hand, open **REIMBURSEMENT INFORMATION** General ♦ See notes on page 286. Medicare ♦ Follow–up Days — 90 ♦ Assistant Surgeon — not paid ♦ Supply Charges — not allowed ♦ Outpatient Limit — does not apply ♦ Major Surgery Rules Apply

CPT CODE	SERVICE	ICD-9-CM
26735	Open treatment of phalangeal shaft fracture, proximal or middle phalanx, finger or thumb, with or without internal or external fixation, each	816.01 Fx mid/prox phalanx, hand, closed 816.03 Fx mult phalanx, hand, closed 816.11 Fx mid/prox phalanx, hand, open 816.13 Fx mult phalanx, hand, open

REIMBURSEMENT INFORMATION

General

- ♦ See notes on page 286.

Medicare

- ♦ Follow-up Days — 90
- ♦ Assistant Surgeon — not paid
- ♦ Supply Charges — not allowed
- ♦ Outpatient Limit — does not apply
- ♦ Major Surgery Rules Apply

CPT CODE	SERVICE	ICD-9-CM
26740	Closed treatment of articular fracture, involving metacarpophalangeal or interphalangeal joint; without manipulation, each	815.04 Fx metacarpal neck, closed 815.14 Fx metacarpal neck, open 816.00 Fx phalanx, hand NOS, closed 816.01 Fx mid/prox phalanx, hand, closed 816.02 Fx distal phalanx, hand, closed 816.03 Fx mult phalanx, hand, closed 816.10 Fx phalanx, hand NOS, open 816.11 Fx mid/prox phalanx, hand, open 816.12 Fx distal phalanx, hand, open 816.13 Fx mult phalanx, hand, open 817.0 Multiple Fx hand, closed
26742	Closed treatment of articular fracture, involving metacarpophalangeal or interphalangeal joint; with manipulation, each	

REIMBURSEMENT INFORMATION

General

- ♦ See notes on page 286.

Medicare

- ♦ Follow-up Days — 90
- ♦ Assistant Surgeon — not paid
- ♦ Supply Charges — not allowed
- ♦ Outpatient Limit
  26740 — applies
  26742 — does not apply
- ♦ Major Surgery Rules Apply

CPT CODE	SERVICE	ICD–9–CM
26746	Open treatment of articular fracture, involving metacarpophalangeal or interphalangeal joint, with or without internal or external fixation, each	815.04 Fx metacarpal neck, closed 815.14 Fx metacarpal neck, open 816.00 Fx phalanx, hand NOS, closed 816.01 Fx mid/prox phalanx, hand, closed 816.02 Fx distal phalanx, hand, closed 816.03 Fx mult phalanx, hand, closed 816.10 Fx phalanx, hand NOS, open 816.11 Fx mid/prox phalanx, hand, open 816.12 Fx distal phalanx, hand, open 816.13 Fx mult phalanx, hand, open 817.0 Multiple Fx hand, closed 817.1 Multiple Fx hand, open

REIMBURSEMENT INFORMATION

General

- See notes on page 286.

Medicare

- Follow–up Days — 90
- Assistant Surgeon — not paid
- Supply Charges — not allowed
- Outpatient Limit — does not apply
- Major Surgery Rules Apply

CPT CODE	SERVICE	ICD–9–CM
26750	Closed treatment of distal phalangeal fracture, finger or thumb; without manipulation, each	816.02 Fx distal phalanx, hand, closed 816.12 Fx distal phalanx, hand, open

REIMBURSEMENT INFORMATION

General

- See notes on page 286.

Medicare

- Follow–up Days — 90
- Assistant Surgeon — not paid
- Supply Charges — not allowed
- Outpatient Limit — does not apply
- Major Surgery Rules Apply

CPT CODE	SERVICE	ICD-9-CM
26755	Closed treatment of distal phalangeal fracture, finger or thumb; with manipulation, each	816.02 Fx distal phalanx, hand, closed 816.03 Fx mult phalanx, hand, closed 816.12 Fx distal phalanx, hand, open 816.13 Fx mult phalanx, hand, open **REIMBURSEMENT INFORMATION** <u>General</u> ♦ See notes on page 286. <u>Medicare</u> ♦ Follow-up Days — 90 ♦ Assistant Surgeon — not paid ♦ Supply Charges — not allowed ♦ Outpatient Limit — does not apply ♦ Major Surgery Rules Apply
26756	Percutaneous skeletal fixation of distal phalangeal fracture, finger or thumb, each	816.02 Fx distal phalanx, hand, closed 816.03 Fx mult phalanx, hand, closed 816.12 Fx distal phalanx, hand, open 816.13 Fx mult phalanx, hand, open **REIMBURSEMENT INFORMATION** <u>General</u> ♦ See notes on page 286. <u>Medicare</u> ♦ Follow-up Days — 90 ♦ Assistant Surgeon — not paid ♦ Supply Charges — not allowed ♦ Outpatient Limit — does not apply ♦ Major Surgery Rules Apply
26765	Open treatment of distal phalangeal fracture, finger or thumb, with or without internal or external fixation, each	816.02 Fx distal phalanx, hand, closed 816.03 Fx mult phalanx, hand, closed 816.12 Fx distal phalanx, hand, open 816.13 Fx mult phalanx, hand, open **REIMBURSEMENT INFORMATION** <u>General</u> ♦ See notes on page 286. <u>Medicare</u> ♦ Follow-up Days — 90 ♦ Assistant Surgeon — not paid ♦ Supply Charges — not allowed ♦ Outpatient Limit — does not apply ♦ Major Surgery Rules Apply

CPT CODE	SERVICE	ICD–9–CM
26770	Closed treatment of interphalangeal joint dislocation, single, with manipulation; without anesthesia	718.34 Recurrent dislocation, hand 834.02 Disloc interphalangeal hand, closed 834.12 Disloc interphalangeal hand, open
26775	Closed treatment of interphalangeal joint dislocation, single, with manipulation; requiring anesthesia	

REIMBURSEMENT INFORMATION

General

- ♦ See notes on page 286.

Medicare

- ♦ Follow–up Days — 90
- ♦ Assistant Surgeon — not paid
- ♦ Supply Charges — not allowed
- ♦ Outpatient Limit — does not apply
- ♦ Major Surgery Rules Apply

CPT CODE	SERVICE	ICD–9–CM
26776	Percutaneous skeletal fixation of interphalangeal joint dislocation, single, with manipulation	718.34 Recurrent dislocation, hand 834.02 Disloc interphalangeal hand, closed 834.12 Disloc interphalangeal hand, open

REIMBURSEMENT INFORMATION

General

- ♦ See notes on page 286.

Medicare

- ♦ Follow–up Days — 90
- ♦ Assistant Surgeon — paid
- ♦ Supply Charges — not allowed
- ♦ Outpatient Limit — does not apply
- ♦ Major Surgery Rules Apply

CPT CODE	SERVICE	ICD–9–CM
26785	Open treatment of interphalangeal joint dislocation, with or without internal or external fixation, single	718.34 Recurrent dislocation, hand 834.02 Disloc interphalangeal hand, closed 834.12 Disloc interphalangeal hand, open

REIMBURSEMENT INFORMATION

General

- ♦ See notes on page 286.

Medicare

- ♦ Follow–up Days — 90
- ♦ Assistant Surgeon — not paid
- ♦ Supply Charges — not allowed
- ♦ Outpatient Limit — does not apply
- ♦ Major Surgery Rules Apply

CPT CODE	SERVICE
26820	Fusion in opposition, thumb, with autogenous graft (includes obtaining graft)

ICD–9–CM

138.	Late effects of acute polio
170.5	M-Neoplasm, Wrist/Hand bones
198.5	M2-Neoplasm, Bone and bone marrow
213.5	B-Neoplasm, Wrist/Hand bones
237.7	UB-Neoplasm, Neurofibromatosis
252.0	Hyperparathyroidism
354.0	Carpal tunnel syndrome
354.1	Lesion of median nerve NEC
354.2	Ulnar nerve lesion
356.1	Peroneal muscular atrophy
711.04	Pyogenic arthritis, hand
711.94	Infect arthritis NOS, hand
714.0	Rheumatoid arthritis
714.30	Juvenile rheumatoid arthritis NOS
714.31	Juvenile acute rheumatoid arthritis
714.32	Pauciarticular juv rheum arthritis
714.33	Monoarticular juv rheum arthritis
714.4	Chronic postrheumatic arthritis
715.14	Loc prim osteoarthritis, hand
715.24	Loc 2nd osteoarthritis, hand
715.34	Loc osteoarthritis NOS, hand
715.94	Osteoarthrosis NOS, hand
716.04	Kaschin-Beck disease, hand
716.14	Traumatic arthropathy, hand
716.24	Allergic arthritis, hand
716.34	Climacteric arthritis, hand
716.44	Transient arthropathy, hand
718.04	Articular cartilage dis, hand
718.24	Pathologic dislocation, hand
718.34	Recurrent dislocation, hand
730.14	Chronic osteomyelitis, hand
733.82	Nonunion of fracture
814.0x	Carpal fracture, closed
814.1x	Carpal fracture, open
815.0x	Metacarpal fracture, closed
815.1x	Metacarpal fracture, open
907.4	Late effect, nerve injury shld/arm
996.66	Reaction, internal joint prosthesis
996.67	Reaction, internal ortho device NEC

REIMBURSEMENT INFORMATION

General

- See notes on page 286.

Medicare

- Follow–up Days — 90
- Assistant Surgeon — paid
- Supply Charges — not allowed
- Outpatient Limit — does not apply
- Major Surgery Rules Apply

CPT CODE	SERVICE
26841	Arthrodesis, carpometacarpal joint, thumb, with or without internal fixation
26842	Arthrodesis, carpometacarpal joint, thumb, with or without internal fixation; with autograft (includes obtaining graft)

ICD–9–CM

138.	Late effects of acute polio
170.5	M-Neoplasm, Wrist/Hand bones
198.5	M2-Neoplasm, Bone and bone marrow
213.5	B-Neoplasm, Wrist/Hand bones
237.7	UB-Neoplasm, Neurofibromatosis
252.0	Hyperparathyroidism
356.1	Peroneal muscular atrophy
711.04	Pyogenic arthritis, hand
711.94	Infect arthritis NOS, hand
714.0	Rheumatoid arthritis
714.3x	Juvenile chronic polyarthritis
714.4	Chronic postrheumatic arthritis
715.14	Loc prim osteoarthritis, hand
715.24	Loc 2nd osteoarthritis, hand
715.34	Loc osteoarthritis NOS, hand
715.94	Osteoarthrosis NOS, hand
716.04	Kaschin-Beck disease, hand
716.14	Traumatic arthropathy, hand
716.24	Allergic arthritis, hand
716.34	Climacteric arthritis, hand
716.44	Transient arthropathy, hand
718.04	Articular cartilage dis, hand
718.24	Pathologic dislocation, hand
718.34	Recurrent dislocation, hand
718.44	Contracture of joint, hand
718.54	Ankylosis of joint, hand
719.44	Pain in joint, hand
730.14	Chronic osteomyelitis, hand
733.82	Nonunion of fracture
814.0x	Carpal fracture, closed
814.1x	Carpal fracture, open
815.0x	Metacarpal fracture, closed
815.1x	Metacarpal fracture, open
905.6	Late effect of dislocation
905.8	Late effect of tendon injury
906.4	Late effect of crushing
906.6	Late effect of wrist/hand burn
996.66	Reaction, internal joint prosthesis
996.67	Reaction, internal ortho device NEC

REIMBURSEMENT INFORMATION

General

- See notes on page 286.

Medicare

- Follow–up Days — 90
- Assistant Surgeon — paid
- Supply Charges — not allowed
- Outpatient Limit — does not apply
- Major Surgery Rules Apply

CPT CODE	SERVICE	ICD–9–CM	
26843	Arthrodesis, carpometacarpal joint, digits, other than thumb	138.	Late effects of acute polio
		170.5	M-Neoplasm, Wrist/Hand bones
		198.5	M2-Neoplasm, Bone and bone marrow
26844	Arthrodesis, carpometacarpal joint, digits, other than thumb; with autograft (includes obtaining graft)	213.5	B-Neoplasm, Wrist/Hand bones
		237.7	UB-Neoplasm, Neurofibromatosis
		252.0	Hyperparathyroidism
		356.1	Peroneal muscular atrophy
		711.04	Pyogenic arthritis, hand
		711.94	Infect arthritis NOS, hand
		714.0	Rheumatoid arthritis
		714.3x	Juvenile chronic polyarthritis
		714.4	Chronic postrheumatic arthritis
		715.14	Loc prim osteoarthritis, hand
		715.24	Loc 2nd osteoarthritis, hand
		715.34	Loc osteoarthritis NOS, hand
		715.94	Osteoarthrosis NOS, hand
		716.04	Kaschin-Beck disease, hand
		716.14	Traumatic arthropathy, hand
		716.24	Allergic arthritis, hand
		716.34	Climacteric arthritis, hand
		716.44	Transient arthropathy, hand
		718.04	Articular cartilage dis, hand
		718.24	Pathologic dislocation, hand
		718.34	Recurrent dislocation, hand
		718.44	Contracture of joint, hand
		718.54	Ankylosis of joint, hand
		719.44	Pain in joint, hand
		730.14	Chronic osteomyelitis, hand
		733.82	Nonunion of fracture
		814.0x	Carpal fracture, closed
		814.1x	Carpal fracture, open
		815.0x	Metacarpal fracture, closed
		815.1x	Metacarpal fracture, open
		905.6	Late effect of dislocation
		905.8	Late effect of tendon injury
		906.4	Late effect of crushing
		906.6	Late effect of wrist/hand burn
		996.66	Reaction, internal joint prosthesis
		996.67	Reaction, internal ortho device NEC

REIMBURSEMENT INFORMATION

General

- See notes on page 286.

Medicare

- Follow–up Days — 90
- Assistant Surgeon — paid
- Supply Charges — not allowed
- Outpatient Limit — does not apply
- Major Surgery Rules Apply

CPT CODE	SERVICE
26850	Arthrodesis, metacarpophalangeal joint, with or without internal fixation
26852	Arthrodesis, metacarpophalangeal joint, with or without internal fixation; with autograft (includes obtaining graft)

ICD–9–CM

138.	Late effects of acute polio
170.5	M-Neoplasm, Wrist/Hand bones
198.5	M2-Neoplasm, Bone and bone marrow
213.5	B-Neoplasm, Wrist/Hand bones
237.7	UB-Neoplasm, Neurofibromatosis
252.0	Hyperparathyroidism
356.1	Peroneal muscular atrophy
711.04	Pyogenic arthritis, hand
711.94	Infect arthritis NOS, hand
714.0	Rheumatoid arthritis
714.3x	Juvenile chronic polyarthritis
714.4	Chronic postrheumatic arthritis
715.14	Loc prim osteoarthritis, hand
715.24	Loc 2nd osteoarthritis, hand
715.34	Loc osteoarthritis NOS, hand
715.94	Osteoarthrosis NOS, hand
716.04	Kaschin-Beck disease, hand
716.14	Traumatic arthropathy, hand
716.24	Allergic arthritis, hand
716.34	Climacteric arthritis, hand
716.44	Transient arthropathy, hand
718.04	Articular cartilage dis, hand
718.24	Pathologic dislocation, hand
718.34	Recurrent dislocation, hand
718.44	Contracture of joint, hand
718.54	Ankylosis of joint, hand
719.44	Pain in joint, hand
729.5	Pain in limb
730.14	Chronic osteomyelitis, hand
733.82	Nonunion of fracture
815.0x	Metacarpal fracture, closed
815.1x	Metacarpal fracture, open
816.0x	Phalanges fracture, closed
816.1x	Phalanges fracture, open
817.0	Multiple Fx hand, closed
817.1	Multiple Fx hand, open
905.6	Late effect of dislocation
905.8	Late effect of tendon injury
906.4	Late effect of crushing
906.6	Late effect of wrist/hand burn
996.66	Reaction, internal joint prosthesis
996.67	Reaction, internal ortho device NEC

REIMBURSEMENT INFORMATION

General

- See notes on page 286.

Medicare

- Follow–up Days — 90
- Assistant Surgeon — paid
- Supply Charges — not allowed
- Outpatient Limit — does not apply
- Major Surgery Rules Apply

CPT CODE	SERVICE
26860	Arthrodesis, interphalangeal joint, with or without internal fixation
26861	Arthrodesis, interphalangeal joint, with or without internal fixation; each additional interphalangeal joint
26862	Arthrodesis, interphalangeal joint, with or without internal fixation; with autograft (includes obtaining graft)
26863	Arthrodesis, interphalangeal joint, with or without internal fixation; with autograft (includes obtaining graft), each additional joint

ICD–9–CM

138.	Late effects of acute polio
170.5	M-Neoplasm, Wrist/Hand bones
198.5	M2-Neoplasm, Bone and bone marrow
213.5	B-Neoplasm, Wrist/Hand bones
237.7	UB-Neoplasm, Neurofibromatosis
252.0	Hyperparathyroidism
356.1	Peroneal muscular atrophy
711.04	Pyogenic arthritis, hand
711.94	Infect arthritis NOS, hand
714.0	Rheumatoid arthritis
714.3x	Juvenile chronic polyarthritis
714.4	Chronic postrheumatic arthritis
715.14	Loc prim osteoarthritis, hand
715.24	Loc 2nd osteoarthritis, hand
715.34	Loc osteoarthritis NOS, hand
715.94	Osteoarthrosis NOS, hand
716.04	Kaschin-Beck disease, hand
716.14	Traumatic arthropathy, hand
716.24	Allergic arthritis, hand
716.34	Climacteric arthritis, hand
716.44	Transient arthropathy, hand
718.04	Articular cartilage dis, hand
718.24	Pathologic dislocation, hand
718.34	Recurrent dislocation, hand
718.44	Contracture of joint, hand
718.54	Ankylosis of joint, hand
719.44	Pain in joint, hand
729.5	Pain in limb
730.14	Chronic osteomyelitis, hand
733.82	Nonunion of fracture
816.0x	Phalanges fracture, closed
816.1x	Phalanges fracture, open
817.0	Multiple Fx hand, closed
817.1	Multiple Fx hand, open
905.6	Late effect of dislocation
905.8	Late effect of tendon injury
906.4	Late effect of crushing
906.6	Late effect of wrist/hand burn
996.66	Reaction, internal joint prosthesis
996.67	Reaction, internal ortho device NEC

REIMBURSEMENT INFORMATION

General

- See notes on page 286.

Medicare

- Follow–up Days
  26860, 26862 — 90
  26861, 26863 — none; falls within global period of another procedure
- Assistant Surgeon
  26860, 26862–26863 — not paid
  26861 — not paid
- Supply Charges — not allowed
- Outpatient Limit — does not apply
- Major Surgery Rules Apply (26860, 26862)

CPT CODE	SERVICE
26910	Amputation, metacarpal, with finger or thumb (ray amputation), single, with or without interosseous transfer

CPT NOTES

- ◆ For hand through metacarpal bones, see 25927.
- ◆ For repositioning, see 26550, 26555.

ICD–9–CM

170.5	M-Neoplasm, Wrist/Hand bones
198.5	M2-Neoplasm, Bone and bone marrow
238.0	UB-Neoplasm, Bone
239.2	Bone/Skin neoplasm NOS
730.13	Chronic osteomyelitis, forearm
733.49	Aseptic necrosis of bone NEC
755.01	Polydactyly, fingers
785.4	Gangrene
883.1	Open wound of finger, complicated
883.2	Open wound of finger w/tendon
885.1	Traumatic thumb amputation, compl
886.1	Traumatic finger amputation, compl
905.2	Late effect, arm fracture
905.8	Late effect of tendon injury
905.9	Late effect of traumatic amputation
906.1	Late effect, open wound extremity
906.6	Late effect of wrist/hand burn
927.3	Crushing injury, finger
944.31	3rd deg burn, finger
944.32	3rd deg burn, thumb
944.33	3rd deg burn, mult fingers
944.34	3rd deg burn, finger w/thumb
944.41	Deep 3rd deg burn, finger
944.42	Deep 3rd deg burn, thumb
944.43	Deep 3rd deg burn, mult fingers
944.44	Deep 3rd deg burn, finger w/thumb
991.1	Frostbite of hand

REIMBURSEMENT INFORMATION

General

- ◆ See notes on page 286.

Medicare

- ◆ Follow–up Days — 90
- ◆ Assistant Surgeon — not paid
- ◆ Supply Charges — not allowed
- ◆ Outpatient Limit — does not apply
- ◆ Major Surgery Rules Apply

CPT CODE	SERVICE
26951	Amputation, finger or thumb, primary or secondary, any joint or phalanx, finger, including neurectomies; with direct closure
26952	Amputation, finger or thumb, primary or secondary, any joint or phalanx, finger, including neurectomies; with local advancement flaps (V-Y, hood)

CPT NOTES

- For hand through metacarpal bones, see 25927.
- For repair of soft tissue defect requiring split or full thickness graft or other pedicle flaps, see 15050-15755.

ICD–9–CM

170.5	M-Neoplasm, Wrist/Hand bones
198.5	M2-Neoplasm, Bone and bone marrow
238.0	UB-Neoplasm, Bone
239.2	Bone/Skin neoplasm NOS
730.13	Chronic osteomyelitis, forearm
733.49	Aseptic necrosis of bone NEC
755.01	Polydactyly, fingers
785.4	Gangrene
883.1	Open wound of finger, complicated
883.2	Open wound of finger w/tendon
885.1	Traumatic thumb amputation, compl
886.1	Traumatic finger amputation, compl
905.2	Late effect, arm fracture
905.8	Late effect of tendon injury
905.9	Late effect of traumatic amputation
906.1	Late effect, open wound extremity
906.6	Late effect of wrist/hand burn
927.3	Crushing injury, finger
944.31	3rd deg burn, finger
944.32	3rd deg burn, thumb
944.33	3rd deg burn, mult fingers
944.34	3rd deg burn, finger w/thumb
944.41	Deep 3rd deg burn, finger
944.42	Deep 3rd deg burn, thumb
944.43	Deep 3rd deg burn, mult fingers
944.44	Deep 3rd deg burn, finger w/thumb
991.1	Frostbite of hand

REIMBURSEMENT INFORMATION

General

- See notes on page 286.

Medicare

- Follow–up Days — 90
- Assistant Surgeon — not paid
- Supply Charges — not allowed
- Outpatient Limit — does not apply
- Major Surgery Rules Apply

CPT CODE	SERVICE	ICD–9–CM

26990 Incision and drainage, pelvis or hip joint area; deep abscess or hematoma

26991 Incision and drainage, pelvis or hip joint area; infected bursa

CPT NOTES

- For incision and drainage procedures, superficial, see 10040-10160.

682.6	Cellulitis of leg
711.05	Pyogenic arthritis, pelvis/thigh
711.95	Infect arthritis NOS, pelvis/thigh
726.5	Enthesopathy of hip
727.2	Occupational bursitis
727.3	Bursitis NOS
727.4x	Ganglion/cyst synovium/tendon/bursa
727.89	Synovium/tendon/bursa disorder NEC
906.3	Late effect of contusion
906.4	Late effect of crushing
909.3	Late effect of surg/med complic
924.0x	Contusion, hip and thigh
928.0x	Crushing injury, hip and thigh
928.8	Multiple crushing injuries, leg

REIMBURSEMENT INFORMATION

General

- See notes on page 286.

Medicare

- Follow–up Days — 90
- Assistant Surgeon — not paid
- Supply Charges — not allowed
- Outpatient Limit — does not apply
- Major Surgery Rules Apply

26992 Incision, deep, with opening of bone cortex (eg, for osteomyelitis or bone abscess), pelvis and/or hip joint

CPT NOTES

- For incision and drainage procedures, superficial, see 10040-10160.

730.05	Acute osteomyelitis, pelvis/thigh
730.15	Chronic osteomyelitis, pelvis/thigh
730.25	Osteomyelitis NOS, pelvis/thigh
730.95	Bone infection NOS, pelvis/thigh

REIMBURSEMENT INFORMATION

General

- See notes on page 286.

Medicare

- Follow–up Days — 90
- Assistant Surgeon — by report
- Supply Charges — not allowed
- Outpatient Limit — does not apply
- Major Surgery Rules Apply

CPT CODE	SERVICE
27035	Hip joint denervation, intrapelvic or extrapelvic intra-articular branches of sciatic, femoral or obturator nerves

CPT NOTES

- ♦ For incision and drainage procedures, superficial, see 10040-10160.
- ♦ For obturator neurectomy, see 64763, 65766.

ICD–9–CM

714.0	Rheumatoid arthritis
715.15	Loc prim osteoarthritis, pelv/thigh
715.25	Loc 2nd osteoarthritis, pelv/thigh
715.35	Loc osteoarthritis NOS, pelv/thigh

REIMBURSEMENT INFORMATION

General

- ♦ See notes on page 286.

Medicare

- ♦ Follow–up Days — 90
- ♦ Assistant Surgeon — paid
- ♦ Supply Charges — not allowed
- ♦ Outpatient Limit — does not apply
- ♦ Major Surgery Rules Apply

27040	Biopsy, soft tissue of pelvis and hip area; superficial
27041	Biopsy, soft tissue of pelvis and hip area; deep

CPT NOTES

- ♦ For needle biopsy of soft tissue, use 20206.

ICD–9–CM

171.3	M-Neoplasm, Soft tissue, leg
171.6	M-Neoplasm, Soft tissue, pelvis
215.3	B-Neoplasm, Soft tissue, leg
215.6	B-Neoplasm, Soft tissue, pelvis
238.1	UB-Neoplasm, Soft tissue
239.2	Bone/Skin neoplasm NOS

REIMBURSEMENT INFORMATION

General

- ♦ See notes on page 286.

Medicare

- ♦ Follow–up Days
  27040 — 10
  27041 — 90
- ♦ Assistant Surgeon — not paid
- ♦ Supply Charges — not allowed
- ♦ Outpatient Limit — does not apply
- ♦ Minor Surgery Rules Apply (27040)
  Major Surgery Rules Apply (27041)

CPT CODE	SERVICE	ICD–9–CM
27047	Excision, tumor, pelvis and hip area; subcutaneous	171.3 M-Neoplasm, Soft tissue, leg 171.6 M-Neoplasm, Soft tissue, pelvis 215.3 B-Neoplasm, Soft tissue, leg 215.6 B-Neoplasm, Soft tissue, pelvis 238.1 UB-Neoplasm, Soft tissue 239.2 Bone/Skin neoplasm NOS
27048	Excision, tumor, pelvis and hip area; deep, subfascial, intramuscular	

REIMBURSEMENT INFORMATION

General

- ♦ See notes on page 286.

Medicare

- ♦ Follow–up Days — 90
- ♦ Assistant Surgeon
  27047 — not paid
  27048 — not paid
- ♦ Supply Charges — not allowed
- ♦ Outpatient Limit — does not apply
- ♦ Major Surgery Rules Apply

CPT CODE	SERVICE	ICD–9–CM
27049	Radical resection of tumor (eg, malignant neoplasm), soft tissue of pelvis and hip area	171.3 M-Neoplasm, Soft tissue, leg 171.6 M-Neoplasm, Soft tissue, pelvis 238.1 UB-Neoplasm, Soft tissue 239.2 Bone/Skin neoplasm NOS

REIMBURSEMENT INFORMATION

General

- ♦ See notes on page 286.

Medicare

- ♦ Follow–up Days — 90
- ♦ Assistant Surgeon — paid
- ♦ Supply Charges — not allowed
- ♦ Outpatient Limit — does not apply
- ♦ Major Surgery Rules Apply

CPT CODE	SERVICE	ICD–9–CM
27060	Excision; ischial bursa	726.5 Enthesopathy of hip
27062	Excision; trochanteric bursa or calcification	

CPT NOTES

- ♦ For arthrocentesis or needling of bursa, see 20610.

REIMBURSEMENT INFORMATION

General

- ♦ See notes on page 286.

Medicare

- ♦ Follow–up Days — 90
- ♦ Assistant Surgeon — paid
- ♦ Supply Charges — not allowed
- ♦ Outpatient Limit — does not apply
- ♦ Major Surgery Rules Apply

CPT CODE	SERVICE	ICD-9-CM
27070	Partial excision (craterization, saucerization) (eg, for osteomyelitis); superficial (eg, wing of ilium, symphysis pubis or greater trochanter of femur)	344.00 Quadriplegia NOS 344.1 Paraplegia NOS 730.05 Acute osteomyelitis, pelvis/thigh 730.15 Chronic osteomyelitis, pelvis/thigh 730.25 Osteomyelitis NOS, pelvis/thigh 730.35 Periostitis, pelvis/thigh 731.0 Osteitis deformans NOS 733.21 Solitary bone cyst 733.22 Aneurysmal bone cyst 733.29 Bone cyst NEC 906.0 Late effect, open wound head/trunk 906.1 Late effect, open wound extremity 996.66 Reaction, internal joint prosthesis **REIMBURSEMENT INFORMATION** General ♦ See notes on page 286. Medicare ♦ Follow-up Days — 90 ♦ Assistant Surgeon — paid ♦ Supply Charges — not allowed ♦ Outpatient Limit — does not apply ♦ Major Surgery Rules Apply
27071	Partial excision (craterization, saucerization) (eg, for osteomyelitis); deep	344.00 Quadriplegia NOS 344.1 Paraplegia NOS 730.05 Acute osteomyelitis, pelvis/thigh 730.15 Chronic osteomyelitis, pelvis/thigh 730.35 Periostitis, pelvis/thigh 731.0 Osteitis deformans NOS 733.21 Solitary bone cyst 733.22 Aneurysmal bone cyst 733.29 Bone cyst NEC **REIMBURSEMENT INFORMATION** General ♦ See notes on page 286. Medicare ♦ Follow-up Days — 90 ♦ Assistant Surgeon — paid ♦ Supply Charges — not allowed ♦ Outpatient Limit — does not apply ♦ Major Surgery Rules Apply

CPT CODE	SERVICE	ICD–9–CM
▲ **27075**	Radical resection of tumor or infection; wing of ilium, one pubic or ischial ramus or symphysis pubis	170.6 M-Neoplasm, Pelvic girdle 238.0 UB-Neoplasm, Bone 239.2 Bone/Skin neoplasm NOS 344.00 Quadriplegia NOS 344.1 Paraplegia NOS 730.05 Acute osteomyelitis, pelvis/thigh 730.15 Chronic osteomyelitis, pelvis/thigh 906.0 Late effect, open wound head/trunk 906.1 Late effect, open wound extremity

REIMBURSEMENT INFORMATION

General

- See notes on page 286.
- Description changed in 1995 CPT.

Medicare

- Follow–up Days — 90
- Assistant Surgeon — paid
- Supply Charges — not allowed
- Outpatient Limit — does not apply
- Major Surgery Rules Apply

CPT CODE	SERVICE	ICD–9–CM
▲ **27076**	Radical resection of tumor or infection; ilium, including acetabulum, both pubic rami, or ischium and acetabulum	170.6 M-Neoplasm, Pelvic girdle 213.6 B-Neoplasm, Pelvic girdle 238.0 UB-Neoplasm, Bone 239.2 Bone/Skin neoplasm NOS 730.05 Acute osteomyelitis, pelvis/thigh 730.15 Chronic osteomyelitis, pelvis/thigh 906.0 Late effect, open wound head/trunk 906.1 Late effect, open wound extremity 996.66 Reaction, internal joint prosthesis

REIMBURSEMENT INFORMATION

General

- See notes on page 286.
- Description changed in 1995 CPT.

Medicare

- Follow–up Days — 90
- Assistant Surgeon — paid
- Supply Charges — not allowed
- Outpatient Limit — does not apply
- Major Surgery Rules Apply

CPT CODE	SERVICE	ICD-9-CM	
▲ 27077	Radical resection of tumor or infection; innominate bone, total	170.6	M-Neoplasm, Pelvic girdle
		213.6	B-Neoplasm, Pelvic girdle
		238.0	UB-Neoplasm, Bone
		239.2	Bone/Skin neoplasm NOS
		344.00	Quadriplegia NOS
		344.1	Paraplegia NOS
		682.2	Cellulitis of trunk
		707.0	Decubitus ulcer
		730.05	Acute osteomyelitis, pelvis/thigh
		730.15	Chronic osteomyelitis, pelvis/thigh
		879.7	Open wound of trunk NEC, complic

REIMBURSEMENT INFORMATION

General

- ♦ See notes on page 286.
- ♦ Description changed in 1995 CPT.

Medicare

- ♦ Follow–up Days — 90
- ♦ Assistant Surgeon — paid
- ♦ Supply Charges — not allowed
- ♦ Outpatient Limit — does not apply
- ♦ Major Surgery Rules Apply

CPT CODE	SERVICE	ICD-9-CM	
▲ 27078	Radical resection of tumor or infection; ischial tuberosity and greater trochanter of femur	170.7	M-Neoplasm, Long bones, lower limb
▲ 27079	Radical resection of tumor or infection; ischial tuberosity and greater trochanter of femur, with skin flaps	213.7	B-Neoplasm, Long bones, lower limb
		238.0	UB-Neoplasm, Bone
		239.2	Bone/Skin neoplasm NOS
		344.00	Quadriplegia NOS
		344.1	Paraplegia NOS
		682.2	Cellulitis of trunk
		682.6	Cellulitis of leg
		707.0	Decubitus ulcer
		730.05	Acute osteomyelitis, pelvis/thigh
		730.15	Chronic osteomyelitis, pelvis/thigh
		879.7	Open wound of trunk NEC, complic

REIMBURSEMENT INFORMATION

General

- ♦ See notes on page 286.
- ♦ Description changed in 1995 CPT.

Medicare

- ♦ Follow–up Days — 90
- ♦ Assistant Surgeon — paid
- ♦ Supply Charges — not allowed
- ♦ Outpatient Limit — does not apply
- ♦ Major Surgery Rules Apply

CPT CODE	SERVICE
27080	Coccygectomy, primary

CPT NOTES

- For pressure (decubitis) ulcer, see 15920, 15922 and 15931-15958.

ICD–9–CM

170.6	M-Neoplasm, Pelvic girdle
213.6	B-Neoplasm, Pelvic girdle
238.0	UB-Neoplasm, Bone
239.2	Bone/Skin neoplasm NOS
344.00	Quadriplegia NOS
344.1	Paraplegia NOS
707.0	Decubitus ulcer
724.79	Disorder of coccyx NEC
730.05	Acute osteomyelitis, pelvis/thigh
730.15	Chronic osteomyelitis, pelvis/thigh
805.6	Fx sacrum/coccyx, closed
805.7	Fx sacrum/coccyx, open
879.7	Open wound of trunk NEC, complic

REIMBURSEMENT INFORMATION

General

- See notes on page 286.

Medicare

- Follow–up Days — 90
- Assistant Surgeon — paid
- Supply Charges — not allowed
- Outpatient Limit — does not apply
- Major Surgery Rules Apply

CPT CODE	SERVICE	ICD-9-CM
27086*	Removal of foreign body, pelvis or hip; subcutaneous tissue	709.4 Foreign body granuloma, skin 729.6 Old foreign body in soft tissue 916.6 Foreign body, hip/leg 916.7 Foreign body, hip/leg, infected

REIMBURSEMENT INFORMATION

General

- ♦ See notes on page 286.
- ♦ Starred procedure.

Medicare

- ♦ Follow-up Days — 10
- ♦ Assistant Surgeon — not paid
- ♦ Supply Charges — not allowed
- ♦ Outpatient Limit — does not apply
- ♦ Minor Surgery Rules Apply

CPT CODE	SERVICE	ICD-9-CM
27087	Removal of foreign body, pelvis or hip; deep	728.82 Foreign body granuloma of muscle 729.6 Old foreign body in soft tissue 733.99 Bone/Cartilage disorder NEC 890.1 Open wound of hip/thigh, complic 996.66 Reaction, internal joint prosthesis 996.77 Complication, int joint prosthesis 998.7 Postop foreign subst acute reaction

REIMBURSEMENT INFORMATION

General

- ♦ See notes on page 286.

Medicare

- ♦ Follow-up Days — 90
- ♦ Assistant Surgeon — paid
- ♦ Supply Charges — not allowed
- ♦ Outpatient Limit — does not apply
- ♦ Major Surgery Rules Apply

CPT CODE	SERVICE	ICD–9–CM
27090	Removal of hip prosthesis; (separate procedure)	996.4 Malfunction, int orthoped dev/graft 996.66 Reaction, internal joint prosthesis 996.67 Reaction, internal ortho device NEC 996.77 Complication, int joint prosthesis 996.78 Complication, oth int ortho device 998.5 Postoperative infection V43.6 Joint replacement NEC V54.0 Removal of internal fixation device

REIMBURSEMENT INFORMATION

General

- ♦ See notes on page 286.
- ♦ Separate procedure rules apply.

Medicare

- ♦ Follow–up Days — 90
- ♦ Assistant Surgeon — paid
- ♦ Supply Charges — not allowed
- ♦ Outpatient Limit — does not apply
- ♦ Major Surgery Rules Apply

CPT CODE	SERVICE	ICD–9–CM
27091	Removal of hip prosthesis; complicated, including "total hip" and methylmethacrylate, when applicable	996.4 Malfunction, int orthoped dev/graft 996.66 Reaction, internal joint prosthesis 996.67 Reaction, internal ortho device NEC 996.77 Complication, int joint prosthesis 996.78 Complication, oth int ortho device 998.5 Postoperative infection V43.6 Joint replacement NEC V54.0 Removal of internal fixation device

REIMBURSEMENT INFORMATION

General

- ♦ See notes on page 286.

Medicare

- ♦ Follow–up Days — 90
- ♦ Assistant Surgeon — paid
- ♦ Supply Charges — not allowed
- ♦ Outpatient Limit — does not apply
- ♦ Major Surgery Rules Apply
- ♦ Fragments — 27090

CPT CODE	SERVICE
27093	Injection procedure for hip arthrography; without anesthesia

CPT NOTES

- ♦ For radiological supervision and interpretation, see 73525.

ICD–9–CM

714.0	Rheumatoid arthritis
715.15	Loc prim osteoarthritis, pelv/thigh
715.25	Loc 2nd osteoarthritis, pelv/thigh
715.35	Loc osteoarthritis NOS, pelv/thigh
716.15	Traumatic arthropathy, pelvis/thigh
716.45	Transient arthropathy, pelvis/thigh
718.05	Articular cartilage dis, pelv/thigh
718.15	Loose body in joint, pelvis/thigh
718.25	Pathologic dislocation, pelv/thigh
718.35	Recurrent dislocation, pelvis/thigh
718.45	Contracture of joint, pelvis/thigh
718.55	Ankylosis of joint, pelvis/thigh
718.85	Joint derangement NEC, pelvis/thigh
719.25	Villonodular synovitis, pelv/thigh
719.45	Pain in joint, pelvis/thigh
719.55	Joint stiffness NEC, pelvis/thigh
719.85	Joint disorder NEC, pelvis/thigh
727.00	Synovitis NOS
729.6	Old foreign body in soft tissue
754.30	Congenital hip dislocation, unilat
754.31	Congenital hip dislocation, bilat
754.32	Congenital hip sublux, unilateral
754.33	Congenital hip sublux, bilateral
754.35	Congenital hip dislocation w/sublux
996.4	Malfunction, int orthoped dev/graft
996.66	Reaction, internal joint prosthesis
996.67	Reaction, internal ortho device NEC
996.77	Complication, int joint prosthesis
996.78	Complication, oth int ortho device

REIMBURSEMENT INFORMATION

General

- ♦ See notes on page 286.

Medicare

- ♦ Follow–up Days — 0
- ♦ Assistant Surgeon — not paid
- ♦ Supply Charges — not allowed
- ♦ Outpatient Limit — does not apply
- ♦ Minor Surgery Rules Apply

CPT CODE	SERVICE	ICD–9–CM

27095 Injection procedure for hip arthrography; with anesthesia

CPT NOTES

- For radiological supervision and interpretation, see 73525.

714.0	Rheumatoid arthritis
715.15	Loc prim osteoarthritis, pelv/thigh
715.35	Loc osteoarthritis NOS, pelv/thigh
754.3	Congenital dislocation of hip
996.4	Malfunction, int orthoped dev/graft
996.66	Reaction, internal joint prosthesis
996.67	Reaction, internal ortho device NEC
996.77	Complication, int joint prosthesis
996.78	Complication, oth int ortho device

REIMBURSEMENT INFORMATION

General

- See notes on page 286.

Medicare

- Follow–up Days — 0
- Assistant Surgeon — not paid
- Supply Charges — not allowed
- Outpatient Limit — does not apply
- Minor Surgery Rules Apply

27301 Incision and drainage of deep abscess, infected bursa, or hematoma, thigh or knee region

CPT NOTES

- For incision and drainage of abscess or hematoma, superficial, see 10040-10160.

682.6	Cellulitis of leg
711.06	Pyogenic arthritis, lower leg
711.96	Infect arthritis NOS, lower leg
726.6x	Enthesopathy of knee
726.8	Peripheral enthesopathy NEC
727.2	Occupational bursitis
727.3	Bursitis NOS
727.4x	Ganglion/cyst synovium/tendon/bursa
727.51	Popliteal synovial cyst
727.89	Synovium/tendon/bursa disorder NEC
906.3	Late effect of contusion
906.4	Late effect of crushing
909.3	Late effect of surg/med complic
924.11	Contusion of knee
928.11	Crushing injury, knee
928.8	Multiple crushing injuries, leg

REIMBURSEMENT INFORMATION

General

- See notes on page 286.

Medicare

- Follow–up Days — 90
- Assistant Surgeon — not paid
- Supply Charges — not allowed
- Outpatient Limit — does not apply
- Major Surgery Rules Apply

CPT CODE	SERVICE	ICD–9–CM

27303 Incision, deep, with opening of bone cortex (eg, for osteomyelitis or bone abscess), femur or knee

CPT NOTES

- ♦ For incision and drainage of abscess or hematoma, superficial, see 10040-10160.

730.06	Acute osteomyelitis, lower leg
730.16	Chronic osteomyelitis, lower leg
730.26	Osteomyelitis NOS, lower leg
730.96	Bone infection NOS, lower leg

REIMBURSEMENT INFORMATION

General

- ♦ See notes on page 286.

Medicare

- ♦ Follow–up Days — 90
- ♦ Assistant Surgeon — paid
- ♦ Supply Charges — not allowed
- ♦ Outpatient Limit — does not apply
- ♦ Major Surgery Rules Apply

27305 Fasciotomy, iliotibial (tenotomy), open

CPT NOTES

- ♦ For incision and drainage of abscess or hematoma, superficial, see 10040-10160.
- ♦ For combined Ober-Yount fasciotomy, see 27025.

343.x	Infantile cerebral palsy
714.0	Rheumatoid arthritis
715.26	Loc 2nd osteoarthritis, lower leg
718.46	Contracture of joint, lower leg
727.81	Contracture of tendon
958.8	Early complications of trauma NEC

REIMBURSEMENT INFORMATION

General

- ♦ See notes on page 286

Medicare

- ♦ Follow–up Days — 90
- ♦ Assistant Surgeon — paid
- ♦ Supply Charges — not allowed
- ♦ Outpatient Limit — does not apply
- ♦ Major Surgery Rules Apply

CPT CODE	SERVICE
27306	Tenotomy, subcutaneous, closed, adductor or hamstring, (separate procedure); single
27307	Tenotomy, subcutaneous, closed, adductor or hamstring, (separate procedure); multiple

CPT NOTES

- For incision and drainage of abscess or hematoma, superficial, see 10040-10160.

ICD–9–CM

343.x	Infantile cerebral palsy
344.00	Quadriplegia NOS
344.1	Paraplegia NOS
714.0	Rheumatoid arthritis
715.26	Loc 2nd osteoarthritis, lower leg
718.46	Contracture of joint, lower leg
727.81	Contracture of tendon
958.8	Early complications of trauma NEC

REIMBURSEMENT INFORMATION

General

- See notes on page 286.
- Separate procedure rules apply.

Medicare

- Follow–up Days — 90
- Assistant Surgeon
  27306 — paid
  27307 — not paid
- Supply Charges — not allowed
- Outpatient Limit — does not apply
- Major Surgery Rules Apply

CPT CODE	SERVICE
27323	Biopsy, soft tissue of thigh or knee area; superficial

CPT NOTES

- ♦ For needle biopsy of soft tissue, use 20206.

ICD–9–CM

170.8	M-Neoplasm, Short bones, lower limb
171.3	M-Neoplasm, Soft tissue, leg
198.89	M2-Neoplasm NEC
213.8	B-Neoplasm, Short bones, lower limb
215.3	B-Neoplasm, Soft tissue, leg
238.0	UB-Neoplasm, Bone
238.1	UB-Neoplasm, Soft tissue
239.2	Bone/Skin neoplasm NOS
711.06	Pyogenic arthritis, lower leg
711.96	Infect arthritis NOS, lower leg
714.0	Rheumatoid arthritis
715.16	Loc prim osteoarthritis, lower leg
715.26	Loc 2nd osteoarthritis, lower leg
715.36	Loc osteoarthritis NOS, lower leg
716.16	Traumatic arthropathy, lower leg
717.6	Loose body in knee
717.9	Internal derangement of knee NOS
719.06	Joint effusion, lower leg
719.26	Villonodular synovitis, lower leg
729.6	Old foreign body in soft tissue
730.06	Acute osteomyelitis, lower leg
730.16	Chronic osteomyelitis, lower leg
730.26	Osteomyelitis NOS, lower leg
732.4	Juvenile osteochondrosis, leg

REIMBURSEMENT INFORMATION

General

- ♦ See notes on page 286.

Medicare

- ♦ Follow–up Days — 10
- ♦ Assistant Surgeon — not paid
- ♦ Supply Charges — not allowed
- ♦ Outpatient Limit — does not apply
- ♦ Minor Surgery Rules Apply

CPT CODE	SERVICE
27324	Biopsy, soft tissue of thigh or knee area; deep

CPT NOTES

- For needle biopsy of soft tissue, use 20206.

ICD–9–CM

170.8	M-Neoplasm, Short bones, lower limb
171.3	M-Neoplasm, Soft tissue, leg
198.89	M2-Neoplasm NEC
213.8	B-Neoplasm, Short bones, lower limb
215.3	B-Neoplasm, Soft tissue, leg
238.0	UB-Neoplasm, Bone
238.1	UB-Neoplasm, Soft tissue
239.2	Bone/Skin neoplasm NOS
711.06	Pyogenic arthritis, lower leg
711.96	Infect arthritis NOS, lower leg
714.0	Rheumatoid arthritis
715.16	Loc prim osteoarthritis, lower leg
715.26	Loc 2nd osteoarthritis, lower leg
715.36	Loc osteoarthritis NOS, lower leg
716.16	Traumatic arthropathy, lower leg
717.6	Loose body in knee
717.9	Internal derangement of knee NOS
719.06	Joint effusion, lower leg
719.26	Villonodular synovitis, lower leg
729.6	Old foreign body in soft tissue
730.06	Acute osteomyelitis, lower leg
730.16	Chronic osteomyelitis, lower leg
730.26	Osteomyelitis NOS, lower leg
732.4	Juvenile osteochondrosis, leg

REIMBURSEMENT INFORMATION

General

- See notes on page 286.

Medicare

- Follow–up Days — 90
- Assistant Surgeon — not paid
- Supply Charges — not allowed
- Outpatient Limit — does not apply
- Major Surgery Rules Apply

CPT CODE	SERVICE	ICD-9-CM
27327	Excision, tumor, thigh or knee area; subcutaneous	171.3 M-Neoplasm, Soft tissue, leg 215.3 B-Neoplasm, Soft tissue, leg 238.1 UB-Neoplasm, Soft tissue 239.2 Bone/Skin neoplasm NOS
27328	Excision, tumor, thigh or knee area; deep, subfascial, or intramuscular	

REIMBURSEMENT INFORMATION

General

- ♦ See notes on page 286.

Medicare

- ♦ Follow-up Days — 90
- ♦ Assistant Surgeon — not paid
- ♦ Supply Charges — not allowed
- ♦ Outpatient Limit — does not apply
- ♦ Major Surgery Rules Apply

27329 Radical resection of tumor (eg, malignant neoplasm), soft tissue of thigh or knee area

171.3 M-Neoplasm, Soft tissue, leg
238.1 UB-Neoplasm, Soft tissue
239.2 Bone/Skin neoplasm NOS

REIMBURSEMENT INFORMATION

General

- ♦ See notes on page 286.

Medicare

- ♦ Follow-up Days — 90
- ♦ Assistant Surgeon — paid
- ♦ Supply Charges — not allowed
- ♦ Outpatient Limit — does not apply
- ♦ Major Surgery Rules Apply

▲ **27365** Radical resection of tumor, femur or knee

CPT NOTES

- ♦ For radical resection of tumor, soft tissue, use 27329.

170.7 M-Neoplasm, Long bones, lower limb
238.0 UB-Neoplasm, Bone
239.2 Bone/Skin neoplasm NOS

REIMBURSEMENT INFORMATION

General

- ♦ See notes on page 286.
- ♦ Description changed in 1995 CPT.

Medicare

- ♦ Follow-up Days — 90
- ♦ Assistant Surgeon — paid
- ♦ Supply Charges — not allowed
- ♦ Outpatient Limit — does not apply
- ♦ Major Surgery Rules Apply

CPT CODE	SERVICE
27590	Amputation, thigh, through femur, any level

ICD–9–CM

170.7	M-Neoplasm, Long bones, lower limb
171.3	M-Neoplasm, Soft tissue, leg
238.0	UB-Neoplasm, Bone
239.2	Bone/Skin neoplasm NOS
443.1	Thromboangiitis obliterans
443.9	Peripheral vascular disease NOS
682.6	Cellulitis of leg
711.05	Pyogenic arthritis, pelvis/thigh
711.06	Pyogenic arthritis, lower leg
711.95	Infect arthritis NOS, pelvis/thigh
711.96	Infect arthritis NOS, lower leg
730.15	Chronic osteomyelitis, pelvis/thigh
730.16	Chronic osteomyelitis, lower leg
733.42	Aseptic necrosis, femur head/neck
785.4	Gangrene
897.2	Amputation above knee, unilateral
897.3	Amputate above knee, unilat, compl
928.0x	Crushing injury, hip and thigh

REIMBURSEMENT INFORMATION

General

- See notes on page 286.

Medicare

- Follow–up Days — 90
- Assistant Surgeon — paid
- Supply Charges — not allowed
- Outpatient Limit — does not apply
- Major Surgery Rules Apply
- Fragments — 27596

CPT CODE	SERVICE	ICD–9–CM	
27592	Amputation, thigh, through femur, any level; open, circular (guillotine)	170.7	M-Neoplasm, Long bones, lower limb
		171.3	M-Neoplasm, Soft tissue, leg
		238.0	UB-Neoplasm, Bone
		239.2	Bone/Skin neoplasm NOS
		443.1	Thromboangiitis obliterans
		443.9	Peripheral vascular disease NOS
		682.6	Cellulitis of leg
		711.05	Pyogenic arthritis, pelvis/thigh
		711.06	Pyogenic arthritis, lower leg
		711.95	Infect arthritis NOS, pelvis/thigh
		711.96	Infect arthritis NOS, lower leg
		730.15	Chronic osteomyelitis, pelvis/thigh
		730.16	Chronic osteomyelitis, lower leg
		733.42	Aseptic necrosis, femur head/neck
		785.4	Gangrene
		897.2	Amputation above knee, unilateral
		897.3	Amputate above knee, unilat, compl
		928.0x	Crushing injury, hip and thigh

REIMBURSEMENT INFORMATION

General

- See notes on page 286.

Medicare

- Follow–up Days — 90
- Assistant Surgeon — paid
- Supply Charges — not allowed
- Outpatient Limit — does not apply
- Major Surgery Rules Apply

CPT CODE	SERVICE
27594	Amputation, thigh, through femur, any level; secondary closure or scar revision

ICD–9–CM

170.7	M-Neoplasm, Long bones, lower limb
171.3	M-Neoplasm, Soft tissue, leg
238.0	UB-Neoplasm, Bone
239.2	Bone/Skin neoplasm NOS
443.1	Thromboangiitis obliterans
443.9	Peripheral vascular disease NOS
730.15	Chronic osteomyelitis, pelvis/thigh
730.16	Chronic osteomyelitis, lower leg
733.42	Aseptic necrosis, femur head/neck
785.4	Gangrene
897.2	Amputation above knee, unilateral
897.3	Amputate above knee, unilat, compl
905.4	Late effect, leg fracture
905.9	Late effect of traumatic amputation
906.1	Late effect, open wound extremity
906.4	Late effect of crushing
928.0x	Crushing injury, hip and thigh
928.10	Crushing injury, lower leg
996.96	Complication, reattached leg NEC
997.60	Late amputation stump complic NOS
997.61	Neuroma of amputation stump
997.62	Infection of amputated stump
997.69	Late amputation stump complic NEC

REIMBURSEMENT INFORMATION

General

- See notes on page 286.

Medicare

- Follow–up Days — 90
- Assistant Surgeon — not paid
- Supply Charges — not allowed
- Outpatient Limit — does not apply
- Major Surgery Rules Apply

CPT CODE	SERVICE
27596	Amputation, thigh, through femur, any level; reamputation

ICD–9–CM

170.7	M-Neoplasm, Long bones, lower limb
171.3	M-Neoplasm, Soft tissue, leg
238.0	UB-Neoplasm, Bone
239.2	Bone/Skin neoplasm NOS
443.1	Thromboangiitis obliterans
443.9	Peripheral vascular disease NOS
730.05	Acute osteomyelitis, pelvis/thigh
730.06	Acute osteomyelitis, lower leg
730.15	Chronic osteomyelitis, pelvis/thigh
730.16	Chronic osteomyelitis, lower leg
733.42	Aseptic necrosis, femur head/neck
785.4	Gangrene
897.2	Amputation above knee, unilateral
897.3	Amputate above knee, unilat, compl
905.9	Late effect of traumatic amputation
928.0x	Crushing injury, hip and thigh
996.96	Complication, reattached leg NEC
997.60	Late amputation stump complic NOS
997.61	Neuroma of amputation stump
997.62	Infection of amputated stump
997.69	Late amputation stump complic NEC

REIMBURSEMENT INFORMATION

General

- See notes on page 286.

Medicare

- Follow–up Days — 90
- Assistant Surgeon — paid
- Supply Charges — not allowed
- Outpatient Limit — does not apply
- Major Surgery Rules Apply
- Fragments — 37618

CPT CODE	SERVICE
27598	Disarticulation at knee

ICD–9–CM

170.7	M-Neoplasm, Long bones, lower limb
171.3	M-Neoplasm, Soft tissue, leg
238.0	UB-Neoplasm, Bone
239.2	Bone/Skin neoplasm NOS
443.1	Thromboangiitis obliterans
443.9	Peripheral vascular disease NOS
730.06	Acute osteomyelitis, lower leg
730.16	Chronic osteomyelitis, lower leg
733.42	Aseptic necrosis, femur head/neck
785.4	Gangrene
897.2	Amputation above knee, unilateral
897.3	Amputate above knee, unilat, compl
905.9	Late effect of traumatic amputation
928.0x	Crushing injury, hip and thigh
928.11	Crushing injury, knee
996.96	Complication, reattached leg NEC
997.60	Late amputation stump complic NOS
997.61	Neuroma of amputation stump
997.62	Infection of amputated stump
997.69	Late amputation stump complic NEC

REIMBURSEMENT INFORMATION

General

- See notes on page 286.

Medicare

- Follow–up Days — 90
- Assistant Surgeon — paid
- Supply Charges — not allowed
- Outpatient Limit — does not apply
- Major Surgery Rules Apply

CPT CODE	SERVICE
27600	Decompression fasciotomy, leg; anterior and/or lateral compartments only
27601	Decompression fasciotomy, leg; posterior compartment(s) only
27602	Decompression fasciotomy, leg; anterior and/or lateral, and posterior compartment(s)

CPT NOTES

- For incision and drainage procedures, superficial, see 10040-10160.
- For decompression fasciotomy with debridement, see 27892-27894.

ICD–9–CM

823.0x	Fracture of tibia and fibula closed
823.1x	Fracture of tibia and fibula, open
823.2x	Fracture of tibia and fibula shaft
823.3x	Fracture of tibia and fibula shaft
837.0	Dislocation ankle, closed
837.1	Dislocation ankle, open
891.x	Open wound of knee, leg, ankle
906.4	Late effect of crushing
928.10	Crushing injury, lower leg
958.6	Volkmann's ischemic contracture
958.8	Early complications of trauma NEC

REIMBURSEMENT INFORMATION

General

- See notes on page 286.

Medicare

- Follow–up Days — 90
- Assistant Surgeon — paid
- Supply Charges — not allowed
- Outpatient Limit — does not apply
- Major Surgery Rules Apply

CPT CODE	SERVICE
27603	Incision and drainage, leg or ankle; deep abscess or hematoma
27604	Incision and drainage, leg or ankle; infected bursa

ICD–9–CM

682.6	Cellulitis of leg
711.06	Pyogenic arthritis, lower leg
711.07	Pyogenic arthritis, ankle/foot
711.96	Infect arthritis NOS, lower leg
711.97	Infect arthritis NOS, ankle/foot
726.7x	Enthesopathy of ankle and tarsus
726.8	Peripheral enthesopathy NEC
727.2	Occupational bursitis
727.3	Bursitis NOS
727.4x	Ganglion/cyst synovium/tendon/bursa
727.89	Synovium/tendon/bursa disorder NEC
906.1	Late effect, open wound extremity
906.3	Late effect of contusion
906.4	Late effect of crushing
909.3	Late effect of surg/med complic
924.10	Contusion of lower leg
924.21	Contusion of ankle
928.10	Crushing injury, lower leg
928.21	Crushing injury, ankle
928.8	Multiple crushing injuries, leg

REIMBURSEMENT INFORMATION

General

- See notes on page 286.

Medicare

- Follow–up Days — 90
- Assistant Surgeon — not paid
- Supply Charges — not allowed
- Outpatient Limit — does not apply
- Major Surgery Rules Apply

CPT CODE	SERVICE	ICD–9–CM
27613	Biopsy, soft tissue of leg or ankle area; superficial	171.3 M-Neoplasm, Soft tissue, leg 215.3 B-Neoplasm, Soft tissue, leg 238.1 UB-Neoplasm, Soft tissue 239.2 Bone/Skin neoplasm NOS
27614	Biopsy, soft tissue of leg or ankle area; deep	

CPT NOTES

- For needle biopsy of soft tissue, use 20206.

REIMBURSEMENT INFORMATION

General

- See notes on page 286.

Medicare

- Follow–up Days
  27613 — 10
  27614 –– 90
- Assistant Surgeon — not paid
- Supply Charges — not allowed
- Outpatient Limit — does not apply
- Minor Surgery Rules Apply (27613)
  Major Surgery Rules Apply 27614)

CPT CODE	SERVICE	ICD–9–CM
27615	Radical resection of tumor (eg, malignant neoplasm), soft tissue of leg or ankle area	171.3 M-Neoplasm, Soft tissue, leg 238.1 UB-Neoplasm, Soft tissue 239.2 Bone/Skin neoplasm NOS

REIMBURSEMENT INFORMATION

General

- See notes on page 286.

Medicare

- Follow–up Days — 90
- Assistant Surgeon — paid
- Supply Charges — not allowed
- Outpatient Limit — does not apply
- Major Surgery Rules Apply

CPT CODE	SERVICE	ICD-9-CM
27618	Excision, tumor, leg or ankle area; subcutaneous	171.3 M-Neoplasm, Soft tissue, leg 215.3 B-Neoplasm, Soft tissue, leg 238.1 UB-Neoplasm, Soft tissue 239.2 Bone/Skin neoplasm NOS

REIMBURSEMENT INFORMATION

General

- ◆ See notes on page 286.

Medicare

- ◆ Follow–up Days — 90
- ◆ Assistant Surgeon — not paid
- ◆ Supply Charges — not allowed
- ◆ Outpatient Limit — does not apply
- ◆ Major Surgery Rules Apply

CPT CODE	SERVICE	ICD-9-CM
27619	Excision, tumor, leg or ankle area; deep, subfascial or intramuscular	171.3 M-Neoplasm, Soft tissue, leg 195.5 M-Neoplasm, Lower limb 215.3 B-Neoplasm, Soft tissue, leg 238.1 UB-Neoplasm, Soft tissue 239.2 Bone/Skin neoplasm NOS

REIMBURSEMENT INFORMATION

General

- ◆ See notes on page 286.

Medicare

- ◆ Follow–up Days — 90
- ◆ Assistant Surgeon — not paid
- ◆ Supply Charges — not allowed
- ◆ Outpatient Limit — does not apply
- ◆ Major Surgery Rules Apply

CPT CODE	SERVICE	ICD-9-CM
27630	Excision of lesion of tendon sheath or capsule (eg, cyst or ganglion), leg and/or ankle	727.40 Synovial cyst NOS 727.42 Ganglion of tendon sheath 727.43 Ganglion NOS

REIMBURSEMENT INFORMATION

General

- See notes on page 286.

Medicare

- Follow-up Days — 90
- Assistant Surgeon — not paid
- Supply Charges — not allowed
- Outpatient Limit — does not apply
- Major Surgery Rules Apply

CPT CODE	SERVICE	ICD-9-CM
27640	Partial excision (craterization, saucerization, or diaphysectomy) of bone (eg, for osteomyelitis or exostosis); tibia	170.7 M-Neoplasm, Long bones, lower limb 198.5 M2-Neoplasm, Bone and bone marrow 726.91 Exostosis, site NOS 728.11 Progressive myositis ossificans 730.07 Acute osteomyelitis, ankle/foot 730.16 Chronic osteomyelitis, lower leg 730.17 Chronic osteomyelitis, ankle/foot 730.26 Osteomyelitis NOS, lower leg 730.36 Periostitis, lower leg 731.0 Osteitis deformans NOS 732.4 Juvenile osteochondrosis, leg 733.21 Solitary bone cyst 733.22 Aneurysmal bone cyst 733.29 Bone cyst NEC 733.49 Aseptic necrosis of bone NEC 756.4 Chondrodystrophy

REIMBURSEMENT INFORMATION

General

- See notes on page 286.

Medicare

- Follow-up Days — 90
- Assistant Surgeon — paid
- Supply Charges — not allowed
- Outpatient Limit — does not apply
- Major Surgery Rules Apply

CPT CODE	SERVICE	ICD–9–CM
27641	Partial excision (craterization, saucerization, or diaphysectomy) of bone (eg, for osteomyelitis or exostosis); fibula	170.7 M-Neoplasm, Long bones, lower limb 198.5 M2-Neoplasm, Bone and bone marrow 726.91 Exostosis, site NOS 728.11 Progressive myositis ossificans 730.07 Acute osteomyelitis, ankle/foot 730.16 Chronic osteomyelitis, lower leg 730.17 Chronic osteomyelitis, ankle/foot 730.26 Osteomyelitis NOS, lower leg 730.36 Periostitis, lower leg 731.0 Osteitis deformans NOS 732.4 Juvenile osteochondrosis, leg 733.21 Solitary bone cyst 733.22 Aneurysmal bone cyst 733.29 Bone cyst NEC 733.49 Aseptic necrosis of bone NEC 756.4 Chondrodystrophy 891.1 Open wound of knee/leg/ankle, compl 905.4 Late effect, leg fracture **REIMBURSEMENT INFORMATION** General ♦ See notes on page 286. Medicare ♦ Follow–up Days — 90 ♦ Assistant Surgeon — paid ♦ Supply Charges — not allowed ♦ Outpatient Limit — does not apply ♦ Major Surgery Rules Apply
27650 **27652**	Repair, primary, open or percutaneous, ruptured Achilles tendon Repair, primary, open or percutaneous, ruptured Achilles tendon; with graft (includes obtaining graft)	726.71 Achilles tendinitis 727.67 Rupture, achilles tendon **REIMBURSEMENT INFORMATION** General ♦ See notes on page 286. Medicare ♦ Follow–up Days — 90 ♦ Assistant Surgeon — paid ♦ Supply Charges — not allowed ♦ Outpatient Limit — does not apply ♦ Major Surgery Rules Apply

CPT CODE	SERVICE	ICD-9-CM
27654	Repair, secondary, ruptured Achilles tendon, with or without graft	726.71 Achilles tendinitis 727.67 Rupture, achilles tendon

REIMBURSEMENT INFORMATION

General

- ◆ See notes on page 286.

Medicare

- ◆ Follow-up Days — 90
- ◆ Assistant Surgeon — paid
- ◆ Supply Charges — not allowed
- ◆ Outpatient Limit — does not apply
- ◆ Major Surgery Rules Apply

CPT CODE	SERVICE	ICD-9-CM
27656	Repair, fascial defect of leg	343.x Infantile cerebral palsy 714.0 Rheumatoid arthritis 715.16 Loc prim osteoarthritis, lower leg 715.26 Loc 2nd osteoarthritis, lower leg 718.46 Contracture of joint, lower leg 727.81 Contracture of tendon 728.89 Muscle/ligament disorder NEC 728.9 Muscle/ligament disorder NOS 909.3 Late effect of surg/med complic 958.8 Early complications of trauma NEC

REIMBURSEMENT INFORMATION

General

- ◆ See notes on page 286.

Medicare

- ◆ Follow-up Days — 90
- ◆ Assistant Surgeon — paid
- ◆ Supply Charges — not allowed
- ◆ Outpatient Limit — does not apply
- ◆ Major Surgery Rules Apply

CPT CODE	SERVICE	ICD-9-CM
27658 **27659**	Repair or suture of flexor tendon of leg; primary, without graft, single, each Repair or suture of flexor tendon of leg; secondary with or without graft, single tendon, each	727.68 Rupture, tendons of foot/ankle NEC 844.3 Sprain superior tibiofibular 844.8 Sprain of knee & leg NEC 891.2 Open wound knee/leg/ankle w/tendon **REIMBURSEMENT INFORMATION** General ♦ See notes on page 286. Medicare ♦ Follow–up Days — 90 ♦ Assistant Surgeon — paid ♦ Supply Charges — not allowed ♦ Outpatient Limit — does not apply ♦ Major Surgery Rules Apply
27664 **27665**	Repair or suture of extensor tendon of leg; primary, without graft, single, each Repair or suture of extensor tendon of leg; secondary with or without graft, single tendon, each	727.68 Rupture, tendons of foot/ankle NEC 844.3 Sprain superior tibiofibular 844.8 Sprain of knee & leg NEC 891.2 Open wound knee/leg/ankle w/tendon **REIMBURSEMENT INFORMATION** General ♦ See notes on page 286. Medicare ♦ Follow–up Days — 90 ♦ Assistant Surgeon 27664 — not paid 27665 — paid ♦ Supply Charges — not allowed ♦ Outpatient Limit — does not apply ♦ Major Surgery Rules Apply
27675 **27676**	Repair for dislocating peroneal tendons; without fibular osteotomy Repair for dislocating peroneal tendons; with fibular osteotomy	727.0 Synovitis and tenosynovitis 839.8 Dislocation NEC, closed **REIMBURSEMENT INFORMATION** General ♦ See notes on page 286. Medicare ♦ Follow–up Days — 90 ♦ Assistant Surgeon — paid ♦ Supply Charges — not allowed ♦ Outpatient Limit — does not apply ♦ Major Surgery Rules Apply

CPT CODE	SERVICE
27680	Tenolysis, including tibia, fibula and ankle flexor; single
27681	Tenolysis, including tibia, fibula and ankle flexor; multiple (through same incision), each

ICD–9–CM

138.	Late effects of acute polio
343.x	Infantile cerebral palsy
436.	Acute CVA, ill-defined
714.0	Rheumatoid arthritis
715.16	Loc prim osteoarthritis, lower leg
715.26	Loc 2nd osteoarthritis, lower leg
718.46	Contracture of joint, lower leg
727.81	Contracture of tendon
736.76	Calcaneus deformity NEC
736.79	Acquired ankle/foot deformity NEC
837.0	Dislocation ankle, closed
837.1	Dislocation ankle, open
844.3	Sprain superior tibiofibular
844.8	Sprain of knee & leg NEC
845.0x	Ankle sprain/strain
905.4	Late effect, leg fracture
906.1	Late effect, open wound extremity
906.4	Late effect of crushing
958.8	Early complications of trauma NEC

REIMBURSEMENT INFORMATION

General

- See notes on page 286.

Medicare

- Follow–up Days — 90
- Assistant Surgeon — paid
- Supply Charges — not allowed
- Outpatient Limit — does not apply
- Major Surgery Rules Apply

CPT CODE	SERVICE
27888	Amputation, ankle, through malleoli of tibia and fibula (Syme, Pirogoff type procedures), with plastic closure and resection of nerves

ICD–9–CM

170.7	M-Neoplasm, Long bones, lower limb
171.3	M-Neoplasm, Soft tissue, leg
238.0	UB-Neoplasm, Bone
239.2	Bone/Skin neoplasm NOS
443.1	Thromboangiitis obliterans
443.9	Peripheral vascular disease NOS
730.06	Acute osteomyelitis, lower leg
730.07	Acute osteomyelitis, ankle/foot
730.16	Chronic osteomyelitis, lower leg
730.27	Osteomyelitis NOS, ankle/foot
733.43	Aseptic necrosis, femoral condyle
785.4	Gangrene
897.0	Amputation below knee, unilateral
897.1	Amputate below knee, unilat, compl
928.10	Crushing injury, lower leg
928.2x	Crushing injury, ankle and foot
996.96	Complication, reattached leg NEC
997.60	Late amputation stump complic NOS
997.61	Neuroma of amputation stump
997.62	Infection of amputated stump
997.69	Late amputation stump complic NEC

REIMBURSEMENT INFORMATION

General

- See notes on page 286.

Medicare

- Follow–up Days — 90
- Assistant Surgeon — paid
- Supply Charges — not allowed
- Outpatient Limit — does not apply
- Major Surgery Rules Apply

CPT CODE	SERVICE
27889	Ankle disarticulation

ICD–9–CM

170.8	M-Neoplasm, Short bones, lower limb
171.3	M-Neoplasm, Soft tissue, leg
238.0	UB-Neoplasm, Bone
239.2	Bone/Skin neoplasm NOS
443.1	Thromboangiitis obliterans
443.9	Peripheral vascular disease NOS
730.06	Acute osteomyelitis, lower leg
730.07	Acute osteomyelitis, ankle/foot
730.16	Chronic osteomyelitis, lower leg
730.27	Osteomyelitis NOS, ankle/foot
733.43	Aseptic necrosis, femoral condyle
785.4	Gangrene
897.0	Amputation below knee, unilateral
897.1	Amputate below knee, unilat, compl
928.2x	Crushing injury, ankle and foot
991.2	Frostbite of foot
996.96	Complication, reattached leg NEC
997.60	Late amputation stump complic NOS
997.61	Neuroma of amputation stump
997.62	Infection of amputated stump
997.69	Late amputation stump complic NEC

REIMBURSEMENT INFORMATION

General

- See notes on page 286.

Medicare

- Follow–up Days — 90
- Assistant Surgeon — paid
- Supply Charges — not allowed
- Outpatient Limit — does not apply
- Major Surgery Rules Apply

CPT CODE	SERVICE	ICD-9-CM

27892 Decompression fasciotomy, leg; anterior and/or lateral compartments only, with debridement of nonviable muscle and/or nerve

CPT NOTES

- For decompression fasciotomy of the leg without debridement, see 27600.

823.0x	Fracture of tibia and fibula closed
823.1x	Fracture of tibia and fibula, open
823.2x	Fracture of tibia and fibula shaft
823.3x	Fracture of tibia and fibula shaft
837.0	Dislocation ankle, closed
837.1	Dislocation ankle, open
891.x	Open wound of knee, leg, ankle
906.4	Late effect of crushing
928.10	Crushing injury, lower leg
958.6	Volkmann's ischemic contracture
958.8	Early complications of trauma NEC

REIMBURSEMENT INFORMATION

General

- See notes on page 286.

Medicare

- Follow-up Days — 90
- Assistant Surgeon — paid
- Supply Charges — not allowed
- Outpatient Limit — does not apply
- Major Surgery Rules Apply

27893 Decompression fasciotomy, leg; posterior compartment(s) only, with debridement of nonviable muscle and/or nerve

CPT NOTES

- For decompression fasciotomy of the leg without debridement, see 27601.

823.0x	Fracture of tibia and fibula closed
823.1x	Fracture of tibia and fibula, open
823.2x	Fracture of tibia and fibula shaft
823.3x	Fracture of tibia and fibula shaft
837.0	Dislocation ankle, closed
837.1	Dislocation ankle, open
891.x	Open wound of knee, leg, ankle
906.4	Late effect of crushing
928.10	Crushing injury, lower leg
958.6	Volkmann's ischemic contracture
958.8	Early complications of trauma NEC

REIMBURSEMENT INFORMATION

General

- See notes on page 286.

Medicare

- Follow-up Days — 90
- Assistant Surgeon — by report
- Supply Charges — not allowed
- Outpatient Limit — does not apply
- Major Surgery Rules Apply

CPT CODE	SERVICE
27894	Decompression fasciotomy, leg; anterior and/or lateral, and posterior compartment(s), with debridement of nonviable muscle and/or nerve

CPT NOTES

- For decompression fasciotomy of the leg without debridement, see 27602.

ICD–9–CM

823.0x	Fracture of tibia and fibula closed
823.1x	Fracture of tibia and fibula, open
823.2x	Fracture of tibia and fibula shaft
823.3x	Fracture of tibia and fibula shaft
837.0	Dislocation ankle, closed
837.1	Dislocation ankle, open
891.x	Open wound of knee, leg, ankle
906.4	Late effect of crushing
928.1x	Crushing injury, knee, lower leg
958.6	Volkmann's ischemic contracture
958.8	Early complications of trauma NEC

REIMBURSEMENT INFORMATION

General

- See notes on page 286.

Medicare

- Follow–up Days — 90
- Assistant Surgeon — paid
- Supply Charges — not allowed
- Outpatient Limit — does not apply
- Major Surgery Rules Apply

CPT CODE	SERVICE
28001*	Incision and drainage, infected bursa, foot

CPT RULES

- For incision and drainage procedures, superficial, see 10040-10160.

ICD–9–CM

681.1x	Cellulitis and abscess, toe
682.7	Cellulitis of foot
711.07	Pyogenic arthritis, ankle/foot
711.97	Infect arthritis NOS, ankle/foot
726.7x	Enthesopathy of ankle and tarsus
726.8	Peripheral enthesopathy NEC
726.91	Exostosis, site NOS
727.2	Occupational bursitis
727.3	Bursitis NOS
727.4x	Ganglion/cyst synovium/tendon/bursa
727.89	Synovium/tendon/bursa disorder NEC
906.3	Late effect of contusion
906.4	Late effect of crushing
909.3	Late effect of surg/med complic
924.20	Contusion of foot
924.3	Contusion of toe
924.4	Multiple contusions of leg
928.20	Crushing injury, foot
928.3	Crushing injury, toe
928.8	Multiple crushing injuries, leg

REIMBURSEMENT INFORMATION

General

- See notes on page 286.
- Starred procedure.

Medicare

- Follow–up Days — 10
- Assistant Surgeon — not paid
- Supply Charges — not allowed
- Outpatient Limit — applies
- Minor Surgery Rules Apply

CPT CODE	SERVICE
28002*	Deep dissection below fascia, for deep infection of foot, with or without tendon sheath involvement; single bursal space, specify
28003	Deep dissection below fascia, for deep infection of foot, with or without tendon sheath involvement; multiple areas

CPT RULES

- For incision and drainage procedures, superficial, see 10040-10160.

ICD-9-CM

681.1x	Cellulitis and abscess, toe
682.7	Cellulitis of foot
711.07	Pyogenic arthritis, ankle/foot
711.97	Infect arthritis NOS, ankle/foot
726.7x	Enthesopathy of ankle and tarsus
726.8	Peripheral enthesopathy NEC
726.91	Exostosis, site NOS
727.2	Occupational bursitis
727.3	Bursitis NOS
727.4x	Ganglion/cyst synovium/tendon/bursa
727.89	Synovium/tendon/bursa disorder NEC
906.3	Late effect of contusion
906.4	Late effect of crushing
909.3	Late effect of surg/med complic
924.20	Contusion of foot
924.3	Contusion of toe
924.4	Multiple contusions of leg
928.20	Crushing injury, foot
928.8	Multiple crushing injuries, leg

REIMBURSEMENT INFORMATION

General

- See notes on page 286.
- Starred procedure. (28002)

Medicare

- Follow–up Days — 10
- Assistant Surgeon — not paid
- Supply Charges — not allowed
- Outpatient Limit — does not apply
- Minor Surgery Rules Apply

CPT CODE	SERVICE	ICD–9–CM

28005 Incision, deep, with opening of bone cortex (eg, for osteomyelitis or bone abscess), foot

CPT RULES

- ◆ For incision and drainage procedures, superficial, see 10040-10160.

730.07	Acute osteomyelitis, ankle/foot
730.17	Chronic osteomyelitis, ankle/foot
730.27	Osteomyelitis NOS, ankle/foot
730.97	Bone infection NOS, ankle/foot

REIMBURSEMENT INFORMATION

General

- ◆ See notes on page 286.

Medicare

- ◆ Follow–up Days — 90
- ◆ Assistant Surgeon — not paid
- ◆ Supply Charges — not allowed
- ◆ Outpatient Limit — does not apply
- ◆ Major Surgery Rules Apply

28008 Fasciotomy, plantar and/or toe

CPT RULES

- ◆ For incision and drainage procedures, superficial, see 10040-10160.
- ◆ See also 28060, 28062, 28250.

343.x	Infantile cerebral palsy
714.0	Rheumatoid arthritis
715.17	Loc prim osteoarthritis, ankle/foot
715.27	Loc 2nd osteoarthritis, ankle/foot
718.47	Contracture of joint, ankle/foot
727.81	Contracture of tendon
728.71	Plantar fascial fibromatosis
728.79	Fibromatosis NEC
958.8	Early complications of trauma NEC

REIMBURSEMENT INFORMATION

General

- ◆ See notes on page 286.

Medicare

- ◆ Follow–up Days — 90
- ◆ Assistant Surgeon — not paid
- ◆ Supply Charges — not allowed
- ◆ Outpatient Limit — does not apply
- ◆ Major Surgery Rules Apply

CPT CODE	SERVICE
28020	Arthrotomy, with exploration, drainage or removal of loose or foreign body; intertarsal or tarsometatarsal joint
28022	Arthrotomy, with exploration, drainage or removal of loose or foreign body; metatarsophalangeal joint
28024	Arthrotomy, with exploration, drainage or removal of loose or foreign body; interphalangeal joint

CPT RULES

- ♦ For incision and drainage procedures, superficial, see 10040-10160.

ICD–9–CM

711.07	Pyogenic arthritis, ankle/foot
711.97	Infect arthritis NOS, ankle/foot
714.0	Rheumatoid arthritis
715.17	Loc prim osteoarthritis, ankle/foot
715.27	Loc 2nd osteoarthritis, ankle/foot
715.37	Loc osteoarthritis NOS, ankle/foot
716.17	Traumatic arthropathy, ankle/foot
718.17	Loose body in joint, ankle/foot
719.07	Joint effusion, ankle/foot
719.27	Villonodular synovitis, ankle/foot
729.6	Old foreign body in soft tissue
730.07	Acute osteomyelitis, ankle/foot
730.17	Chronic osteomyelitis, ankle/foot
730.27	Osteomyelitis NOS, ankle/foot
732.5	Juvenile osteochondrosis, foot
892.1	Open wound of foot, complicated
917.7	Foreign body, foot/toe, infected
996.66	Reaction, internal joint prosthesis
998.4.	Foreign body left during procedure
998.5	Postoperative infection

REIMBURSEMENT INFORMATION

General

- ♦ See notes on page 286.

Medicare

- ♦ Follow–up Days — 90
- ♦ Assistant Surgeon
  28020 — paid
  28022–28024 — not paid
- ♦ Supply Charges — not allowed
- ♦ Outpatient Limit — does not apply
- ♦ Major Surgery Rules Apply

28030 Neurectomy of intrinsic musculature of foot

CPT RULES

- ♦ For incision and drainage procedures, superficial, see 10040-10160.

215.3	B-Neoplasm, Soft tissue, leg
343.x	Infantile cerebral palsy
355.3	Lateral popliteal nerve lesion
355.6	Plantar nerve lesion
907.5	Late effect, nerve inj pelvis/leg
997.61	Neuroma of amputation stump

REIMBURSEMENT INFORMATION

General

- ♦ See notes on page 286.

Medicare

- ♦ Follow–up Days — 90
- ♦ Assistant Surgeon — by report
- ♦ Supply Charges — not allowed
- ♦ Outpatient Limit — does not apply
- ♦ Major Surgery Rules Apply

CPT CODE	SERVICE	ICD-9-CM
28035	Tarsal tunnel release (posterior tibial nerve decompression)	355.5 Tarsal tunnel syndrome

CPT RULES

- For incision and drainage procedures, superficial, see 10040-10160.
- For other nerve entrapments, see 64704, 64722.

REIMBURSEMENT INFORMATION

General

- See notes on page 286.

Medicare

- Follow-up Days — 90
- Assistant Surgeon — paid
- Supply Charges — not allowed
- Outpatient Limit — does not apply
- Major Surgery Rules Apply

28043 Excision, tumor, foot; subcutaneous

28045 Excision, tumor, foot; deep, subfascial, intramuscular

171.3	M-Neoplasm, Soft tissue, leg
215.3	B-Neoplasm, Soft tissue, leg
238.1	UB-Neoplasm, Soft tissue
239.2	Bone/Skin neoplasm NOS
355.6	Plantar nerve lesion
782.2	Localized superficial swelling

REIMBURSEMENT INFORMATION

General

- See notes on page 286.

Medicare

- Follow-up Days — 90
- Assistant Surgeon
  28043 — not paid
  28045 — by report
- Supply Charges — not allowed
- Outpatient Limit — does not apply
- Major Surgery Rules Apply

28046 Radical resection of tumor (eg, malignant neoplasm), soft tissue of foot

171.3	M-Neoplasm, Soft tissue, leg
238.1	UB-Neoplasm, Soft tissue
239.2	Bone/Skin neoplasm NOS

REIMBURSEMENT INFORMATION

General

- See notes on page 286.

Medicare

- Follow-up Days — 90
- Assistant Surgeon — paid
- Supply Charges — not allowed
- Outpatient Limit — does not apply
- Major Surgery Rules Apply

CPT CODE	SERVICE
28050	Arthrotomy for synovial biopsy; intertarsal or tarsometatarsal joint
28052	Arthrotomy for synovial biopsy; metatarsophalangeal joint
28054	Arthrotomy for synovial biopsy; interphalangeal joint

ICD–9–CM

170.8	M-Neoplasm, Short bones, lower limb
171.3	M-Neoplasm, Soft tissue, leg
198.89	M2-Neoplasm NEC
213.8	B-Neoplasm, Short bones, lower limb
215.3	B-Neoplasm, Soft tissue, leg
238.0	UB-Neoplasm, Bone
238.1	UB-Neoplasm, Soft tissue
239.2	Bone/Skin neoplasm NOS
711.07	Pyogenic arthritis, ankle/foot
711.97	Infect arthritis NOS, ankle/foot
714.0	Rheumatoid arthritis
715.17	Loc prim osteoarthritis, ankle/foot
715.27	Loc 2nd osteoarthritis, ankle/foot
715.37	Loc osteoarthritis NOS, ankle/foot
716.17	Traumatic arthropathy, ankle/foot
718.17	Loose body in joint, ankle/foot
719.07	Joint effusion, ankle/foot
719.27	Villonodular synovitis, ankle/foot
727.06	Tenosynovitis of foot/ankle
729.6	Old foreign body in soft tissue
730.07	Acute osteomyelitis, ankle/foot
730.17	Chronic osteomyelitis, ankle/foot
730.27	Osteomyelitis NOS, ankle/foot
732.5	Juvenile osteochondrosis, foot
892.1	Open wound of foot, complicated
917.7	Foreign body, foot/toe, infected
996.66	Reaction, internal joint prosthesis
998.4	Foreign body left during procedure
998.5	Postoperative infection

REIMBURSEMENT INFORMATION

General

- See notes on page 286.

Medicare

- Follow–up Days — 90
- Assistant Surgeon
  28050–28052 — paid
  28054 — by report
- Supply Charges — not allowed
- Outpatient Limit
  28050, 28054 — does not apply
  28052 — applies
- Major Surgery Rules Apply

CPT CODE	SERVICE	ICD-9-CM
28060	Fasciectomy, excision of plantar fascia; partial (separate procedure)	343.x Infantile cerebral palsy 714.0 Rheumatoid arthritis 715.17 Loc prim osteoarthritis, ankle/foot 715.27 Loc 2nd osteoarthritis, ankle/foot 718.47 Contracture of joint, ankle/foot 727.81 Contracture of tendon 728.71 Plantar fascial fibromatosis 728.79 Fibromatosis NEC 958.8 Early complications of trauma NEC
28062	Fasciectomy, excision of plantar fascia; radical (separate procedure)	

CPT NOTES

- For plantar fasciotomy, see 28008, 28250.

REIMBURSEMENT INFORMATION

General

- See notes on page 286.
- Separate procedure rules apply.

Medicare

- Follow-up Days — 90
- Assistant Surgeon — paid
- Supply Charges — not allowed
- Outpatient Limit — does not apply
- Major Surgery Rules Apply

CPT CODE	SERVICE	ICD-9-CM
28070	Synovectomy; intertarsal or tarsometatarsal joint, each	343.x Infantile cerebral palsy 714.0 Rheumatoid arthritis 715.17 Loc prim osteoarthritis, ankle/foot 715.27 Loc 2nd osteoarthritis, ankle/foot 716.17 Traumatic arthropathy, ankle/foot 718.47 Contracture of joint, ankle/foot 718.57 Ankylosis of joint, ankle/foot 719.27 Villonodular synovitis, ankle/foot 727.00 Synovitis NOS 727.81 Contracture of tendon 728.79 Fibromatosis NEC 958.8 Early complications of trauma NEC
28072	Synovectomy; metatarsophalangeal joint, each	

REIMBURSEMENT INFORMATION

General

- See notes on page 286.

Medicare

- Follow-up Days — 90
- Assistant Surgeon — paid
- Supply Charges — not allowed
- Outpatient Limit — does not apply
- Major Surgery Rules Apply

CPT CODE	SERVICE	ICD-9-CM
28080	Excision of interdigital (Morton) neuroma, single, each	355.6 Plantar nerve lesion

REIMBURSEMENT INFORMATION

General

- See notes on page 286.

Medicare

- Follow-up Days — 90
- Assistant Surgeon — by report
- Supply Charges — not allowed
- Outpatient Limit — does not apply
- Major Surgery Rules Apply

CPT CODE	SERVICE	ICD-9-CM	
28086	Synovectomy, tendon sheath, foot; flexor	343.x	Infantile cerebral palsy
28088	Synovectomy, tendon sheath, foot; extensor	714.0	Rheumatoid arthritis
		715.17	Loc prim osteoarthritis, ankle/foot
		715.27	Loc 2nd osteoarthritis, ankle/foot
		716.17	Traumatic arthropathy, ankle/foot
		718.47	Contracture of joint, ankle/foot
		718.57	Ankylosis of joint, ankle/foot
		719.27	Villonodular synovitis, ankle/foot
		727.00	Synovitis NOS
		727.81	Contracture of tendon
		728.79	Fibromatosis NEC
		958.8	Early complications of trauma NEC

REIMBURSEMENT INFORMATION

General

- See notes on page 286.

Medicare

- Follow-up Days — 90
- Assistant Surgeon
  28086 — paid
  28088 — not paid
- Supply Charges — not allowed
- Outpatient Limit — does not apply
- Major Surgery Rules Apply

CPT CODE	SERVICE	ICD–9–CM
28090	Excision of lesion of tendon or fibrous sheath or capsule (including synovectomy) (cyst or ganglion); foot	727.40 Synovial cyst NOS 727.41 Ganglion of joint 727.42 Ganglion of tendon sheath 727.43 Ganglion NOS 727.49 Bursal cyst NEC
28092	Excision of lesion of tendon or fibrous sheath or capsule (including synovectomy) (cyst or ganglion); toes	

REIMBURSEMENT INFORMATION

General

- ♦ See notes on page 286.

Medicare

- ♦ Follow–up Days — 90
- ♦ Assistant Surgeon — not paid
- ♦ Supply Charges — not allowed
- ♦ Outpatient Limit — does not apply
- ♦ Major Surgery Rules Apply

CPT CODE	SERVICE	ICD–9–CM
28100	Excision or curettage of bone cyst or benign tumor, talus or calcaneus	213.8 B-Neoplasm, Short bones, lower limb 733.20 Cyst of bone NOS 733.21 Solitary bone cyst 733.22 Aneurysmal bone cyst 733.29 Bone cyst NEC
28102	Excision or curettage of bone cyst or benign tumor, talus or calcaneus; with iliac or other autograft (includes obtaining graft)	
28103	Excision or curettage of bone cyst or benign tumor, talus or calcaneus; with allograft	

REIMBURSEMENT INFORMATION

General

- ♦ See notes on page 286.

Medicare

- ♦ Follow–up Days — 90
- ♦ Assistant Surgeon — paid
- ♦ Supply Charges — not allowed
- ♦ Outpatient Limit — does not apply
- ♦ Major Surgery Rules Apply

CPT CODE	SERVICE	ICD-9-CM
28104	Excision or curettage of bone cyst or benign tumor, tarsal or metatarsal bones, except talus or calcaneus	
28106	Excision or curettage of bone cyst or benign tumor, tarsal or metatarsal bones, except talus or calcaneus; with iliac or other autograft (includes obtaining graft)	
28107	Excision or curettage of bone cyst or benign tumor, tarsal or metatarsal bones, except talus or calcaneus; with allograft	

ICD-9-CM

213.8 B-Neoplasm, Short bones, lower limb
733.20 Cyst of bone NOS
733.21 Solitary bone cyst
733.22 Aneurysmal bone cyst
733.29 Bone cyst NEC

REIMBURSEMENT INFORMATION

General

- ♦ See notes on page 286.

Medicare

- ♦ Follow-up Days — 90
- ♦ Assistant Surgeon — paid
- ♦ Supply Charges — not allowed
- ♦ Outpatient Limit — does not apply
- ♦ Major Surgery Rules Apply

28108 Excision or curettage of bone cyst or benign tumor, phalanges of foot

CPT NOTES

- ♦ For ostectomy, partial (e.g., hallux valgus, Silver type procedure), see 28290.

ICD-9-CM

213.8 B-Neoplasm, Short bones, lower limb
733.20 Cyst of bone NOS
733.21 Solitary bone cyst
733.22 Aneurysmal bone cyst
733.29 Bone cyst NEC

REIMBURSEMENT INFORMATION

General

- ♦ See notes on page 286.

Medicare

- ♦ Follow-up Days — 90
- ♦ Assistant Surgeon — not paid
- ♦ Supply Charges — not allowed
- ♦ Outpatient Limit — applies
- ♦ Major Surgery Rules Apply

CPT CODE	SERVICE
28110	Ostectomy, partial excision, fifth metatarsal head (bunionette) (separate procedure)

ICD–9–CM

170.8	M-Neoplasm, Short bones, lower limb
198.5	M2-Neoplasm, Bone and bone marrow
213.8	B-Neoplasm, Short bones, lower limb
238.0	UB-Neoplasm, Bone
239.2	Bone/Skin neoplasm NOS
250.8x	Diabetes w/manifestations
714.0	Rheumatoid arthritis
714.3x	Juvenile chronic polyarthritis
715.27	Loc 2nd osteoarthritis, ankle/foot
727.1	Bunion
730.17	Chronic osteomyelitis, ankle/foot
731.8	Bone involvement in other diseases
755.67	Anomalies of foot NEC

REIMBURSEMENT INFORMATION

General

- See notes on page 286.
- Separate procedure rules apply.

Medicare

- Follow–up Days — 90
- Assistant Surgeon — paid
- Supply Charges — not allowed
- Outpatient Limit — does not apply
- Major Surgery Rules Apply

CPT CODE	SERVICE
28111	Ostectomy, complete excision; first metatarsal head
28112	Ostectomy, complete excision; other metatarsal head (second, third or fourth)
28113	Ostectomy, complete excision; fifth metatarsal head
28114	Ostectomy, complete excision; all metatarsal heads, with partial proximal phalangectomy, excluding first metatarsal (Clayton type procedure)

ICD–9–CM

170.8	M-Neoplasm, Short bones, lower limb
198.5	M2-Neoplasm, Bone and bone marrow
213.8	B-Neoplasm, Short bones, lower limb
238.0	UB-Neoplasm, Bone
239.2	Bone/Skin neoplasm NOS
250.8x	Diabetes w/manifestations
714.0	Rheumatoid arthritis
714.3x	Juvenile chronic polyarthritis
715.27	Loc 2nd osteoarthritis, ankle/foot
727.1	Bunion
730.17	Chronic osteomyelitis, ankle/foot
731.8	Bone involvement in other diseases
755.67	Anomalies of foot NEC

REIMBURSEMENT INFORMATION

General

- See notes on page 286.

Medicare

- Follow-up Days — 90
- Assistant Surgeon
  28111–28112, 28114 — paid
  28113 — by report
- Supply Charges — not allowed
- Outpatient Limit — does not apply
- Major Surgery Rules Apply

CPT CODE	SERVICE	ICD-9-CM
28116	Ostectomy, excision of tarsal coalition	170.8 M-Neoplasm, Short bones, lower limb 198.5 M2-Neoplasm, Bone and bone marrow 213.8 B-Neoplasm, Short bones, lower limb 238.0 UB-Neoplasm, Bone 239.2 Bone/Skin neoplasm NOS 250.8x Diabetes w/manifestations 714.0 Rheumatoid arthritis 714.3x Juvenile chronic polyarthritis 715.27 Loc 2nd osteoarthritis, ankle/foot 727.1 Bunion 730.17 Chronic osteomyelitis, ankle/foot 731.8 Bone involvement in other diseases 755.67 Anomalies of foot NEC **REIMBURSEMENT INFORMATION** General ◆ See notes on page 286. Medicare ◆ Follow-up Days — 90 ◆ Assistant Surgeon — paid ◆ Supply Charges — not allowed ◆ Outpatient Limit — does not apply ◆ Major Surgery Rules Apply
28118	Ostectomy, calcaneus	170.8 M-Neoplasm, Short bones, lower limb 198.5 M2-Neoplasm, Bone and bone marrow 213.8 B-Neoplasm, Short bones, lower limb 238.0 UB-Neoplasm, Bone 239.2 Bone/Skin neoplasm NOS 250.8x Diabetes w/manifestations 707.x Chronic ulcer of skin 714.0 Rheumatoid arthritis 714.3x Juvenile chronic polyarthritis 715.27 Loc 2nd osteoarthritis, ankle/foot 727.1 Bunion 730.17 Chronic osteomyelitis, ankle/foot 731.8 Bone involvement in other diseases 755.67 Anomalies of foot NEC 892.1 Open wound of foot, complicated **REIMBURSEMENT INFORMATION** General ◆ See notes on page 286. Medicare ◆ Follow-up Days — 90 ◆ Assistant Surgeon — paid ◆ Supply Charges — not allowed ◆ Outpatient Limit — does not apply ◆ Major Surgery Rules Apply

CPT CODE	SERVICE	ICD-9-CM
28119	Ostectomy, calcaneus; for spur, with or without plantar fascial release	726.73 Calcaneal spur 726.91 Exostosis, site NOS

REIMBURSEMENT INFORMATION

General

- See notes on page 286.

Medicare

- Follow-up Days — 90
- Assistant Surgeon — paid
- Supply Charges — not allowed
- Outpatient Limit — does not apply
- Major Surgery Rules Apply
- Fragments — 28118

28120 Partial excision (craterization, saucerization, sequestrectomy, or diaphysectomy) of bone (eg, for osteomyelitis or talar bossing), talus or calcaneus

707.x	Chronic ulcer of skin
726.91	Exostosis, site NOS
730.07	Acute osteomyelitis, ankle/foot
730.17	Chronic osteomyelitis, ankle/foot
730.27	Osteomyelitis NOS, ankle/foot
731.0	Osteitis deformans NOS
732.5	Juvenile osteochondrosis, foot
733.21	Solitary bone cyst
733.22	Aneurysmal bone cyst
733.29	Bone cyst NEC
733.49	Aseptic necrosis of bone NEC
756.4	Chondrodystrophy
892.1	Open wound of foot, complicated

REIMBURSEMENT INFORMATION

General

- See notes on page 286.

Medicare

- Follow-up Days — 90
- Assistant Surgeon — paid
- Supply Charges — not allowed
- Outpatient Limit — does not apply
- Major Surgery Rules Apply

CPT CODE	SERVICE	ICD-9-CM
28122	Partial excision (craterization, saucerization, or diaphysectomy) of bone (eg, for osteomyelitis or tarsal bossing), tarsal or metatarsal bone, except talus or calcaneus	726.91 Exostosis, site NOS 730.07 Acute osteomyelitis, ankle/foot 730.17 Chronic osteomyelitis, ankle/foot 730.27 Osteomyelitis NOS, ankle/foot 731.0 Osteitis deformans NOS 732.5 Juvenile osteochondrosis, foot 733.21 Solitary bone cyst 733.22 Aneurysmal bone cyst 733.29 Bone cyst NEC 733.44 Aseptic necrosis, talus 756.4 Chondrodystrophy **REIMBURSEMENT INFORMATION** General ◆ See notes on page 286. Medicare ◆ Follow-up Days — 90 ◆ Assistant Surgeon — paid ◆ Supply Charges — not allowed ◆ Outpatient Limit — does not apply ◆ Major Surgery Rules Apply
28124	Partial excision (craterization, saucerization, or diaphysectomy) of bone (eg, for osteomyelitis or dorsal bossing), phalanx of toe	726.91 Exostosis, site NOS 730.07 Acute osteomyelitis, ankle/foot 730.17 Chronic osteomyelitis, ankle/foot 730.27 Osteomyelitis NOS, ankle/foot 731.0 Osteitis deformans NOS 732.5 Juvenile osteochondrosis, foot 733.21 Solitary bone cyst 733.22 Aneurysmal bone cyst 733.29 Bone cyst NEC 733.44 Aseptic necrosis, talus 756.4 Chondrodystrophy **REIMBURSEMENT INFORMATION** General ◆ See notes on page 286. Medicare ◆ Follow-up Days — 90 ◆ Assistant Surgeon — not paid ◆ Supply Charges — not allowed ◆ Outpatient Limit — applies ◆ Major Surgery Rules Apply

CPT CODE	SERVICE	ICD-9-CM
▲ 28126	Resection, partial or complete, phalangeal base, single toe, each	

700.	Corns and callosities
714.0	Rheumatoid arthritis
714.3x	Juvenile chronic polyarthritis
715.17	Loc prim osteoarthritis, ankle/foot
715.27	Loc 2nd osteoarthritis, ankle/foot
735.5	Claw toe

REIMBURSEMENT INFORMATION

General

- ♦ See notes on page 286.
- ♦ Description changed in 1995 CPT.

Medicare

- ♦ Follow–up Days — 90
- ♦ Assistant Surgeon — not paid
- ♦ Supply Charges — not allowed
- ♦ Outpatient Limit — applies
- ♦ Major Surgery Rules Apply

28140 Metatarsectomy

170.8	M-Neoplasm, Short bones, lower limb
198.5	M2-Neoplasm, Bone and bone marrow
213.8	B-Neoplasm, Short bones, lower limb
238.0	UB-Neoplasm, Bone
239.2	Bone/Skin neoplasm NOS
250.80	Diabetes w/manifest NEC, type II
250.81	Diabetes w/manifest NEC, type I
714.0	Rheumatoid arthritis
714.3x	Juvenile chronic polyarthritis
715.17	Loc prim osteoarthritis, ankle/foot
715.27	Loc 2nd osteoarthritis, ankle/foot
730.07	Acute osteomyelitis, ankle/foot
730.17	Chronic osteomyelitis, ankle/foot
731.8	Bone involvement in other diseases
892.1	Open wound of foot, complicated

REIMBURSEMENT INFORMATION

General

- ♦ See notes on page 286.

Medicare

- ♦ Follow–up Days — 90
- ♦ Assistant Surgeon — paid
- ♦ Supply Charges — not allowed
- ♦ Outpatient Limit — does not apply
- ♦ Major Surgery Rules Apply

CPT CODE	SERVICE
28150	Phalangectomy of toe, single, each

ICD–9–CM

170.8	M-Neoplasm, Short bones, lower limb
198.5	M2-Neoplasm, Bone and bone marrow
213.8	B-Neoplasm, Short bones, lower limb
238.0	UB-Neoplasm, Bone
239.2	Bone/Skin neoplasm NOS
250.80	Diabetes w/manifest NEC, type II
250.81	Diabetes w/manifest NEC, type I
714.0	Rheumatoid arthritis
714.3x	Juvenile chronic polyarthritis
715.17	Loc prim osteoarthritis, ankle/foot
715.27	Loc 2nd osteoarthritis, ankle/foot
730.07	Acute osteomyelitis, ankle/foot
730.17	Chronic osteomyelitis, ankle/foot
731.8	Bone involvement in other diseases
735.x	Acquired deformities of toe

REIMBURSEMENT INFORMATION

General

- See notes on page 286.

Medicare

- Follow–up Days — 90
- Assistant Surgeon — not paid
- Supply Charges — not allowed
- Outpatient Limit — does not apply
- Major Surgery Rules Apply

CPT CODE	SERVICE
28153	Resection, head of phalanx, toe

ICD-9-CM

170.8	M-Neoplasm, Short bones, lower limb
198.5	M2-Neoplasm, Bone and bone marrow
213.8	B-Neoplasm, Short bones, lower limb
238.0	UB-Neoplasm, Bone
239.2	Bone/Skin neoplasm NOS
250.80	Diabetes w/manifest NEC, type II
250.81	Diabetes w/manifest NEC, type I
714.0	Rheumatoid arthritis
714.3x	Juvenile chronic polyarthritis
715.17	Loc prim osteoarthritis, ankle/foot
715.27	Loc 2nd osteoarthritis, ankle/foot
730.07	Acute osteomyelitis, ankle/foot
730.17	Chronic osteomyelitis, ankle/foot
731.8	Bone involvement in other diseases
735.x	Acquired deformities of toe

REIMBURSEMENT INFORMATION

General

- See notes on page 286.

Medicare

- Follow–up Days — 90
- Assistant Surgeon — not paid
- Supply Charges — not allowed
- Outpatient Limit — applies
- Major Surgery Rules Apply

CPT CODE	SERVICE	ICD-9-CM	
28160	Hemiphalangectomy or interphalangeal joint excision, toe, single, each	170.8	M-Neoplasm, Short bones, lower limb
		198.5	M2-Neoplasm, Bone and bone marrow
		213.8	B-Neoplasm, Short bones, lower limb
		238.0	UB-Neoplasm, Bone
		239.2	Bone/Skin neoplasm NOS
		250.80	Diabetes w/manifest NEC, type II
		250.81	Diabetes w/manifest NEC, type I
		714.0	Rheumatoid arthritis
		714.3x	Juvenile chronic polyarthritis
		715.17	Loc prim osteoarthritis, ankle/foot
		715.27	Loc 2nd osteoarthritis, ankle/foot
		730.07	Acute osteomyelitis, ankle/foot
		730.17	Chronic osteomyelitis, ankle/foot
		731.8	Bone involvement in other diseases
		735.x	Acquired deformities of toe

REIMBURSEMENT INFORMATION

General

- ♦ See notes on page 286.

Medicare

- ♦ Follow–up Days — 90
- ♦ Assistant Surgeon — not paid
- ♦ Supply Charges — not allowed
- ♦ Outpatient Limit — applies
- ♦ Major Surgery Rules Apply

CPT CODE	SERVICE	ICD-9-CM	
▲ **28171**	Radical resection of tumor, bone; tarsal (except talus or calcaneus)	170.8	M-Neoplasm, Short bones, lower limb
▲ **28173**	Radical resection of tumor (bone); metatarsal	238.0	UB-Neoplasm, Bone
▲ **28175**	Radical resection of tumor, bone; phalanx of toe	239.2	Bone/Skin neoplasm NOS

CPT NOTES

- ♦ For talus or calcaneus, see 27647.

REIMBURSEMENT INFORMATION

General

- ♦ See notes on page 286.
- ♦ Description changed in 1995 CPT.

Medicare

- ♦ Follow–up Days — 90
- ♦ Assistant Surgeon — paid
- ♦ Supply Charges — not allowed
- ♦ Outpatient Limit — does not apply
- ♦ Major Surgery Rules Apply

CPT CODE	SERVICE	ICD-9-CM
28190*	Removal of foreign body, foot; subcutaneous	709.4 Foreign body granuloma, skin 728.82 Foreign body granuloma of muscle 892.1 Open wound of foot, complicated 917.6 Foreign body, foot/toe 917.7 Foreign body, foot/toe, infected V54.0 Removal of internal fixation device

REIMBURSEMENT INFORMATION

General

- ♦ See notes on page 286.
- ♦ Starred procedure.

Medicare

- ♦ Follow-up Days — 10
- ♦ Assistant Surgeon — not paid
- ♦ Supply Charges — not allowed
- ♦ Outpatient Limit — applies
- ♦ Minor Surgery Rules Apply

CPT CODE	SERVICE	ICD-9-CM
28192	Removal of foreign body, foot; deep	728.82 Foreign body granuloma of muscle 729.6 Old foreign body in soft tissue 733.99 Bone/Cartilage disorder NEC 892.1 Open wound of foot, complicated 996.66 Reaction, internal joint prosthesis 996.77 Complication, int joint prosthesis 998.7 Postop foreign subst acute reaction
28193	Removal of foreign body, foot; complicated	

REIMBURSEMENT INFORMATION

General

- ♦ See notes on page 286.

Medicare

- ♦ Follow-up Days — 90
- ♦ Assistant Surgeon — not paid
- ♦ Supply Charges — not allowed
- ♦ Outpatient Limit — does not apply
- ♦ Major Surgery Rules Apply

CPT CODE	SERVICE	ICD–9–CM
28200	Repair or suture of tendon, foot, flexor, single; primary or secondary, without free graft, each tendon	727.67 Rupture, achilles tendon 727.68 Rupture, tendons of foot/ankle NEC 844.3 Sprain superior tibiofibular 844.8 Sprain of knee & leg NEC 845.1x Foot sprain/strain 892.2 Open wound of foot w/tendon **REIMBURSEMENT INFORMATION** General ◆ See notes on page 286. Medicare ◆ Follow–up Days — 90 ◆ Assistant Surgeon — paid ◆ Supply Charges — not allowed ◆ Outpatient Limit — does not apply ◆ Major Surgery Rules Apply
28202	Repair or suture of tendon, foot, flexor, single; secondary with free graft, each tendon (includes obtaining graft)	727.67 Rupture, achilles tendon 727.68 Rupture, tendons of foot/ankle NEC 845.1x Foot sprain/strain 892.2 Open wound of foot w/tendon **REIMBURSEMENT INFORMATION** General ◆ See notes on page 286. Medicare ◆ Follow–up Days — 90 ◆ Assistant Surgeon — paid ◆ Supply Charges — not allowed ◆ Outpatient Limit — does not apply ◆ Major Surgery Rules Apply
28208 **28210**	Repair or suture of tendon, foot, extensor, single; primary or secondary, each tendon Repair of suture or tendon, foot, extensor, single; secondary with free graft, each tendon (includes obtaining graft)	727.67 Rupture, achilles tendon 727.68 Rupture, tendons of foot/ankle NEC 845.1x Foot sprain/strain 892.2 Open wound of foot w/tendon **REIMBURSEMENT INFORMATION** General ◆ See notes on page 286. Medicare ◆ Follow–up Days — 90 ◆ Assistant Surgeon — paid ◆ Supply Charges — not allowed ◆ Outpatient Limit — does not apply ◆ Major Surgery Rules Apply

CPT CODE	SERVICE	ICD-9-CM
28220	Tenolysis, flexor, foot; single	727.06 Tenosynovitis of foot/ankle 735.8 Acquired deformities of toe NEC
28222	Tenolysis, flexor, foot; multiple (through same incision)	

REIMBURSEMENT INFORMATION

General

- ♦ See notes on page 286.

Medicare

- ♦ Follow-up Days — 90
- ♦ Assistant Surgeon — not paid
- ♦ Supply Charges — not allowed
- ♦ Outpatient Limit
  28220 — applies
  28222 — does not apply
- ♦ Major Surgery Rules Apply

CPT CODE	SERVICE	ICD-9-CM
28225	Tenolysis, extensor, foot; single	727.06 Tenosynovitis of foot/ankle 735.8 Acquired deformities of toe NEC
28226	Tenolysis, extensor, foot; multiple (through same incision)	

REIMBURSEMENT INFORMATION

General

- ♦ See notes on page 286.

Medicare

- ♦ Follow-up Days — 90
- ♦ Assistant Surgeon — paid
- ♦ Supply Charges — not allowed
- ♦ Outpatient Limit — does not apply
- ♦ Major Surgery Rules Apply

CPT CODE	SERVICE	ICD-9-CM
28230	Tenotomy, open, flexor; foot, single or multiple (separate procedure)	735.4 Other hammer toe 735.5 Claw toe 754.51 Talipes equinovarus 754.70 Talipes NOS 754.71 Talipes cavus 754.79 Congenital foot deformity NEC 755.66 Anomalies of toes NEC
28232	Tenotomy, open, flexor; toe, single, (separate procedure)	

REIMBURSEMENT INFORMATION

General

- ♦ See notes on page 286.
- ♦ Separate procedure rules apply.

Medicare

- ♦ Follow-up Days — 90
- ♦ Assistant Surgeon — not paid
- ♦ Supply Charges — not allowed
- ♦ Outpatient Limit — applies
- ♦ Major Surgery Rules Apply

CPT CODE	SERVICE	ICD–9–CM
28234	Tenotomy, open, extensor, foot or toe	735.4 Other hammer toe 735.5 Claw toe 754.51 Talipes equinovarus 754.70 Talipes NOS 754.71 Talipes cavus 754.79 Congenital foot deformity NEC 755.66 Anomalies of toes NEC

REIMBURSEMENT INFORMATION

General

- ♦ See notes on page 286.

Medicare

- ♦ Follow–up Days — 90
- ♦ Assistant Surgeon — not paid
- ♦ Supply Charges — not allowed
- ♦ Outpatient Limit — applies
- ♦ Major Surgery Rules Apply

CPT CODE	SERVICE	ICD–9–CM
28250	Division of plantar fascia and muscle ("Steindler stripping") (separate procedure)	736.73 Cavus deformity of foot 754.51 Talipes equinovarus 754.71 Talipes cavus 754.79 Congenital foot deformity NEC

REIMBURSEMENT INFORMATION

General

- ♦ See notes on page 286.
- ♦ Separate procedure rules apply.

Medicare

- ♦ Follow–up Days — 90
- ♦ Assistant Surgeon — paid
- ♦ Supply Charges — not allowed
- ♦ Outpatient Limit — does not apply
- ♦ Major Surgery Rules Apply

CPT CODE	SERVICE	ICD–9–CM
▲ 28270	Capsulotomy; metatarsophalangeal joint, with or without tenorrhaphy, single, each joint (separate procedure)	718.47 Contracture of joint, ankle/foot 735.4 Other hammer toe 735.5 Claw toe 735.8 Acquired deformities of toe NEC
▲ 28272	Capsulotomy; interphalangeal joint, single, each joint (separate procedure)	

REIMBURSEMENT INFORMATION

General

- ♦ See notes on page 286.
- ♦ Separate procedure rules apply.
- ♦ Description changed in 1995 CPT.

Medicare

- ♦ Follow–up Days — 90
- ♦ Assistant Surgeon — not paid
- ♦ Supply Charges — not allowed
- ♦ Outpatient Limit — applies
- ♦ Major Surgery Rules Apply

CPT CODE	SERVICE	ICD–9–CM
▲ 28280	Webbing operation (create syndactylism of toes) (Kelikian type procedure)	700. Corns and callosities 735.x Acquired deformities of toe

REIMBURSEMENT INFORMATION

General

- ♦ See notes on page 286.
- ♦ Description changed in 1995 CPT.

Medicare

- ♦ Follow–up Days — 90
- ♦ Assistant Surgeon — by report
- ♦ Supply Charges — not allowed
- ♦ Outpatient Limit — does not apply
- ♦ Major Surgery Rules Apply

CPT CODE	SERVICE	ICD–9–CM
▲ 28285	Hammertoe operation, one toe (eg, interphalangeal fusion, filleting, phalangectomy)	755.66 Anomalies of toes NEC

REIMBURSEMENT INFORMATION

General

- ♦ See notes on page 286.
- ♦ Description changed in 1995 CPT.

Medicare

- ♦ Follow–up Days — 90
- ♦ Assistant Surgeon — paid
- ♦ Supply Charges — not allowed
- ♦ Outpatient Limit — does not apply
- ♦ Major Surgery Rules Apply
- ♦ Fragments — 28153, 28160

CPT CODE	SERVICE	ICD–9–CM
▲ 28286	Cock-up fifth toe operation with plastic skin closure, (Ruiz-Mora type procedure)	735.4 Other hammer toe 735.5 Claw toe 755.66 Anomalies of toes NEC

REIMBURSEMENT INFORMATION

General

- ♦ See notes on page 286.
- ♦ Description changed in 1995 CPT.

Medicare

- ♦ Follow–up Days — 90
- ♦ Assistant Surgeon — not paid
- ♦ Supply Charges — not allowed
- ♦ Outpatient Limit — does not apply
- ♦ Major Surgery Rules Apply

CPT CODE	SERVICE	ICD-9-CM
28288	Ostectomy, partial, exostectomy or condylectomy, single, metatarsal head, first through fifth, each metatarsal head	700. Corns and callosities 714.0 Rheumatoid arthritis 714.3x Juvenile chronic polyarthritis 715.27 Loc 2nd osteoarthritis, ankle/foot 727.1 Bunion 730.17 Chronic osteomyelitis, ankle/foot 731.8 Bone involvement in other diseases 755.67 Anomalies of foot NEC 892.1 Open wound of foot, complicated

REIMBURSEMENT INFORMATION

General

- See notes on page 286.

Medicare

- Follow-up Days — 90
- Assistant Surgeon — not paid
- Supply Charges — not allowed
- Outpatient Limit — does not apply
- Major Surgery Rules Apply

CPT CODE	SERVICE	ICD-9-CM
28470	Closed treatment of metatarsal fracture; without manipulation, each	825.25 Fx metatarsal, closed 825.35 Fx metatarsal, open
28475	Closed treatment of metatarsal fracture; with manipulation, each	

REIMBURSEMENT INFORMATION

General

- See notes on page 286.

Medicare

- Follow-up Days — 90
- Assistant Surgeon — not paid
- Supply Charges — not allowed
- Outpatient Limit — applies
- Major Surgery Rules Apply

CPT CODE	SERVICE	ICD-9-CM
28485	Open treatment of metatarsal fracture, with or without internal or external fixation, each	825.25 Fx metatarsal, closed 825.35 Fx metatarsal, open **REIMBURSEMENT INFORMATION** <u>General</u> ◆ See notes on page 286. <u>Medicare</u> ◆ Follow–up Days — 90 ◆ Assistant Surgeon — paid ◆ Supply Charges — not allowed ◆ Outpatient Limit — does not apply ◆ Major Surgery Rules Apply
28490 **28495**	Closed treatment of fracture great toe, phalanx or phalanges; without manipulation Closed treatment of fracture great toe, phalanx or phalanges; with manipulation	826.0 Fx phalanx, foot, closed 826.1 Fx phalanx, foot, open **REIMBURSEMENT INFORMATION** <u>General</u> ◆ See notes on page 286. <u>Medicare</u> ◆ Follow–up Days — 90 ◆ Assistant Surgeon — not paid ◆ Supply Charges — not allowed ◆ Outpatient Limit — applies ◆ Major Surgery Rules Apply
28505	Open treatment of fracture great toe, phalanx or phalanges, with or without internal or external fixation	826.0 Fx phalanx, foot, closed 826.1 Fx phalanx, foot, open **REIMBURSEMENT INFORMATION** <u>General</u> ◆ See notes on page 286. <u>Medicare</u> ◆ Follow–up Days — 90 ◆ Assistant Surgeon — not paid ◆ Supply Charges — not allowed ◆ Outpatient Limit — does not apply ◆ Major Surgery Rules Apply

CPT CODE	SERVICE	ICD-9-CM
28510	Closed treatment of fracture, phalanx or phalanges, other than great toe; without manipulation, each	826.0 Fx phalanx, foot, closed 826.1 Fx phalanx, foot, open
28515	Closed treatment of fracture, phalanx or phalanges, other than great toe; with manipulation, each	

REIMBURSEMENT INFORMATION

General

- See notes on page 286.

Medicare

- Follow-up Days — 90
- Assistant Surgeon — not paid
- Supply Charges — not allowed
- Outpatient Limit — applies
- Major Surgery Rules Apply

CPT CODE	SERVICE	ICD-9-CM
28525	Open treatment of fracture, phalanx or phalanges, other than great toe, with or without internal or external fixation, each	826.0 Fx phalanx, foot, closed 826.1 Fx phalanx, foot, open

REIMBURSEMENT INFORMATION

General

- See notes on page 286.

Medicare

- Follow-up Days — 90
- Assistant Surgeon — not paid
- Supply Charges — not allowed
- Outpatient Limit — does not apply
- Major Surgery Rules Apply

CPT CODE	SERVICE	ICD-9-CM
28530	Closed treatment of sesamoid fracture	825.29 Fx foot bone NEC, closed

REIMBURSEMENT INFORMATION

General

- See notes on page 286.

Medicare

- Follow-up Days — 90
- Assistant Surgeon — by report
- Supply Charges — not allowed
- Outpatient Limit — applies
- Major Surgery Rules Apply

CPT CODE	SERVICE	ICD–9–CM
28630*	Closed treatment of metatarsophalangeal joint dislocation; without anesthesia	718.27 Pathologic dislocation, ankle/foot 718.37 Recurrent dislocation, ankle/foot 838.05 Disloc metatarsophalangeal, closed 838.15 Disloc metatarsophalangeal, open
28635*	Closed treatment of metatarsophalangeal joint dislocation; requiring anesthesia	

REIMBURSEMENT INFORMATION

General

- See notes on page 286.
- Starred procedure.

Medicare

- Follow–up Days — 10
- Assistant Surgeon — not paid
- Supply Charges — not allowed
- Outpatient Limit
  28630 — applies
  28635 — does not apply
- Minor Surgery Rules Apply

CPT CODE	SERVICE	ICD–9–CM
28636	Percutaneous skeletal fixation of metatarsophalangeal joint dislocation, with manipulation	718.27 Pathologic dislocation, ankle/foot 718.37 Recurrent dislocation, ankle/foot 838.05 Disloc metatarsophalangeal, closed 838.15 Disloc metatarsophalangeal, open

REIMBURSEMENT INFORMATION

General

- See notes on page 286.

Medicare

- Follow–up Days — 10
- Assistant Surgeon — not paid
- Supply Charges — not allowed
- Outpatient Limit — does not apply
- Minor Surgery Rules Apply

CPT CODE	SERVICE	ICD-9-CM
28645	Open treatment of metatarsophalangeal joint dislocation, with or without internal or external fixation	718.27 Pathologic dislocation, ankle/foot 718.37 Recurrent dislocation, ankle/foot 838.05 Disloc metatarsophalangeal, closed 838.15 Disloc metatarsophalangeal, open

REIMBURSEMENT INFORMATION

General

- ♦ See notes on page 286.

Medicare

- ♦ Follow-up Days — 90
- ♦ Assistant Surgeon — not paid
- ♦ Supply Charges — not allowed
- ♦ Outpatient Limit — does not apply
- ♦ Major Surgery Rules Apply

CPT CODE	SERVICE	ICD-9-CM
28660*	Closed treatment of interphalangeal joint dislocation; without anesthesia	718.27 Pathologic dislocation, ankle/foot 718.37 Recurrent dislocation, ankle/foot 838.06 Disloc interphalangeal foot, closed 838.16 Disloc interphalangeal foot, open
28665*	Closed treatment of interphalangeal joint dislocation; requiring anesthesia	

REIMBURSEMENT INFORMATION

General

- ♦ See notes on page 286.
- ♦ Starred procedure.

Medicare

- ♦ Follow-up Days — 10
- ♦ Assistant Surgeon — not paid
- ♦ Supply Charges — not allowed
- ♦ Outpatient Limit — does not apply
- ♦ Minor Surgery Rules Apply

CPT CODE	SERVICE	ICD–9–CM
28666	Percutaneous skeletal fixation of interphalangeal joint dislocation, with manipulation	718.27 Pathologic dislocation, ankle/foot 718.37 Recurrent dislocation, ankle/foot 838.06 Disloc interphalangeal foot, closed 838.16 Disloc interphalangeal foot, open **REIMBURSEMENT INFORMATION** General ◆ See notes on page 286. Medicare ◆ Follow–up Days — 10 ◆ Assistant Surgeon — paid ◆ Supply Charges — not allowed ◆ Outpatient Limit — does not apply ◆ Minor Surgery Rules Apply
28675	Open treatment of interphalangeal joint dislocation, with or without internal or external fixation	718.27 Pathologic dislocation, ankle/foot 718.37 Recurrent dislocation, ankle/foot 838.06 Disloc interphalangeal foot, closed 838.16 Disloc interphalangeal foot, open **REIMBURSEMENT INFORMATION** General ◆ See notes on page 286. Medicare ◆ Follow–up Days — 90 ◆ Assistant Surgeon — paid ◆ Supply Charges — not allowed ◆ Outpatient Limit — does not apply ◆ Major Surgery Rules Apply

CPT CODE	SERVICE
28800	Amputation, foot; midtarsal (Chopart type procedure)
28805	Amputation, foot; transmetatarsal

ICD–9–CM

170.8	M-Neoplasm, Short bones, lower limb
198.5	M2-Neoplasm, Bone and bone marrow
238.0	UB-Neoplasm, Bone
239.2	Bone/Skin neoplasm NOS
250.60	Diabetes w/neuro manifest, type II
250.70	Diabetes circulat disord, type II
443.1	Thromboangiitis obliterans
443.81	Peripheral angiopathy in other dis
443.9	Peripheral vascular disease NOS
730.07	Acute osteomyelitis, ankle/foot
730.27	Osteomyelitis NOS, ankle/foot
733.49	Aseptic necrosis of bone NEC
785.4	Gangrene
892.1	Open wound of foot, complicated
896.0	Amputation of foot, unilateral
896.1	Amputation of foot, unilat, compl
928.20	Crushing injury, foot
991.2	Frostbite of foot
996.95	Complication, reattached foot/toe
997.60	Late amputation stump complic NOS
997.61	Neuroma of amputation stump
997.62	Infection of amputated stump
997.69	Late amputation stump complic NEC

REIMBURSEMENT INFORMATION

General

- See notes on page 286.

Medicare

- Follow–up Days — 90
- Assistant Surgeon — paid
- Supply Charges — not allowed
- Outpatient Limit — does not apply
- Major Surgery Rules Apply

CPT CODE	SERVICE
28810	Amputation, metatarsal, with toe, single

ICD–9–CM

170.8	M-Neoplasm, Short bones, lower limb
198.5	M2-Neoplasm, Bone and bone marrow
238.0	UB-Neoplasm, Bone
239.2	Bone/Skin neoplasm NOS
250.60	Diabetes w/neuro manifest, type II
250.70	Diabetes circulat disord, type II
443.1	Thromboangiitis obliterans
443.81	Peripheral angiopathy in other dis
443.9	Peripheral vascular disease NOS
730.07	Acute osteomyelitis, ankle/foot
730.27	Osteomyelitis NOS, ankle/foot
733.49	Aseptic necrosis of bone NEC
785.4	Gangrene
893.1	Open wound of toe, complicated
895.x	Traumatic amputation of toe(s)
896.0	Amputation of foot, unilateral
896.1	Amputation of foot, unilat, compl
928.20	Crushing injury, foot
928.3	Crushing injury, toe
991.2	Frostbite of foot
996.95	Complication, reattached foot/toe
997.60	Late amputation stump complic NOS
997.61	Neuroma of amputation stump
997.62	Infection of amputated stump
997.69	Late amputation stump complic NEC

REIMBURSEMENT INFORMATION

General

- See notes on page 286.

Medicare

- Follow–up Days — 90
- Assistant Surgeon — by report
- Supply Charges — not allowed
- Outpatient Limit — does not apply
- Major Surgery Rules Apply

CPT CODE **SERVICE**

28820 Amputation, toe; metatarsophalangeal joint

28825 Amputation, toe; interphalangeal joint

CPT NOTES

- For amputation of tuft of distal phalanx, use 11752.

ICD–9–CM

170.8	M-Neoplasm, Short bones, lower limb
198.5	M2-Neoplasm, Bone and bone marrow
238.0	UB-Neoplasm, Bone
239.2	Bone/Skin neoplasm NOS
250.60	Diabetes w/neuro manifest, type II
250.70	Diabetes circulat disord, type II
443.1	Thromboangiitis obliterans
443.81	Peripheral angiopathy in other dis
443.9	Peripheral vascular disease NOS
730.07	Acute osteomyelitis, ankle/foot
730.27	Osteomyelitis NOS, ankle/foot
733.49	Aseptic necrosis of bone NEC
755.02	Polydactyly, toes
785.4	Gangrene
893.1	Open wound of toe, complicated
895.x	Traumatic amputation of toe(s)
928.3	Crushing injury, toe
991.2	Frostbite of foot
996.95	Complication, reattached foot/toe
997.60	Late amputation stump complic NOS
997.61	Neuroma of amputation stump
997.62	Infection of amputated stump
997.69	Late amputation stump complic NEC

REIMBURSEMENT INFORMATION

General

- See notes on page 286.

Medicare

- Follow–up Days — 90
- Assistant Surgeon — not paid
- Supply Charges — not allowed
- Outpatient Limit — does not apply
- Major Surgery Rules Apply

CPT CODE	SERVICE
29049	Application; plaster figure of eight

CPT NOTES

- This procedure applies when the cast application or strapping is a replacement procedure used during or after the period of follow-up care. Additional visits are reportable only if significant identifiable further services are provided at the time of the cast application or strapping.
- If cast application or strapping is provided as an initial procedure in which no surgery is performed (e.g., casting of a sprained ankle or knee), use the appropriate office evaluation and management in addition to 99070 for supplies.
- The procedure includes removal of cast or strapping.

ICD–9–CM

810.0x	Clavicle fracture, closed
810.1x	Clavicle fracture, open
811.0x	Scapula fracture, closed
811.1x	Scapula fracture, open

REIMBURSEMENT INFORMATION

General

- See notes on page 286.

Medicare

- Follow–up Days — 0
- Assistant Surgeon — not paid
- Supply Charges — not allowed
- Outpatient Limit — applies
- Minor Surgery Rules Apply

CPT CODE	SERVICE
29065	Application; shoulder to hand (long arm)

CPT NOTES

- This procedure applies when the cast application or strapping is a replacement procedure used during or after the period of follow-up care. Additional visits are reportable only if significant identifiable further services are provided at the time of the cast application or strapping.
- If cast application or strapping is provided as an initial procedure in which no surgery is performed (e.g., casting of a sprained ankle or knee), use the appropriate office evaluation and management in addition to 99070 for supplies.
- The procedure includes removal of cast or strapping.

ICD–9–CM

195.4	M-Neoplasm, Upper limb
213.4	B-Neoplasm, Long bones, arm
213.5	B-Neoplasm, Wrist/Hand bones
239.2	Bone/Skin neoplasm NOS
343.x	Infantile cerebral palsy
354.2	Ulnar nerve lesion
354.3	Radial nerve lesion
358.0	Myasthenia gravis
707.0	Decubitus ulcer
716.02	Kaschin-Beck disease, upper arm
716.03	Kaschin-Beck disease, forearm
716.22	Allergic arthritis, upper arm
719.23	Villonodular synovitis, forearm
719.42	Pain in joint, upper arm
719.43	Pain in joint, forearm
719.62	Joint symptom NEC, upper arm
719.63	Joint symptom NEC, forearm
719.82	Joint disorder NEC, upper arm
719.83	Joint disorder NEC, forearm
725.	Polymyalgia rheumatica
726.3x	Enthesopathy of elbow region
726.4	Enthesopathy of wrist/carpus
727.04	Radial styloid tenosynovitis
727.05	Tenosynovitis of hand/wrist NEC
728.6	Contracture of palmar fascia
729.2	Neuralgia/neuritis NOS
733.81	Malunion of fracture
733.82	Nonunion of fracture
755.59	Upper limb anomaly NEC
812.0x	Humerus fracture, upper end, closed
812.1x	Humerus fracture, upper end, open
812.21	Fx humerus shaft, closed
812.31	Fx humerus shaft, open
812.4x	Humerus fracture, lower end, closed
812.5x	Humerus fracture, lower end, open
813.0x	Fracture of radius/ulna, upper end
813.1x	Fracture of radius/ulna, lower end
813.2x	Fracture of radius and ulna shaft
813.3x	Fracture of radius and ulna shaft
813.4x	Fracture of radius/ulna, lower end
813.5x	Fracture of radius/ulna, lower end
814.0x	Carpal fracture, closed
814.1x	Carpal fracture, open
832.0x	Elbow dislocation, closed
832.1x	Elbow dislocation, open
833.0x	Wrist dislocation, closed
833.1x	Wrist dislocation, open
905.2	Late effect, arm fracture
927.03	Crushing injury, upper arm
927.1x	Crushing injury, elbow and forearm
927.21	Crushing injury, wrist
955.2	Injury ulnar nerve
955.3	Injury radial nerve
V54.0	Removal of internal fixation device
V54.8	Orthopedic aftercare NEC
V67.0	Surgery follow-up

CPT CODE	SERVICE	ICD–9–CM
29065 (Cont'd.)		V67.4 Fracture follow-up
		V67.5 Follow-up exam, following treatment

REIMBURSEMENT INFORMATION

General

- See notes on page 286.

Medicare

- Follow–up Days — 0
- Assistant Surgeon — not paid
- Supply Charges — not allowed
- Outpatient Limit — applies
- Minor Surgery Rules Apply

CPT CODE	SERVICE
29075	Application; elbow to finger (short arm)

CPT NOTES

- This procedure applies when the cast application or strapping is a replacement procedure used during or after the period of follow-up care. Additional visits are reportable only if significant identifiable further services are provided at the time of the cast application or strapping.
- If cast application or strapping is provided as an initial procedure in which no surgery is performed (e.g., casting of a sprained ankle or knee), use the appropriate office evaluation and management in addition to 99070 for supplies.
- The procedure includes removal of cast or strapping.

ICD–9–CM

195.4	M-Neoplasm, Upper limb
213.4	B-Neoplasm, Long bones, arm
213.5	B-Neoplasm, Wrist/Hand bones
239.2	Bone/Skin neoplasm NOS
343.x	Infantile cerebral palsy
354.0	Carpal tunnel syndrome
354.2	Ulnar nerve lesion
354.3	Radial nerve lesion
358.0	Myasthenia gravis
443.0	Raynaud's syndrome
707.0	Decubitus ulcer
714.0	Rheumatoid arthritis
715.12	Loc prim osteoarthritis, upper arm
715.13	Loc prim osteoarthritis, forearm
715.14	Loc prim osteoarthritis, hand
715.22	Loc 2nd osteoarthritis, upper arm
715.23	Loc 2nd osteoarthritis, forearm
715.24	Loc 2nd osteoarthritis, hand
715.32	Loc osteoarthritis NOS, upper arm
715.33	Loc osteoarthritis NOS, forearm
715.34	Loc osteoarthritis NOS, hand
716.02	Kaschin-Beck disease, upper arm
716.03	Kaschin-Beck disease, forearm
716.04	Kaschin-Beck disease, hand
716.42	Transient arthropathy, upper arm
716.43	Transient arthropathy, forearm
716.44	Transient arthropathy, hand
718.52	Ankylosis of joint, upper arm
718.53	Ankylosis of joint, forearm
718.54	Ankylosis of joint, hand
718.82	Joint derangement NEC, upper arm
718.83	Joint derangement NEC, forearm
718.84	Joint derangement NEC, hand
719.22	Villonodular synovitis, upper arm
719.23	Villonodular synovitis, forearm
719.24	Villonodular synovitis, hand
719.42	Pain in joint, upper arm
719.43	Pain in joint, forearm
719.44	Pain in joint, hand
719.62	Joint symptom NEC, upper arm
719.63	Joint symptom NEC, forearm
719.64	Joint symptom NEC, hand
719.82	Joint disorder NEC, upper arm
719.83	Joint disorder NEC, forearm
719.84	Joint disorder NEC, hand
726.3x	Enthesopathy of elbow region
726.4	Enthesopathy of wrist/carpus
727.04	Radial styloid tenosynovitis
727.05	Tenosynovitis of hand/wrist NEC
728.6	Contracture of palmar fascia
729.2	Neuralgia/neuritis NOS
730.02	Acute osteomyelitis, upper arm
730.03	Acute osteomyelitis, forearm
730.04	Acute osteomyelitis, hand
730.12	Chronic osteomyelitis, upper arm
730.13	Chronic osteomyelitis, forearm

CPT CODE	SERVICE	ICD–9–CM	
29075 (Cont'd.)		730.14	Chronic osteomyelitis, hand
		730.22	Osteomyelitis NOS, upper arm
		730.23	Osteomyelitis NOS, forearm
		730.24	Osteomyelitis NOS, hand
		733.10	Pathologic fracture, site NOS
		733.12	Pathologic Fx distal radius/ulna
		733.19	Pathologic fracture, site NEC
		733.81	Malunion of fracture
		733.82	Nonunion of fracture
		736.2x	Acquired deformity of finger
		813.0x	Fracture of radius/ulna, upper end
		813.1x	Fracture of radius/ulna, lower end
		813.2x	Fracture of radius and ulna shaft
		813.3x	Fracture of radius and ulna shaft
		813.4x	Fracture of radius/ulna, lower end
		813.5x	Fracture of radius/ulna, lower end
		814.0x	Carpal fracture, closed
		814.1x	Carpal fracture, open
		815.0x	Metacarpal fracture, closed
		815.1x	Metacarpal fracture, open
		816.0x	Phalanges fracture, closed
		816.1x	Phalanges fracture, open
		833.0x	Wrist dislocation, closed
		833.1x	Wrist dislocation, open
		834.01	Disloc metacarpophalangeal, closed
		834.02	Disloc interphalangeal hand, closed
		834.11	Disloc metacarpophalangeal, open
		834.12	Disloc interphalangeal hand, open
		905.2	Late effect, arm fracture
		927.10	Crushing injury, forearm
		927.2x	Crushing injury, wrist and hand
		955.2	Injury ulnar nerve
		955.3	Injury radial nerve
		955.4	Injury musculocutaneous nerve
		955.5	Injury cutaneous sensory nerve/arm
		955.6	Injury digital nerve
		V54.0	Removal of internal fixation device
		V54.8	Orthopedic aftercare NEC
		V67.4	Fracture follow-up

REIMBURSEMENT INFORMATION

General

- See notes on page 286.

Medicare

- Follow–up Days — 0
- Assistant Surgeon — not paid
- Supply Charges — not allowed
- Outpatient Limit — applies
- Minor Surgery Rules Apply

CPT CODE **SERVICE**

29085 Application; hand to lower forearm (gauntlet)

CPT NOTES

- This procedure applies when the cast application or strapping is a replacement procedure used during or after the period of follow-up care. Additional visits are reportable only if significant identifiable further services are provided at the time of the cast application or strapping.
- If cast application or strapping is provided as an initial procedure in which no surgery is performed (e.g., casting of a sprained ankle or knee), use the appropriate office evaluation and management in addition to 99070 for supplies.
- The procedure includes removal of cast or strapping.

ICD–9–CM

195.4	M-Neoplasm, Upper limb
213.4	B-Neoplasm, Long bones, arm
213.5	B-Neoplasm, Wrist/Hand bones
239.2	Bone/Skin neoplasm NOS
343.x	Infantile cerebral palsy
354.0	Carpal tunnel syndrome
354.2	Ulnar nerve lesion
354.3	Radial nerve lesion
358.0	Myasthenia gravis
443.0	Raynaud's syndrome
707.0	Decubitus ulcer
714.0	Rheumatoid arthritis
715.13	Loc prim osteoarthritis, forearm
715.14	Loc prim osteoarthritis, hand
715.23	Loc 2nd osteoarthritis, forearm
715.24	Loc 2nd osteoarthritis, hand
715.33	Loc osteoarthritis NOS, forearm
715.34	Loc osteoarthritis NOS, hand
716.03	Kaschin-Beck disease, forearm
716.04	Kaschin-Beck disease, hand
716.43	Transient arthropathy, forearm
716.44	Transient arthropathy, hand
718.53	Ankylosis of joint, forearm
718.54	Ankylosis of joint, hand
718.83	Joint derangement NEC, forearm
718.84	Joint derangement NEC, hand
719.23	Villonodular synovitis, forearm
719.24	Villonodular synovitis, hand
719.43	Pain in joint, forearm
719.44	Pain in joint, hand
719.63	Joint symptom NEC, forearm
719.64	Joint symptom NEC, hand
719.83	Joint disorder NEC, forearm
719.84	Joint disorder NEC, hand
726.3x	Enthesopathy of elbow region
726.4	Enthesopathy of wrist/carpus
727.04	Radial styloid tenosynovitis
727.05	Tenosynovitis of hand/wrist NEC
728.6	Contracture of palmar fascia
729.2	Neuralgia/neuritis NOS
730.03	Acute osteomyelitis, forearm
730.04	Acute osteomyelitis, hand
730.13	Chronic osteomyelitis, forearm
730.14	Chronic osteomyelitis, hand
730.23	Osteomyelitis NOS, forearm
730.24	Osteomyelitis NOS, hand
733.10	Pathologic fracture, site NOS
733.12	Pathologic Fx distal radius/ulna
733.19	Pathologic fracture, site NEC
733.81	Malunion of fracture
733.82	Nonunion of fracture
736.2x	Acquired deformity of finger
813.4x	Fracture of radius/ulna, lower end
813.5x	Fracture of radius/ulna, lower end
814.0x	Carpal fracture, closed
814.1x	Carpal fracture, open

CPT CODE	SERVICE
29085 (Cont'd.)	

ICD–9–CM

815.0x	Metacarpal fracture, closed
815.1x	Metacarpal fracture, open
816.0x	Phalanges fracture, closed
816.1x	Phalanges fracture, open
833.0x	Wrist dislocation, closed
833.1x	Wrist dislocation, open
834.01	Disloc metacarpophalangeal, closed
834.02	Disloc interphalangeal hand, closed
834.11	Disloc metacarpophalangeal, open
834.12	Disloc interphalangeal hand, open
905.2	Late effect, arm fracture
927.10	Crushing injury, forearm
927.2x	Crushing injury, wrist and hand
955.2	Injury ulnar nerve
955.3	Injury radial nerve
955.4	Injury musculocutaneous nerve
955.5	Injury cutaneous sensory nerve/arm
955.6	Injury digital nerve
V54.0	Removal of internal fixation device
V54.8	Orthopedic aftercare NEC
V67.4	Fracture follow-up

REIMBURSEMENT INFORMATION

General

- See notes on page 286.

Medicare

- Follow–up Days — 0
- Assistant Surgeon — not paid
- Supply Charges — not allowed
- Outpatient Limit — applies
- Minor Surgery Rules Apply

CPT CODE	SERVICE
29105	Application of long arm splint (shoulder to hand)

CPT NOTES

- This procedure applies when the cast application or strapping is a replacement procedure used during or after the period of follow-up care. Additional visits are reportable only if significant identifiable further services are provided at the time of the cast application or strapping.
- If cast application or strapping is provided as an initial procedure in which no surgery is performed (e.g., casting of a sprained ankle or knee), use the appropriate office evaluation and management in addition to 99070 for supplies.
- The procedure includes removal of cast or strapping.

ICD–9–CM

195.4	M-Neoplasm, Upper limb
213.4	B-Neoplasm, Long bones, arm
213.5	B-Neoplasm, Wrist/Hand bones
239.2	Bone/Skin neoplasm NOS
343.x	Infantile cerebral palsy
354.2	Ulnar nerve lesion
354.3	Radial nerve lesion
358.0	Myasthenia gravis
707.0	Decubitus ulcer
716.02	Kaschin-Beck disease, upper arm
716.03	Kaschin-Beck disease, forearm
716.22	Allergic arthritis, upper arm
718.42	Contracture of joint, upper arm
718.52	Ankylosis of joint, upper arm
719.23	Villonodular synovitis, forearm
719.42	Pain in joint, upper arm
719.43	Pain in joint, forearm
719.52	Joint stiffness NEC, upper arm
719.62	Joint symptom NEC, upper arm
719.63	Joint symptom NEC, forearm
719.82	Joint disorder NEC, upper arm
719.83	Joint disorder NEC, forearm
725.	Polymyalgia rheumatica
726.3x	Enthesopathy of elbow region
726.4	Enthesopathy of wrist/carpus
727.04	Radial styloid tenosynovitis
727.05	Tenosynovitis of hand/wrist NEC
728.6	Contracture of palmar fascia
729.2	Neuralgia/neuritis NOS
733.81	Malunion of fracture
733.82	Nonunion of fracture
755.59	Upper limb anomaly NEC
812.0x	Humerus fracture, upper end, closed
812.1x	Humerus fracture, upper end, open
812.21	Fx humerus shaft, closed
812.31	Fx humerus shaft, open
812.4x	Humerus fracture, lower end, closed
812.5x	Humerus fracture, lower end, open
813.0x	Fracture of radius/ulna, upper end
813.1x	Fracture of radius/ulna, lower end
813.2x	Fracture of radius and ulna shaft
813.3x	Fracture of radius and ulna shaft
813.4x	Fracture of radius/ulna, lower end
813.5x	Fracture of radius/ulna, lower end
814.0x	Carpal fracture, closed
814.1x	Carpal fracture, open
832.0x	Elbow dislocation, closed
832.1x	Elbow dislocation, open
833.0x	Wrist dislocation, closed
833.1x	Wrist dislocation, open
841.x	Elbow/forearm sprain and strain
842.00	Sprain of wrist NOS
842.1x	Hand sprain/strain
880.03	Open wound of upper arm
880.13	Open wound of upper arm, complic
880.23	Open wound upper arm w/tendon

CPT CODE	SERVICE
29105 (Cont'd.)	

ICD–9–CM

881.0x	Elbow/forearm/wrist open wound
881.1x	Elbow/forearm/wrist complex wound
881.2x	Elbow/forearm/wrist, tendon wound
905.2	Late effect, arm fracture
927.03	Crushing injury, upper arm
927.1x	Crushing injury, elbow and forearm
927.21	Crushing injury, wrist
955.2	Injury ulnar nerve
955.3	Injury radial nerve
V54.0	Removal of internal fixation device
V54.8	Orthopedic aftercare NEC
V67.0	Surgery follow-up
V67.4	Fracture follow-up
V67.5	Follow-up exam, following treatment

REIMBURSEMENT INFORMATION

General

- See notes on page 286.

Medicare

- Follow–up Days — 0
- Assistant Surgeon — not paid
- Supply Charges — not allowed
- Outpatient Limit — applies
- Minor Surgery Rules Apply

CPT CODE	SERVICE
29125	Application of short arm splint (forearm to hand); static
29126	Application of short arm splint (forearm to hand); dynamic

CPT NOTES

- This procedure applies when the cast application or strapping is a replacement procedure used during or after the period of follow-up care. Additional visits are reportable only if significant identifiable further services are provided at the time of the cast application or strapping.
- If cast application or strapping is provided as an initial procedure in which no surgery is performed (e.g., casting of a sprained ankle or knee), use the appropriate office evaluation and management in addition to 99070 for supplies.
- Listed procedures include removal of cast or strapping.

ICD–9–CM

195.4	M-Neoplasm, Upper limb
213.4	B-Neoplasm, Long bones, arm
213.5	B-Neoplasm, Wrist/Hand bones
239.2	Bone/Skin neoplasm NOS
343.x	Infantile cerebral palsy
354.	Mononeuritis of upper limb
354.0	Carpal tunnel syndrome
354.2	Ulnar nerve lesion
354.3	Radial nerve lesion
358.0	Myasthenia gravis
443.0	Raynaud's syndrome
707.0	Decubitus ulcer
714.0	Rheumatoid arthritis
715.12	Loc prim osteoarthritis, upper arm
715.13	Loc prim osteoarthritis, forearm
715.14	Loc prim osteoarthritis, hand
715.22	Loc 2nd osteoarthritis, upper arm
715.23	Loc 2nd osteoarthritis, forearm
715.24	Loc 2nd osteoarthritis, hand
715.32	Loc osteoarthritis NOS, upper arm
715.33	Loc osteoarthritis NOS, forearm
715.34	Loc osteoarthritis NOS, hand
716.02	Kaschin-Beck disease, upper arm
716.03	Kaschin-Beck disease, forearm
716.04	Kaschin-Beck disease, hand
716.42	Transient arthropathy, upper arm
716.43	Transient arthropathy, forearm
716.44	Transient arthropathy, hand
718.33	Recurrent dislocation, forearm
718.43	Contracture of joint, forearm
718.52	Ankylosis of joint, upper arm
718.53	Ankylosis of joint, forearm
718.54	Ankylosis of joint, hand
718.82	Joint derangement NEC, upper arm
718.83	Joint derangement NEC, forearm
718.84	Joint derangement NEC, hand
719.22	Villonodular synovitis, upper arm
719.23	Villonodular synovitis, forearm
719.24	Villonodular synovitis, hand
719.42	Pain in joint, upper arm
719.43	Pain in joint, forearm
719.44	Pain in joint, hand
719.53	Joint stiffness NEC, forearm
719.62	Joint symptom NEC, upper arm
719.63	Joint symptom NEC, forearm
719.64	Joint symptom NEC, hand
719.82	Joint disorder NEC, upper arm
719.83	Joint disorder NEC, forearm
719.84	Joint disorder NEC, hand
726.30	Elbow enthesopathy NOS
726.31	Medial epicondylitis
726.32	Lateral epicondylitis
726.33	Olecranon bursitis
726.39	Elbow enthesopathy NEC
726.4	Enthesopathy of wrist/carpus
727.04	Radial styloid tenosynovitis

CPT CODE	SERVICE	ICD–9–CM	
29125, 29126 (Cont'd.)		727.05	Tenosynovitis of hand/wrist NEC
		728.6	Contracture of palmar fascia
		729.2	Neuralgia/neuritis NOS
		730.02	Acute osteomyelitis, upper arm
		730.03	Acute osteomyelitis, forearm
		730.04	Acute osteomyelitis, hand
		730.12	Chronic osteomyelitis, upper arm
		730.13	Chronic osteomyelitis, forearm
		730.14	Chronic osteomyelitis, hand
		730.22	Osteomyelitis NOS, upper arm
		730.23	Osteomyelitis NOS, forearm
		730.24	Osteomyelitis NOS, hand
		733.10	Pathologic fracture, site NOS
		733.12	Pathologic Fx distal radius/ulna
		733.19	Pathologic fracture, site NEC
		733.81	Malunion of fracture
		733.82	Nonunion of fracture
		736.2x	Acquired deformity of finger
		813.0x	Fracture of radius/ulna, upper end
		813.1x	Fracture of radius/ulna, lower end
		813.2x	Fracture of radius and ulna shaft
		813.3x	Fracture of radius and ulna shaft
		813.4x	Fracture of radius/ulna, lower end
		813.5x	Fracture of radius/ulna, lower end
		814.0x	Carpal fracture, closed
		814.1x	Carpal fracture, open
		815.0x	Metacarpal fracture, closed
		815.1x	Metacarpal fracture, open
		816.0x	Phalanges fracture, closed
		816.1x	Phalanges fracture, open
		833.0x	Wrist dislocation, closed
		833.1x	Wrist dislocation, open
		834.0x	Finger dislocation, closed
		834.1x	Finger dislocation, open
		842.0x	Wrist sprain/strain
		842.1x	Hand sprain/strain
		881.00	Open wound of forearm
		881.02	Open wound of wrist
		881.10	Open wound of forearm, complicated
		881.12	Open wound of wrist, complicated
		881.20	Open wound of forearm w/tendon
		881.22	Open wound of wrist w/tendon
		882.x	Open wound of hand
		905.2	Late effect, arm fracture
		927.10	Crushing injury, forearm
		927.2x	Crushing injury, wrist and hand
		955.2	Injury ulnar nerve
		955.3	Injury radial nerve
		955.4	Injury musculocutaneous nerve
		955.5	Injury cutaneous sensory nerve/arm
		955.6	Injury digital nerve
		V54.0	Removal of internal fixation device
		V54.8	Orthopedic aftercare NEC

CPT CODE	SERVICE	ICD-9-CM
29125, 29126 (Cont'd.)		V67.4 Fracture follow-up

REIMBURSEMENT INFORMATION

General

- ♦ See notes on page 286.

Medicare

- ♦ Follow-up Days — 0
- ♦ Assistant Surgeon — not paid
- ♦ Supply Charges — not allowed
- ♦ Outpatient Limit — applies
- ♦ Minor Surgery Rules Apply

CPT CODE	SERVICE
29130	Application of finger splint; static
29131	Application of finger splint; dynamic

CPT NOTES

- This procedure applies when the cast application or strapping is a replacement procedure used during or after the period of follow-up care. Additional visits are reportable only if significant identifiable further services are provided at the time of the cast application or strapping.
- If cast application or strapping is provided as an initial procedure in which no surgery is performed (e.g., casting of a sprained ankle or knee), use the appropriate office evaluation and management in addition to 99070 for supplies.
- Listed procedures include removal of cast or strapping.

ICD–9–CM

195.4	M-Neoplasm, Upper limb
213.4	B-Neoplasm, Long bones, arm
213.5	B-Neoplasm, Wrist/Hand bones
239.2	Bone/Skin neoplasm NOS
443.0	Raynaud's syndrome
714.0	Rheumatoid arthritis
715.14	Loc prim osteoarthritis, hand
715.24	Loc 2nd osteoarthritis, hand
715.34	Loc osteoarthritis NOS, hand
716.04	Kaschin-Beck disease, hand
716.44	Transient arthropathy, hand
718.44	Contracture of joint, hand
718.54	Ankylosis of joint, hand
718.84	Joint derangement NEC, hand
719.24	Villonodular synovitis, hand
719.44	Pain in joint, hand
719.64	Joint symptom NEC, hand
719.84	Joint disorder NEC, hand
727.03	Trigger finger
727.04	Radial styloid tenosynovitis
730.04	Acute osteomyelitis, hand
730.14	Chronic osteomyelitis, hand
730.24	Osteomyelitis NOS, hand
733.10	Pathologic fracture, site NOS
733.12	Pathologic Fx distal radius/ulna
733.19	Pathologic fracture, site NEC
733.81	Malunion of fracture
733.82	Nonunion of fracture
736.21	Boutonniere deformity, finger
736.22	Swan-neck deformity, finger
736.29	Acquired finger deformity NEC
816.01	Fx mid/prox phalanx, hand, closed
816.02	Fx distal phalanx, hand, closed
816.03	Fx mult phalanx, hand, closed
816.11	Fx mid/prox phalanx, hand, open
816.12	Fx distal phalanx, hand, open
816.13	Fx mult phalanx, hand, open
833.0x	Wrist dislocation, closed
833.1x	Wrist dislocation, open
834.01	Disloc metacarpophalangeal, closed
834.02	Disloc interphaiangeal hand, closed
834.11	Disloc metacarpophalangeal, open
834.12	Disloc interphalangeal hand, open
927.3	Crushing injury, finger
955.6	Injury digital nerve
V54.0	Removal of internal fixation device
V54.8	Orthopedic aftercare NEC
V67.4	Fracture follow-up

CPT CODE **SERVICE**

29130, 29131 (Cont'd.)

ICD–9–CM

REIMBURSEMENT INFORMATION

General

- See notes on page 286.

Medicare

- Follow–up Days — 0
- Assistant Surgeon — not paid
- Supply Charges — not allowed
- Outpatient Limit — applies
- Minor Surgery Rules Apply

CPT CODE	SERVICE	ICD–9–CM

29260 Strapping; elbow or wrist

CPT NOTES

- This procedure applies when the cast application or strapping is a replacement procedure used during or after the period of follow-up care. Additional visits are reportable only if significant identifiable further services are provided at the time of the cast application or strapping.
- If cast application or strapping is provided as an initial procedure in which no surgery is performed (e.g., casting of a sprained ankle or knee), use the appropriate office evaluation and management in addition to 99070 for supplies.
- The procedure includes removal of cast or strapping.

014.04	TB peritonitis, culture dx
726.3x	Enthesopathy of elbow region
726.4	Enthesopathy of wrist/carpus
813.4x	Fracture of radius/ulna, lower end
813.5x	Fracture of radius/ulna, lower end
814.0x	Carpal fracture, closed
814.1x	Carpal fracture, open
841.x	Elbow/forearm sprain and strain
842.1x	Hand sprain/strain
923.1x	Contusion, elbow and forearm
923.21	Contusion of wrist
V67.4	Fracture follow-up

REIMBURSEMENT INFORMATION

General

- See notes on page 286.

Medicare

- Follow–up Days — 0
- Assistant Surgeon — not paid
- Supply Charges — not allowed
- Outpatient Limit — applies
- Minor Surgery Rules Apply

29280 Strapping; hand or finger

CPT NOTES

- This procedure applies when the cast application or strapping is a replacement procedure used during or after the period of follow-up care. Additional visits are reportable only if significant identifiable further services are provided at the time of the cast application or strapping.
- If cast application or strapping is provided as an initial procedure in which no surgery is performed (e.g., casting of a sprained ankle or knee), use the appropriate office evaluation and management in addition to 99070 for supplies.
- The procedure includes removal of cast or strapping.

354.0	Carpal tunnel syndrome
715.14	Loc prim osteoarthritis, hand
715.24	Loc 2nd osteoarthritis, hand
715.34	Loc osteoarthritis NOS, hand
816.01	Fx mid/prox phalanx, hand, closed
816.02	Fx distal phalanx, hand, closed
816.03	Fx mult phalanx, hand, closed
816.11	Fx mid/prox phalanx, hand, open
816.12	Fx distal phalanx, hand, open
816.13	Fx mult phalanx, hand, open
V67.4	Fracture follow-up

REIMBURSEMENT INFORMATION

General

- See notes on page 286.

Medicare

- Follow–up Days — 0
- Assistant Surgeon — not paid
- Supply Charges — not allowed
- Outpatient Limit — applies
- Minor Surgery Rules Apply

CPT CODE	SERVICE
29305	Application of hip spica cast; one leg
29325	Application of hip spica cast; one and one-half spica or both legs

CPT NOTES

- This procedure applies when the cast application or strapping is a replacement procedure used during or after the period of follow-up care. Additional visits are reportable only if significant identifiable further services are provided at the time of the cast application or strapping.
- If cast application or strapping is provided as an initial procedure in which no surgery is performed (e.g., casting of a sprained ankle or knee), use the appropriate office evaluation and management in addition to 99070 for supplies.
- The procedure includes removal of cast or strapping.

ICD–9–CM

343.x	Infantile cerebral palsy
707.0	Decubitus ulcer
718.45	Contracture of joint, pelvis/thigh
754.3x	Congenital dislocation of hip
820.0x	Transcervical femur fracture closed
820.1x	Transcervical femur fracture, open
820.2x	Pertrochanteric femur fracture
820.3x	Pertrochanteric femur fracture
835.0x	Hip dislocation, closed
835.1x	Hip dislocation, open
V54.0	Removal of internal fixation device
V54.8	Orthopedic aftercare NEC
V67.4	Fracture follow-up

REIMBURSEMENT INFORMATION

General

- See notes on page 286.

Medicare

- Follow–up Days — 0
- Assistant Surgeon — not paid
- Supply Charges — not allowed
- Outpatient Limit — does not apply
- Minor Surgery Rules Apply

CPT CODE **SERVICE**

29345 Application of long leg cast (thigh to toes)

CPT NOTES

- This procedure applies when the cast application or strapping is a replacement procedure used during or after the period of follow-up care. Additional visits are reportable only if significant identifiable further services are provided at the time of the cast application or strapping.
- If cast application or strapping is provided as an initial procedure in which no surgery is performed (e.g., casting of a sprained ankle or knee), use the appropriate office evaluation and management in addition to 99070 for supplies.
- The procedure includes removal of cast or strapping.

ICD–9–CM

213.6	B-Neoplasm, Pelvic girdle
213.7	B-Neoplasm, Long bones, lower limb
213.8	B-Neoplasm, Short bones, lower limb
215.3	B-Neoplasm, Soft tissue, leg
707.0	Decubitus ulcer
719.46	Pain in joint, lower leg
727.81	Contracture of tendon
728.71	Plantar fascial fibromatosis
730.06	Acute osteomyelitis, lower leg
730.16	Chronic osteomyelitis, lower leg
730.26	Osteomyelitis NOS, lower leg
732.4	Juvenile osteochondrosis, leg
732.7	Osteochondritis dissecans
733.16	Pathologic fracture of tibia/fibula
735.0	Hallux valgus
754.7x	Deformities of feet
755.02	Polydactyly, toes
755.13	Syndactyly of toes, no fusion
755.14	Syndactyly of toes, w/fusion
755.6x	Anomaly of lower limb
821.01	Fx femur shaft, closed
821.11	Fx femur shaft, open
821.2x	Femur fracture, lower end, closed
821.3x	Femur fracture, lower end, open
822.0	Fracture of patella, closed
822.1	Fracture of patella, open
823.0x	Fracture of tibia and fibula closed
823.1x	Fracture of tibia and fibula, open
823.3x	Fracture of tibia and fibula shaft
823.8x	Tibia/fibula fracture NOS, closed
824.x	Fracture of ankle
825.0	Fx calcaneus, closed
825.1	Fx calcaneus, open
825.2x	Tarsal/metatarsal fracture, closed
825.3x	Tarsal/metatarsal fracture, open
836.0	Tear medial meniscus knee, current
836.1	Tear lateral meniscus knee, current
836.2	Tear meniscus NEC, current
836.3	Dislocation patella, closed
836.4	Dislocation patella, open
836.5x	Knee dislocation, closed
836.6x	Knee dislocation, open
837.0	Dislocation ankle, closed
837.1	Dislocation ankle, open
844.x	Sprains and strains of knee and leg
845.0x	Ankle sprain/strain
845.1x	Foot sprain/strain
V43.6	Joint replacement NEC
V54.0	Removal of internal fixation device
V54.8	Orthopedic aftercare NEC
V67.4	Fracture follow-up

CPT CODE	SERVICE	ICD–9–CM
29345 (Cont'd.)		

REIMBURSEMENT INFORMATION

General

- ♦ See notes on page 286.

Medicare

- ♦ Follow–up Days — 0
- ♦ Assistant Surgeon — not paid
- ♦ Supply Charges — not allowed
- ♦ Outpatient Limit — applies
- ♦ Minor Surgery Rules Apply

CPT CODE	SERVICE
29355	Application of long leg cast (thigh to toes); walker or ambulatory type

CPT NOTES

- This procedure applies when the cast application or strapping is a replacement procedure used during or after the period of follow-up care. Additional visits are reportable only if significant identifiable further services are provided at the time of the cast application or strapping.
- If cast application or strapping is provided as an initial procedure in which no surgery is performed (e.g., casting of a sprained ankle or knee), use the appropriate office evaluation and management in addition to 99070 for supplies.
- The procedure includes removal of cast or strapping.

ICD–9–CM

213.6	B-Neoplasm, Pelvic girdle
213.7	B-Neoplasm, Long bones, lower limb
213.8	B-Neoplasm, Short bones, lower limb
215.3	B-Neoplasm, Soft tissue, leg
707.0	Decubitus ulcer
719.46	Pain in joint, lower leg
727.81	Contracture of tendon
728.71	Plantar fascial fibromatosis
730.06	Acute osteomyelitis, lower leg
730.16	Chronic osteomyelitis, lower leg
730.26	Osteomyelitis NOS, lower leg
732.4	Juvenile osteochondrosis, leg
732.7	Osteochondritis dissecans
733.16	Pathologic fracture of tibia/fibula
735.0	Hallux valgus
754.7x	Deformities of feet
755.02	Polydactyly, toes
755.13	Syndactyly of toes, no fusion
755.14	Syndactyly of toes, w/fusion
755.61	Congenital coxa valga
755.62	Congenital coxa vara
755.63	Congenital hip deformity NEC
755.64	Congenital knee deformity
755.65	Macrodactylia of toes
755.66	Anomalies of toes NEC
755.67	Anomalies of foot NEC
755.69	Lower limb anomaly NEC
821.01	Fx femur shaft, closed
821.11	Fx femur shaft, open
821.2x	Femur fracture, lower end, closed
821.3x	Femur fracture, lower end, open
822.0	Fracture of patella, closed
822.1	Fracture of patella, open
823.0x	Fracture of tibia and fibula closed
823.1x	Fracture of tibia and fibula, open
823.3x	Fracture of tibia and fibula shaft
823.8x	Tibia/fibula fracture NOS, closed
824.x	Fracture of ankle
825.0	Fx calcaneus, closed
825.1	Fx calcaneus, open
825.2x	Tarsal/metatarsal fracture, closed
825.3x	Tarsal/metatarsal fracture, open
836.0	Tear medial meniscus knee, current
836.1	Tear lateral meniscus knee, current
836.2	Tear meniscus NEC, current
836.3	Dislocation patella, closed
836.4	Dislocation patella, open
836.5x	Knee dislocation, closed
836.6x	Knee dislocation, open
837.0	Dislocation ankle, closed
837.1	Dislocation ankle, open
844.x	Sprains and strains of knee and leg
845.0x	Ankle sprain/strain
845.1x	Foot sprain/strain
V43.6	Joint replacement NEC
V54.0	Removal of internal fixation device

CPT CODE	SERVICE	ICD–9–CM
29355 (Cont'd.)		V54.8 Orthopedic aftercare NEC V67.4 Fracture follow-up

REIMBURSEMENT INFORMATION

General

- ♦ See notes on page 286.

Medicare

- ♦ Follow–up Days — 0
- ♦ Assistant Surgeon — not paid
- ♦ Supply Charges — not allowed
- ♦ Outpatient Limit — applies
- ♦ Minor Surgery Rules Apply

CPT CODE **SERVICE**

29358 Application of long leg cast brace

CPT NOTES

- This procedure applies when the cast application or strapping is a replacement procedure used during or after the period of follow-up care. Additional visits are reportable only if significant identifiable further services are provided at the time of the cast application or strapping.
- If cast application or strapping is provided as an initial procedure in which no surgery is performed (e.g., casting of a sprained ankle or knee), use the appropriate office evaluation and management in addition to 99070 for supplies.
- The procedure includes removal of cast or strapping.

ICD–9–CM

213.6	B-Neoplasm, Pelvic girdle
213.7	B-Neoplasm, Long bones, lower limb
213.8	B-Neoplasm, Short bones, lower limb
215.3	B-Neoplasm, Soft tissue, leg
707.0	Decubitus ulcer
719.46	Pain in joint, lower leg
727.81	Contracture of tendon
728.71	Plantar fascial fibromatosis
730.06	Acute osteomyelitis, lower leg
730.16	Chronic osteomyelitis, lower leg
730.26	Osteomyelitis NOS, lower leg
732.4	Juvenile osteochondrosis, leg
732.7	Osteochondritis dissecans
733.16	Pathologic fracture of tibia/fibula
735.0	Hallux valgus
754.7x	Deformities of feet
755.02	Polydactyly, toes
755.13	Syndactyly of toes, no fusion
755.14	Syndactyly of toes, w/fusion
755.6x	Anomaly of lower limb
821.01	Fx femur shaft, closed
821.11	Fx femur shaft, open
821.2x	Femur fracture, lower end, closed
821.3x	Femur fracture, lower end, open
822.0	Fracture of patella, closed
822.1	Fracture of patella, open
823.0x	Fracture of tibia and fibula closed
823.1x	Fracture of tibia and fibula, open
823.3x	Fracture of tibia and fibula shaft
823.8x	Tibia/fibula fracture NOS, closed
824.x	Fracture of ankle
825.0	Fx calcaneus, closed
825.1	Fx calcaneus, open
825.2x	Tarsal/metatarsal fracture, closed
825.3x	Tarsal/metatarsal fracture, open
836.0	Tear medial meniscus knee, current
836.1	Tear lateral meniscus knee, current
836.2	Tear meniscus NEC, current
836.3	Dislocation patella, closed
836.4	Dislocation patella, open
836.5x	Knee dislocation, closed
836.6x	Knee dislocation, open
837.0	Dislocation ankle, closed
837.1	Dislocation ankle, open
844.x	Sprains and strains of knee and leg
845.0x	Ankle sprain/strain
845.1x	Foot sprain/strain
V43.6	Joint replacement NEC
V54.0	Removal of internal fixation device
V54.8	Orthopedic aftercare NEC
V67.4	Fracture follow-up

CPT CODE	SERVICE	ICD–9–CM
29358 (Cont'd.)		

REIMBURSEMENT INFORMATION

General

- See notes on page 286.

Medicare

- Follow–up Days — 0
- Assistant Surgeon — not paid
- Supply Charges — not allowed
- Outpatient Limit — applies
- Minor Surgery Rules Apply

CPT CODE	SERVICE
29365	Application of cylinder cast (thigh to ankle)

CPT NOTES

- This procedure applies when the cast application or strapping is a replacement procedure used during or after the period of follow-up care. Additional visits are reportable only if significant identifiable further services are provided at the time of the cast application or strapping.
- If cast application or strapping is provided as an initial procedure in which no surgery is performed (e.g., casting of a sprained ankle or knee), use the appropriate office evaluation and management in addition to 99070 for supplies.
- The procedure includes removal of cast or strapping.

ICD–9–CM

213.7	B-Neoplasm, Long bones, lower limb
213.8	B-Neoplasm, Short bones, lower limb
682.6	Cellulitis of leg
707.0	Decubitus ulcer
715.15	Loc prim osteoarthritis, pelv/thigh
715.16	Loc prim osteoarthritis, lower leg
717.0	Old bucket tear, medial meniscus
717.1	Derange anterior medial meniscus
717.2	Derange posterior medial meniscus
717.3	Derangement medial meniscus NEC
717.4x	Derangement of lateral meniscus
717.5	Derangement of meniscus NEC
717.8x	Internal derangement of knee
718.46	Contracture of joint, lower leg
727.81	Contracture of tendon
732.7	Osteochondritis dissecans
733.16	Pathologic fracture of tibia/fibula
821.01	Fx femur shaft, closed
821.11	Fx femur shaft, open
821.2x	Femur fracture, lower end, closed
821.3x	Femur fracture, lower end, open
822.0	Fracture of patella, closed
822.1	Fracture of patella, open
823.0x	Fracture of tibia and fibula closed
823.1x	Fracture of tibia and fibula, open
823.3x	Fracture of tibia and fibula shaft
823.8x	Tibia/fibula fracture NOS, closed
836.0	Tear medial meniscus knee, current
836.1	Tear lateral meniscus knee, current
836.2	Tear meniscus NEC, current
836.3	Dislocation patella, closed
836.4	Dislocation patella, open
836.5x	Knee dislocation, closed
836.6x	Knee dislocation, open
844.x	Sprains and strains of knee and leg
V67.4	Fracture follow-up

REIMBURSEMENT INFORMATION

General

- See notes on page 286.

Medicare

- Follow–up Days — 0
- Assistant Surgeon — not paid
- Supply Charges — not allowed
- Outpatient Limit — applies
- Minor Surgery Rules Apply

CPT CODE	SERVICE
29405	Application of short leg cast (below knee to toes)

CPT NOTES

- This procedure applies when the cast application or strapping is a replacement procedure used during or after the period of follow-up care. Additional visits are reportable only if significant identifiable further services are provided at the time of the cast application or strapping.
- If cast application or strapping is provided as an initial procedure in which no surgery is performed (e.g., casting of a sprained ankle or knee), use the appropriate office evaluation and management in addition to 99070 for supplies.
- The procedure includes removal of cast or strapping.

ICD–9–CM

170.7	M-Neoplasm, Long bones, lower limb
170.8	M-Neoplasm, Short bones, lower limb
195.5	M-Neoplasm, Lower limb
213.7	B-Neoplasm, Long bones, lower limb
213.8	B-Neoplasm, Short bones, lower limb
355.5	Tarsal tunnel syndrome
707.x	Chronic ulcer of skin
715.16	Loc prim osteoarthritis, lower leg
715.17	Loc prim osteoarthritis, ankle/foot
715.25	Loc 2nd osteoarthritis, pelv/thigh
715.27	Loc 2nd osteoarthritis, ankle/foot
715.35	Loc osteoarthritis NOS, pelv/thigh
715.37	Loc osteoarthritis NOS, ankle/foot
715.96	Osteoarthrosis NOS, lower leg
715.97	Osteoarthrosis NOS, ankle/foot
718.46	Contracture of joint, lower leg
718.47	Contracture of joint, ankle/foot
718.56	Ankylosis of joint, lower leg
718.57	Ankylosis of joint, ankle/foot
718.86	Joint derangement NEC, lower leg
718.87	Joint derangement NEC, ankle/foot
719.66	Joint symptom NEC, lower leg
719.67	Joint symptom NEC, ankle/foot
726.7x	Enthesopathy of ankle and tarsus
727.06	Tenosynovitis of foot/ankle
727.81	Contracture of tendon
728.71	Plantar fascial fibromatosis
730.06	Acute osteomyelitis, lower leg
730.07	Acute osteomyelitis, ankle/foot
730.16	Chronic osteomyelitis, lower leg
730.17	Chronic osteomyelitis, ankle/foot
730.26	Osteomyelitis NOS, lower leg
730.27	Osteomyelitis NOS, ankle/foot
733.16	Pathologic fracture of tibia/fibula
733.22	Aneurysmal bone cyst
735.x	Acquired deformities of toe
736.7x	Acquired deformity, ankle and foot
754.5x	Varus deformities of feet
754.6x	Valgus deformity of feet
754.7x	Deformities of feet
755.67	Anomalies of foot NEC
755.69	Lower limb anomaly NEC
823.0x	Fracture of tibia and fibula closed
823.1x	Fracture of tibia and fibula, open
823.3x	Fracture of tibia and fibula shaft
823.8x	Tibia/fibula fracture NOS, closed
824.x	Fracture of ankle
825.0	Fx calcaneus, closed
825.1	Fx calcaneus, open
825.2x	Tarsal/metatarsal fracture, closed
825.3x	Tarsal/metatarsal fracture, open
826.0	Fx phalanx, foot, closed
826.1	Fx phalanx, foot, open
837.0	Dislocation ankle, closed
837.1	Dislocation ankle, open
838.0x	Foot dislocation, closed

CPT CODE	SERVICE	ICD-9-CM
29405 (Cont'd.)		838.1x Foot dislocation, open 845.0x Ankle sprain/strain 845.1x Foot sprain/strain 892.x Open wound of foot V54.0 Removal of internal fixation device V67.4 Fracture follow-up

REIMBURSEMENT INFORMATION

General

- See notes on page 286.

Medicare

- Follow-up Days — 0
- Assistant Surgeon — not paid
- Supply Charges — not allowed
- Outpatient Limit — applies
- Minor Surgery Rules Apply

CPT CODE	SERVICE
29425	Application of short leg cast (below knee to toes); walking or ambulatory type

CPT NOTES

- This procedure applies when the cast application or strapping is a replacement procedure used during or after the period of follow-up care. Additional visits are reportable only if significant identifiable further services are provided at the time of the cast application or strapping.
- If cast application or strapping is provided as an initial procedure in which no surgery is performed (e.g., casting of a sprained ankle or knee), use the appropriate office evaluation and management in addition to 99070 for supplies.
- The procedure includes removal of cast or strapping.

ICD–9–CM

170.7	M-Neoplasm, Long bones, lower limb
170.8	M-Neoplasm, Short bones, lower limb
195.5	M-Neoplasm, Lower limb
213.7	B-Neoplasm, Long bones, lower limb
213.8	B-Neoplasm, Short bones, lower limb
355.5	Tarsal tunnel syndrome
707.x	Chronic ulcer of skin
715.16	Loc prim osteoarthritis, lower leg
715.17	Loc prim osteoarthritis, ankle/foot
715.25	Loc 2nd osteoarthritis, pelv/thigh
715.27	Loc 2nd osteoarthritis, ankle/foot
715.35	Loc osteoarthritis NOS, pelv/thigh
715.37	Loc osteoarthritis NOS, ankle/foot
715.96	Osteoarthrosis NOS, lower leg
715.97	Osteoarthrosis NOS, ankle/foot
718.46	Contracture of joint, lower leg
718.47	Contracture of joint, ankle/foot
718.56	Ankylosis of joint, lower leg
718.57	Ankylosis of joint, ankle/foot
718.86	Joint derangement NEC, lower leg
718.87	Joint derangement NEC, ankle/foot
719.66	Joint symptom NEC, lower leg
719.67	Joint symptom NEC, ankle/foot
726.7x	Enthesopathy of ankle and tarsus
727.06	Tenosynovitis of foot/ankle
727.81	Contracture of tendon
728.71	Plantar fascial fibromatosis
730.06	Acute osteomyelitis, lower leg
730.07	Acute osteomyelitis, ankle/foot
730.16	Chronic osteomyelitis, lower leg
730.17	Chronic osteomyelitis, ankle/foot
730.26	Osteomyelitis NOS, lower leg
730.27	Osteomyelitis NOS, ankle/foot
733.16	Pathologic fracture of tibia/fibula
733.22	Aneurysmal bone cyst
735.x	Acquired deformities of toe
736.7x	Acquired deformity, ankle and foot
754.5x	Varus deformities of feet
754.6x	Valgus deformity of feet
754.7x	Deformities of feet
755.67	Anomalies of foot NEC
755.69	Lower limb anomaly NEC
823.0x	Fracture of tibia and fibula closed
823.1x	Fracture of tibia and fibula, open
823.3x	Fracture of tibia and fibula shaft
823.8x	Tibia/fibula fracture NOS, closed
824.x	Fracture of ankle
825.0	Fx calcaneus, closed
825.1	Fx calcaneus, open
825.2x	Tarsal/metatarsal fracture, closed
825.3x	Tarsal/metatarsal fracture, open
826.0	Fx phalanx, foot, closed
826.1	Fx phalanx, foot, open
837.0	Dislocation ankle, closed
837.1	Dislocation ankle, open
838.0x	Foot dislocation, closed

CPT CODE	SERVICE	ICD–9–CM	
29425 (Cont'd.)		838.1x	Foot dislocation, open
		845.0x	Ankle sprain/strain
		845.1x	Foot sprain/strain
		892.x	Open wound of foot
		V54.0	Removal of internal fixation device
		V67.4	Fracture follow-up

REIMBURSEMENT INFORMATION

General

- See notes on page 286.

Medicare

- Follow–up Days — 0
- Assistant Surgeon — not paid
- Supply Charges — not allowed
- Outpatient Limit — applies
- Minor Surgery Rules Apply

CPT CODE	SERVICE
29435	Application of patellar tendon bearing (PTB) cast

CPT NOTES

- This procedure applies when the cast application or strapping is a replacement procedure used during or after the period of follow-up care. Additional visits are reportable only if significant identifiable further services are provided at the time of the cast application or strapping.
- If cast application or strapping is provided as an initial procedure in which no surgery is performed (e.g., casting of a sprained ankle or knee), use the appropriate office evaluation and management in addition to 99070 for supplies.
- The procedure includes removal of cast or strapping.

ICD–9–CM

213.8	B-Neoplasm, Short bones, lower limb
707.0	Decubitus ulcer
730.17	Chronic osteomyelitis, ankle/foot
733.16	Pathologic fracture of tibia/fibula
822.0	Fracture of patella, closed
822.1	Fracture of patella, open
823.0x	Fracture of tibia and fibula closed
823.1x	Fracture of tibia and fibula, open
823.3x	Fracture of tibia and fibula shaft
823.8x	Tibia/fibula fracture NOS, closed
824.x	Fracture of ankle
825.0	Fx calcaneus, closed
825.1	Fx calcaneus, open
825.2x	Tarsal/metatarsal fracture, closed
825.3x	Tarsal/metatarsal fracture, open
V67.4	Fracture follow-up

REIMBURSEMENT INFORMATION

General

- See notes on page 286.

Medicare

- Follow–up Days — 0
- Assistant Surgeon — not paid
- Supply Charges — not allowed
- Outpatient Limit — applies
- Minor Surgery Rules Apply

CPT CODE	SERVICE	ICD–9–CM
29440	Adding walker to previously applied cast	V67.4 Fracture follow-up

CPT NOTES

- This procedure applies when the cast application or strapping is a replacement procedure used during or after the period of follow-up care. Additional visits are reportable only if significant identifiable further services are provided at the time of the cast application or strapping.
- If cast application or strapping is provided as an initial procedure in which no surgery is performed (e.g., casting of a sprained ankle or knee), use the appropriate office evaluation and management in addition to 99070 for supplies.
- The procedure includes removal of cast or strapping.

REIMBURSEMENT INFORMATION

General

- See notes on page 286.

Medicare

- Follow–up Days — 0
- Assistant Surgeon — not paid
- Supply Charges — not allowed
- Outpatient Limit — applies
- Minor Surgery Rules Apply

● **29445** Application of rigid total contact leg cast

250.6x	Diabetes w/neurologic manifestation
250.8x	Diabetes w/manifestations
355.8	Mononeuritis of leg NOS
356.1	Peroneal muscular atrophy
356.9	Idiopathic periph neuropathy NOS

CPT NOTES

- This procedure applies when the cast application or strapping is a replacement procedure used during or after the period of follow-up care. Additional visits are reportable only if significant identifiable further services are provided at the time of the cast application or strapping.
- If cast application or strapping is provided as an initial procedure in which no surgery is performed (e.g., casting of a sprained ankle or knee), use the appropriate office evaluation and management in addition to 99070 for supplies.
- The procedure includes removal of cast or strapping.

REIMBURSEMENT INFORMATION

General

- See notes on page 286.
- New procedure 1995 CPT.

Medicare

- Follow–up Days — 0
- Assistant Surgeon — not paid
- Supply Charges — not allowed
- Outpatient Limit — applies
- Minor Surgery Rules Apply

CPT CODE	SERVICE
29505	Application of long leg splint (thigh to ankle or toes)

CPT NOTES

- This procedure applies when the cast application or strapping is a replacement procedure used during or after the period of follow-up care. Additional visits are reportable only if significant identifiable further services are provided at the time of the cast application or strapping.
- If cast application or strapping is provided as an initial procedure in which no surgery is performed (e.g., casting of a sprained ankle or knee), use the appropriate office evaluation and management in addition to 99070 for supplies.
- The procedure includes removal of cast or strapping.

ICD-9-CM

213.6	B-Neoplasm, Pelvic girdle
213.7	B-Neoplasm, Long bones, lower limb
213.8	B-Neoplasm, Short bones, lower limb
215.3	B-Neoplasm, Soft tissue, leg
707.0	Decubitus ulcer
719.46	Pain in joint, lower leg
727.81	Contracture of tendon
728.71	Plantar fascial fibromatosis
730.06	Acute osteomyelitis, lower leg
730.16	Chronic osteomyelitis, lower leg
730.26	Osteomyelitis NOS, lower leg
732.4	Juvenile osteochondrosis, leg
732.7	Osteochondritis dissecans
733.16	Pathologic fracture of tibia/fibula
735.0	Hallux valgus
754.7x	Deformities of feet
755.02	Polydactyly, toes
755.13	Syndactyly of toes, no fusion
755.14	Syndactyly of toes, w/fusion
755.6x	Anomaly of lower limb
821.01	Fx femur shaft, closed
821.11	Fx femur shaft, open
821.2x	Femur fracture, lower end, closed
821.3x	Femur fracture, lower end, open
822.0	Fracture of patella, closed
822.1	Fracture of patella, open
823.0x	Fracture of tibia and fibula closed
823.1x	Fracture of tibia and fibula, open
823.3x	Fracture of tibia and fibula shaft
823.8x	Tibia/fibula fracture NOS, closed
824.x	Fracture of ankle
825.0	Fx calcaneus, closed
825.1	Fx calcaneus, open
825.2x	Tarsal/metatarsal fracture, closed
825.3x	Tarsal/metatarsal fracture, open
836.0	Tear medial meniscus knee, current
836.1	Tear lateral meniscus knee, current
836.2	Tear meniscus NEC, current
836.3	Dislocation patella, closed
836.4	Dislocation patella, open
836.5x	Knee dislocation, closed
836.6x	Knee dislocation, open
837.0	Dislocation ankle, closed
837.1	Dislocation ankle, open
844.x	Sprains and strains of knee and leg
845.0x	Ankle sprain/strain
845.1x	Foot sprain/strain
V43.6	Joint replacement NEC
V54.0	Removal of internal fixation device
V54.8	Orthopedic aftercare NEC
V67.4	Fracture follow-up

CPT CODE	SERVICE	ICD–9–CM

29505 (Cont'd.)

REIMBURSEMENT INFORMATION

General

- ♦ See notes on page 286.

Medicare

- ♦ Follow–up Days — 0
- ♦ Assistant Surgeon — not paid
- ♦ Supply Charges — not allowed
- ♦ Outpatient Limit — does not apply
- ♦ Minor Surgery Rules Apply

CPT CODE	SERVICE
29515	Application of short leg splint (calf to foot)

CPT NOTES

- This procedure applies when the cast application or strapping is a replacement procedure used during or after the period of follow-up care. Additional visits are reportable only if significant identifiable further services are provided at the time of the cast application or strapping.
- If cast application or strapping is provided as an initial procedure in which no surgery is performed (e.g., casting of a sprained ankle or knee), use the appropriate office evaluation and management in addition to 99070 for supplies.
- The procedure includes removal of cast or strapping.

ICD–9–CM

170.7	M-Neoplasm, Long bones, lower limb
170.8	M-Neoplasm, Short bones, lower limb
195.5	M-Neoplasm, Lower limb
213.7	B-Neoplasm, Long bones, lower limb
213.8	B-Neoplasm, Short bones, lower limb
355.5	Tarsal tunnel syndrome
707.x	Chronic ulcer of skin
715.16	Loc prim osteoarthritis, lower leg
715.17	Loc prim osteoarthritis, ankle/foot
715.25	Loc 2nd osteoarthritis, pelv/thigh
715.27	Loc 2nd osteoarthritis, ankle/foot
715.35	Loc osteoarthritis NOS, pelv/thigh
715.37	Loc osteoarthritis NOS, ankle/foot
715.96	Osteoarthrosis NOS, lower leg
715.97	Osteoarthrosis NOS, ankle/foot
718.46	Contracture of joint, lower leg
718.47	Contracture of joint, ankle/foot
718.56	Ankylosis of joint, lower leg
718.57	Ankylosis of joint, ankle/foot
718.86	Joint derangement NEC, lower leg
718.87	Joint derangement NEC, ankle/foot
719.66	Joint symptom NEC, lower leg
719.67	Joint symptom NEC, ankle/foot
726.7x	Enthesopathy of ankle and tarsus
727.06	Tenosynovitis of foot/ankle
727.81	Contracture of tendon
728.71	Plantar fascial fibromatosis
730.06	Acute osteomyelitis, lower leg
730.07	Acute osteomyelitis, ankle/foot
730.16	Chronic osteomyelitis, lower leg
730.17	Chronic osteomyelitis, ankle/foot
730.26	Osteomyelitis NOS, lower leg
730.27	Osteomyelitis NOS, ankle/foot
733.16	Pathologic fracture of tibia/fibula
733.22	Aneurysmal bone cyst
735.x	Acquired deformities of toe
736.7x	Acquired deformity, ankle and foot
754.5x	Varus deformities of feet
754.6x	Valgus deformity of feet
754.7x	Deformities of feet
755.67	Anomalies of foot NEC
755.69	Lower limb anomaly NEC
823.0x	Fracture of tibia and fibula closed
823.1x	Fracture of tibia and fibula, open
823.3x	Fracture of tibia and fibula shaft
823.8x	Tibia/fibula fracture NOS, closed
824.x	Fracture of ankle
825.0	Fx calcaneus, closed
825.1	Fx calcaneus, open
825.2x	Tarsal/metatarsal fracture, closed
825.3x	Tarsal/metatarsal fracture, open
826.0	Fx phalanx, foot, closed
826.1	Fx phalanx, foot, open
837.0	Dislocation ankle, closed
837.1	Dislocation ankle, open
838.0x	Foot dislocation, closed

CPT CODE	SERVICE	ICD–9–CM

29515 (Cont'd.)

838.1x Foot dislocation, open
845.0x Ankle sprain/strain
845.1x Foot sprain/strain
892.x Open wound of foot
V54.0 Removal of internal fixation device
V67.4 Fracture follow-up

REIMBURSEMENT INFORMATION

General

- See notes on page 286.

Medicare

- Follow–up Days — 0
- Assistant Surgeon — not paid
- Supply Charges — not allowed
- Outpatient Limit — applies
- Minor Surgery Rules Apply

29520 Strapping; hip

CPT NOTES

- This procedure applies when the cast application or strapping is a replacement procedure used during or after the period of follow-up care. Additional visits are reportable only if significant identifiable further services are provided at the time of the cast application or strapping.
- If cast application or strapping is provided as an initial procedure in which no surgery is performed (e.g., casting of a sprained ankle or knee), use the appropriate office evaluation and management in addition to 99070 for supplies.
- The procedure includes removal of cast or strapping.

707.x Chronic ulcer of skin
754.3x Congenital dislocation of hip
820.0x Transcervical femur fracture closed
820.1x Transcervical femur fracture, open
820.2x Pertrochanteric femur fracture
820.3x Pertrochanteric femur fracture
835.0x Hip dislocation, closed
835.1x Hip dislocation, open
V54.0 Removal of internal fixation device
V54.8 Orthopedic aftercare NEC
V67.4 Fracture follow-up

REIMBURSEMENT INFORMATION

General

- See notes on page 286.

Medicare

- Follow–up Days — 0
- Assistant Surgeon — not paid
- Supply Charges — not allowed
- Outpatient Limit — applies
- Minor Surgery Rules Apply

CPT CODE	SERVICE
29550	Strapping; toes

CPT NOTES

- This procedure applies when the cast application or strapping is a replacement procedure used during or after the period of follow-up care. Additional visits are reportable only if significant identifiable further services are provided at the time of the cast application or strapping.
- If cast application or strapping is provided as an initial procedure in which no surgery is performed (e.g., casting of a sprained ankle or knee), use the appropriate office evaluation and management in addition to 99070 for supplies.
- The procedure includes removal of cast or strapping.

ICD–9–CM

707.x	Chronic ulcer of skin
726.8	Peripheral enthesopathy NEC
728.71	Plantar fascial fibromatosis
730.07	Acute osteomyelitis, ankle/foot
730.17	Chronic osteomyelitis, ankle/foot
730.27	Osteomyelitis NOS, ankle/foot
735.0	Hallux valgus
735.1	Hallux varus
735.2	Hallux rigidus
735.3	Hallux malleus
735.4	Other hammer toe
825.0	Fx calcaneus, closed
825.1	Fx calcaneus, open
825.20	Fx foot bone NOS, closed
825.21	Fx astragalus, closed
825.22	Fx navicular, foot, closed
825.23	Fx cuboid, closed
825.24	Fx cuneiform, foot, closed
825.25	Fx metatarsal, closed
825.29	Fx foot bone NEC, closed
825.30	Fx foot bone NOS, open
825.31	Fx astragalus, open
825.32	Fx navicular, foot, open
825.33	Fx cuboid, open
825.34	Fx cuneiform, foot, open
825.35	Fx metatarsal, open
825.39	Fx foot bone NEC, open
826.0	Fx phalanx, foot, closed
826.1	Fx phalanx, foot, open
893.x	Open wound of toe(s)
924.3	Contusion of toe
928.3	Crushing injury, toe
V67.4	Fracture follow-up

REIMBURSEMENT INFORMATION

General

- See notes on page 286.

Medicare

- Follow–up Days — 0
- Assistant Surgeon — not paid
- Supply Charges — not allowed
- Outpatient Limit — applies
- Minor Surgery Rules Apply

CPT CODE **SERVICE**

29580 Strapping; Unna boot

CPT NOTES

- This procedure applies when the cast application or strapping is a replacement procedure used during or after the period of follow-up care. Additional visits are reportable only if significant identifiable further services are provided at the time of the cast application or strapping.
- If cast application or strapping is provided as an initial procedure in which no surgery is performed (e.g., casting of a sprained ankle or knee), use the appropriate office evaluation and management in addition to 99070 for supplies.
- The procedure includes removal of cast or strapping.

ICD–9–CM

094.0	Tabes dorsalis
250.6	Diabetes w/neurologic manifestation
336.0	Syringomyelia
355.6	Plantar nerve lesion
355.7	Mononeuritis of leg NEC
355.8	Mononeuritis of leg NOS
443.0	Raynaud's syndrome
443.1	Thromboangiitis obliterans
443.9	Peripheral vascular disease NOS
454.	Varicose veins of lower extremity
681.1x	Cellulitis and abscess, toe
701.8	Hypertrophic/atrophic skin NEC
707.x	Chronic ulcer of skin
713.5	Arthropathy w/neurological disorder
714.0	Rheumatoid arthritis
726.7x	Enthesopathy of ankle and tarsus
727.06	Tenosynovitis of foot/ankle
727.3	Bursitis NOS
728.6	Contracture of palmar fascia
730.07	Acute osteomyelitis, ankle/foot
730.17	Chronic osteomyelitis, ankle/foot
730.27	Osteomyelitis NOS, ankle/foot
735.2	Hallux rigidus
782.0	Skin sensation disturbance
845.0x	Ankle sprain/strain
845.1x	Foot sprain/strain

REIMBURSEMENT INFORMATION

General

- See notes on page 286.

Medicare

- Follow–up Days — 0
- Assistant Surgeon — not paid
- Supply Charges — not allowed
- Outpatient Limit — applies
- Minor Surgery Rules Apply

CPT CODE	SERVICE
29700	Removal or bivalving; gauntlet, boot or body cast
29705	Removal or bivalving; full arm or full leg cast

CPT NOTES

- This procedure applies when the cast application or strapping is a replacement procedure used during or after the period of follow-up care. Additional visits are reportable only if significant identifiable further services are provided at the time of the cast application or strapping.
- If cast application or strapping is provided as an initial procedure in which no surgery is performed (e.g., casting of a sprained ankle or knee), use the appropriate office evaluation and management in addition to 99070 for supplies.
- The procedure includes removal of cast or strapping.
- Codes for cast removal should be employed only for cast applied by another physician.

ICD–9–CM

V54.8	Orthopedic aftercare NEC
V67.4	Fracture follow-up

REIMBURSEMENT INFORMATION

General

- See notes on page 286.

Medicare

- Follow–up Days — 0
- Assistant Surgeon — not paid
- Supply Charges — not allowed
- Outpatient Limit — applies
- Minor Surgery Rules Apply

CPT CODE	SERVICE
29730	Windowing of cast

CPT NOTES

- This procedure applies when the cast application or strapping is a replacement procedure used during or after the period of follow-up care. Additional visits are reportable only if significant identifiable further services are provided at the time of the cast application or strapping.
- If cast application or strapping is provided as an initial procedure in which no surgery is performed (e.g., casting of a sprained ankle or knee), use the appropriate office evaluation and management in addition to 99070 for supplies.
- The procedure includes removal of cast or strapping.
- Codes for cast removal should be employed only for cast applied by another physician.

ICD–9–CM

880.0x	Shoulder/upper arm, open wound
880.1x	Shoulder/upper arm, cplx open wound
880.2x	Shoulder/upper arm, w/tendon
881.0x	Elbow/forearm/wrist open wound
881.1x	Elbow/forearm/wrist complex wound
881.2x	Elbow/forearm/wrist, tendon wound
882.x	Open wound of hand
883.x	Open wound of finger(s)
884.x	Open wound of upper limb
885.x	Traumatic amputation of thumb
886.x	Traumatic finger amputation
887.x	Traumatic arm/hand amputation
890.x	Open wound of hip and thigh
891.x	Open wound of knee, leg, ankle
892.x	Open wound of foot
893.x	Open wound of toe(s)
894.x	Open wound of lower limb
895.x	Traumatic amputation of toe(s)
896.x	Traumatic amputation of foot
897.x	Traumatic amputation of leg(s)
V54.8	Orthopedic aftercare NEC
V67.4	Fracture follow-up

REIMBURSEMENT INFORMATION

General

- See notes on page 286.

Medicare

- Follow–up Days — 0
- Assistant Surgeon — not paid
- Supply Charges — not allowed
- Outpatient Limit — applies
- Minor Surgery Rules Apply

CPT CODE	SERVICE
29848	Arthroscopy, wrist, surgical; with release of transverse carpal ligament

CPT NOTES

- ♦ Surgical arthroscopy always includes a diagnostic arthroscopy.
- ♦ When arthroscopy is performed in conjunction with arthrotomy, add modifier -51 or 09951.
- ♦ For open procedure, see 64721.

ICD–9–CM

354.0	Carpal tunnel syndrome
711.03	Pyogenic arthritis, forearm
711.93	Infect arthritis NOS, forearm
714.0	Rheumatoid arthritis
715.13	Loc prim osteoarthritis, forearm
715.23	Loc 2nd osteoarthritis, forearm
715.33	Loc osteoarthritis NOS, forearm
716.13	Traumatic arthropathy, forearm
716.93	Arthropathy NOS, forearm
718.13	Loose body in joint, forearm
718.83	Joint derangement NEC, forearm
719.03	Joint effusion, forearm
719.23	Villonodular synovitis, forearm
719.43	Pain in joint, forearm
727.00	Synovitis NOS
729.6	Old foreign body in soft tissue
730.03	Acute osteomyelitis, forearm
730.13	Chronic osteomyelitis, forearm
730.23	Osteomyelitis NOS, forearm
732.3	Juvenile osteochondrosis, arm
814.0x	Carpal fracture, closed
814.1x	Carpal fracture, open
833.0x	Wrist dislocation, closed
833.1x	Wrist dislocation, open
842.0x	Wrist sprain/strain
881.00	Open wound of forearm
881.02	Open wound of wrist
881.10	Open wound of forearm, complicated
881.12	Open wound of wrist, complicated
881.20	Open wound of forearm w/tendon
881.22	Open wound of wrist w/tendon
996.66	Reaction, internal joint prosthesis

REIMBURSEMENT INFORMATION

General

- ♦ See notes on page 286.

Medicare

- ♦ Follow–up Days — 90
- ♦ Assistant Surgeon — not paid
- ♦ Supply Charges — not allowed
- ♦ Outpatient Limit — does not apply
- ♦ Major Surgery Rules Apply

CPT CODE	SERVICE	ICD-9-CM	
30000*	Drainage abscess or hematoma, nasal, internal approach	461.1	Acute frontal sinusitis
		473.8	Chronic sinusitis NEC
		478.1	Nasal and sinus disease NEC
		682.0	Cellulitis of face
		920.	Contusion face/scalp/neck
		998.1	Hemorrhage complicating a procedure
		998.5	Postoperative infection

CPT NOTES

- For external approach, see 10060, 10140.

REIMBURSEMENT INFORMATION

General

- Starred procedure.

Medicare

- Follow-up Days — 10
- Assistant Surgeon — not paid
- Supply Charges — not allowed
- Outpatient Limit — applies
- Minor Surgery Rules Apply

CPT CODE	SERVICE	ICD-9-CM	
30020*	Drainage abscess or hematoma, nasal septum	461.1	Acute frontal sinusitis
		478.1	Nasal and sinus disease NEC
		682.0	Cellulitis of face
		738.0	Acquired nose deformity
		905.0	Late effect, skull/face fracture
		906.0	Late effect, open wound head/trunk
		920.	Contusion face/scalp/neck
		998.1	Hemorrhage complicating a procedure
		998.5	Postoperative infection

CPT NOTES

- For lateral rhinotomy, see specific application (e.g., 30118, 30320).

REIMBURSEMENT INFORMATION

General

- Starred procedure.

Medicare

- Follow-up Days — 10
- Assistant Surgeon — not paid
- Supply Charges — not allowed
- Outpatient Limit — applies
- Minor Surgery Rules Apply

CPT CODE **SERVICE** | **ICD–9–CM**

30100 Biopsy, intranasal

CPT NOTES

- For biopsy skin of nose, see 11100, 11101.

160.0	M-Neoplasm, Nasal cavities
160.2	M-Neoplasm, Maxillary sinus
160.3	M-Neoplasm, Ethmoidal sinus
160.4	M-Neoplasm, Frontal sinus
160.5	M-Neoplasm, Sphenoidal sinus
212.0	B-Neoplasm, Nasal cavity/sinus
235.9	UB-Neoplasm, Respiratory system NOS
239.1	Respiratory system neoplasm NOS
471.0	Polyp of nasal cavity
471.8	Nasal sinus polyp NEC
478.1	Nasal and sinus disease NEC
784.2	Swelling in head/neck

REIMBURSEMENT INFORMATION

Medicare

- Follow–up Days — 0
- Assistant Surgeon — not paid
- Supply Charges — not allowed
- Outpatient Limit — applies
- Minor Surgery Rules Apply

30110 Excision, nasal polyp(s), simple

CPT NOTES

- Normally completed in an office setting.

471.0	Polyp of nasal cavity
471.8	Nasal sinus polyp NEC

REIMBURSEMENT INFORMATION

Medicare

- Follow–up Days — 10
- Assistant Surgeon — not paid
- Supply Charges — not allowed
- Outpatient Limit — applies
- Minor Surgery Rules Apply

30115 Excision, nasal polyp(s), extensive

CPT NOTES

- Normally requires the facilities available in a hospital setting.

471.0	Polyp of nasal cavity
471.8	Nasal sinus polyp NEC
471.9	Nasal polyp NOS
478.1	Nasal and sinus disease NEC

REIMBURSEMENT INFORMATION

Medicare

- Follow–up Days — 90
- Assistant Surgeon — not paid
- Supply Charges — not allowed
- Outpatient Limit — does not apply
- Major Surgery Rules Apply

CPT CODE	SERVICE	ICD–9–CM
30117	Excision or destruction, any method (including laser), intranasal lesion; internal approach	160.0 M-Neoplasm, Nasal cavities 210.7 B-Neoplasm, Nasopharynx 212.0 B-Neoplasm, Nasal cavity/sinus 461.0 Acute maxillary sinusitis 478.1 Nasal and sinus disease NEC **REIMBURSEMENT INFORMATION** Medicare ◆ Follow–up Days — 90 ◆ Assistant Surgeon 30117 — not paid 30118 — paid ◆ Supply Charges — not allowed ◆ Outpatient Limit — does not apply ◆ Major Surgery Rules Apply
30118	Excision or destruction, any method (including laser), intranasal lesion; external approach (lateral rhinotomy)	
30120	Excision or surgical planing of skin of nose for rhinophyma	695.3 Rosacea **REIMBURSEMENT INFORMATION** Medicare ◆ Follow–up Days — 90 ◆ Assistant Surgeon — not paid ◆ Supply Charges — not allowed ◆ Outpatient Limit — does not apply ◆ Major Surgery Rules Apply
30124	Excision dermoid cyst, nose; simple, skin, subcutaneous	213.0 B-Neoplasm, Skull/Face bone 709.8 Skin disorders NEC **REIMBURSEMENT INFORMATION** Medicare ◆ Follow–up Days — 90 ◆ Assistant Surgeon — not paid ◆ Supply Charges — not allowed ◆ Outpatient Limit — does not apply ◆ Major Surgery Rules Apply

CPT CODE	SERVICE	ICD–9–CM
30125	Excision dermoid cyst, nose; complex, under bone or cartilage	212.0 B-Neoplasm, Nasal cavity/sinus

REIMBURSEMENT INFORMATION

Medicare

- Follow–up Days — 90
- Assistant Surgeon — paid
- Supply Charges — not allowed
- Outpatient Limit — does not apply
- Major Surgery Rules Apply

30130 Excision turbinate, partial or complete

375.22	Epiphora d/t insufficient drainage
375.53	Lacrimal canaliculi stenosis
375.55	Neonatal nasolacrimal obstruction
375.56	Acquired nasolacrimal duct stenosis
461.x	Acute sinusitis
470.	Deviated nasal septum
473.x	Chronic sinusitis
478.0	Hypertrophy of nasal turbinates
478.1	Nasal and sinus disease NEC
738.0	Acquired nose deformity
V51.	Aftercare w/plastic surgery

REIMBURSEMENT INFORMATION

Medicare

- Follow–up Days — 90
- Assistant Surgeon — not paid
- Supply Charges — not allowed
- Outpatient Limit — does not apply
- Major Surgery Rules Apply

30140 Submucous resection turbinate, partial or complete

CPT RULES

- For submucous resection of nasal septum, use 30520.
- For reduction of turbinates, use 30140 with modifier -52.

461.x	Acute sinusitis
470.	Deviated nasal septum
473.x	Chronic sinusitis
478.0	Hypertrophy of nasal turbinates
478.1	Nasal and sinus disease NEC
738.0	Acquired nose deformity
V51.	Aftercare w/plastic surgery

REIMBURSEMENT INFORMATION

Medicare

- Follow–up Days — 90
- Assistant Surgeon — not paid
- Supply Charges — not allowed
- Outpatient Limit — does not apply
- Major Surgery Rules Apply

CPT CODE / SERVICE	ICD–9–CM
30150 Rhinectomy; partial **30160** Rhinectomy; total **CPT NOTES** ◆ For closure and/or reconstruction, primary or delayed, see Integumentary System, 13150-13152, 14060-14300, 15120, 15121, 15260, 15261, 15760, 20900-20912.	160.0 M-Neoplasm, Nasal cavities 173.3 M-Neoplasm, Skin of face NEC 195.0 M-Neoplasm, Head/face/neck **REIMBURSEMENT INFORMATION** Medicare ◆ Follow–up Days — 90 ◆ Assistant Surgeon — paid ◆ Supply Charges — not allowed ◆ Outpatient Limit — does not apply ◆ Major Surgery Rules Apply
30200* Injection into turbinate(s), therapeutic	461.x Acute sinusitis 470. Deviated nasal septum 478.0 Hypertrophy of nasal turbinates 478.1 Nasal and sinus disease NEC 784.0 Headache **REIMBURSEMENT INFORMATION** General ◆ Starred procedure. Medicare ◆ Follow–up Days — 0 ◆ Assistant Surgeon — not paid ◆ Supply Charges — not allowed ◆ Outpatient Limit — applies ◆ Minor Surgery Rules Apply
30210* Displacement therapy (Proetz type)	381.81 Dysfunction of Eustachian tube 460. Acute nasopharyngitis 461.0 Acute maxillary sinusitis 470. Deviated nasal septum 478.1 Nasal and sinus disease NEC 784.7 Epistaxis **REIMBURSEMENT INFORMATION** General ◆ Starred procedure. Medicare ◆ Follow–up Days — 10 ◆ Assistant Surgeon — not paid ◆ Supply Charges — not allowed ◆ Outpatient Limit — applies ◆ Minor Surgery Rules Apply

CPT CODE	SERVICE	ICD–9–CM
30220	Insertion, nasal septal prosthesis (button)	470. Deviated nasal septum 478.0 Hypertrophy of nasal turbinates 905.0 Late effect, skull/face fracture 906.0 Late effect, open wound head/trunk 909.3 Late effect of surg/med complic 909.5 Late effect of adverse drug effect 998.5 Postoperative infection V51. Aftercare w/plastic surgery **REIMBURSEMENT INFORMATION** Medicare ♦ Follow–up Days — 10 ♦ Assistant Surgeon — not paid ♦ Supply Charges — not allowed ♦ Outpatient Limit — applies ♦ Minor Surgery Rules Apply
30300*	Removal foreign body, intranasal; office type procedure	932. Foreign body in nose **REIMBURSEMENT INFORMATION** General ♦ Starred procedure. (30300) Medicare ♦ Follow–up Days 30300–30310 — 10 30320 — 90 ♦ Assistant Surgeon 30300 — not paid 30310–30320 — by report ♦ Supply Charges — not allowed ♦ Outpatient Limit 30300 — applies 30310–30320 — does not apply ♦ Minor Surgery Rules Apply (30300–30310) Major Surgery Rules Apply (30320)
30310	Removal foreign body, intranasal; requiring general anesthesia	
30320	Removal foreign body, intranasal; by lateral rhinotomy	

CPT CODE SERVICE	ICD–9–CM
30400 Rhinoplasty, primary; lateral and alar cartilages and/or elevation of nasal tip **CPT NOTES** ♦ For obtaining tissues for graft, see 20900-20926, 21210. ♦ For columellar reconstruction, see 13150 et seq.	470. Deviated nasal septum 478.1 Nasal and sinus disease NEC 716.08 Kaschin-Beck disease NEC 738.0 Acquired nose deformity 748.1 Congenital nose anomaly NEC V51. Aftercare w/plastic surgery **REIMBURSEMENT INFORMATION** <u>Medicare</u> ♦ Follow–up Days — 90 ♦ Assistant Surgeon — not paid ♦ Supply Charges — not allowed ♦ Outpatient Limit — does not apply ♦ Major Surgery Rules Apply
30410 Rhinoplasty, primary; complete, external parts including bony pyramid, lateral and alar cartilages, and/or elevation of nasal tip **CPT NOTES** ♦ For obtaining tissues for graft, see 20900-20926, 21210.	470. Deviated nasal septum 716.08 Kaschin-Beck disease NEC 738.0 Acquired nose deformity 754.0 Congen skull/face/jaw deformity V51. Aftercare w/plastic surgery **REIMBURSEMENT INFORMATION** <u>Medicare</u> ♦ Follow–up Days — 90 ♦ Assistant Surgeon — paid ♦ Supply Charges — not allowed ♦ Outpatient Limit — does not apply ♦ Major Surgery Rules Apply
30420 Rhinoplasty, primary; including major septal repair **CPT NOTES** ♦ For obtaining tissues for graft, see 20900-20926, 21210.	195.0 M-Neoplasm, Head/face/neck 470. Deviated nasal septum 478.1 Nasal and sinus disease NEC 738.0 Acquired nose deformity 748.1 Congenital nose anomaly NEC 754.0 Congen skull/face/jaw deformity 802.0 Nasal bone Fx, closed 802.6 Fx orbital floor, closed 905.0 Late effect, skull/face fracture V51. Aftercare w/plastic surgery **REIMBURSEMENT INFORMATION** <u>Medicare</u> ♦ Follow–up Days — 90 ♦ Assistant Surgeon — not paid ♦ Supply Charges — not allowed ♦ Outpatient Limit — does not apply ♦ Major Surgery Rules Apply

CPT CODE	SERVICE	ICD–9–CM

30430 Rhinoplasty, secondary; minor revision (small amount of nasal tip work)

CPT NOTES

- For obtaining tissues for graft, see 20900-20926, 21210.

160.0	M-Neoplasm, Nasal cavities
212.0	B-Neoplasm, Nasal cavity/sinus
216.3	B-Neoplasm, Skin of face NEC
470.	Deviated nasal septum
738.0	Acquired nose deformity
748.1	Congenital nose anomaly NEC
V50.1	Plastic surgery NEC

REIMBURSEMENT INFORMATION

Medicare

- Follow–up Days — 90
- Assistant Surgeon — paid
- Supply Charges — not allowed
- Outpatient Limit — does not apply
- Major Surgery Rules Apply

30435 Rhinoplasty, secondary; intermediate revision (bony work with osteotomies)

CPT NOTES

- For obtaining tissues for graft, see 20900-20926, 21210.

160.0	M-Neoplasm, Nasal cavities
212.0	B-Neoplasm, Nasal cavity/sinus
478.1	Nasal and sinus disease NEC
716.08	Kaschin-Beck disease NEC
905.0	Late effect, skull/face fracture
V50.1	Plastic surgery NEC

REIMBURSEMENT INFORMATION

Medicare

- Follow–up Days — 90
- Assistant Surgeon — paid
- Supply Charges — not allowed
- Outpatient Limit — does not apply
- Major Surgery Rules Apply

CPT CODE	SERVICE	ICD–9–CM	
30450	Rhinoplasty, secondary; major revision (nasal tip work and osteotomies)	160.0	M-Neoplasm, Nasal cavities
		173.3	M-Neoplasm, Skin of face NEC
		212.0	B-Neoplasm, Nasal cavity/sinus
		216.3	B-Neoplasm, Skin of face NEC
		478.1	Nasal and sinus disease NEC
		716.08	Kaschin-Beck disease NEC
		905.0	Late effect, skull/face fracture
		V50.1	Plastic surgery NEC

CPT NOTES

- For obtaining tissues for graft, see 20900-20926, 21210.

REIMBURSEMENT INFORMATION

Medicare

- Follow–up Days — 90
- Assistant Surgeon — paid
- Supply Charges — not allowed
- Outpatient Limit — does not apply
- Major Surgery Rules Apply

CPT CODE	SERVICE	ICD–9–CM	
30460	Rhinoplasty for nasal deformity secondary to congenital cleft lip and/or palate, including columellar lengthening; tip only	748.1	Congenital nose anomaly NEC
30462	Rhinoplasty for nasal deformity secondary to congenital cleft lip and/or palate, including columellar lengthening; tip, septum, osteotomies	749.0x	Cleft palate
		749.1x	Cleft lip
		749.2x	Cleft palate w/cleft lip
		V13.6	Hx of congenital malformation

CPT NOTES

- For obtaining tissues for graft, see 20900-20926, 21210.

REIMBURSEMENT INFORMATION

Medicare

- Follow–up Days — 90
- Assistant Surgeon — paid
- Supply Charges — not allowed
- Outpatient Limit — does not apply
- Major Surgery Rules Apply

CPT CODE	SERVICE	ICD–9–CM

30520 Septoplasty or submucous resection, with or without cartilage scoring, contouring or replacement with graft

CPT NOTES

- For obtaining tissues for graft, see 20900-20926, 21210.
- For submucous resection of turbinates, use 30140.

ICD–9–CM

461.0	Acute maxillary sinusitis
461.8	Other acute sinusitis
470.	Deviated nasal septum
473.0	Chronic maxillary sinusitis
473.2	Chronic ethmoidal sinusitis
473.8	Chronic sinusitis NEC
477.9	Allergic rhinitis NOS
478.0	Hypertrophy of nasal turbinates
478.1	Nasal and sinus disease NEC
738.0	Acquired nose deformity
748.1	Congenital nose anomaly NEC
754.0	Congen skull/face/jaw deformity
802.0	Nasal bone Fx, closed
802.1	Nasal bone Fx, open

REIMBURSEMENT INFORMATION

Medicare

- Follow–up Days — 90
- Assistant Surgeon — not paid
- Supply Charges — not allowed
- Outpatient Limit — does not apply
- Major Surgery Rules Apply

30540 Repair choanal atresia; intranasal

30545 Repair choanal atresia; transpalatine

CPT NOTES

- For obtaining tissues for graft, see 20900-20926, 21210.

ICD–9–CM

748.0	Congenital choanal atresia

REIMBURSEMENT INFORMATION

Medicare

- Follow–up Days — 90
- Assistant Surgeon — paid
- Supply Charges — not allowed
- Outpatient Limit — does not apply
- Major Surgery Rules Apply

CPT CODE / SERVICE	ICD–9–CM
30560* Lysis intranasal synechia	

30560* Lysis intranasal synechia

CPT NOTES

- For obtaining tissues for graft, see 20900-20926, 21210.

ICD–9–CM

461.0	Acute maxillary sinusitis
470.	Deviated nasal septum
471.0	Polyp of nasal cavity
471.8	Nasal sinus polyp NEC
473.2	Chronic ethmoidal sinusitis
473.3	Chronic sphenoidal sinusitis
473.8	Chronic sinusitis NEC
478.1	Nasal and sinus disease NEC
519.8	Respiratory system disease NEC
905.0	Late effect, skull/face fracture
906.0	Late effect, open wound head/trunk

REIMBURSEMENT INFORMATION

General

- Starred procedure.

Medicare

- Follow–up Days — 10
- Assistant Surgeon — not paid
- Supply Charges — not allowed
- Outpatient Limit — does not apply
- Minor Surgery Rules Apply

30580 Repair fistula; oromaxillary (combine with 31030 if antrotomy is included)

CPT NOTES

- For obtaining tissues for graft, see 20900-20926, 21210.

ICD–9–CM

461.0	Acute maxillary sinusitis
473.0	Chronic maxillary sinusitis
522.7	Periapical abscess w/sinus
524.3	Tooth position anomaly
526.0	Developmental odontogenic cysts
526.2	Jaw cysts NEC
526.3	Jaw, central giant cell granuloma
526.4	Inflammation of jaw
528.3	Cellulitis/abscess of mouth
905.0	Late effect, skull/face fracture
906.0	Late effect, open wound head/trunk
909.2	Late effect of radiation
V13.6	Hx of congenital malformation

REIMBURSEMENT INFORMATION

Medicare

- Follow–up Days — 90
- Assistant Surgeon — not paid
- Supply Charges — not allowed
- Outpatient Limit — does not apply
- Major Surgery Rules Apply

CPT CODE SERVICE	ICD-9-CM
30600 Repair fistula; oronasal **CPT NOTES** ◆ For obtaining tissues for graft, see 20900-20926, 21210.	473.0 Chronic maxillary sinusitis 524.3 Tooth position anomaly 526.0 Developmental odontogenic cysts 526.2 Jaw cysts NEC 526.3 Jaw, central giant cell granuloma 526.4 Inflammation of jaw 528.3 Cellulitis/abscess of mouth 749.0x Cleft palate 749.2x Cleft palate w/cleft lip 909.2 Late effect of radiation V13.6 Hx of congenital malformation **REIMBURSEMENT INFORMATION** Medicare ◆ Follow-up Days — 90 ◆ Assistant Surgeon — not paid ◆ Supply Charges — not allowed ◆ Outpatient Limit — does not apply ◆ Major Surgery Rules Apply
30620 Septal or other intranasal dermatoplasty (does not include obtaining graft) **CPT NOTES** ◆ For obtaining tissues for graft, see 20900-20926, 21210.	461.0 Acute maxillary sinusitis 470. Deviated nasal septum 471.0 Polyp of nasal cavity 471.8 Nasal sinus polyp NEC 473.8 Chronic sinusitis NEC 478.1 Nasal and sinus disease NEC 738.0 Acquired nose deformity 748.1 Congenital nose anomaly NEC 754.0 Congen skull/face/jaw deformity 784.7 Epistaxis 802.0 Nasal bone Fx, closed 802.1 Nasal bone Fx, open 909.3 Late effect of surg/med complic 959.0 Face and neck injury NOS V51. Aftercare w/plastic surgery **REIMBURSEMENT INFORMATION** Medicare ◆ Follow-up Days — 90 ◆ Assistant Surgeon — not paid ◆ Supply Charges — not allowed ◆ Outpatient Limit — does not apply ◆ Major Surgery Rules Apply

CPT CODE SERVICE	ICD–9–CM
30630 Repair nasal septal perforations **CPT NOTES** ◆ For obtaining tissues for graft, see 20900-20926, 21210.	470. Deviated nasal septum 478.1 Nasal and sinus disease NEC 802.1 Nasal bone Fx, open 905.0 Late effect, skull/face fracture 906.0 Late effect, open wound head/trunk 909.3 Late effect of surg/med complic 909.5 Late effect of adverse drug effect 998.5 Postoperative infection V51. Aftercare w/plastic surgery **REIMBURSEMENT INFORMATION** Medicare ◆ Follow–up Days — 90 ◆ Assistant Surgeon — not paid ◆ Supply Charges — not allowed ◆ Outpatient Limit — does not apply ◆ Major Surgery Rules Apply
30801* Cauterization and/or ablation, mucosa of turbinates, unilateral or bilateral, any method, (separate procedure); superficial **30802** Cauterization and/or ablation, mucosa of turbinates, unilateral or bilateral, any method, (separate procedure); intramural	473.2 Chronic ethmoidal sinusitis 473.8 Chronic sinusitis NEC 473.9 Chronic sinusitis NOS 478.0 Hypertrophy of nasal turbinates 478.1 Nasal and sinus disease NEC 519.8 Respiratory system disease NEC 784.0 Headache 784.7 Epistaxis **REIMBURSEMENT INFORMATION** General ◆ Starred procedure. (30801) ◆ Separate procedure rules apply. Medicare ◆ Follow–up Days — 10 ◆ Assistant Surgeon — not paid ◆ Supply Charges — not allowed ◆ Outpatient Limit — does not apply ◆ Minor Surgery Rules Apply

CPT CODE	SERVICE	ICD-9-CM
30901*	Control nasal hemorrhage, anterior, simple (limited cautery and/or packing) any method	160.0 M-Neoplasm, Nasal cavities 212.0 B-Neoplasm, Nasal cavity/sinus 401.9 Essential hypertension NOS 784.7 Epistaxis 959.0 Face and neck injury NOS

REIMBURSEMENT INFORMATION

General

- ♦ Starred procedure.

Medicare

- ♦ Follow–up Days — 0
- ♦ Assistant Surgeon — not paid
- ♦ Supply Charges — not allowed
- ♦ Outpatient Limit — applies
- ♦ Minor Surgery Rules Apply

CPT CODE	SERVICE	ICD-9-CM
30903*	Control nasal hemorrhage, anterior, complex (extensive cautery and/or packing) any method	375.56 Acquired nasolacrimal duct stenosis 784.7 Epistaxis 802.0 Nasal bone Fx, closed 959.0 Face and neck injury NOS 998.1 Hemorrhage complicating a procedure

REIMBURSEMENT INFORMATION

General

- ♦ Starred procedure.

Medicare

- ♦ Follow–up Days — 0
- ♦ Assistant Surgeon — not paid
- ♦ Supply Charges — not allowed
- ♦ Outpatient Limit — does not apply
- ♦ Minor Surgery Rules Apply

CPT CODE	SERVICE	ICD–9–CM
30905*	Control nasal hemorrhage, posterior, with posterior nasal packs and/or cauterization, any method; initial	478.1 Nasal and sinus disease NEC 784.7 Epistaxis 959.0 Face and neck injury NOS 998.1 Hemorrhage complicating a procedure **REIMBURSEMENT INFORMATION** General ◆ Starred procedure. Medicare ◆ Follow–up Days — 0 ◆ Assistant Surgeon — not paid ◆ Supply Charges — not allowed ◆ Outpatient Limit — does not apply ◆ Minor Surgery Rules Apply
30906*	Control nasal hemorrhage, posterior, with posterior nasal packs and/or cauterization, any method; subsequent	478.1 Nasal and sinus disease NEC 784.7 Epistaxis 802.0 Nasal bone Fx, closed 802.1 Nasal bone Fx, open 802.4 Fx malar/maxillary, closed 802.5 Fx malar/maxillary, open 959.0 Face and neck injury NOS 998.1 Hemorrhage complicating a procedure **REIMBURSEMENT INFORMATION** General ◆ Starred procedure. Medicare ◆ Follow–up Days — 0 ◆ Assistant Surgeon — not paid ◆ Supply Charges — not allowed ◆ Outpatient Limit — does not apply ◆ Minor Surgery Rules Apply
30915	Ligation arteries; ethmoidal **CPT NOTES** ◆ For ligation external carotid artery, see 37600.	473.2 Chronic ethmoidal sinusitis 784.7 Epistaxis **REIMBURSEMENT INFORMATION** Medicare ◆ Follow–up Days — 90 ◆ Assistant Surgeon — not paid ◆ Supply Charges — not allowed ◆ Outpatient Limit — does not apply ◆ Major Surgery Rules Apply

CPT CODE	SERVICE	ICD-9-CM
30920	Ligation arteries; internal maxillary artery, transantral **CPT NOTES** ♦ For ligation external carotid artery, see 37600.	784.7 Epistaxis 801.x Fracture of base of skull 873.20 Open wound of nose NOS 873.21 Open wound of nasal septum 873.22 Open wound of nasal cavity 873.23 Open wound of nasal sinus 873.29 Multiple open nose wounds 873.30 Open wound of nose NOS, complicated 873.31 Open wound nasal septum, complic 873.32 Open wound nasal cavity, complic 873.33 Open wound nasal sinus, complic 873.39 Multiple open nose wounds, complic **REIMBURSEMENT INFORMATION** Medicare ♦ Follow–up Days — 90 ♦ Assistant Surgeon — not paid ♦ Supply Charges — not allowed ♦ Outpatient Limit — does not apply ♦ Major Surgery Rules Apply
30930	Fracture nasal turbinate(s), therapeutic	470. Deviated nasal septum 471.0 Polyp of nasal cavity 472.0 Chronic rhinitis 473.3 Chronic sphenoidal sinusitis 473.8 Chronic sinusitis NEC 478.0 Hypertrophy of nasal turbinates 478.1 Nasal and sinus disease NEC 738.0 Acquired nose deformity 754.0 Congen skull/face/jaw deformity 959.0 Face and neck injury NOS **REIMBURSEMENT INFORMATION** Medicare ♦ Follow–up Days — 10 ♦ Assistant Surgeon — not paid ♦ Supply Charges — not allowed ♦ Outpatient Limit — does not apply ♦ Minor Surgery Rules Apply

CPT CODE	SERVICE	ICD-9-CM
30999	Unlisted procedure, nose	231.8 CA in situ, Respiratory system NEC 461.0 Acute maxillary sinusitis 470. Deviated nasal septum 473.9 Chronic sinusitis NOS 474.10 Hypertrophy of tonsils/adenoids 478.0 Hypertrophy of nasal turbinates 478.1 Nasal and sinus disease NEC 738.0 Acquired nose deformity 784.7 Epistaxis 802.0 Nasal bone Fx, closed 932. Foreign body in nose 959.0 Face and neck injury NOS **REIMBURSEMENT INFORMATION** Medicare ◆ Follow-up Days — determined by local carrier ◆ Assistant Surgeon — determined by local carrier ◆ Supply Charges — determined by local carrier ◆ Outpatient Limit — determined by local carrier
31000*	Lavage by cannulation; maxillary sinus (antrum puncture or natural ostium)	461.0 Acute maxillary sinusitis 461.8 Other acute sinusitis 461.9 Acute sinusitis NOS 471.8 Nasal sinus polyp NEC 473.0 Chronic maxillary sinusitis 473.2 Chronic ethmoidal sinusitis 473.8 Chronic sinusitis NEC 473.9 Chronic sinusitis NOS 802.4 Fx malar/maxillary, closed 802.5 Fx malar/maxillary, open 905.0 Late effect, skull/face fracture **REIMBURSEMENT INFORMATION** General ◆ Starred procedure. Medicare ◆ Follow-up Days — 10 ◆ Assistant Surgeon — not paid ◆ Supply Charges — not allowed ◆ Outpatient Limit — applies ◆ Minor Surgery Rules Apply

CPT CODE	SERVICE	ICD–9–CM
31002*	Lavage by cannulation; sphenoid sinus	473.3 Chronic sphenoidal sinusitis 905.0 Late effect, skull/face fracture

REIMBURSEMENT INFORMATION

General

- ♦ Starred procedure.

Medicare

- ♦ Follow–up Days — 10
- ♦ Assistant Surgeon — by report
- ♦ Supply Charges — not allowed
- ♦ Outpatient Limit — applies
- ♦ Minor Surgery Rules Apply

31020 Sinusotomy, maxillary (antrotomy); intranasal

376.21	Thyrotoxic exophthalmos
461.0	Acute maxillary sinusitis
461.8	Other acute sinusitis
473.0	Chronic maxillary sinusitis
473.8	Chronic sinusitis NEC
473.9	Chronic sinusitis NOS
682.0	Cellulitis of face
754.0	Congen skull/face/jaw deformity
802.35	Fx angle of jaw, open
905.0	Late effect, skull/face fracture
932.	Foreign body in nose

REIMBURSEMENT INFORMATION

Medicare

- ♦ Follow–up Days — 90
- ♦ Assistant Surgeon — not paid
- ♦ Supply Charges — not allowed
- ♦ Outpatient Limit — does not apply
- ♦ Major Surgery Rules Apply

CPT CODE	SERVICE	ICD-9-CM
31030	Sinusotomy, maxillary (antrotomy); radical (Caldwell-Luc) without removal of antrochoanal polyps	376.01 Orbital cellulitis 461.0 Acute maxillary sinusitis 461.8 Other acute sinusitis 470. Deviated nasal septum 473.0 Chronic maxillary sinusitis 473.8 Chronic sinusitis NEC 478.1 Nasal and sinus disease NEC 526.4 Inflammation of jaw 527.6 Salivary gland mucocele 754.0 Congen skull/face/jaw deformity 802.35 Fx angle of jaw, open 802.5 Fx malar/maxillary, open 802.7 Fx orbital floor, open 905.0 Late effect, skull/face fracture 932. Foreign body in nose **REIMBURSEMENT INFORMATION** <u>Medicare</u> ◆ Follow–up Days — 90 ◆ Assistant Surgeon — not paid ◆ Supply Charges — not allowed ◆ Outpatient Limit — does not apply ◆ Major Surgery Rules Apply
31032	Sinusotomy, maxillary (antrotomy); radical (Caldwell-Luc) with removal of antrochoanal polyps	461.0 Acute maxillary sinusitis 471.8 Nasal sinus polyp NEC 473.0 Chronic maxillary sinusitis 905.0 Late effect, skull/face fracture **REIMBURSEMENT INFORMATION** <u>Medicare</u> ◆ Follow–up Days — 90 ◆ Assistant Surgeon — not paid ◆ Supply Charges — not allowed ◆ Outpatient Limit — does not apply ◆ Major Surgery Rules Apply

CPT CODE	SERVICE	ICD–9–CM
31040	Pterygomaxillary fossa surgery, any approach **CPT NOTES** ◆ For transantral ligation of internal maxillary artery, see 30920.	784.7 Epistaxis 935.0 Foreign body in mouth **REIMBURSEMENT INFORMATION** Medicare ◆ Follow–up Days — 90 ◆ Assistant Surgeon — not paid ◆ Supply Charges — not allowed ◆ Outpatient Limit — does not apply ◆ Major Surgery Rules Apply
31050	Sinusotomy, sphenoid, with or without biopsy	461.3 Acute sphenoidal sinusitis 461.8 Other acute sinusitis 473.3 Chronic sphenoidal sinusitis 473.8 Chronic sinusitis NEC 473.9 Chronic sinusitis NOS **REIMBURSEMENT INFORMATION** Medicare ◆ Follow–up Days — 90 ◆ Assistant Surgeon — not paid ◆ Supply Charges — not allowed ◆ Outpatient Limit — does not apply ◆ Major Surgery Rules Apply
31051	Sinusotomy, sphenoid, with or without biopsy; with mucosal stripping or removal of polyp(s)	461.3 Acute sphenoidal sinusitis 461.8 Other acute sinusitis 473.3 Chronic sphenoidal sinusitis 473.8 Chronic sinusitis NEC 473.9 Chronic sinusitis NOS 905.0 Late effect, skull/face fracture **REIMBURSEMENT INFORMATION** Medicare ◆ Follow–up Days — 90 ◆ Assistant Surgeon — not paid ◆ Supply Charges — not allowed ◆ Outpatient Limit — does not apply ◆ Major Surgery Rules Apply

CPT CODE	SERVICE	ICD–9–CM
31070	Sinusotomy frontal; external, simple (trephine operation)	461.1 Acute frontal sinusitis 461.8 Other acute sinusitis 473.1 Chronic frontal sinusitis 473.8 Chronic sinusitis NEC **REIMBURSEMENT INFORMATION** Medicare ◆ Follow–up Days — 90 ◆ Assistant Surgeon 31070 — not paid 31075 — not paid ◆ Supply Charges — not allowed ◆ Outpatient Limit — does not apply ◆ Major Surgery Rules Apply
31075	Sinusotomy frontal; transorbital, unilateral (for mucocele or osteoma, Lynch type)	
31080	Sinusotomy frontal; obliterative without osteoplastic flap, brow incision (includes ablation)	213.0 B-Neoplasm, Skull/Face bone 473.1 Chronic frontal sinusitis 801.x Fracture of base of skull 905.0 Late effect, skull/face fracture **REIMBURSEMENT INFORMATION** Medicare ◆ Follow–up Days — 90 ◆ Assistant Surgeon — paid ◆ Supply Charges — not allowed ◆ Outpatient Limit — does not apply ◆ Major Surgery Rules Apply
31081	Sinusotomy frontal; obliterative without osteoplastic flap, coronal incision (includes ablation)	
31084	Sinusotomy frontal; obliterative, with osteoplastic flap, brow incision	
31085	Sinusotomy frontal; obliterative, with osteoplastic flap, coronal incision	
31086	Sinusotomy frontal; nonobliterative, with osteoplastic flap, brow incision	
31087	Sinusotomy frontal; nonobliterative, with osteoplastic flap, coronal incision	
31090	Sinusotomy combined, three or more sinuses	461.x Acute sinusitis 473.x Chronic sinusitis **REIMBURSEMENT INFORMATION** Medicare ◆ Follow–up Days — 90 ◆ Assistant Surgeon — not paid ◆ Supply Charges — not allowed ◆ Outpatient Limit — does not apply ◆ Major Surgery Rules Apply

CPT CODE	SERVICE	ICD–9–CM
31200	Ethmoidectomy; intranasal, anterior	375.22 Epiphora d/t insufficient drainage 375.32 Acute dacryocystitis 375.56 Acquired nasolacrimal duct stenosis 461.2 Acute ethmoidal sinusitis 461.8 Other acute sinusitis 473.2 Chronic ethmoidal sinusitis 473.8 Chronic sinusitis NEC 478.0 Hypertrophy of nasal turbinates **REIMBURSEMENT INFORMATION** <u>Medicare</u> ◆ Follow–up Days — 90 ◆ Assistant Surgeon — not paid ◆ Supply Charges — not allowed ◆ Outpatient Limit — does not apply ◆ Major Surgery Rules Apply
31201	Ethmoidectomy; intranasal, total	461.2 Acute ethmoidal sinusitis 461.8 Other acute sinusitis 473.2 Chronic ethmoidal sinusitis 473.8 Chronic sinusitis NEC **REIMBURSEMENT INFORMATION** <u>Medicare</u> ◆ Follow–up Days — 90 ◆ Assistant Surgeon — not paid ◆ Supply Charges — not allowed ◆ Outpatient Limit — does not apply ◆ Major Surgery Rules Apply
31205	Ethmoidectomy; extranasal, total	375.54 Lacrimal sac stenosis 375.56 Acquired nasolacrimal duct stenosis 376.01 Orbital cellulitis 461.2 Acute ethmoidal sinusitis 461.8 Other acute sinusitis 473.2 Chronic ethmoidal sinusitis 473.8 Chronic sinusitis NEC **REIMBURSEMENT INFORMATION** <u>Medicare</u> ◆ Follow–up Days — 90 ◆ Assistant Surgeon — paid ◆ Supply Charges — not allowed ◆ Outpatient Limit — does not apply ◆ Major Surgery Rules Apply

CPT CODE	SERVICE	ICD–9–CM

31225 Maxillectomy; without orbital exenteration

CPT NOTES

- For orbital exenteration only, see 65110 et seq.
- For skin grafts, see 15120 et seq.

160.2	M-Neoplasm, Maxillary sinus
170.0	M-Neoplasm, Skull/Face bone
195.0	M-Neoplasm, Head/face/neck
199.1	M-Neoplasm NOS
200.01	Reticulosarcoma, head/neck/face
200.11	Lymphosarcoma, head/neck/face
200.21	Burkitt's tumor, head/neck face
200.81	Mixed lymphosarcoma, head/neck/face
235.1	UB-Neoplasm, Oral cavity/pharynx
238.0	UB-Neoplasm, Bone
239.2	Bone/Skin neoplasm NOS

REIMBURSEMENT INFORMATION

Medicare

- Follow–up Days — 90
- Assistant Surgeon — paid
- Supply Charges — not allowed
- Outpatient Limit — does not apply
- Major Surgery Rules Apply

31230 Maxillectomy; with orbital exenteration (en bloc)

CPT NOTES

- For orbital exenteration only, see 65110 et seq.
- For skin grafts, see 15120 et seq.

170.0	M-Neoplasm, Skull/Face bone
195.0	M-Neoplasm, Head/face/neck
199.1	M-Neoplasm NOS
200.01	Reticulosarcoma, head/neck/face
200.11	Lymphosarcoma, head/neck/face
200.21	Burkitt's tumor, head/neck face
200.81	Mixed lymphosarcoma, head/neck/face
235.1	UB-Neoplasm, Oral cavity/pharynx
238.0	UB-Neoplasm, Bone
239.2	Bone/Skin neoplasm NOS

REIMBURSEMENT INFORMATION

Medicare

- Follow–up Days — 90
- Assistant Surgeon — paid
- Supply Charges — not allowed
- Outpatient Limit — does not apply
- Major Surgery Rules Apply

CPT CODE	SERVICE
31231	Nasal endoscopy, diagnostic, unilateral or bilateral (separate procedure)

CPT NOTES

- A surgical sinus endoscopy always includes a sinusotomy and diagnostic endoscopy.
- This code is used to report a unilateral procedure unless otherwise specified.
- Diagnostic evaluation refers to employing a nasal/sinus endoscope to inspect the interior of the nasal cavity and the middle and superior meatus, the turbinates, and the spheno-ethomoid recess. Any time a diagnostic evaluation is performed all these areas would be inspected and a separate code is not reported for each area.

ICD–9–CM

160.0	M-Neoplasm, Nasal cavities
161.0	M-Neoplasm, Glottis
212.0	B-Neoplasm, Nasal cavity/sinus
229.8	Benign neoplasm NEC
231.8	CA in situ, Respiratory system NEC
374.11	Senile ectropion
375.53	Lacrimal canaliculi stenosis
375.56	Acquired nasolacrimal duct stenosis
380.22	Acute otitis externa NEC
381.81	Dysfunction of Eustachian tube
461.x	Acute sinusitis
470.	Deviated nasal septum
471.0	Polyp of nasal cavity
471.1	Polypoid sinus degeneration
471.8	Nasal sinus polyp NEC
472.0	Chronic rhinitis
472.1	Chronic pharyngitis
472.2	Chronic nasopharyngitis
473.x	Chronic sinusitis
477.0	Allergic rhinitis d/t pollen
478.0	Hypertrophy of nasal turbinates
478.1	Nasal and sinus disease NEC
738.0	Acquired nose deformity
748.1	Congenital nose anomaly NEC
749.0x	Cleft palate
749.2x	Cleft palate w/cleft lip
781.1	Smell/taste sensation disturbance
784.49	Voice disturbance NEC
784.7	Epistaxis
941.05	Burn NOS, nose

REIMBURSEMENT INFORMATION

General

- Separate procedure rules apply.

Medicare

- Follow–up Days — 0
- Assistant Surgeon — not paid
- Supply Charges — not allowed
- Outpatient Limit — does not apply
- Minor Surgery Rules Apply

CPT CODE	SERVICE
31233	Nasal/sinus endoscopy, diagnostic with maxillary sinusoscopy (via inferior meatus or canine fossa puncture)

CPT NOTES

- A surgical sinus endoscopy always includes a sinusotomy and diagnostic endoscopy.
- This code is used to report a unilateral procedure unless otherwise specified.
- Diagnostic evaluation refers to employing a nasal/sinus endoscope to inspect the interior of the nasal cavity and the middle and superior meatus, the turbinates, and the spheno-ethomoid recess. Any time a diagnostic evaluation is performed all these areas would be inspected and a separate code is not reported for each area.

ICD–9–CM

160.0	M-Neoplasm, Nasal cavities
161.0	M-Neoplasm, Glottis
212.0	B-Neoplasm, Nasal cavity/sinus
229.8	Benign neoplasm NEC
231.8	CA in situ, Respiratory system NEC
374.11	Senile ectropion
375.53	Lacrimal canaliculi stenosis
375.56	Acquired nasolacrimal duct stenosis
380.22	Acute otitis externa NEC
381.81	Dysfunction of Eustachian tube
461.0	Acute maxillary sinusitis
461.1	Acute frontal sinusitis
461.2	Acute ethmoidal sinusitis
461.3	Acute sphenoidal sinusitis
461.8	Other acute sinusitis
461.9	Acute sinusitis NOS
470.	Deviated nasal septum
471.0	Polyp of nasal cavity
471.1	Polypoid sinus degeneration
471.8	Nasal sinus polyp NEC
472.0	Chronic rhinitis
472.1	Chronic pharyngitis
472.2	Chronic nasopharyngitis
473.x	Chronic sinusitis
477.0	Allergic rhinitis d/t pollen
478.0	Hypertrophy of nasal turbinates
478.1	Nasal and sinus disease NEC
738.0	Acquired nose deformity
748.1	Congenital nose anomaly NEC
781.1	Smell/taste sensation disturbance
784.7	Epistaxis
941.05	Burn NOS, nose

REIMBURSEMENT INFORMATION

Medicare

- Follow–up Days — 0
- Assistant Surgeon — not paid
- Supply Charges — not allowed
- Outpatient Limit — does not apply
- Minor Surgery Rules Apply

CPT CODE	SERVICE
31235	Nasal/sinus endoscopy, diagnostic with sphenoid sinusoscopy (via puncture of sphenoidal face or cannulation of osteum)

CPT NOTES

- A surgical sinus endoscopy always includes a sinusotomy and diagnostic endoscopy.
- This code is used to report a unilateral procedure unless otherwise specified.
- Diagnostic evaluation refers to employing a nasal/sinus endoscope to inspect the interior of the nasal cavity and the middle and superior meatus, the turbinates, and the spheno-ethomoid recess. Any time a diagnostic evaluation is performed all these areas would be inspected and a separate code is not reported for each area.

ICD–9–CM

160.0	M-Neoplasm, Nasal cavities
161.0	M-Neoplasm, Glottis
212.0	B-Neoplasm, Nasal cavity/sinus
229.8	Benign neoplasm NEC
231.8	CA in situ, Respiratory system NEC
374.11	Senile ectropion
375.53	Lacrimal canaliculi stenosis
375.56	Acquired nasolacrimal duct stenosis
380.22	Acute otitis externa NEC
381.81	Dysfunction of Eustachian tube
461.x	Acute sinusitis
470.	Deviated nasal septum
471.0	Polyp of nasal cavity
471.1	Polypoid sinus degeneration
471.8	Nasal sinus polyp NEC
472.0	Chronic rhinitis
472.1	Chronic pharyngitis
472.2	Chronic nasopharyngitis
473.x	Chronic sinusitis
477.0	Allergic rhinitis d/t pollen
478.0	Hypertrophy of nasal turbinates
478.1	Nasal and sinus disease NEC
738.0	Acquired nose deformity
748.1	Congenital nose anomaly NEC
781.1	Smell/taste sensation disturbance
784.7	Epistaxis
941.05	Burn NOS, nose

REIMBURSEMENT INFORMATION

Medicare

- Follow–up Days — 0
- Assistant Surgeon — not paid
- Supply Charges — not allowed
- Outpatient Limit — does not apply
- Minor Surgery Rules Apply

CPT CODE	SERVICE	ICD–9–CM

31237 Nasal/sinus endoscopy, surgical; with biopsy, polypectomy or debridement (separate procedure)

CPT NOTES

- A surgical sinus endoscopy always includes a sinusotomy and diagnostic endoscopy.
- This code is used to report a unilateral procedure unless otherwise specified.

471.0	Polyp of nasal cavity
471.1	Polypoid sinus degeneration
471.8	Nasal sinus polyp NEC
471.9	Nasal polyp NOS
478.1	Nasal and sinus disease NEC
932.	Foreign body in nose

REIMBURSEMENT INFORMATION

General

- Separate procedure rules apply.

Medicare

- Follow–up Days — 0
- Assistant Surgeon — not paid
- Supply Charges — not allowed
- Outpatient Limit — does not apply
- Minor Surgery Rules Apply

31238 Nasal/sinus endoscopy, surgical; with control of epistaxis

31239 Nasal/sinus endoscopy, surgical; with dacryocystorhinostomy

31240 Nasal/sinus endoscopy, surgical; with concha bullosa resection

CPT NOTES

- A surgical sinus endoscopy always includes a sinusotomy and diagnostic endoscopy.
- This code is used to report a unilateral procedure unless otherwise specified.

471.0	Polyp of nasal cavity
471.1	Polypoid sinus degeneration
471.8	Nasal sinus polyp NEC
471.9	Nasal polyp NOS
478.1	Nasal and sinus disease NEC

REIMBURSEMENT INFORMATION

Medicare

- Follow–up Days — 0
- Assistant Surgeon — by report
- Supply Charges — not allowed
- Outpatient Limit — does not apply
- Minor Surgery Rules Apply

CPT CODE **SERVICE**

- ● **31254** Nasal/sinus endoscopy, surgical; with ethmoidectomy, partial (anterior)
- ● **31255** Nasal/sinus endoscopy, surgical; with ethmoidectomy, total (anterior and posterior)

CPT NOTES

- ♦ A surgical sinus endoscopy always includes a sinusotomy and diagnostic endoscopy.
- ♦ This code is used to report a unilateral procedure unless otherwise specified.

ICD–9–CM

212.0	B-Neoplasm, Nasal cavity/sinus
229.8	Benign neoplasm NEC
375.56	Acquired nasolacrimal duct stenosis
461.0	Acute maxillary sinusitis
461.2	Acute ethmoidal sinusitis
461.8	Other acute sinusitis
461.9	Acute sinusitis NOS
471.0	Polyp of nasal cavity
471.1	Polypoid sinus degeneration
471.8	Nasal sinus polyp NEC
471.9	Nasal polyp NOS
473.0	Chronic maxillary sinusitis
473.2	Chronic ethmoidal sinusitis
473.8	Chronic sinusitis NEC
473.9	Chronic sinusitis NOS
478.1	Nasal and sinus disease NEC
519.8	Respiratory system disease NEC

REIMBURSEMENT INFORMATION

General

- ♦ New procedure, 1995 CPT.

Medicare

- ♦ Follow–up Days — 0
- ♦ Assistant Surgeon — not paid
- ♦ Supply Charges — not allowed
- ♦ Outpatient Limit — does not apply
- ♦ Minor Surgery Rules Apply

CPT CODE **SERVICE**

● **31256** Nasal/sinus endoscopy, surgical with maxillary antrostomy

● **31267** Nasal/sinus endoscopy, surgical, with maxillary antrostomy; with removal of tissue from maxillary sinus

CPT NOTES

- ♦ A surgical sinus endoscopy always includes a sinusotomy and diagnostic endoscopy.
- ♦ This code is used to report a unilateral procedure unless otherwise specified.

ICD–9–CM

212.0	B-Neoplasm, Nasal cavity/sinus
229.8	Benign neoplasm NEC
235.9	UB-Neoplasm, Respiratory system NOS
461.0	Acute maxillary sinusitis
461.1	Acute frontal sinusitis
461.8	Other acute sinusitis
461.9	Acute sinusitis NOS
471.0	Polyp of nasal cavity
471.1	Polypoid sinus degeneration
471.8	Nasal sinus polyp NEC
471.9	Nasal polyp NOS
473.0	Chronic maxillary sinusitis
473.2	Chronic ethmoidal sinusitis
473.8	Chronic sinusitis NEC
473.9	Chronic sinusitis NOS
478.1	Nasal and sinus disease NEC
519.8	Respiratory system disease NEC

REIMBURSEMENT INFORMATION

General

- ♦ New procedure, 1995 CPT.

Medicare

- ♦ Follow–up Days — 0
- ♦ Assistant Surgeon — not paid
- ♦ Supply Charges — not allowed
- ♦ Outpatient Limit — does not apply
- ♦ Minor Surgery Rules Apply

● **31276** Nasal/sinus endoscopy, surgical with frontal sinus exploration, with or without removal of tissue from frontal sinus

CPT NOTES

- ♦ A surgical sinus endoscopy always includes a sinusotomy and diagnostic endoscopy.
- ♦ This code is used to report a unilateral procedure unless otherwise specified.

212.0	B-Neoplasm, Nasal cavity/sinus
461.1	Acute frontal sinusitis
461.2	Acute ethmoidal sinusitis
461.8	Other acute sinusitis
471.8	Nasal sinus polyp NEC
471.9	Nasal polyp NOS
473.1	Chronic frontal sinusitis
473.2	Chronic ethmoidal sinusitis
473.8	Chronic sinusitis NEC
478.1	Nasal and sinus disease NEC

REIMBURSEMENT INFORMATION

General

- ♦ New procedure, 1995 CPT.

Medicare

- ♦ Follow–up Days — 0
- ♦ Assistant Surgeon — not paid
- ♦ Supply Charges — not allowed
- ♦ Outpatient Limit — does not apply
- ♦ Minor Surgery Rules Apply

CPT CODE	SERVICE	ICD–9–CM

31288 Nasal/sinus endoscopy, surgical, with sphenoidotomy; with removal of tissue from the sphenoid sinus

CPT NOTES

- ♦ A surgical sinus endoscopy always includes a sinusotomy and diagnostic endoscopy.
- ♦ This code is used to report a unilateral procedure unless otherwise specified.

461.3 Acute sphenoidal sinusitis
461.8 Other acute sinusitis
470. Deviated nasal septum
473.3 Chronic sphenoidal sinusitis
473.8 Chronic sinusitis NEC

REIMBURSEMENT INFORMATION

Medicare

- ♦ Follow–up Days — 0
- ♦ Assistant Surgeon — not paid
- ♦ Supply Charges — not allowed
- ♦ Outpatient Limit — does not apply
- ♦ Minor Surgery Rules Apply

31290 Nasal/sinus endoscopy, surgical, with repair of cerebrospinal fluid leak; ethmoid region

CPT NOTES

- ♦ A surgical sinus endoscopy always includes a sinusotomy and diagnostic endoscopy.
- ♦ This code is used to report a unilateral procedure unless otherwise specified.

461.2 Acute ethmoidal sinusitis
461.8 Other acute sinusitis
470. Deviated nasal septum
473.2 Chronic ethmoidal sinusitis
473.8 Chronic sinusitis NEC
905.0 Late effect, skull/face fracture

REIMBURSEMENT INFORMATION

Medicare

- ♦ Follow–up Days — 10
- ♦ Assistant Surgeon — by report
- ♦ Supply Charges — not allowed
- ♦ Outpatient Limit — does not apply
- ♦ Minor Surgery Rules Apply

31291 Nasal/sinus endoscopy, surgical, with repair of cerebrospinal fluid leak; sphenoid region

CPT NOTES

- ♦ A surgical sinus endoscopy always includes a sinusotomy and diagnostic endoscopy.
- ♦ This code is used to report a unilateral procedure unless otherwise specified.

461.3 Acute sphenoidal sinusitis
461.8 Other acute sinusitis
470. Deviated nasal septum
473.3 Chronic sphenoidal sinusitis
473.8 Chronic sinusitis NEC
905.0 Late effect, skull/face fracture

REIMBURSEMENT INFORMATION

Medicare

- ♦ Follow–up Days — 10
- ♦ Assistant Surgeon — by report
- ♦ Supply Charges — not allowed
- ♦ Outpatient Limit — does not apply
- ♦ Minor Surgery Rules Apply

CPT CODE	SERVICE	ICD–9–CM	
31292	Nasal/sinus endoscopy, surgical; with medial or inferior orbital wall decompression	376.21	Thyrotoxic exophthalmos
31293	Nasal/sinus endoscopy, surgical; with medial orbital wall and inferior orbital wall decompression	376.22	Exophthalmic ophthalmoplegia
31294	Nasal/sinus endoscopy, surgical; with optic nerve decompression	376.31	Constant exophthalmos
		376.32	Orbital hemorrhage
		376.33	Orbital edema
		376.36	Lateral globe displacement
		376.42	Exostosis of orbit
		376.43	Orbit deformity d/t bone disease
		376.47	Orbit deformity d/t trauma/surgery
		461.x	Acute sinusitis
		473.x	Chronic sinusitis
		801.x	Fracture of base of skull
		905.0	Late effect, skull/face fracture
		921.2	Contusion of orbital tissue

CPT NOTES

- A surgical sinus endoscopy always includes a sinusotomy and diagnostic endoscopy.
- This code is used to report a unilateral procedure unless otherwise specified.

REIMBURSEMENT INFORMATION

Medicare

- Follow–up Days
  31292 — 0
  31293–31294 — 10
- Assistant Surgeon
  31292 — not paid
  31293–31294 — by report
- Supply Charges — not allowed
- Outpatient Limit — does not apply
- Minor Surgery Rules Apply

CPT CODE	SERVICE	ICD–9–CM	
31299	Unlisted procedure, accessory sinuses	375.56	Acquired nasolacrimal duct stenosis
		461.0	Acute maxillary sinusitis
		461.1	Acute frontal sinusitis
		461.8	Other acute sinusitis
		461.9	Acute sinusitis NOS
		471.8	Nasal sinus polyp NEC
		471.9	Nasal polyp NOS
		473.0	Chronic maxillary sinusitis
		473.2	Chronic ethmoidal sinusitis
		473.8	Chronic sinusitis NEC
		478.0	Hypertrophy of nasal turbinates
		478.1	Nasal and sinus disease NEC
		519.8	Respiratory system disease NEC
		738.0	Acquired nose deformity
		784.0	Headache

CPT NOTES

- For hypophysectomy, transantral or transeptal approach, see 61548.
- For transcranial hypophysectomy, see 61546.

REIMBURSEMENT INFORMATION

Medicare

- Follow–up Days — determined by local carrier
- Assistant Surgeon — determined by local carrier
- Supply Charges — determined by local carrier
- Outpatient Limit — determined by local carrier

CPT CODE	SERVICE	ICD-9-CM
31300	Laryngotomy (thyrotomy, laryngofissure); with removal of tumor or laryngocele, cordectomy	161.0 M-Neoplasm, Glottis 161.3 M-Neoplasm, Laryngeal cartilages 161.9 M-Neoplasm, Larynx NOS
31320	Laryngotomy (thyrotomy, laryngofissure); diagnostic	

REIMBURSEMENT INFORMATION

Medicare

- Follow-up Days — 90
- Assistant Surgeon
  31300 — paid
  31320 — by report
- Supply Charges — not allowed
- Outpatient Limit — does not apply
- Major Surgery Rules Apply

CPT CODE	SERVICE	ICD-9-CM
31360	Laryngectomy; total, without radical neck dissection	161.0 M-Neoplasm, Glottis 161.9 M-Neoplasm, Larynx NOS 231.0 CA in situ, Larynx
31365	Laryngectomy; total, with radical neck dissection	
31367	Laryngectomy; subtotal supraglottic, without radical neck dissection	
31368	Laryngectomy; subtotal supraglottic, with radical neck dissection	

REIMBURSEMENT INFORMATION

Medicare

- Follow-up Days — 90
- Assistant Surgeon — paid
- Supply Charges — not allowed
- Outpatient Limit — does not apply
- Major Surgery Rules Apply

CPT CODE	SERVICE	ICD-9-CM
31370	Partial laryngectomy (hemilaryngectomy); horizontal	161.0 M-Neoplasm, Glottis 161.1 M-Neoplasm, Supraglottis 161.2 M-Neoplasm, Subglottis 161.3 M-Neoplasm, Laryngeal cartilages 161.8 M-Neoplasm, Larynx NEC 231.0 CA in situ, Larynx
31375	Partial laryngectomy (hemilaryngectomy); laterovertical	
31380	Partial laryngectomy (hemilaryngectomy); anterovertical	
31382	Partial laryngectomy (hemilaryngectomy); antero-latero-vertical	

REIMBURSEMENT INFORMATION

Medicare

- Follow-up Days — 90
- Assistant Surgeon — paid
- Supply Charges — not allowed
- Outpatient Limit — does not apply
- Major Surgery Rules Apply

CPT CODE	SERVICE	ICD–9–CM
31390	Pharyngolaryngectomy, with radical neck dissection; without reconstruction	161.0 M-Neoplasm, Glottis 161.1 M-Neoplasm, Supraglottis 161.2 M-Neoplasm, Subglottis 161.3 M-Neoplasm, Laryngeal cartilages 161.8 M-Neoplasm, Larynx NEC 231.0 CA in situ, Larynx
31395	Pharyngolaryngectomy, with radical neck dissection; with reconstruction	

REIMBURSEMENT INFORMATION

Medicare

- Follow–up Days — 90
- Assistant Surgeon — paid
- Supply Charges — not allowed
- Outpatient Limit — does not apply
- Major Surgery Rules Apply

31400 Arytenoidectomy or arytenoidopexy, external approach

CPT NOTES

- For endoscopic arytenoidectomy, see 31560.

161.0 M-Neoplasm, Glottis
161.1 M-Neoplasm, Supraglottis
161.2 M-Neoplasm, Subglottis
161.3 M-Neoplasm, Laryngeal cartilages
161.8 M-Neoplasm, Larynx NEC
212.1 B-Neoplasm, Larynx

REIMBURSEMENT INFORMATION

Medicare

- Follow–up Days — 90
- Assistant Surgeon — paid
- Supply Charges — not allowed
- Outpatient Limit — does not apply
- Major Surgery Rules Apply

31420 Epiglottidectomy

161.0 M-Neoplasm, Glottis
161.1 M-Neoplasm, Supraglottis
161.2 M-Neoplasm, Subglottis
161.3 M-Neoplasm, Laryngeal cartilages
161.8 M-Neoplasm, Larynx NEC
212.1 B-Neoplasm, Larynx

REIMBURSEMENT INFORMATION

Medicare

- Follow–up Days — 90
- Assistant Surgeon — paid
- Supply Charges — not allowed
- Outpatient Limit — does not apply
- Major Surgery Rules Apply

CPT CODE	SERVICE	ICD–9–CM
31500	Intubation, endotracheal, emergency procedure	427.5 Cardiac arrest 478.6 Edema of larynx 482.1 Pseudomonal pneumonia 518.5 Post traum pulmonary insufficiency 518.81 Respiratory failure 518.82 Other pulmonary insufficiency 748.3 Congenital laryngotrach anomaly NEC 770.0 NB Congenital pneumonia 770.1 NB meconium aspiration syndrome 770.2 NB interstitial emphysema 770.6 NB transitory tachypnea 770.8 Post-birth resp problem NEC 770.9 NB respiratory condition NOS 776.1 Neonatal thrombocytopenia 799.1 Respiratory arrest

CPT NOTES

- For injection procedure for bronchography, see 31656, 31708, 31710.

REIMBURSEMENT INFORMATION

Medicare

- Follow–up Days — 0
- Assistant Surgeon — not paid
- Supply Charges — not allowed
- Outpatient Limit — does not apply
- Minor Surgery Rules Apply

CPT CODE	SERVICE	ICD–9–CM
31502	Tracheotomy tube change prior to establishment of fistula tract	519.8 Respiratory system disease NEC V55.0 Attention to tracheostomy

REIMBURSEMENT INFORMATION

Medicare

- Follow–up Days — 0
- Assistant Surgeon — not paid
- Supply Charges — not allowed
- Outpatient Limit — does not apply
- Minor Surgery Rules Apply

CPT CODE **SERVICE**

31505 Laryngoscopy, indirect (separate procedure); diagnostic

CPT NOTES

- For endoscopic procedures, code appropriate endoscopy of each anatomic site examined.

ICD–9–CM

148.1	M-Neoplasm, Pyriform sinus
161.0	M-Neoplasm, Glottis
231.0	CA in situ, Larynx
235.1	UB-Neoplasm, Oral cavity/pharynx
235.6	UB-Neoplasm, Larynx
461.8	Other acute sinusitis
464.0	Acute laryngitis
464.10	Acute tracheitis, no obstruction
464.11	Acute tracheitis w/obstruction
464.20	Acute laryngotracheitis no obstruct
464.21	Acute laryngotracheitis w/obstruct
464.30	Acute epiglottitis, no obstruction
464.31	Acute epiglottitis w/obstruction
472.1	Chronic pharyngitis
472.2	Chronic nasopharyngitis
473.8	Chronic sinusitis NEC
474.0	Chronic tonsillitis
475.	Peritonsillar abscess
476.0	Chronic laryngitis
476.1	Chronic laryngotracheitis
478.1	Nasal and sinus disease
478.4	Polyp of vocal cord/larynx
478.5	Vocal cord disease NEC
478.6	Edema of larynx
478.7x	Disease of larynx NOS
519.0	Tracheostomy complication
527.2	Sialoadenitis
530.6	Acquired esophageal diverticulum
784.1	Throat pain
784.40	Voice disturbance NOS
784.41	Aphonia
784.49	Voice disturbance NEC
787.2	Dysphagia
933.0	Foreign body in pharynx
935.0	Foreign body in mouth
V10.02	Hx of oral/pharynx malignancy NEC

REIMBURSEMENT INFORMATION

General

- Separate procedure rules apply.

Medicare

- Follow–up Days — 0
- Assistant Surgeon — not paid
- Supply Charges — not allowed
- Outpatient Limit — applies
- Minor Surgery Rules Apply

CPT CODE	SERVICE	ICD–9–CM

31510 Laryngoscopy, indirect (separate procedure); with biopsy

CPT NOTES

- ♦ For endoscopic procedures, code appropriate endoscopy of each anatomic site examined.

ICD–9–CM

148.1	M-Neoplasm, Pyriform sinus
161.0	M-Neoplasm, Glottis
231.0	CA in situ, Larynx
235.1	UB-Neoplasm, Oral cavity/pharynx
235.6	UB-Neoplasm, Larynx
461.8	Other acute sinusitis
464.0	Acute laryngitis
464.10	Acute tracheitis, no obstruction
464.11	Acute tracheitis w/obstruction
464.20	Acute laryngotracheitis no obstruct
464.21	Acute laryngotracheitis w/obstruct
464.30	Acute epiglottitis, no obstruction
464.31	Acute epiglottitis w/obstruction
472.1	Chronic pharyngitis
472.2	Chronic nasopharyngitis

REIMBURSEMENT INFORMATION

General

- ♦ Separate procedure rules apply.

Medicare

- ♦ Follow–up Days — 0
- ♦ Assistant Surgeon — not paid
- ♦ Supply Charges — not allowed
- ♦ Outpatient Limit — does not apply
- ♦ Minor Surgery Rules Apply

31511 Laryngoscopy, indirect (separate procedure); with removal of foreign body

CPT NOTES

- ♦ For endoscopic procedures, code appropriate endoscopy of each anatomic site examined.

933.1	Foreign body in larynx
935.0	Foreign body in mouth
935.1	Foreign body in esophagus

REIMBURSEMENT INFORMATION

General

- ♦ Separate procedure rules apply.

Medicare

- ♦ Follow–up Days — 0
- ♦ Assistant Surgeon — not paid
- ♦ Supply Charges — not allowed
- ♦ Outpatient Limit — does not apply
- ♦ Minor Surgery Rules Apply

CPT CODE	SERVICE	ICD–9–CM

31512 Laryngoscopy, indirect (separate procedure); with removal of lesion

CPT NOTES

- For endoscopic procedures, code appropriate endoscopy of each anatomic site examined.

148.1 M-Neoplasm, Pyriform sinus
161.0 M-Neoplasm, Glottis
231.0 CA in situ, Larynx
235.1 UB-Neoplasm, Oral cavity/pharynx
235.6 UB-Neoplasm, Larynx
748.3 Congenital laryngotrach anomaly NEC

REIMBURSEMENT INFORMATION

General

- Separate procedure rules apply.

Medicare

- Follow–up Days — 0
- Assistant Surgeon — by report
- Supply Charges — not allowed
- Outpatient Limit — does not apply
- Minor Surgery Rules Apply

31513 Laryngoscopy, indirect (separate procedure); with vocal cord injection

CPT NOTES

- For endoscopic procedures, code appropriate endoscopy of each anatomic site examined.

478.30 Vocal cord/larynx paralysis NOS
478.5 Vocal cord disease NEC

REIMBURSEMENT INFORMATION

General

- Separate procedure rules apply.

Medicare

- Follow–up Days — 0
- Assistant Surgeon — not paid
- Supply Charges — not allowed
- Outpatient Limit — does not apply
- Minor Surgery Rules Apply

31515 Laryngoscopy, direct, with or without tracheoscopy; for aspiration

CPT NOTES

- For endoscopic procedures, code appropriate endoscopy of each anatomic site examined.

466.0 Acute bronchitis
478.30 Vocal cord/larynx paralysis NOS
478.4 Polyp of vocal cord/larynx
478.74 Stenosis of larynx
518.81 Respiratory failure
787.2 Dysphagia
933.1 Foreign body in larynx
934.1 Foreign body, main bronchus

REIMBURSEMENT INFORMATION

Medicare

- Follow–up Days — 0
- Assistant Surgeon — not paid
- Supply Charges — not allowed
- Outpatient Limit — does not apply
- Minor Surgery Rules Apply

CPT CODE	SERVICE
31520	Laryngoscopy, direct, with or without tracheoscopy; diagnostic, newborn

CPT NOTES

- For endoscopic procedures, code appropriate endoscopy of each anatomic site examined.

ICD–9–CM

478.74	Stenosis of larynx
786.09	Respiratory abnormality NEC

REIMBURSEMENT INFORMATION

Medicare

- Follow–up Days — 0
- Assistant Surgeon — not paid
- Supply Charges — not allowed
- Outpatient Limit — does not apply
- Minor Surgery Rules Apply

CPT CODE **SERVICE**

31525 Laryngoscopy, direct, with or without tracheoscopy; diagnostic, except newborn

CPT NOTES

- For endoscopic procedures, code appropriate endoscopy of each anatomic site examined.

ICD–9–CM

112.89	Candidiasis site NEC
141.0	M-Neoplasm, Tongue base
141.1	M-Neoplasm, Tongue dorsal surface
150.0	M-Neoplasm, Cervical esophagus
196.0	M-Neoplasm, Lymph head/neck/face
210.4	B-Neoplasm, Mouth NEC/NOS
210.8	B-Neoplasm, Hypopharynx
212.1	B-Neoplasm, Larynx
229.8	Benign neoplasm NEC
235.1	UB-Neoplasm, Oral cavity/pharynx
464.0	Acute laryngitis
464.30	Acute epiglottitis, no obstruction
470.	Deviated nasal septum
472.1	Chronic pharyngitis
474.0	Chronic tonsillitis
474.11	Hypertrophy of tonsils
475.	Peritonsillar abscess
478.2x	Diseases of pharynx NEC
478.3x	Paralysis of vocal cords or larynx
478.4	Polyp of vocal cord/larynx
478.5	Vocal cord disease NEC
478.6	Edema of larynx
478.7x	Disease of larynx NEC
501.	Asbestosis
519.1	Trachea/bronchus disease NEC
519.8	Respiratory system disease NEC
528.7	Oral epithelium disturbance NEC
780.56	Sleep stage dysfunctions
784.2	Swelling in head/neck
784.40	Voice disturbance NOS
784.41	Aphonia
784.49	Voice disturbance NEC
784.8	Hemorrhage from throat
786.1	Stridor
787.2	Dysphagia
933.0	Foreign body in pharynx
935.1	Foreign body in esophagus
947.2	Burn of Esophagus

REIMBURSEMENT INFORMATION

Medicare

- Follow–up Days — 0
- Assistant Surgeon — not paid
- Supply Charges — not allowed
- Outpatient Limit — does not apply
- Minor Surgery Rules Apply

CPT CODE	SERVICE	ICD–9–CM	
31526	Laryngoscopy, direct, with or without tracheoscopy; diagnostic, with operating microscope	231.0	CA in situ, Larynx
		465.0	Acute laryngopharyngitis
		476.0	Chronic laryngitis
		478.26	Cyst of pharynx/nasopharynx
		519.0	Tracheostomy complication
		530.6	Acquired esophageal diverticulum
		784.40	Voice disturbance NOS
		784.41	Aphonia
		784.49	Voice disturbance NEC
		786.09	Respiratory abnormality NEC
		786.1	Stridor
		787.2	Dysphagia

CPT NOTES

- For endoscopic procedures, code appropriate endoscopy of each anatomic site examined.

REIMBURSEMENT INFORMATION

Medicare

- Follow–up Days — 0
- Assistant Surgeon — not paid
- Supply Charges — not allowed
- Outpatient Limit — does not apply
- Minor Surgery Rules Apply

CPT CODE	SERVICE	ICD–9–CM	
31527	Laryngoscopy, direct, with or without tracheoscopy; with insertion of obturator	231.0	CA in situ, Larynx
		465.0	Acute laryngopharyngitis
		476.0	Chronic laryngitis
		478.26	Cyst of pharynx/nasopharynx
		519.0	Tracheostomy complication
		530.6	Acquired esophageal diverticulum
		784.40	Voice disturbance NOS
		784.41	Aphonia
		784.49	Voice disturbance NEC
		786.09	Respiratory abnormality NEC
		786.1	Stridor
		787.2	Dysphagia

CPT NOTES

- For endoscopic procedures, code appropriate endoscopy of each anatomic site examined.

REIMBURSEMENT INFORMATION

Medicare

- Follow–up Days — 0
- Assistant Surgeon — by report
- Supply Charges — not allowed
- Outpatient Limit — does not apply
- Minor Surgery Rules Apply

CPT CODE	SERVICE	ICD–9–CM
31528	Laryngoscopy, direct, with or without tracheoscopy; with dilatation, initial	478.74 Stenosis of larynx

CPT NOTES

- For endoscopic procedures, code appropriate endoscopy of each anatomic site examined.

REIMBURSEMENT INFORMATION

Medicare

- Follow–up Days — 0
- Assistant Surgeon — not paid
- Supply Charges — not allowed
- Outpatient Limit — does not apply
- Minor Surgery Rules Apply

31529 Laryngoscopy, direct, with or without tracheoscopy; with dilatation, subsequent

519.1 Trachea/bronchus disease NEC

CPT NOTES

- For endoscopic procedures, code appropriate endoscopy of each anatomic site examined.

REIMBURSEMENT INFORMATION

Medicare

- Follow–up Days — 0
- Assistant Surgeon — by report
- Supply Charges — not allowed
- Outpatient Limit — does not apply
- Minor Surgery Rules Apply

31530 Laryngoscopy, direct, operative, with foreign body removal

31531 Laryngoscopy, direct, operative, with foreign body removal; with operating microscope

933.0 Foreign body in pharynx
933.1 Foreign body in larynx
934.0 Foreign body, trachea
935.1 Foreign body in esophagus

CPT NOTES

- For endoscopic procedures, code appropriate endoscopy of each anatomic site examined.

REIMBURSEMENT INFORMATION

Medicare

- Follow–up Days — 0
- Assistant Surgeon — not paid
- Supply Charges — not allowed
- Outpatient Limit — does not apply
- Minor Surgery Rules Apply

CPT CODE **SERVICE**

31535 Laryngoscopy, direct, operative, with biopsy

CPT NOTES

- For endoscopic procedures, code appropriate endoscopy of each anatomic site examined.

ICD–9–CM

141.0	M-Neoplasm, Tongue base
141.9	M-Neoplasm, Tongue NOS
142.0	M-Neoplasm, Parotid gland
145.0	M-Neoplasm, Cheek mucosa
145.3	M-Neoplasm, Soft palate
146.0	M-Neoplasm, Tonsil
148.9	M-Neoplasm, Hypopharynx NOS
149.0	M-Neoplasm, Pharynx NOS
161.0	M-Neoplasm, Glottis
161.1	M-Neoplasm, Supraglottis
161.8	M-Neoplasm, Larynx NEC
195.0	M-Neoplasm, Head/face/neck
196.0	M-Neoplasm, Lymph head/neck/face
210.4	B-Neoplasm, Mouth NEC/NOS
210.6	B-Neoplasm, Oropharynx NEC
210.8	B-Neoplasm, Hypopharynx
212.1	B-Neoplasm, Larynx
231.0	CA in situ, Larynx
235.1	UB-Neoplasm, Oral cavity/pharynx
235.6	UB-Neoplasm, Larynx
464.0	Acute laryngitis
476.0	Chronic laryngitis
478.4	Polyp of vocal cord/larynx
478.5	Vocal cord disease NEC
478.74	Stenosis of larynx
478.79	Disease of larynx NEC
528.6	Leukoplakia of oral mucosa/tongue
784.1	Throat pain
784.2	Swelling in head/neck
784.49	Voice disturbance NEC
787.2	Dysphagia

REIMBURSEMENT INFORMATION

Medicare

- Follow–up Days — 0
- Assistant Surgeon — not paid
- Supply Charges — not allowed
- Outpatient Limit — does not apply
- Minor Surgery Rules Apply

CPT CODE	SERVICE
31536	Laryngoscopy, direct, operative, with biopsy; with operating microscope

CPT NOTES

- For endoscopic procedures, code appropriate endoscopy of each anatomic site examined.

ICD–9–CM

141.0	M-Neoplasm, Tongue base
141.9	M-Neoplasm, Tongue NOS
142.0	M-Neoplasm, Parotid gland
145.0	M-Neoplasm, Cheek mucosa
145.3	M-Neoplasm, Soft palate
146.0	M-Neoplasm, Tonsil
148.9	M-Neoplasm, Hypopharynx NOS
149.0	M-Neoplasm, Pharynx NOS
161.0	M-Neoplasm, Glottis
161.1	M-Neoplasm, Supraglottis
161.8	M-Neoplasm, Larynx NEC
195.0	M-Neoplasm, Head/face/neck
196.0	M-Neoplasm, Lymph head/neck/face
210.4	B-Neoplasm, Mouth NEC/NOS
210.6	B-Neoplasm, Oropharynx NEC
210.8	B-Neoplasm, Hypopharynx
212.1	B-Neoplasm, Larynx
231.0	CA in situ, Larynx
235.1	UB-Neoplasm, Oral cavity/pharynx
235.6	UB-Neoplasm, Larynx
464.0	Acute laryngitis
476.0	Chronic laryngitis
478.4	Polyp of vocal cord/larynx
478.5	Vocal cord disease NEC
478.74	Stenosis of larynx
478.79	Disease of larynx NEC
528.6	Leukoplakia of oral mucosa/tongue
784.1	Throat pain
784.2	Swelling in head/neck
784.49	Voice disturbance NEC
787.2	Dysphagia

REIMBURSEMENT INFORMATION

Medicare

- Follow–up Days — 0
- Assistant Surgeon — not paid
- Supply Charges — not allowed
- Outpatient Limit — does not apply
- Minor Surgery Rules Apply
- Fragments — 31535

CPT CODE	SERVICE
31540	Laryngoscopy, direct, operative, with excision of tumor and/or stripping of vocal cords or epiglottis

CPT NOTES

- For endoscopic procedures, code appropriate endoscopy of each anatomic site examined.

ICD–9–CM

141.0	M-Neoplasm, Tongue base
141.9	M-Neoplasm, Tongue NOS
142.0	M-Neoplasm, Parotid gland
145.0	M-Neoplasm, Cheek mucosa
145.3	M-Neoplasm, Soft palate
146.0	M-Neoplasm, Tonsil
148.9	M-Neoplasm, Hypopharynx NOS
149.0	M-Neoplasm, Pharynx NOS
161.0	M-Neoplasm, Glottis
161.1	M-Neoplasm, Supraglottis
161.8	M-Neoplasm, Larynx NEC
195.0	M-Neoplasm, Head/face/neck
196.0	M-Neoplasm, Lymph head/neck/face
210.2	B-Neoplasm, Major salivary glands
210.4	B-Neoplasm, Mouth NEC/NOS
210.6	B-Neoplasm, Oropharynx NEC
210.8	B-Neoplasm, Hypopharynx
210.9	B-Neoplasm, Pharynx NOS
212.1	B-Neoplasm, Larynx
231.0	CA in situ, Larynx
235.1	UB-Neoplasm, Oral cavity/pharynx
235.6	UB-Neoplasm, Larynx
476.0	Chronic laryngitis
478.4	Polyp of vocal cord/larynx
478.70	Disease of larynx NOS
478.74	Stenosis of larynx
528.6	Leukoplakia of oral mucosa/tongue

REIMBURSEMENT INFORMATION

Medicare

- Follow–up Days — 0
- Assistant Surgeon — not paid
- Supply Charges — not allowed
- Outpatient Limit — does not apply
- Minor Surgery Rules Apply

CPT CODE	SERVICE
31541	Laryngoscopy, direct, operative, with excision of tumor and/or stripping of vocal cords or epiglottis; with operating microscope

CPT NOTES

- For endoscopic procedures, code appropriate endoscopy of each anatomic site examined.

ICD–9–CM

141.0	M-Neoplasm, Tongue base
141.9	M-Neoplasm, Tongue NOS
142.0	M-Neoplasm, Parotid gland
145.0	M-Neoplasm, Cheek mucosa
145.3	M-Neoplasm, Soft palate
146.0	M-Neoplasm, Tonsil
148.9	M-Neoplasm, Hypopharynx NOS
149.0	M-Neoplasm, Pharynx NOS
161.0	M-Neoplasm, Glottis
161.1	M-Neoplasm, Supraglottis
161.8	M-Neoplasm, Larynx NEC
195.0	M-Neoplasm, Head/face/neck
196.0	M-Neoplasm, Lymph head/neck/face
210.2	B-Neoplasm, Major salivary glands
210.4	B-Neoplasm, Mouth NEC/NOS
210.6	B-Neoplasm, Oropharynx NEC
210.8	B-Neoplasm, Hypopharynx
210.9	B-Neoplasm, Pharynx NOS
212.1	B-Neoplasm, Larynx
231.0	CA in situ, Larynx
235.1	UB-Neoplasm, Oral cavity/pharynx
235.6	UB-Neoplasm, Larynx
476.0	Chronic laryngitis
478.4	Polyp of vocal cord/larynx
478.70	Disease of larynx NOS
478.74	Stenosis of larynx
528.6	Leukoplakia of oral mucosa/tongue

REIMBURSEMENT INFORMATION

Medicare

- Follow–up Days — 0
- Assistant Surgeon — not paid
- Supply Charges — not allowed
- Outpatient Limit — does not apply
- Minor Surgery Rules Apply
- Fragments — 31525, 31540

CPT CODE	SERVICE

31560 Laryngoscopy, direct, operative, with arytenoidectomy

31561 Laryngoscopy, direct, operative, with arytenoidectomy; with operating microscope

CPT NOTES

- For endoscopic procedures, code appropriate endoscopy of each anatomic site examined.

ICD–9–CM

161.0	M-Neoplasm, Glottis
161.1	M-Neoplasm, Supraglottis
161.2	M-Neoplasm, Subglottis
161.3	M-Neoplasm, Laryngeal cartilages
210.1	B-Neoplasm, Tongue
212.1	B-Neoplasm, Larynx
231.0	CA in situ, Larynx
235.1	UB-Neoplasm, Oral cavity/pharynx
235.6	UB-Neoplasm, Larynx

REIMBURSEMENT INFORMATION

Medicare

- Follow–up Days — 0
- Assistant Surgeon
  31560 — by report
  31561 — not paid
- Supply Charges — not allowed
- Outpatient Limit — does not apply
- Minor Surgery Rules Apply

31570 Laryngoscopy, direct, with injection into vocal cord(s), therapeutic

CPT NOTES

- For endoscopic procedures, code appropriate endoscopy of each anatomic site examined.

478.33	Vocal cord paralysis, bilat, part
784.49	Voice disturbance NEC

REIMBURSEMENT INFORMATION

Medicare

- Follow–up Days — 0
- Assistant Surgeon — not paid
- Supply Charges — not allowed
- Outpatient Limit — does not apply
- Minor Surgery Rules Apply

CPT CODE **SERVICE**

31571 Laryngoscopy, direct, with injection into vocal cord(s), therapeutic; with operating microscope

CPT NOTES

- For endoscopic procedures, code appropriate endoscopy of each anatomic site examined.

ICD–9–CM

161.0	M-Neoplasm, Glottis
161.1	M-Neoplasm, Supraglottis
161.2	M-Neoplasm, Subglottis
161.3	M-Neoplasm, Laryngeal cartilages
210.1	B-Neoplasm, Tongue
212.1	B-Neoplasm, Larynx
231.0	CA in situ, Larynx
235.1	UB-Neoplasm, Oral cavity/pharynx
235.6	UB-Neoplasm, Larynx

REIMBURSEMENT INFORMATION

Medicare

- Follow–up Days — 0
- Assistant Surgeon — not paid
- Supply Charges — not allowed
- Outpatient Limit — does not apply
- Minor Surgery Rules Apply

CPT CODE **SERVICE**

31575 Laryngoscopy, flexible fiberscopic; diagnostic

CPT NOTES

- For endoscopic procedures, code appropriate endoscopy of each anatomic site examined.

ICD–9–CM

161.0	M-Neoplasm, Glottis
161.1	M-Neoplasm, Supraglottis
161.2	M-Neoplasm, Subglottis
161.3	M-Neoplasm, Laryngeal cartilages
210.1	B-Neoplasm, Tongue
212.1	B-Neoplasm, Larynx
231.0	CA in situ, Larynx
235.1	UB-Neoplasm, Oral cavity/pharynx
235.6	UB-Neoplasm, Larynx
464.0	Acute laryngitis
464.10	Acute tracheitis, no obstruction
464.11	Acute tracheitis w/obstruction
464.20	Acute laryngotracheitis no obstruct
464.21	Acute laryngotracheitis w/obstruct
464.30	Acute epiglottitis, no obstruction
464.31	Acute epiglottitis w/obstruction
472.1	Chronic pharyngitis
472.2	Chronic nasopharyngitis
476.0	Chronic laryngitis
478.2x	Diseases of pharynx NEC
478.3x	Paralysis of vocal cords or larynx
478.4	Polyp of vocal cord/larynx
478.5	Vocal cord disease NEC
478.7x	Disease of larynx NEC
522.7	Periapical abscess w/sinus
527.6	Salivary gland mucocele
528.6	Leukoplakia of oral mucosa/tongue
748.2	Congenital laryngeal web anomaly
748.3	Congenital laryngotrach anomaly NEC
784.1	Throat pain
784.40	Voice disturbance NOS
784.49	Voice disturbance NEC
787.2	Dysphagia
933.0	Foreign body in pharynx
933.1	Foreign body in larynx

REIMBURSEMENT INFORMATION

Medicare

- Follow–up Days — 0
- Assistant Surgeon — not paid
- Supply Charges — not allowed
- Outpatient Limit — applies
- Minor Surgery Rules Apply

CPT CODE	SERVICE
31576	Laryngoscopy, flexible fiberscopic; with biopsy

CPT NOTES

- For endoscopic procedures, code appropriate endoscopy of each anatomic site examined.

ICD–9–CM

141.0	M-Neoplasm, Tongue base
141.9	M-Neoplasm, Tongue NOS
142.0	M-Neoplasm, Parotid gland
145.0	M-Neoplasm, Cheek mucosa
145.3	M-Neoplasm, Soft palate
146.0	M-Neoplasm, Tonsil
148.9	M-Neoplasm, Hypopharynx NOS
149.0	M-Neoplasm, Pharynx NOS
161.0	M-Neoplasm, Glottis
161.1	M-Neoplasm, Supraglottis
161.3	M-Neoplasm, Laryngeal cartilages
161.8	M-Neoplasm, Larynx NEC
195.0	M-Neoplasm, Head/face/neck
196.0	M-Neoplasm, Lymph head/neck/face
210.4	B-Neoplasm, Mouth NEC/NOS
210.6	B-Neoplasm, Oropharynx NEC
210.8	B-Neoplasm, Hypopharynx
212.1	B-Neoplasm, Larynx
231.0	CA in situ, Larynx
235.1	UB-Neoplasm, Oral cavity/pharynx
235.6	UB-Neoplasm, Larynx
464.0	Acute laryngitis
476.0	Chronic laryngitis
478.4	Polyp of vocal cord/larynx
478.5	Vocal cord disease NEC
478.74	Stenosis of larynx
478.79	Disease of larynx NEC
528.6	Leukoplakia of oral mucosa/tongue
784.1	Throat pain
784.2	Swelling in head/neck
784.49	Voice disturbance NEC
787.2	Dysphagia

REIMBURSEMENT INFORMATION

Medicare

- Follow–up Days — 0
- Assistant Surgeon — not paid
- Supply Charges — not allowed
- Outpatient Limit — does not apply
- Minor Surgery Rules Apply

CPT CODE SERVICE	ICD–9–CM
31577 Laryngoscopy, flexible fiberscopic; with removal of foreign body **CPT NOTES** ♦ For endoscopic procedures, code appropriate endoscopy of each anatomic site examined.	933.0 Foreign body in pharynx 933.1 Foreign body in larynx **REIMBURSEMENT INFORMATION** Medicare ♦ Follow–up Days — 0 ♦ Assistant Surgeon — not paid ♦ Supply Charges — not allowed ♦ Outpatient Limit — does not apply ♦ Minor Surgery Rules Apply
31578 Laryngoscopy, flexible fiberscopic; with removal of lesion **CPT NOTES** ♦ For endoscopic procedures, code appropriate endoscopy of each anatomic site examined.	161.3 M-Neoplasm, Laryngeal cartilages 212.1 B-Neoplasm, Larynx **REIMBURSEMENT INFORMATION** Medicare ♦ Follow–up Days — 0 ♦ Assistant Surgeon — by report ♦ Supply Charges — not allowed ♦ Outpatient Limit — does not apply ♦ Minor Surgery Rules Apply
31579 Laryngoscopy, flexible fiberoptic; with stroboscopy **CPT NOTES** ♦ For endoscopic procedures, code appropriate endoscopy of each anatomic site examined.	141.0 M-Neoplasm, Tongue base 235.1 UB-Neoplasm, Oral cavity/pharynx 464.20 Acute laryngotracheitis no obstruct 476.0 Chronic laryngitis 478.20 Disease of pharynx NOS 478.30 Vocal cord/larynx paralysis NOS 478.4 Polyp of vocal cord/larynx 478.6 Edema of larynx 478.70 Disease of larynx NOS 784.49 Voice disturbance NEC **REIMBURSEMENT INFORMATION** Medicare ♦ Follow–up Days — 0 ♦ Assistant Surgeon — not paid ♦ Supply Charges — not allowed ♦ Outpatient Limit — applies ♦ Minor Surgery Rules Apply

CPT CODE	SERVICE	ICD–9–CM
31580	Laryngoplasty; for laryngeal web, two stage, with keel insertion and removal	748.2 Congenital laryngeal web anomaly **REIMBURSEMENT INFORMATION** Medicare ◆ Follow–up Days — 90 ◆ Assistant Surgeon — paid ◆ Supply Charges — not allowed ◆ Outpatient Limit — does not apply ◆ Major Surgery Rules Apply
31582	Laryngoplasty; for laryngeal stenosis, with graft or core mold, including tracheotomy	478.74 Stenosis of larynx **REIMBURSEMENT INFORMATION** Medicare ◆ Follow–up Days — 90 ◆ Assistant Surgeon — paid ◆ Supply Charges — not allowed ◆ Outpatient Limit — does not apply ◆ Major Surgery Rules Apply
31584	Laryngoplasty; with open reduction of fracture	807.6 Fracture larynx/trachea-open **REIMBURSEMENT INFORMATION** Medicare ◆ Follow–up Days — 90 ◆ Assistant Surgeon — paid ◆ Supply Charges — not allowed ◆ Outpatient Limit — does not apply ◆ Major Surgery Rules Apply
31585 **31586**	Treatment of closed laryngeal fracture; without manipulation Treatment of closed laryngeal fracture; with closed manipulative reduction	807.5 Fracture larynx/trachea-closed **REIMBURSEMENT INFORMATION** Medicare ◆ Follow–up Days — 90 ◆ Assistant Surgeon — by report ◆ Supply Charges — not allowed ◆ Outpatient Limit — does not apply ◆ Major Surgery Rules Apply

CPT CODE	SERVICE	ICD-9-CM
31587	Laryngoplasty, cricoid split	478.74 Stenosis of larynx **REIMBURSEMENT INFORMATION** Medicare ♦ Follow-up Days — 90 ♦ Assistant Surgeon — paid ♦ Supply Charges — not allowed ♦ Outpatient Limit — does not apply ♦ Major Surgery Rules Apply
31588	Laryngoplasty, not otherwise specified (eg, for burns, reconstruction after partial laryngectomy)	478.32 Vocal cord paralysis, unilat, total 478.33 Vocal cord paralysis, bilat, part 784.49 Voice disturbance NEC 947.1 Burn of larynx, trachea, and lung **REIMBURSEMENT INFORMATION** Medicare ♦ Follow-up Days — 90 ♦ Assistant Surgeon — paid ♦ Supply Charges — not allowed ♦ Outpatient Limit — does not apply ♦ Major Surgery Rules Apply
31590	Laryngeal reinnervation by neuromuscular pedicle	478.32 Vocal cord paralysis, unilat, total 478.33 Vocal cord paralysis, bilat, part **REIMBURSEMENT INFORMATION** Medicare ♦ Follow-up Days — 90 ♦ Assistant Surgeon — paid ♦ Supply Charges — not allowed ♦ Outpatient Limit — does not apply ♦ Major Surgery Rules Apply

CPT CODE	SERVICE
31599	Unlisted procedure, larynx

ICD–9–CM

193.	M-Neoplasm, Thyroid gland
226.	B-Neoplasm, Thyroid gland
246.9	Disorder of thyroid NOS
464.0	Acute laryngitis
478.32	Vocal cord paralysis, unilat, total

REIMBURSEMENT INFORMATION

Medicare

- Follow–up Days — determined by local carrier
- Assistant Surgeon — determined by local carrier
- Supply Charges — determined by local carrier
- Outpatient Limit — determined by local carrier

CPT CODE	SERVICE	ICD–9–CM	
31600	Tracheostomy, planned (separate procedure)	141.0	M-Neoplasm, Tongue base
		146.0	M-Neoplasm, Tonsil
		148.9	M-Neoplasm, Hypopharynx NOS
		161.0	M-Neoplasm, Glottis
		161.1	M-Neoplasm, Supraglottis
		161.8	M-Neoplasm, Larynx NEC
		212.1	B-Neoplasm, Larynx
		235.1	UB-Neoplasm, Oral cavity/pharynx
		239.1	Respiratory system neoplasm NOS
		416.9	Chronic pulmonary heart disease NOS
		478.5	Vocal cord disease NEC
		478.6	Edema of larynx
		478.74	Stenosis of larynx
		478.79	Disease of larynx NEC
		486.	Pneumonia, organism NOS
		518.5	Post traum pulmonary insufficiency
		518.8	Diseases of lung
		518.81	Respiratory failure
		518.82	Other pulmonary insufficiency
		519.0	Tracheostomy complication
		519.1	Trachea/bronchus disease NEC
		519.8	Respiratory system disease NEC
		519.9	Respiratory system disease NOS
		786.09	Respiratory abnormality NEC
		799.0	Asphyxia
		799.1	Respiratory arrest
		852.20	Traumatic subdural hemorrhage
		V46.1	Respirator dependence

REIMBURSEMENT INFORMATION

General

- Separate procedure rules apply.

Medicare

- Follow–up Days — 0
- Assistant Surgeon — not paid
- Supply Charges — not allowed
- Outpatient Limit — does not apply
- Minor Surgery Rules Apply

CPT CODE	SERVICE	ICD–9–CM
31601	Tracheostomy, planned (separate procedure); under two years	478.6 Edema of larynx 478.74 Stenosis of larynx 478.79 Disease of larynx NEC 519.0 Tracheostomy complication 519.1 Trachea/bronchus disease NEC 786.09 Respiratory abnormality NEC V46.1 Respirator dependence **REIMBURSEMENT INFORMATION** <u>General</u> ◆ Separate procedure rules apply. <u>Medicare</u> ◆ Follow–up Days — 0 ◆ Assistant Surgeon — paid ◆ Supply Charges — not allowed ◆ Outpatient Limit — does not apply ◆ Minor Surgery Rules Apply
31603 **31605**	Tracheostomy, emergency procedure; transtracheal Tracheostomy, emergency procedure; cricothyroid membrane	518.81 Respiratory failure 518.82 Other pulmonary insufficiency 519.0 Tracheostomy complication 519.8 Respiratory system disease NEC 784.8 Hemorrhage from throat 786.09 Respiratory abnormality NEC 799.0 Asphyxia 799.1 Respiratory arrest 874.8 Open wound of neck NEC 933.0 Foreign body in pharynx 933.1 Foreign body in larynx 934.0 Foreign body, trachea 959.0 Face and neck injury NOS 989.5 Toxic effect of venom **REIMBURSEMENT INFORMATION** <u>Medicare</u> ◆ Follow–up Days — 0 ◆ Assistant Surgeon — not paid ◆ Supply Charges — not allowed ◆ Outpatient Limit — does not apply ◆ Minor Surgery Rules Apply

CPT CODE	SERVICE	ICD–9–CM

31610 Tracheostomy, fenestration procedure with skin flaps

CPT NOTES

- For endotracheal intubation, see 31500.
- For tracheal aspiration under direct vision, see 31515.

212.1	B-Neoplasm, Larynx
480.1	Respiratory syncytial viral pneum
486.	Pneumonia, organism NOS
519.0	Tracheostomy complication
519.1	Trachea/bronchus disease NEC
748.3	Congenital laryngotrach anomaly NEC
786.09	Respiratory abnormality NEC

REIMBURSEMENT INFORMATION

Medicare

- Follow–up Days — 90
- Assistant Surgeon — not paid
- Supply Charges — not allowed
- Outpatient Limit — does not apply
- Major Surgery Rules Apply

31611 Construction of tracheoesophageal fistula and subsequent insertion of an alaryngeal speech prosthesis (eg, voice button, Blom-Singer prosthesis)

161.0	M-Neoplasm, Glottis
161.1	M-Neoplasm, Supraglottis
161.2	M-Neoplasm, Subglottis
161.3	M-Neoplasm, Laryngeal cartilages
161.8	M-Neoplasm, Larynx NEC
161.9	M-Neoplasm, Larynx NOS
162.0	M-Neoplasm, Trachea
V52.8	Fit/adjust prosthetic device NEC

REIMBURSEMENT INFORMATION

Medicare

- Follow–up Days — 90
- Assistant Surgeon — paid
- Supply Charges — not allowed
- Outpatient Limit — does not apply
- Major Surgery Rules Apply

▲ **31612** Tracheal puncture, percutaneous with transtracheal aspiration and/or injection

486.	Pneumonia, organism NOS
519.0	Tracheostomy complication

REIMBURSEMENT INFORMATION

General

- Description changed in 1995 CPT.

Medicare

- Follow–up Days — 0
- Assistant Surgeon — not paid
- Supply Charges — not allowed
- Outpatient Limit — does not apply
- Minor Surgery Rules Apply

CPT CODE	SERVICE	ICD–9–CM
31613	Tracheostoma revision; simple, without flap rotation	519.0 Tracheostomy complication 519.8 Respiratory system disease NEC V55.0 Attention to tracheostomy **REIMBURSEMENT INFORMATION** Medicare ◆ Follow–up Days — 90 ◆ Assistant Surgeon — not paid ◆ Supply Charges — not allowed ◆ Outpatient Limit — does not apply ◆ Major Surgery Rules Apply
31614	Tracheostoma revision; complex, with flap rotation	478.79 Disease of larynx NEC 519.0 Tracheostomy complication 519.8 Respiratory system disease NEC V55.0 Attention to tracheostomy **REIMBURSEMENT INFORMATION** Medicare ◆ Follow–up Days — 90 ◆ Assistant Surgeon — not paid ◆ Supply Charges — not allowed ◆ Outpatient Limit — does not apply ◆ Major Surgery Rules Apply

CPT CODE **SERVICE**

31700 Catheterization, transglottic (separate procedure)

CPT RULES

- For endotracheal intubation, see 31500.
- For tracheal aspiration under direct vision, see 31515.

ICD–9–CM

427.5	Cardiac arrest
466.0	Acute bronchitis
466.1	Acute bronchiolitis
478.30	Vocal cord/larynx paralysis NOS
478.6	Edema of larynx
478.74	Stenosis of larynx
482.1	Pseudomonal pneumonia
518.5	Post traum pulmonary insufficiency
518.81	Respiratory failure
518.82	Other pulmonary insufficiency
748.3	Congenital laryngotrach anomaly NEC
770.0	NB Congenital pneumonia
770.1	NB meconium aspiration syndrome
770.2	NB interstitial emphysema
770.6	NB transitory tachypnea
770.8	Post-birth resp problem NEC
770.9	NB respiratory condition NOS
776.1	Neonatal thrombocytopenia
799.1	Respiratory arrest

REIMBURSEMENT INFORMATION

General

- Separate procedure rules apply.

Medicare

- Follow–up Days — 0
- Assistant Surgeon — not paid
- Supply Charges — not allowed
- Outpatient Limit — does not apply
- Minor Surgery Rules Apply

31730 Transtracheal (percutaneous) introduction of needle wire dilator/stent or indwelling tube for oxygen therapy

CPT NOTES

- For endotracheal intubation, see 31500.
- For tracheal aspiration under direct vision, see 31515.

478.74	Stenosis of larynx
478.79	Disease of larynx NEC

REIMBURSEMENT INFORMATION

Medicare

- Follow–up Days — 0
- Assistant Surgeon — paid
- Supply Charges — not allowed
- Outpatient Limit — does not apply
- Minor Surgery Rules Apply

CPT CODE	SERVICE	ICD–9–CM
31750	Tracheoplasty; cervical	161.0 M-Neoplasm, Glottis 161.1 M-Neoplasm, Supraglottis 161.2 M-Neoplasm, Subglottis 161.3 M-Neoplasm, Laryngeal cartilages 161.8 M-Neoplasm, Larynx NEC 162.0 M-Neoplasm, Trachea
31755	Tracheoplasty; tracheopharyngeal fistulization, each stage	

REIMBURSEMENT INFORMATION

Medicare

- Follow–up Days — 90
- Assistant Surgeon — paid
- Supply Charges — not allowed
- Outpatient Limit — does not apply
- Major Surgery Rules Apply

CPT CODE	SERVICE	ICD–9–CM
31766	Carinal reconstruction	162.2 M-Neoplasm, Main bronchus 197.3 M2-Neoplasm, Respiratory NEC

REIMBURSEMENT INFORMATION

Medicare

- Follow–up Days — 90
- Assistant Surgeon — paid
- Supply Charges — not allowed
- Outpatient Limit — does not apply
- Major Surgery Rules Apply

CPT CODE	SERVICE	ICD–9–CM
▲ **31800**	Suture of tracheal wound or injury; cervical	874.00 Open wound of larynx w/trachea 874.01 Open wound of larynx 874.02 Open wound of trachea 874.10 Open wound larynx w/trachea, compl 874.12 Open wound of trachea, complicated 874.8 Open wound of neck NEC 874.9 Open wound of neck NEC, complicated
▲ **31805**	Suture of tracheal wound or injury; intrathoracic	

REIMBURSEMENT INFORMATION

General

- Description changed in 1995 CPT.

Medicare

- Follow–up Days — 90
- Assistant Surgeon
  31800 — by report
  31805 — paid
- Supply Charges — not allowed
- Outpatient Limit — does not apply
- Major Surgery Rules Apply

CPT CODE	SERVICE	ICD-9-CM
31820	Surgical closure tracheostomy or fistula; without plastic repair	519.0 Tracheostomy complication 748.3 Congenital laryngotrach anomaly NEC 786.09 Respiratory abnormality NEC
31825	Surgical closure tracheostomy or fistula; with plastic repair	

CPT NOTES

- For repair tracheosophageal fistula, see 43305, 43312.

REIMBURSEMENT INFORMATION

Medicare

- Follow-up Days — 90
- Assistant Surgeon — not paid
- Supply Charges — not allowed
- Outpatient Limit — does not apply
- Major Surgery Rules Apply

31830 Revision of tracheostomy scar

519.0 Tracheostomy complication
701.4 Keloid scar
709.2 Scar/fibrosis of skin

REIMBURSEMENT INFORMATION

Medicare

- Follow-up Days — 90
- Assistant Surgeon — not paid
- Supply Charges — not allowed
- Outpatient Limit — does not apply
- Major Surgery Rules Apply

31899 Unlisted procedure, trachea, bronchi

464.10 Acute tracheitis, no obstruction
476.0 Chronic laryngitis
478.34 Vocal cord paralysis, bilat, total
478.74 Stenosis of larynx
478.79 Disease of larynx NEC
508.9 Respiratory cond, ext agent NOS
519.0 Tracheostomy complication
786.09 Respiratory abnormality NEC
787.2 Dysphagia
V55.0 Attention to tracheostomy

REIMBURSEMENT INFORMATION

Medicare

- Follow-up Days — determined by local carrier
- Assistant Surgeon — determined by local carrier
- Supply Charges — determined by local carrier
- Outpatient Limit — determined by local carrier

CPT CODE	SERVICE	ICD–9–CM	
32820	Major reconstruction, chest wall (post-traumatic)	875.0	Open wound of chest
		875.1	Open wound of chest, complicated

REIMBURSEMENT INFORMATION

Medicare

- Follow–up Days — 90
- Assistant Surgeon — paid
- Supply Charges — not allowed
- Outpatient Limit — does not apply
- Major Surgery Rules Apply

CPT CODE	SERVICE
35800	Exploration for postoperative hemorrhage, thrombosis or infection; neck

CPT NOTES

- Selective vascular catheterizations should be coded to include introduction and all lesser order selective catheterizations used in the approach (e.g., the description for a selective right middle cerebral artery catheterization includes the introduction and placement catheterization of the right common and internal carotid arteries).
- Additional second and/or third order arterial catheterizations within the same family of arteries supplied by a single first order artery should be expressed by 36218 or 36248. Additional first order or higher catheterizations in vascular families supplied by a first order vessel different from a previously selected and coded family should be separately coded using the conventions described above.
- For monitoring, operation of pump and other nonsurgical services, see 99190-99192, 99291, 99292, 99354-99360.
- For other medical or laboratory related services, see appropriate section.
- For radiological supervision and interpretation, see 75600-75978.
- Primary vascular procedure listings include establishing both inflow and outflow by whatever procedures necessary. Also included is that portion of the operative arteriogram performed by the surgeon, as indicated. Sympathectomy, when done, is included in the listed aortic procedures. For unlisted vascular procedure, use 37799.

ICD–9–CM

874.8	Open wound of neck NEC
874.9	Open wound of neck NEC, complicated
998.1	Hemorrhage complicating a procedure

REIMBURSEMENT INFORMATION

Medicare

- Follow–up Days — 90
- Assistant Surgeon — paid
- Supply Charges — not allowed
- Outpatient Limit — does not apply
- Major Surgery Rules Apply

CPT CODE	SERVICE	ICD-9-CM	
35820	Exploration for postoperative hemorrhage, thrombosis or infection; chest	875.1	Open wound of chest, complicated
		998.1	Hemorrhage complicating a procedure

CPT NOTES

- Selective vascular catheterizations should be coded to include introduction and all lesser order selective catheterizations used in the approach (e.g., the description for a selective right middle cerebral artery catheterization includes the introduction and placement catheterization of the right common and internal carotid arteries).
- Additional second and/or third order arterial catheterizations within the same family of arteries supplied by a single first order artery should be expressed by 36218 or 36248. Additional first order or higher catheterizations in vascular families supplied by a first order vessel different from a previously selected and coded family should be separately coded using the conventions described above.
- For monitoring, operation of pump and other nonsurgical services, see 99190-99192, 99291, 99292, 99354-99360.
- For other medical or laboratory related services, see appropriate section.
- For radiological supervision and interpretation, see 75600-75978.
- Primary vascular procedure listings include establishing both inflow and outflow by whatever procedures necessary. Also included is that portion of the operative arteriogram performed by the surgeon, as indicated. Sympathectomy, when done, is included in the listed aortic procedures. For unlisted vascular procedure, use 37799.

REIMBURSEMENT INFORMATION

Medicare

- Follow–up Days — 90
- Assistant Surgeon — paid
- Supply Charges — not allowed
- Outpatient Limit — does not apply
- Major Surgery Rules Apply

CPT CODE **SERVICE**

35840 Exploration for postoperative hemorrhage, thrombosis or infection; abdomen

CPT NOTES

- Selective vascular catheterizations should be coded to include introduction and all lesser order selective catheterizations used in the approach (e.g., the description for a selective right middle cerebral artery catheterization includes the introduction and placement catheterization of the right common and internal carotid arteries).
- Additional second and/or third order arterial catheterizations within the same family of arteries supplied by a single first order artery should be expressed by 36218 or 36248. Additional first order or higher catheterizations in vascular families supplied by a first order vessel different from a previously selected and coded family should be separately coded using the conventions described above.
- For monitoring, operation of pump and other nonsurgical services, see 99190-99192, 99291, 99292, 99354-99360.
- For other medical or laboratory related services, see appropriate section.
- For radiological supervision and interpretation, see 75600-75978.
- Primary vascular procedure listings include establishing both inflow and outflow by whatever procedures necessary. Also included is that portion of the operative arteriogram performed by the surgeon, as indicated. Sympathectomy, when done, is included in the listed aortic procedures. For unlisted vascular procedure, use 37799.

ICD-9-CM

998.1 Hemorrhage complicating a procedure

REIMBURSEMENT INFORMATION

Medicare

- Follow-up Days — 90
- Assistant Surgeon — paid
- Supply Charges — not allowed
- Outpatient Limit — does not apply
- Major Surgery Rules Apply

CPT CODE	SERVICE
35860	Exploration for postoperative hemorrhage, thrombosis or infection; extremity

CPT NOTES

- Selective vascular catheterizations should be coded to include introduction and all lesser order selective catheterizations used in the approach (e.g., the description for a selective right middle cerebral artery catheterization includes the introduction and placement catheterization of the right common and internal carotid arteries).
- Additional second and/or third order arterial catheterizations within the same family of arteries supplied by a single first order artery should be expressed by 36218 or 36248. Additional first order or higher catheterizations in vascular families supplied by a first order vessel different from a previously selected and coded family should be separately coded using the conventions described above.
- For monitoring, operation of pump and other nonsurgical services, see 99190-99192, 99291, 99292, 99354-99360.
- For other medical or laboratory related services, see appropriate section.
- For radiological supervision and interpretation, see 75600-75978.
- Primary vascular procedure listings include establishing both inflow and outflow by whatever procedures necessary. Also included is that portion of the operative arteriogram performed by the surgeon, as indicated. Sympathectomy, when done, is included in the listed aortic procedures. For unlisted vascular procedure, use 37799.

ICD–9–CM

996.91	Complication, reattached forearm
996.92	Complication, reattached hand
996.93	Complication, reattached finger
996.94	Complication, reattached arm NEC
996.95	Complication, reattached foot/toe
996.96	Complication, reattached leg NEC
998.1	Hemorrhage complicating a procedure

REIMBURSEMENT INFORMATION

Medicare

- Follow–up Days — 90
- Assistant Surgeon — paid
- Supply Charges — not allowed
- Outpatient Limit — does not apply
- Major Surgery Rules Apply

CPT CODE **SERVICE**

35875 Thrombectomy of arterial or venous graft

CPT NOTES

- Selective vascular catheterizations should be coded to include introduction and all lesser order selective catheterizations used in the approach (e.g., the description for a selective right middle cerebral artery catheterization includes the introduction and placement catheterization of the right common and internal carotid arteries).
- Additional second and/or third order arterial catheterizations within the same family of arteries supplied by a single first order artery should be expressed by 36218 or 36248. Additional first order or higher catheterizations in vascular families supplied by a first order vessel different from a previously selected and coded family should be separately coded using the conventions described above.
- For monitoring, operation of pump and other nonsurgical services, see 99190-99192, 99291, 99292, 99354-99360.
- For other medical or laboratory related services, see appropriate section.
- For radiological supervision and interpretation, see 75600-75978.
- Primary vascular procedure listings include establishing both inflow and outflow by whatever procedures necessary. Also included is that portion of the operative arteriogram performed by the surgeon, as indicated. Sympathectomy, when done, is included in the listed aortic procedures. For unlisted vascular procedure, use 37799.

ICD–9–CM

443.9	Peripheral vascular disease NOS
444.21	Upper extremity embolism
444.22	Lower extremity embolism
996.52	Other tissue graft malfunction
996.62	Reaction to oth vascular dev/graft

REIMBURSEMENT INFORMATION

Medicare

- Follow–up Days — 90
- Assistant Surgeon — paid
- Supply Charges — not allowed
- Outpatient Limit — does not apply
- Major Surgery Rules Apply

CPT CODE	SERVICE
40490	Biopsy of lip

CPT NOTES

- For procedures on skin of lips, see 10040 et seq.

ICD–9–CM

079.9	Viral/chlamydial infection NOS
140.0	M-Neoplasm, Upper lip, vermilion
140.1	M-Neoplasm, Lower lip, vermilion
140.3	M-Neoplasm, Upper lip, inner aspect
140.4	M-Neoplasm, Lower lip, inner aspect
140.5	M-Neoplasm, Lip NOS, inner NOS
140.6	M-Neoplasm, lip, commissure
140.8	M-Neoplasm, Lip NEC
140.9	M-Neoplasm, Lip/vermilion NOS
149.8	M-Neoplasm, Oral cavity/pharynx NEC
172.0	Malignant melanoma, Lip
173.0	M-Neoplasm, Skin of lip
210.0	B-Neoplasm, Lip
210.1	B-Neoplasm, Tongue
210.4	B-Neoplasm, Mouth NEC/NOS
216.0	B-Neoplasm, Skin of lip
228.01	Hemangioma, Skin
230.0	CA in situ, Oral cavity/pharynx
232.0	CA in situ, Skin of lip
235.1	UB-Neoplasm, Oral cavity/pharynx
238.2	UB-Neoplasm, Skin
239.0	Digestive neoplasm NOS
527.2	Sialoadenitis
527.6	Salivary gland mucocele
527.7	Salivary secretion disturbance
528.0	Stomatitis
528.5	Diseases of lips
528.6	Leukoplakia of oral mucosa/tongue
528.7	Oral epithelium disturbance NEC
528.9	Oral soft tissue disease NEC
706.2	Sebaceous cyst
710.2	Sicca syndrome

REIMBURSEMENT INFORMATION

Medicare

- Follow–up Days — 0
- Assistant Surgeon — not paid
- Supply Charges — not allowed
- Outpatient Limit — applies
- Minor Surgery Rules Apply

CPT CODE	SERVICE	ICD–9–CM

40500 Vermilionectomy (lip shave), with mucosal advancement

CPT NOTES

- ♦ For procedures on skin of lips, see 10040 et seq.

140.0	M-Neoplasm, Upper lip, vermilion
172.0	Malignant melanoma, Lip
210.0	B-Neoplasm, Lip
216.0	B-Neoplasm, Skin of lip
230.0	CA in situ, Oral cavity/pharynx
232.0	CA in situ, Skin of lip
235.1	UB-Neoplasm, Oral cavity/pharynx
528.6	Leukoplakia of oral mucosa/tongue

REIMBURSEMENT INFORMATION

Medicare

- ♦ Follow–up Days — 90
- ♦ Assistant Surgeon — not paid
- ♦ Supply Charges — not allowed
- ♦ Outpatient Limit — does not apply
- ♦ Major Surgery Rules Apply

40510 Excision of lip; transverse wedge excision with primary closure

CPT NOTES

- ♦ For procedures on skin of lips, see 10040 et seq.
- ♦ For excision of mucous lesions, see 40810-40816.

140.0	M-Neoplasm, Upper lip, vermilion
140.1	M-Neoplasm, Lower lip, vermilion
140.3	M-Neoplasm, Upper lip, inner aspect
140.4	M-Neoplasm, Lower lip, inner aspect
140.5	M-Neoplasm, Lip NOS, inner NOS
140.6	M-Neoplasm, lip, commissure
140.8	M-Neoplasm, Lip NEC
140.9	M-Neoplasm, Lip/vermilion NOS
172.0	Malignant melanoma, Lip
173.0	M-Neoplasm, Skin of lip
195.0	M-Neoplasm, Head/face/neck
210.0	B-Neoplasm, Lip
216.0	B-Neoplasm, Skin of lip
228.01	Hemangioma, Skin
230.0	CA in situ, Oral cavity/pharynx
235.1	UB-Neoplasm, Oral cavity/pharynx
528.5	Diseases of lips

REIMBURSEMENT INFORMATION

Medicare

- ♦ Follow–up Days — 90
- ♦ Assistant Surgeon — not paid
- ♦ Supply Charges — not allowed
- ♦ Outpatient Limit — does not apply
- ♦ Major Surgery Rules Apply

CPT CODE	SERVICE	ICD–9–CM

40520 Excision of lip; V-excision with primary direct linear closure

CPT NOTES

- ♦ For procedures on skin of lips, see 10040 et seq.
- ♦ For excision of mucous lesions, see 40810-40816.

140.0	M-Neoplasm, Upper lip, vermilion
140.1	M-Neoplasm, Lower lip, vermilion
140.3	M-Neoplasm, Upper lip, inner aspect
140.4	M-Neoplasm, Lower lip, inner aspect
140.5	M-Neoplasm, Lip NOS, inner NOS
140.6	M-Neoplasm, lip, commissure
140.8	M-Neoplasm, Lip NEC
140.9	M-Neoplasm, Lip/vermilion NOS
172.0	Malignant melanoma, Lip
173.0	M-Neoplasm, Skin of lip
195.0	M-Neoplasm, Head/face/neck
228.01	Hemangioma, Skin
235.1	UB-Neoplasm, Oral cavity/pharynx
710.2	Sicca syndrome

REIMBURSEMENT INFORMATION

Medicare

- ♦ Follow–up Days — 90
- ♦ Assistant Surgeon — not paid
- ♦ Supply Charges — not allowed
- ♦ Outpatient Limit — does not apply
- ♦ Major Surgery Rules Apply

40525 Excision of lip; full thickness, reconstruction with local flap (eg, Estlander or fan)

40527 Excision of lip; full thickness, reconstruction with cross lip flap (Abbe-Estlander)

CPT NOTES

- ♦ For procedures on skin of lips, see 10040 et seq.

140.0	M-Neoplasm, Upper lip, vermilion
140.1	M-Neoplasm, Lower lip, vermilion
140.3	M-Neoplasm, Upper lip, inner aspect
140.4	M-Neoplasm, Lower lip, inner aspect
140.5	M-Neoplasm, Lip NOS, inner NOS
140.6	M-Neoplasm, lip, commissure
140.8	M-Neoplasm, Lip NEC
140.9	M-Neoplasm, Lip/vermilion NOS
172.0	Malignant melanoma, Lip
173.0	M-Neoplasm, Skin of lip
195.0	M-Neoplasm, Head/face/neck
235.1	UB-Neoplasm, Oral cavity/pharynx
873.53	Open wound of lip, complicated

REIMBURSEMENT INFORMATION

Medicare

- ♦ Follow–up Days — 90
- ♦ Assistant Surgeon — not paid
- ♦ Supply Charges — not allowed
- ♦ Outpatient Limit — does not apply
- ♦ Major Surgery Rules Apply

CPT CODE	SERVICE	ICD–9–CM

40530 Resection of lip, more than one-fourth, without reconstruction

CPT NOTES

- For procedures on skin of lips, see 10040 et seq.
- For reconstruction, see 13131 et seq.

140.0	M-Neoplasm, Upper lip, vermilion
140.1	M-Neoplasm, Lower lip, vermilion
140.3	M-Neoplasm, Upper lip, inner aspect
140.4	M-Neoplasm, Lower lip, inner aspect
140.5	M-Neoplasm, Lip NOS, inner NOS
140.6	M-Neoplasm, lip, commissure
140.8	M-Neoplasm, Lip NEC
140.9	M-Neoplasm, Lip/vermilion NOS
172.0	Malignant melanoma, Lip
173.0	M-Neoplasm, Skin of lip
195.0	M-Neoplasm, Head/face/neck
210.0	B-Neoplasm, Lip
235.1	UB-Neoplasm, Oral cavity/pharynx

REIMBURSEMENT INFORMATION

Medicare

- Follow–up Days — 90
- Assistant Surgeon — not paid
- Supply Charges — not allowed
- Outpatient Limit — does not apply
- Major Surgery Rules Apply

40650 Repair lip, full thickness; vermilion only

CPT NOTES

- For procedures on skin of lips, see 10040 et seq.

140.0	M-Neoplasm, Upper lip, vermilion
140.1	M-Neoplasm, Lower lip, vermilion
140.9	M-Neoplasm, Lip/vermilion NOS
173.0	M-Neoplasm, Skin of lip
873.43	Open wound of lip
873.53	Open wound of lip, complicated
873.59	Open wound of face NEC, complicated
941.33	3rd deg burn, lip
998.2	Accidental op laceration/puncture
998.3	Postop wound disruption

REIMBURSEMENT INFORMATION

Medicare

- Follow–up Days — 90
- Assistant Surgeon — not paid
- Supply Charges — not allowed
- Outpatient Limit — does not apply
- Major Surgery Rules Apply

CPT CODE	SERVICE	ICD-9-CM
40652	Repair lip, full thickness; up to half vertical height	
40654	Repair lip, full thickness; over one half vertical height, or complex	

140.0 M-Neoplasm, Upper lip, vermilion
140.1 M-Neoplasm, Lower lip, vermilion
140.3 M-Neoplasm, Upper lip, inner aspect
140.4 M-Neoplasm, Lower lip, inner aspect
140.5 M-Neoplasm, Lip NOS, inner NOS
140.6 M-Neoplasm, lip, commissure
140.8 M-Neoplasm, Lip NEC
173.0 M-Neoplasm, Skin of lip
873.43 Open wound of lip
873.53 Open wound of lip, complicated
873.59 Open wound of face NEC, complicated
941.33 3rd deg burn, lip
998.2 Accidental op laceration/puncture
998.3 Postop wound disruption

CPT NOTES

- For procedures on skin of lips, see 10040 et seq.

REIMBURSEMENT INFORMATION

Medicare

- Follow–up Days — 90
- Assistant Surgeon — not paid
- Supply Charges — not allowed
- Outpatient Limit — does not apply
- Major Surgery Rules Apply

40700 Plastic repair of cleft lip/nasal deformity; primary, partial or complete, unilateral

40701 Plastic repair of cleft lip/nasal deformity; primary bilateral, one stage procedure

749.10 Cleft lip NOS
749.11 Unilateral cleft lip, complete
749.12 Unilateral cleft lip, incomplete
749.20 Cleft palate w/cleft lip NOS
749.21 Unilat cleft palate/lip, complete
749.22 Unilat cleft palate/lip, incomplete
749.25 Cleft palate w/cleft lip NEC
V13.6 Hx of congenital malformation

CPT NOTES

- For procedures on skin of lips, see 10040 et seq.
- To report rhinoplasty only for nasal deformity secondary to congenital cleft lip, see 30460, 30462.
- For repiar cleft palate, see 42000 et seq.
- For other reconstructive procedures, see 14060, 14061, 15120-15261, 15574, 15576, 15630.

REIMBURSEMENT INFORMATION

Medicare

- Follow–up Days — 90
- Assistant Surgeon — not paid
- Supply Charges — not allowed
- Outpatient Limit — does not apply
- Major Surgery Rules Apply

CPT CODE	SERVICE	ICD-9-CM

40702 Plastic repair of cleft lip/nasal deformity; primary bilateral, one of two stages

CPT NOTES

- For procedures on skin of lips, see 10040 et seq.
- To report rhinoplasty only for nasal deformity secondary to congenital cleft lip, see 30460, 30462.
- For repair cleft palate, see 42000 et seq.
- For other reconstructive procedures, see 14060, 14061, 15120-15261, 15574, 15576, 15630.

749.10	Cleft lip NOS
749.13	Bilateral cleft lip, complete
749.14	Bilateral cleft lip, incomplete
749.2x	Cleft palate w/cleft lip
V13.6	Hx of congenital malformation

REIMBURSEMENT INFORMATION

Medicare

- Follow–up Days — 90
- Assistant Surgeon — paid
- Supply Charges — not allowed
- Outpatient Limit — does not apply
- Major Surgery Rules Apply

40720 Plastic repair of cleft lip/nasal deformity; secondary, by recreation of defect and reclosure

CPT NOTES

- For procedures on skin of lips, see 10040 et seq.
- To report rhinoplasty only for nasal deformity secondary to congenital cleft lip, see 30460, 30462.
- For repair cleft palate, see 42000 et seq.
- For other reconstructive procedures, see 14060, 14061, 15120-15261, 15574, 15576, 15630.

749.10	Cleft lip NOS
749.11	Unilateral cleft lip, complete
749.12	Unilateral cleft lip, incomplete
749.25	Cleft palate w/cleft lip NEC
749.2x	Cleft palate w/cleft lip
V13.6	Hx of congenital malformation

REIMBURSEMENT INFORMATION

Medicare

- Follow–up Days — 90
- Assistant Surgeon — by report
- Supply Charges — not allowed
- Outpatient Limit — does not apply
- Major Surgery Rules Apply

CPT CODE	SERVICE	ICD–9–CM

40761 Plastic repair of cleft lip; with cross lip pedicle flap (Abbe- Estlander type), including sectioning and inserting of pedicle

CPT NOTES

- ♦ For procedures on skin of lips, see 10040 et seq.
- ♦ For repair cleft palate, see 42000 et seq.
- ♦ For other reconstructive procedures, see 14060, 14061, 15120-15261, 15574, 15576, 15630.

749.10 Cleft lip NOS
749.11 Unilateral cleft lip, complete
749.13 Bilateral cleft lip, complete
749.14 Bilateral cleft lip, incomplete
749.20 Cleft palate w/cleft lip NOS
749.21 Unilat cleft palate/lip, complete
749.23 Bilat cleft palate/lip, complete
749.24 Bilat cleft palate/lip, incomplete
749.25 Cleft palate w/cleft lip NEC
V13.6 Hx of congenital malformation

REIMBURSEMENT INFORMATION

Medicare

- ♦ Follow–up Days — 90
- ♦ Assistant Surgeon — paid
- ♦ Supply Charges — not allowed
- ♦ Outpatient Limit — does not apply
- ♦ Major Surgery Rules Apply

40799 Unlisted procedure, lips

CPT NOTES

- ♦ For procedures on skin of lips, see 10040 et seq.

144.0 M-Neoplasm, Anterior floor of mouth
160.2 M-Neoplasm, Maxillary sinus
228.00 Hemangioma NOS
229.8 Benign neoplasm NEC

REIMBURSEMENT INFORMATION

Medicare

- ♦ Follow–up Days — determined by local carrier
- ♦ Assistant Surgeon — determined by local carrier
- ♦ Supply Charges — determined by local carrier
- ♦ Outpatient Limit — determined by local carrier

CPT CODE **SERVICE**

40800* Drainage of abscess, cyst, hematoma, vestibule of mouth; simple

CPT NOTES

- The vestibule is the part of the oral cavity outside the dentoalveolar structures; it includes the mucosal and submucosal tissue of lips and cheeks.

ICD–9–CM

522.0	Pulpitis
522.5	Periapical abscess w/o sinus
522.7	Periapical abscess w/sinus
522.8	Radicular cyst
523.3	Acute periodontitis
525.2	Atrophy, edentulous alveolar ridge
526.0	Developmental odontogenic cysts
526.1	Fissural cysts of jaw
526.2	Jaw cysts NEC
526.4	Inflammation of jaw
527.2	Sialoadenitis
527.3	Salivary gland abscess
527.4	Salivary gland fistula
527.6	Salivary gland mucocele
528.3	Cellulitis/abscess of mouth
528.4	Oral soft tissue cyst
528.5	Diseases of lips
528.7	Oral epithelium disturbance NEC
528.9	Oral soft tissue disease NEC
920.	Contusion face/scalp/neck

REIMBURSEMENT INFORMATION

General

- Starred procedure.

Medicare

- Follow–up Days — 10
- Assistant Surgeon — not paid
- Supply Charges — not allowed
- Outpatient Limit — applies
- Minor Surgery Rules Apply

CPT CODE	SERVICE
40801	Drainage of abscess, cyst, hematoma, vestibule of mouth; complicated

CPT NOTES

- The vestibule is the part of the oral cavity outside the dentoalveolar structures; it includes the mucosal and submucosal tissue of lips and cheeks.

ICD–9–CM

522.0	Pulpitis
522.5	Periapical abscess w/o sinus
522.7	Periapical abscess w/sinus
522.8	Radicular cyst
523.3	Acute periodontitis
525.2	Atrophy, edentulous alveolar ridge
526.0	Developmental odontogenic cysts
526.1	Fissural cysts of jaw
526.2	Jaw cysts NEC
526.4	Inflammation of jaw
527.3	Salivary gland abscess
527.4	Salivary gland fistula
527.6	Salivary gland mucocele
528.3	Cellulitis/abscess of mouth
528.4	Oral soft tissue cyst
528.5	Diseases of lips
528.9	Oral soft tissue disease NEC
680.0	Carbuncle of face
682.0	Cellulitis of face
730.08	Acute osteomyelitis NEC
920.	Contusion face/scalp/neck

REIMBURSEMENT INFORMATION

Medicare

- Follow–up Days — 10
- Assistant Surgeon — not paid
- Supply Charges — not allowed
- Outpatient Limit — does not apply
- Minor Surgery Rules Apply

CPT CODE	SERVICE	ICD-9-CM

40804* Removal of embedded foreign body, vestibule of mouth; simple

40805 Removal of embedded foreign body, vestibule of mouth; complicated

CPT NOTES

- ♦ The vestibule is the part of the oral cavity outside the dentoalveolar structures; it includes the mucosal and submucosal tissue of lips and cheeks.

935.0 Foreign body in mouth

REIMBURSEMENT INFORMATION

General

- ♦ Starred procedure. (40804)

Medicare

- ♦ Follow-up Days — 10
- ♦ Assistant Surgeon
  40804 — not paid
  40805 — by report
- ♦ Supply Charges — not allowed
- ♦ Outpatient Limit
  40804 — applies
  40805 — does not apply
- ♦ Minor Surgery Rules Apply

40806 Incision of labial frenum (frenotomy)

CPT NOTES

- ♦ The vestibule is the part of the oral cavity outside the dentoalveolar structures; it includes the mucosal and submucosal tissue of lips and cheeks.

210.0 B-Neoplasm, Lip
524.5 Dentofacial functional abnormality
528.9 Oral soft tissue disease NEC
744.9 Congenital face/neck anomaly NOS
750.0 Tongue tie

REIMBURSEMENT INFORMATION

Medicare

- ♦ Follow-up Days — 0
- ♦ Assistant Surgeon — by report
- ♦ Supply Charges — not allowed
- ♦ Outpatient Limit — does not apply
- ♦ Minor Surgery Rules Apply

CPT CODE	SERVICE
40808	Biopsy, vestibule of mouth

CPT NOTES

- The vestibule is the part of the oral cavity outside the dentoalveolar structures; it includes the mucosal and submucosal tissue of lips and cheeks.

ICD–9–CM

145.0	M-Neoplasm, Cheek mucosa
145.1	M-Neoplasm, Mouth vestibule
145.9	M-Neoplasm, Mouth NOS
210.0	B-Neoplasm, Lip
210.4	B-Neoplasm, Mouth NEC/NOS
230.0	CA in situ, Oral cavity/pharynx
235.1	UB-Neoplasm, Oral cavity/pharynx
239.0	Digestive neoplasm NOS
358.0	Myasthenia gravis
523.1	Chronic gingivitis
523.8	Periodontal disease NEC
523.9	Gingival/periodontal disease NOS
525.9	Dental disorder NOS
526.0	Developmental odontogenic cysts
527.2	Sialoadenitis
527.5	Sialolithiasis
527.9	Salivary gland disease NOS
528.0	Stomatitis
528.4	Oral soft tissue cyst
528.5	Diseases of lips
528.6	Leukoplakia of oral mucosa/tongue
528.7	Oral epithelium disturbance NEC
528.8	Oral submucosal fibrosis, tongue
528.9	Oral soft tissue disease NEC
697.0	Lichen planus
701.5	Abnormal granulation tissue NEC
706.2	Sebaceous cyst

REIMBURSEMENT INFORMATION

Medicare

- Follow–up Days — 10
- Assistant Surgeon — not paid
- Supply Charges — not allowed
- Outpatient Limit — applies
- Minor Surgery Rules Apply

CPT CODE	SERVICE
40810	Excision of lesion of mucosa and submucosa, vestibule of mouth; without repair

CPT NOTES

- The vestibule is the part of the oral cavity outside the dentoalveolar structures; it includes the mucosal and submucosal tissue of lips and cheeks.

ICD–9–CM

145.0	M-Neoplasm, Cheek mucosa
145.1	M-Neoplasm, Mouth vestibule
145.8	M-Neoplasm, Mouth NEC
145.9	M-Neoplasm, Mouth NOS
171.0	M-Neoplasm, Soft tissue, head
171.8	M-Neoplasm, Soft tissue NEC
171.9	M-Neoplasm, Soft tissue NOS
195.0	M-Neoplasm, Head/face/neck
210.0	B-Neoplasm, Lip
210.4	B-Neoplasm, Mouth NEC/NOS
215.0	B-Neoplasm, Soft tissue, head
230.0	CA in situ, Oral cavity/pharynx
235.1	UB-Neoplasm, Oral cavity/pharynx
238.1	UB-Neoplasm, Soft tissue
522.6	Chronic apical periodontitis
526.4	Inflammation of jaw
527.6	Salivary gland mucocele
527.8	Salivary gland disease NEC
528.5	Diseases of lips
528.6	Leukoplakia of oral mucosa/tongue
528.7	Oral epithelium disturbance NEC
528.8	Oral submucosal fibrosis, tongue
528.9	Oral soft tissue disease NEC
706.2	Sebaceous cyst

REIMBURSEMENT INFORMATION

Medicare

- Follow–up Days — 10
- Assistant Surgeon — not paid
- Supply Charges — not allowed
- Outpatient Limit — applies
- Minor Surgery Rules Apply

CPT CODE	SERVICE
40812	Excision of lesion of mucosa and submucosa, vestibule of mouth; with simple repair

CPT NOTES

- The vestibule is the part of the oral cavity outside the dentoalveolar structures; it includes the mucosal and submucosal tissue of lips and cheeks.

ICD–9–CM

145.0	M-Neoplasm, Cheek mucosa
145.1	M-Neoplasm, Mouth vestibule
145.8	M-Neoplasm, Mouth NEC
145.9	M-Neoplasm, Mouth NOS
171.0	M-Neoplasm, Soft tissue, head
171.8	M-Neoplasm, Soft tissue NEC
171.9	M-Neoplasm, Soft tissue NOS
195.0	M-Neoplasm, Head/face/neck
210.0	B-Neoplasm, Lip
210.1	B-Neoplasm, Tongue
210.2	B-Neoplasm, Major salivary glands
210.3	B-Neoplasm, Floor of mouth
210.4	B-Neoplasm, Mouth NEC/NOS
215.0	B-Neoplasm, Soft tissue, head
230.0	CA in situ, Oral cavity/pharynx
235.1	UB-Neoplasm, Oral cavity/pharynx
238.1	UB-Neoplasm, Soft tissue
239.2	Bone/Skin neoplasm NOS
520.8	Tooth devel/eruption disorder NEC
523.8	Periodontal disease NEC
526.4	Inflammation of jaw
527.2	Sialoadenitis
527.5	Sialolithiasis
527.6	Salivary gland mucocele
527.8	Salivary gland disease NEC
528.0	Stomatitis
528.6	Leukoplakia of oral mucosa/tongue
528.7	Oral epithelium disturbance NEC
528.8	Oral submucosal fibrosis, tongue
528.9	Oral soft tissue disease NEC
697.0	Lichen planus
706.2	Sebaceous cyst

REIMBURSEMENT INFORMATION

Medicare

- Follow–up Days — 10
- Assistant Surgeon — not paid
- Supply Charges — not allowed
- Outpatient Limit — applies
- Minor Surgery Rules Apply

CPT CODE **SERVICE**

40814 Excision of lesion of mucosa and submucosa, vestibule of mouth; with complex repair

CPT NOTES

- The vestibule is the part of the oral cavity outside the dentoalveolar structures; it includes the mucosal and submucosal tissue of lips and cheeks.

ICD–9–CM

140.4	M-Neoplasm, Lower lip, inner aspect
145.0	M-Neoplasm, Cheek mucosa
145.1	M-Neoplasm, Mouth vestibule
145.8	M-Neoplasm, Mouth NEC
145.9	M-Neoplasm, Mouth NOS
171.0	M-Neoplasm, Soft tissue, head
171.8	M-Neoplasm, Soft tissue NEC
171.9	M-Neoplasm, Soft tissue NOS
195.0	M-Neoplasm, Head/face/neck
210.0	B-Neoplasm, Lip
210.4	B-Neoplasm, Mouth NEC/NOS
213.0	B-Neoplasm, Skull/Face bone
215.0	B-Neoplasm, Soft tissue, head
230.0	CA in situ, Oral cavity/pharynx
235.1	UB-Neoplasm, Oral cavity/pharynx
238.1	UB-Neoplasm, Soft tissue
239.2	Bone/Skin neoplasm NOS
525.2	Atrophy, edentulous alveolar ridge
526.1	Fissural cysts of jaw
526.3	Jaw, central giant cell granuloma
526.4	Inflammation of jaw
527.2	Sialoadenitis
527.6	Salivary gland mucocele
527.8	Salivary gland disease NEC
528.4	Oral soft tissue cyst
528.5	Diseases of lips
528.6	Leukoplakia of oral mucosa/tongue
528.7	Oral epithelium disturbance NEC
528.8	Oral submucosal fibrosis, tongue
528.9	Oral soft tissue disease NEC
706.2	Sebaceous cyst

REIMBURSEMENT INFORMATION

Medicare

- Follow–up Days — 90
- Assistant Surgeon — not paid
- Supply Charges — not allowed
- Outpatient Limit — does not apply
- Major Surgery Rules Apply

CPT CODE	SERVICE
40816	Excision of lesion of mucosa and submucosa, vestibule of mouth; complex, with excision of underlying muscle

CPT NOTES

- The vestibule is the part of the oral cavity outside the dentoalveolar structures; it includes the mucosal and submucosal tissue of lips and cheeks.

ICD–9–CM

145.0	M-Neoplasm, Cheek mucosa
145.1	M-Neoplasm, Mouth vestibule
145.8	M-Neoplasm, Mouth NEC
145.9	M-Neoplasm, Mouth NOS
171.0	M-Neoplasm, Soft tissue, head
171.8	M-Neoplasm, Soft tissue NEC
171.9	M-Neoplasm, Soft tissue NOS
195.0	M-Neoplasm, Head/face/neck
210.0	B-Neoplasm, Lip
210.3	B-Neoplasm, Floor of mouth
210.4	B-Neoplasm, Mouth NEC/NOS
214.0	Lipoma, Skin of face
215.0	B-Neoplasm, Soft tissue, head
216.0	B-Neoplasm, Skin of lip
230.0	CA in situ, Oral cavity/pharynx
235.1	UB-Neoplasm, Oral cavity/pharynx
238.1	UB-Neoplasm, Soft tissue
523.1	Chronic gingivitis
523.8	Periodontal disease NEC
526.4	Inflammation of jaw
527.6	Salivary gland mucocele
527.8	Salivary gland disease NEC
528.6	Leukoplakia of oral mucosa/tongue
528.7	Oral epithelium disturbance NEC
528.8	Oral submucosal fibrosis, tongue
528.9	Oral soft tissue disease NEC
706.2	Sebaceous cyst

REIMBURSEMENT INFORMATION

Medicare

- Follow–up Days — 90
- Assistant Surgeon — not paid
- Supply Charges — not allowed
- Outpatient Limit — does not apply
- Major Surgery Rules Apply

CPT CODE	SERVICE	ICD–9–CM

40818 Excision of mucosa of vestibule of mouth as donor graft

CPT NOTES

- The vestibule is the part of the oral cavity outside the dentoalveolar structures; it includes the mucosal and submucosal tissue of lips and cheeks.

145.9	M-Neoplasm, Mouth NOS
210.0	B-Neoplasm, Lip
210.3	B-Neoplasm, Floor of mouth
210.4	B-Neoplasm, Mouth NEC/NOS
230.0	CA in situ, Oral cavity/pharynx
235.1	UB-Neoplasm, Oral cavity/pharynx
522.8	Radicular cyst
523.8	Periodontal disease NEC
528.7	Oral epithelium disturbance NEC
528.8	Oral submucosal fibrosis, tongue
528.9	Oral soft tissue disease NEC

REIMBURSEMENT INFORMATION

Medicare

- Follow–up Days — 90
- Assistant Surgeon — not paid
- Supply Charges — not allowed
- Outpatient Limit — does not apply
- Major Surgery Rules Apply

40819 Excision of frenum, labial or buccal (frenumectomy, frenulectomy, frenectomy)

CPT NOTES

- The vestibule is the part of the oral cavity outside the dentoalveolar structures; it includes the mucosal and submucosal tissue of lips and cheeks.

140.3	M-Neoplasm, Upper lip, inner aspect
140.4	M-Neoplasm, Lower lip, inner aspect
140.5	M-Neoplasm, Lip NOS, inner NOS
140.8	M-Neoplasm, Lip NEC
210.0	B-Neoplasm, Lip
210.4	B-Neoplasm, Mouth NEC/NOS
235.1	UB-Neoplasm, Oral cavity/pharynx
523.9	Gingival/periodontal disease NOS
528.9	Oral soft tissue disease NEC
744.9	Congenital face/neck anomaly NOS
750.0	Tongue tie

REIMBURSEMENT INFORMATION

Medicare

- Follow–up Days — 90
- Assistant Surgeon — not paid
- Supply Charges — not allowed
- Outpatient Limit — does not apply
- Major Surgery Rules Apply

CPT CODE	SERVICE	ICD-9-CM

40820 Destruction of lesion or scar of vestibule of mouth by physical methods (eg, laser, thermal, cryo, chemical)

CPT NOTES

- The vestibule is the part of the oral cavity outside the dentoalveolar structures; it includes the mucosal and submucosal tissue of lips and cheeks.

210.4	B-Neoplasm, Mouth NEC/NOS
228.00	Hemangioma NOS
230.0	CA in situ, Oral cavity/pharynx
232.0	CA in situ, Skin of lip
235.1	UB-Neoplasm, Oral cavity/pharynx
239.2	Bone/Skin neoplasm NOS
523.8	Periodontal disease NEC
701.4	Keloid scar

REIMBURSEMENT INFORMATION

Medicare

- Follow–up Days — 10
- Assistant Surgeon — not paid
- Supply Charges — not allowed
- Outpatient Limit — does not apply
- Minor Surgery Rules Apply

40830 Closure of laceration, vestibule of mouth; 2.5 cm or less

CPT NOTES

- The vestibule is the part of the oral cavity outside the dentoalveolar structures; it includes the mucosal and submucosal tissue of lips and cheeks.

145.1	M-Neoplasm, Mouth vestibule
198.89	M2-Neoplasm NEC
873.60	Open wound of mouth NOS
873.61	Open wound of buccal mucosa
873.62	Open wound of gum
873.64	Open wound of tongue/mouth floor
873.69	Open wound of mouth NEC
873.71	Open wound of buccal mucosa, compl
873.72	Open wound of gum, complicated
873.74	Open wound of tongue, complicated
873.79	Open wound of mouth NEC, complic
998.3	Postop wound disruption

REIMBURSEMENT INFORMATION

Medicare

- Follow–up Days — 10
- Assistant Surgeon — not paid
- Supply Charges — not allowed
- Outpatient Limit — does not apply
- Minor Surgery Rules Apply

CPT CODE	SERVICE	ICD-9-CM
40831	Closure of laceration, vestibule of mouth; over 2.5 cm or complex	

CPT NOTES

- The vestibule is the part of the oral cavity outside the dentoalveolar structures; it includes the mucosal and submucosal tissue of lips and cheeks.

ICD-9-CM

145.1	M-Neoplasm, Mouth vestibule
198.89	M2-Neoplasm NEC
873.61	Open wound of buccal mucosa
873.62	Open wound of gum
873.64	Open wound of tongue/mouth floor
873.69	Open wound of mouth NEC
873.70	Open wound of mouth NOS, complic
873.71	Open wound of buccal mucosa, compl
873.72	Open wound of gum, complicated
873.74	Open wound of tongue, complicated
873.79	Open wound of mouth NEC, complic
998.3	Postop wound disruption

REIMBURSEMENT INFORMATION

Medicare

- Follow-up Days — 10
- Assistant Surgeon — not paid
- Supply Charges — not allowed
- Outpatient Limit — does not apply
- Minor Surgery Rules Apply

40840 Vestibuloplasty; anterior

CPT NOTES

- The vestibule is the part of the oral cavity outside the dentoalveolar structures; it includes the mucosal and submucosal tissue of lips and cheeks.
- For skin grafts, see 15000 et seq.

145.1	M-Neoplasm, Mouth vestibule
198.89	M2-Neoplasm NEC
524.9	Dentofacial anomaly NOS
525.2	Atrophy, edentulous alveolar ridge
749.2x	Cleft palate w/cleft lip
905.0	Late effect, skull/face fracture
906.0	Late effect, open wound head/trunk
906.5	Late effect of head/neck burn
908.9	Late effect of injury NOS
947.0	Burn of mouth and pharynx

REIMBURSEMENT INFORMATION

Medicare

- Follow-up Days — 90
- Assistant Surgeon — paid
- Supply Charges — not allowed
- Outpatient Limit — does not apply
- Major Surgery Rules Apply

CPT CODE	SERVICE	ICD–9–CM
40842	Vestibuloplasty; posterior, unilateral	145.1 M-Neoplasm, Mouth vestibule 198.89 M2-Neoplasm NEC 525.2 Atrophy, edentulous alveolar ridge 749.21 Unilat cleft palate/lip, complete 749.22 Unilat cleft palate/lip, incomplete 905.0 Late effect, skull/face fracture 906.0 Late effect, open wound head/trunk 906.5 Late effect of head/neck burn 908.9 Late effect of injury NOS 909.3 Late effect of surg/med complic 947.0 Burn of mouth and pharynx
40843	Vestibuloplasty; posterior, bilateral	
40844	Vestibuloplasty; entire arch	

CPT NOTES

- The vestibule is the part of the oral cavity outside the dentoalveolar structures; it includes the mucosal and submucosal tissue of lips and cheeks.
- For skin grafts, see 15000 et seq.

REIMBURSEMENT INFORMATION

Medicare

- Follow–up Days — 90
- Assistant Surgeon
  40842 — by report
  40843–40844 — paid
- Supply Charges — not allowed
- Outpatient Limit — does not apply
- Major Surgery Rules Apply

40845 Vestibuloplasty; complex (including ridge extension, muscle repositioning)

CPT NOTES

- The vestibule is the part of the oral cavity outside the dentoalveolar structures; it includes the mucosal and submucosal tissue of lips and cheeks.
- For skin grafts, see 15000 et seq.

145.1	M-Neoplasm, Mouth vestibule
198.89	M2-Neoplasm NEC
524.x	Dentofacial anomaly, malocclusion
525.2	Atrophy, edentulous alveolar ridge
749.2x	Cleft palate w/cleft lip
905.0	Late effect, skull/face fracture
906.0	Late effect, open wound head/trunk
906.5	Late effect of head/neck burn
908.9	Late effect of injury NOS
909.3	Late effect of surg/med complic
947.0	Burn of mouth and pharynx

REIMBURSEMENT INFORMATION

Medicare

- Follow–up Days — 90
- Assistant Surgeon — by report
- Supply Charges — not allowed
- Outpatient Limit — does not apply
- Major Surgery Rules Apply

CPT CODE	SERVICE	ICD–9–CM

40899 Unlisted procedure, vestibule of mouth

CPT NOTES

- The vestibule is the part of the oral cavity outside the dentoalveolar structures; it includes the mucosal and submucosal tissue of lips and cheeks.

210.4	B-Neoplasm, Mouth NEC/NOS
520.6	Tooth eruption disturbances
526.81	Exostosis of jaw

REIMBURSEMENT INFORMATION

Medicare

- Follow–up Days — determined by local carrier
- Assistant Surgeon — determined by local carrier
- Supply Charges — determined by local carrier
- Outpatient Limit — determined by local carrier

41000* Intraoral incision and drainage of abscess, cyst, or hematoma of tongue or floor of mouth; lingual

522.0	Pulpitis
522.5	Periapical abscess w/o sinus
522.7	Periapical abscess w/sinus
522.8	Radicular cyst
523.3	Acute periodontitis
526.0	Developmental odontogenic cysts
526.1	Fissural cysts of jaw
526.2	Jaw cysts NEC
526.4	Inflammation of jaw
527.3	Salivary gland abscess
527.6	Salivary gland mucocele
528.3	Cellulitis/abscess of mouth
528.4	Oral soft tissue cyst
528.5	Diseases of lips
529.0	Glossitis
529.8	Tongue disorder NEC

REIMBURSEMENT INFORMATION

General

- Starred procedure.

Medicare

- Follow–up Days — 10
- Assistant Surgeon — not paid
- Supply Charges — not allowed
- Outpatient Limit — does not apply
- Minor Surgery Rules Apply

CPT CODE	SERVICE
41005*	Intraoral incision and drainage of abscess, cyst, or hematoma of tongue or floor of mouth; sublingual, superficial

ICD–9–CM

210.3	B-Neoplasm, Floor of mouth
522.0	Pulpitis
522.5	Periapical abscess w/o sinus
522.7	Periapical abscess w/sinus
522.8	Radicular cyst
523.3	Acute periodontitis
526.0	Developmental odontogenic cysts
526.1	Fissural cysts of jaw
526.2	Jaw cysts NEC
526.4	Inflammation of jaw
527.3	Salivary gland abscess
527.6	Salivary gland mucocele
528.3	Cellulitis/abscess of mouth
528.4	Oral soft tissue cyst
528.5	Diseases of lips
528.9	Oral soft tissue disease NEC
529.0	Glossitis
529.8	Tongue disorder NEC

REIMBURSEMENT INFORMATION

General

- Starred procedure.

Medicare

- Follow–up Days — 10
- Assistant Surgeon — by report
- Supply Charges — not allowed
- Outpatient Limit — does not apply
- Minor Surgery Rules Apply

CPT CODE	SERVICE
41006	Intraoral incision and drainage of abscess, cyst, or hematoma of tongue or floor of mouth; sublingual, deep, supramylohyoid

ICD–9–CM

230.0	CA in situ, Oral cavity/pharynx
522.0	Pulpitis
522.5	Periapical abscess w/o sinus
522.7	Periapical abscess w/sinus
522.8	Radicular cyst
523.3	Acute periodontitis
526.0	Developmental odontogenic cysts
526.1	Fissural cysts of jaw
526.2	Jaw cysts NEC
526.4	Inflammation of jaw
527.3	Salivary gland abscess
527.6	Salivary gland mucocele
528.3	Cellulitis/abscess of mouth
528.4	Oral soft tissue cyst
528.5	Diseases of lips
529.0	Glossitis
529.8	Tongue disorder NEC

REIMBURSEMENT INFORMATION

Medicare

- ♦ Follow–up Days — 90
- ♦ Assistant Surgeon — by report
- ♦ Supply Charges — not allowed
- ♦ Outpatient Limit — does not apply
- ♦ Major Surgery Rules Apply

CPT CODE	SERVICE	ICD–9–CM
41007	Intraoral incision and drainage of abscess, cyst, or hematoma of tongue or floor of mouth; submental space	522.0 Pulpitis 522.5 Periapical abscess w/o sinus 522.7 Periapical abscess w/sinus 522.8 Radicular cyst 523.3 Acute periodontitis 526.0 Developmental odontogenic cysts 526.1 Fissural cysts of jaw 526.2 Jaw cysts NEC 526.4 Inflammation of jaw 527.3 Salivary gland abscess 527.6 Salivary gland mucocele 528.3 Cellulitis/abscess of mouth 528.4 Oral soft tissue cyst 528.5 Diseases of lips 529.0 Glossitis 529.8 Tongue disorder NEC **REIMBURSEMENT INFORMATION** Medicare ◆ Follow–up Days — 90 ◆ Assistant Surgeon — by report ◆ Supply Charges — not allowed ◆ Outpatient Limit — does not apply ◆ Major Surgery Rules Apply
41008	Intraoral incision and drainage of abscess, cyst, or hematoma of tongue or floor of mouth; submandibular space	
41009	Intraoral incision and drainage of abscess, cyst, or hematoma of tongue or floor of mouth; masticator space	
41010	Incision of lingual frenum (frenotomy)	141.3 M-Neoplasm, Tongue ventral surface 141.8 M-Neoplasm, Tongue NEC 524.5 Dentofacial functional abnormality 750.0 Tongue tie **REIMBURSEMENT INFORMATION** Medicare ◆ Follow–up Days — 10 ◆ Assistant Surgeon — by report ◆ Supply Charges — not allowed ◆ Outpatient Limit — does not apply ◆ Minor Surgery Rules Apply

CPT CODE	SERVICE	ICD–9–CM
41015	Extraoral incision and drainage of abscess, cyst, or hematoma of floor of mouth; sublingual	522.0 Pulpitis 522.5 Periapical abscess w/o sinus 522.7 Periapical abscess w/sinus 522.8 Radicular cyst 523.3 Acute periodontitis 526.0 Developmental odontogenic cysts 526.1 Fissural cysts of jaw 526.2 Jaw cysts NEC 526.4 Inflammation of jaw 527.3 Salivary gland abscess 527.6 Salivary gland mucocele 528.3 Cellulitis/abscess of mouth 528.4 Oral soft tissue cyst 528.5 Diseases of lips 529.0 Glossitis 529.8 Tongue disorder NEC
41016	Extraoral incision and drainage of abscess, cyst, or hematoma of floor of mouth; submental	

CPT NOTES

- For frenoplasty, see 41520.

REIMBURSEMENT INFORMATION

Medicare

- Follow–up Days — 90
- Assistant Surgeon — by report
- Supply Charges — not allowed
- Outpatient Limit — does not apply
- Major Surgery Rules Apply

CPT CODE	SERVICE	ICD–9–CM
41017	Extraoral incision and drainage of abscess, cyst, or hematoma of floor of mouth; submandibular	210.4 B-Neoplasm, Mouth NEC/NOS 522.0 Pulpitis 522.5 Periapical abscess w/o sinus 522.7 Periapical abscess w/sinus 522.8 Radicular cyst 523.3 Acute periodontitis 526.0 Developmental odontogenic cysts 526.1 Fissural cysts of jaw 526.2 Jaw cysts NEC 526.4 Inflammation of jaw 527.3 Salivary gland abscess 527.6 Salivary gland mucocele 528.3 Cellulitis/abscess of mouth 528.4 Oral soft tissue cyst 528.5 Diseases of lips 529.0 Glossitis 529.8 Tongue disorder NEC

CPT NOTES

- For frenoplasty, see 41520.

REIMBURSEMENT INFORMATION

Medicare

- Follow–up Days — 90
- Assistant Surgeon — not paid
- Supply Charges — not allowed
- Outpatient Limit — does not apply
- Major Surgery Rules Apply

CPT CODE **SERVICE**

41018 Extraoral incision and drainage of abscess, cyst, or hematoma of floor of mouth; masticator space

CPT NOTES

- For frenoplasty, see 41520.

ICD–9–CM

522.0	Pulpitis
522.5	Periapical abscess w/o sinus
522.7	Periapical abscess w/sinus
522.8	Radicular cyst
523.3	Acute periodontitis
526.0	Developmental odontogenic cysts
526.1	Fissural cysts of jaw
526.2	Jaw cysts NEC
526.4	Inflammation of jaw
527.3	Salivary gland abscess
527.6	Salivary gland mucocele
528.3	Cellulitis/abscess of mouth
528.4	Oral soft tissue cyst
528.5	Diseases of lips
529.0	Glossitis
529.8	Tongue disorder NEC

REIMBURSEMENT INFORMATION

Medicare

- Follow–up Days — 90
- Assistant Surgeon — by report
- Supply Charges — not allowed
- Outpatient Limit — does not apply
- Major Surgery Rules Apply

CPT CODE	SERVICE
41100	Biopsy of tongue; anterior two-thirds

ICD–9–CM

141.1	M-Neoplasm, Tongue dorsal surface
141.2	M-Neoplasm, Tongue tip/lat border
141.3	M-Neoplasm, Tongue ventral surface
141.4	M-Neoplasm, Tongue anterior 2/3 NOS
141.5	M-Neoplasm, Tongue junctional zone
141.8	M-Neoplasm, Tongue NEC
141.9	M-Neoplasm, Tongue NOS
198.89	M2-Neoplasm NEC
210.0	B-Neoplasm, Lip
210.1	B-Neoplasm, Tongue
210.4	B-Neoplasm, Mouth NEC/NOS
230.0	CA in situ, Oral cavity/pharynx
235.1	UB-Neoplasm, Oral cavity/pharynx
239.0	Digestive neoplasm NOS
526.89	Jaw disease NEC
528.6	Leukoplakia of oral mucosa/tongue
528.7	Oral epithelium disturbance NEC
528.8	Oral submucosal fibrosis, tongue
528.9	Oral soft tissue disease NEC
529.0	Glossitis
529.8	Tongue disorder NEC
529.9	Tongue disorder NOS

REIMBURSEMENT INFORMATION

Medicare

- Follow–up Days — 10
- Assistant Surgeon — not paid
- Supply Charges — not allowed
- Outpatient Limit — applies
- Minor Surgery Rules Apply

CPT CODE	SERVICE
41105	Biopsy of tongue; posterior one-third

ICD–9–CM

141.0	M-Neoplasm, Tongue base
141.5	M-Neoplasm, Tongue junctional zone
141.6	M-Neoplasm, Lingual tonsil
141.8	M-Neoplasm, Tongue NEC
141.9	M-Neoplasm, Tongue NOS
198.89	M2-Neoplasm NEC
210.1	B-Neoplasm, Tongue
230.0	CA in situ, Oral cavity/pharynx
235.1	UB-Neoplasm, Oral cavity/pharynx
239.0	Digestive neoplasm NOS
526.89	Jaw disease NEC
528.6	Leukoplakia of oral mucosa/tongue
528.7	Oral epithelium disturbance NEC
528.8	Oral submucosal fibrosis, tongue
528.9	Oral soft tissue disease NEC
529.0	Glossitis
529.1	Geographic tongue
529.9	Tongue disorder NOS

REIMBURSEMENT INFORMATION

Medicare

- ♦ Follow–up Days — 10
- ♦ Assistant Surgeon — not paid
- ♦ Supply Charges — not allowed
- ♦ Outpatient Limit — does not apply
- ♦ Minor Surgery Rules Apply

CPT CODE	SERVICE	ICD–9–CM	
41108	Biopsy of floor of mouth	144.0	M-Neoplasm, Anterior floor of mouth
		144.1	M-Neoplasm, Lateral floor of mouth
		144.8	M-Neoplasm, Floor of mouth NEC
		144.9	M-Neoplasm, Floor of mouth NOS
		145.9	M-Neoplasm, Mouth NOS
		170.1	M-Neoplasm, Mandible
		210.3	B-Neoplasm, Floor of mouth
		214.0	Lipoma, Skin of face
		230.0	CA in situ, Oral cavity/pharynx
		235.1	UB-Neoplasm, Oral cavity/pharynx
		239.0	Digestive neoplasm NOS
		527.6	Salivary gland mucocele
		528.4	Oral soft tissue cyst
		528.6	Leukoplakia of oral mucosa/tongue
		528.7	Oral epithelium disturbance NEC
		528.8	Oral submucosal fibrosis, tongue
		528.9	Oral soft tissue disease NEC
		697.0	Lichen planus
		701.1	Keratoderma, acquired

REIMBURSEMENT INFORMATION

Medicare

- Follow–up Days — 10
- Assistant Surgeon — not paid
- Supply Charges — not allowed
- Outpatient Limit — applies
- Minor Surgery Rules Apply

CPT CODE	SERVICE	ICD–9–CM
41110	Excision of lesion of tongue without closure	141.x Malignant neoplasm of tongue 210.1 B-Neoplasm, Tongue 210.4 B-Neoplasm, Mouth NEC/NOS 230.0 CA in situ, Oral cavity/pharynx 235.1 UB-Neoplasm, Oral cavity/pharynx 239.0 Digestive neoplasm NOS 528.6 Leukoplakia of oral mucosa/tongue 528.7 Oral epithelium disturbance NEC 528.8 Oral submucosal fibrosis, tongue 528.9 Oral soft tissue disease NEC 529.8 Tongue disorder NEC 529.9 Tongue disorder NOS **REIMBURSEMENT INFORMATION** Medicare ♦ Follow–up Days — 10 ♦ Assistant Surgeon — not paid ♦ Supply Charges — not allowed ♦ Outpatient Limit — does not apply ♦ Minor Surgery Rules Apply
41112	Excision of lesion of tongue with closure; anterior two-thirds	141.1 M-Neoplasm, Tongue dorsal surface 141.2 M-Neoplasm, Tongue tip/lat border 141.3 M-Neoplasm, Tongue ventral surface 141.4 M-Neoplasm, Tongue anterior 2/3 NOS 141.8 M-Neoplasm, Tongue NEC 141.9 M-Neoplasm, Tongue NOS 210.1 B-Neoplasm, Tongue 210.4 B-Neoplasm, Mouth NEC/NOS 230.0 CA in situ, Oral cavity/pharynx 235.1 UB-Neoplasm, Oral cavity/pharynx 239.0 Digestive neoplasm NOS 528.0 Stomatitis 528.6 Leukoplakia of oral mucosa/tongue 528.7 Oral epithelium disturbance NEC 528.8 Oral submucosal fibrosis, tongue 528.9 Oral soft tissue disease NEC 529.0 Glossitis 529.9 Tongue disorder NOS **REIMBURSEMENT INFORMATION** Medicare ♦ Follow–up Days — 90 ♦ Assistant Surgeon — not paid ♦ Supply Charges — not allowed ♦ Outpatient Limit — does not apply ♦ Major Surgery Rules Apply

CPT CODE	SERVICE	ICD–9–CM	
41113	Excision of lesion of tongue with closure; posterior one-third	141.0	M-Neoplasm, Tongue base
		141.1	M-Neoplasm, Tongue dorsal surface
		141.3	M-Neoplasm, Tongue ventral surface
		141.5	M-Neoplasm, Tongue junctional zone
		141.6	M-Neoplasm, Lingual tonsil
		141.8	M-Neoplasm, Tongue NEC
		141.9	M-Neoplasm, Tongue NOS
		210.0	B-Neoplasm, Lip
		210.1	B-Neoplasm, Tongue
		210.4	B-Neoplasm, Mouth NEC/NOS
		230.0	CA in situ, Oral cavity/pharynx
		235.1	UB-Neoplasm, Oral cavity/pharynx
		239.0	Digestive neoplasm NOS
		528.6	Leukoplakia of oral mucosa/tongue
		528.7	Oral epithelium disturbance NEC
		528.8	Oral submucosal fibrosis, tongue
		528.9	Oral soft tissue disease NEC
		529.0	Glossitis
		529.9	Tongue disorder NOS

REIMBURSEMENT INFORMATION

Medicare

- Follow–up Days — 90
- Assistant Surgeon — not paid
- Supply Charges — not allowed
- Outpatient Limit — does not apply
- Major Surgery Rules Apply

CPT CODE	SERVICE	ICD-9-CM	
41114	Excision of lesion of tongue with closure; with local tongue flap	141.0	M-Neoplasm, Tongue base
		141.1	M-Neoplasm, Tongue dorsal surface
		141.2	M-Neoplasm, Tongue tip/lat border
		141.3	M-Neoplasm, Tongue ventral surface
		141.4	M-Neoplasm, Tongue anterior 2/3 NOS
		141.5	M-Neoplasm, Tongue junctional zone
		141.6	M-Neoplasm, Lingual tonsil
		141.8	M-Neoplasm, Tongue NEC
		141.9	M-Neoplasm, Tongue NOS
		210.1	B-Neoplasm, Tongue
		230.0	CA in situ, Oral cavity/pharynx
		239.0	Digestive neoplasm NOS
		528.6	Leukoplakia of oral mucosa/tongue
		528.7	Oral epithelium disturbance NEC
		528.8	Oral submucosal fibrosis, tongue
		528.9	Oral soft tissue disease NEC
		529.9	Tongue disorder NOS

CPT NOTES

- List in addition to code 41112 or 41113.

REIMBURSEMENT INFORMATION

Medicare

- Follow-up Days — 90
- Assistant Surgeon — not paid
- Supply Charges — not allowed
- Outpatient Limit — does not apply
- Major Surgery Rules Apply

CPT CODE	SERVICE	ICD-9-CM	
41115	Excision of lingual frenum (frenectomy)	141.3	M-Neoplasm, Tongue ventral surface
		141.8	M-Neoplasm, Tongue NEC
		524.2	Dental arch relationship anomaly
		528.7	Oral epithelium disturbance NEC
		750.0	Tongue tie
		V13.6	Hx of congenital malformation

REIMBURSEMENT INFORMATION

Medicare

- Follow-up Days — 10
- Assistant Surgeon — by report
- Supply Charges — not allowed
- Outpatient Limit — does not apply
- Minor Surgery Rules Apply

CPT CODE	SERVICE
41116	Excision, lesion of floor of mouth

ICD–9–CM

141.0	M-Neoplasm, Tongue base
143.1	M-Neoplasm, Lower gum
144.0	M-Neoplasm, Anterior floor of mouth
144.1	M-Neoplasm, Lateral floor of mouth
144.8	M-Neoplasm, Floor of mouth NEC
144.9	M-Neoplasm, Floor of mouth NOS
145.8	M-Neoplasm, Mouth NEC
210.2	B-Neoplasm, Major salivary glands
210.3	B-Neoplasm, Floor of mouth
210.4	B-Neoplasm, Mouth NEC/NOS
214.1	Lipoma, Skin NEC
230.0	CA in situ, Oral cavity/pharynx
235.1	UB-Neoplasm, Oral cavity/pharynx
239.0	Digestive neoplasm NOS
520.6	Tooth eruption disturbances
527.6	Salivary gland mucocele
528.6	Leukoplakia of oral mucosa/tongue
528.7	Oral epithelium disturbance NEC
528.8	Oral submucosal fibrosis, tongue
528.9	Oral soft tissue disease NEC

REIMBURSEMENT INFORMATION

Medicare

- ♦ Follow–up Days — 90
- ♦ Assistant Surgeon — not paid
- ♦ Supply Charges — not allowed
- ♦ Outpatient Limit — does not apply
- ♦ Major Surgery Rules Apply

CPT CODE	SERVICE
41120	Glossectomy; less than one-half tongue

ICD–9–CM

141.0	M-Neoplasm, Tongue base
141.1	M-Neoplasm, Tongue dorsal surface
141.2	M-Neoplasm, Tongue tip/lat border
141.3	M-Neoplasm, Tongue ventral surface
141.4	M-Neoplasm, Tongue anterior 2/3 NOS
141.5	M-Neoplasm, Tongue junctional zone
141.6	M-Neoplasm, Lingual tonsil
141.8	M-Neoplasm, Tongue NEC
141.9	M-Neoplasm, Tongue NOS
144.0	M-Neoplasm, Anterior floor of mouth
144.1	M-Neoplasm, Lateral floor of mouth
144.8	M-Neoplasm, Floor of mouth NEC
144.9	M-Neoplasm, Floor of mouth NOS
145.8	M-Neoplasm, Mouth NEC
149.1	M-Neoplasm, Waldeyer's ring
149.8	M-Neoplasm, Oral cavity/pharynx NEC
750.19	Tongue anomaly NEC
758.0	Down's syndrome
V13.6	Hx of congenital malformation

REIMBURSEMENT INFORMATION

Medicare

- Follow–up Days — 90
- Assistant Surgeon — paid
- Supply Charges — not allowed
- Outpatient Limit — does not apply
- Major Surgery Rules Apply

CPT CODE	SERVICE
41130	Glossectomy; hemiglossectomy

ICD–9–CM

141.0	M-Neoplasm, Tongue base
141.1	M-Neoplasm, Tongue dorsal surface
141.2	M-Neoplasm, Tongue tip/lat border
141.3	M-Neoplasm, Tongue ventral surface
141.4	M-Neoplasm, Tongue anterior 2/3 NOS
141.5	M-Neoplasm, Tongue junctional zone
141.6	M-Neoplasm, Lingual tonsil
141.8	M-Neoplasm, Tongue NEC
141.9	M-Neoplasm, Tongue NOS
144.0	M-Neoplasm, Anterior floor of mouth
144.1	M-Neoplasm, Lateral floor of mouth
144.8	M-Neoplasm, Floor of mouth NEC
144.9	M-Neoplasm, Floor of mouth NOS
145.8	M-Neoplasm, Mouth NEC
149.1	M-Neoplasm, Waldeyer's ring
149.8	M-Neoplasm, Oral cavity/pharynx NEC

REIMBURSEMENT INFORMATION

Medicare

- ♦ Follow–up Days — 90
- ♦ Assistant Surgeon — paid
- ♦ Supply Charges — not allowed
- ♦ Outpatient Limit — does not apply
- ♦ Major Surgery Rules Apply

CPT CODE	SERVICE	ICD–9–CM	
41135	Glossectomy; partial, with unilateral radical neck dissection	141.0	M-Neoplasm, Tongue base
		141.1	M-Neoplasm, Tongue dorsal surface
		141.3	M-Neoplasm, Tongue ventral surface
		141.4	M-Neoplasm, Tongue anterior 2/3 NOS
		141.5	M-Neoplasm, Tongue junctional zone
		141.8	M-Neoplasm, Tongue NEC
		141.9	M-Neoplasm, Tongue NOS

REIMBURSEMENT INFORMATION

Medicare

- Follow–up Days — 90
- Assistant Surgeon — paid
- Supply Charges — not allowed
- Outpatient Limit — does not apply
- Major Surgery Rules Apply

CPT CODE	SERVICE	ICD–9–CM	
41140	Glossectomy; complete or total, with or without tracheostomy, without radical neck dissection	141.0	M-Neoplasm, Tongue base
		141.1	M-Neoplasm, Tongue dorsal surface
		141.2	M-Neoplasm, Tongue tip/lat border
		141.3	M-Neoplasm, Tongue ventral surface
		141.4	M-Neoplasm, Tongue anterior 2/3 NOS
		141.5	M-Neoplasm, Tongue junctional zone
		141.6	M-Neoplasm, Lingual tonsil
		141.8	M-Neoplasm, Tongue NEC
		141.9	M-Neoplasm, Tongue NOS
		144.0	M-Neoplasm, Anterior floor of mouth
		144.1	M-Neoplasm, Lateral floor of mouth
		144.8	M-Neoplasm, Floor of mouth NEC
		144.9	M-Neoplasm, Floor of mouth NOS
		145.8	M-Neoplasm, Mouth NEC
		149.1	M-Neoplasm, Waldeyer's ring
		149.8	M-Neoplasm, Oral cavity/pharynx NEC

REIMBURSEMENT INFORMATION

Medicare

- Follow–up Days — 90
- Assistant Surgeon — paid
- Supply Charges — not allowed
- Outpatient Limit — does not apply
- Major Surgery Rules Apply

CPT CODE	SERVICE	ICD-9-CM
41145	Glossectomy; complete or total, with or without tracheostomy, with unilateral radical neck dissection	141.0 M-Neoplasm, Tongue base 141.1 M-Neoplasm, Tongue dorsal surface 141.3 M-Neoplasm, Tongue ventral surface 141.4 M-Neoplasm, Tongue anterior 2/3 NOS 141.5 M-Neoplasm, Tongue junctional zone 141.8 M-Neoplasm, Tongue NEC 141.9 M-Neoplasm, Tongue NOS **REIMBURSEMENT INFORMATION** Medicare ♦ Follow-up Days — 90 ♦ Assistant Surgeon — paid ♦ Supply Charges — not allowed ♦ Outpatient Limit — does not apply ♦ Major Surgery Rules Apply
41150	Glossectomy; composite procedure with resection floor of mouth and mandibular resection, without radical neck dissection	144.0 M-Neoplasm, Anterior floor of mouth 144.1 M-Neoplasm, Lateral floor of mouth 144.8 M-Neoplasm, Floor of mouth NEC 144.9 M-Neoplasm, Floor of mouth NOS **REIMBURSEMENT INFORMATION** Medicare ♦ Follow-up Days — 90 ♦ Assistant Surgeon — paid ♦ Supply Charges — not allowed ♦ Outpatient Limit — does not apply ♦ Major Surgery Rules Apply

CPT CODE	SERVICE	ICD-9-CM	
41153	Glossectomy; composite procedure with resection floor of mouth, with suprahyoid neck dissection	141.0	M-Neoplasm, Tongue base
		141.1	M-Neoplasm, Tongue dorsal surface
		141.2	M-Neoplasm, Tongue tip/lat border
		141.3	M-Neoplasm, Tongue ventral surface
		141.4	M-Neoplasm, Tongue anterior 2/3 NOS
		141.5	M-Neoplasm, Tongue junctional zone
		141.6	M-Neoplasm, Lingual tonsil
		141.8	M-Neoplasm, Tongue NEC
		141.9	M-Neoplasm, Tongue NOS
		144.0	M-Neoplasm, Anterior floor of mouth
		144.1	M-Neoplasm, Lateral floor of mouth
		144.8	M-Neoplasm, Floor of mouth NEC
		144.9	M-Neoplasm, Floor of mouth NOS
		230.0	CA in situ, Oral cavity/pharynx

REIMBURSEMENT INFORMATION

Medicare

- Follow–up Days — 90
- Assistant Surgeon — paid
- Supply Charges — not allowed
- Outpatient Limit — does not apply
- Major Surgery Rules Apply

CPT CODE	SERVICE	ICD-9-CM	
41155	Glossectomy; composite procedure with resection floor of mouth, mandibular resection, and radical neck dissection (Commando type)	141.0	M-Neoplasm, Tongue base
		141.1	M-Neoplasm, Tongue dorsal surface
		141.2	M-Neoplasm, Tongue tip/lat border
		141.3	M-Neoplasm, Tongue ventral surface
		141.4	M-Neoplasm, Tongue anterior 2/3 NOS
		141.5	M-Neoplasm, Tongue junctional zone
		141.6	M-Neoplasm, Lingual tonsil
		141.8	M-Neoplasm, Tongue NEC
		141.9	M-Neoplasm, Tongue NOS
		144.0	M-Neoplasm, Anterior floor of mouth
		144.1	M-Neoplasm, Lateral floor of mouth
		144.8	M-Neoplasm, Floor of mouth NEC
		144.9	M-Neoplasm, Floor of mouth NOS

REIMBURSEMENT INFORMATION

Medicare

- Follow–up Days — 90
- Assistant Surgeon — paid
- Supply Charges — not allowed
- Outpatient Limit — does not apply
- Major Surgery Rules Apply

CPT CODE	SERVICE	ICD–9–CM
41250*	Repair of laceration 2.5 cm or less; floor of mouth and/or anterior two-thirds of tongue	873.64 Open wound of tongue/mouth floor 873.69 Open wound of mouth NEC 873.74 Open wound of tongue, complicated 873.79 Open wound of mouth NEC, complic 998.3 Postop wound disruption
41251*	Repair of laceration 2.5 cm or less; floor of mouth and/or posterior one-third of tongue	

REIMBURSEMENT INFORMATION

General

- ♦ Starred procedure.

Medicare

- ♦ Follow–up Days — 10
- ♦ Assistant Surgeon
  41250 — not paid
  41251 — by report
- ♦ Supply Charges — not allowed
- ♦ Outpatient Limit — does not apply
- ♦ Minor Surgery Rules Apply

CPT CODE	SERVICE	ICD–9–CM
41252*	Repair of laceration of tongue, floor of mouth, over 2.6 cm or complex	873.64 Open wound of tongue/mouth floor 873.69 Open wound of mouth NEC 873.70 Open wound of mouth NOS, complic 873.71 Open wound of buccal mucosa, compl 873.72 Open wound of gum, complicated 873.74 Open wound of tongue, complicated 873.79 Open wound of mouth NEC, complic 998.3 Postop wound disruption

REIMBURSEMENT INFORMATION

General

- ♦ Starred procedure.

Medicare

- ♦ Follow–up Days — 10
- ♦ Assistant Surgeon — not paid
- ♦ Supply Charges — not allowed
- ♦ Outpatient Limit — does not apply
- ♦ Minor Surgery Rules Apply

CPT CODE	SERVICE	ICD–9–CM
41500	Fixation of tongue, mechanical, other than suture (eg, K-wire)	524.04 Mandibular hypoplasia 750.0 Tongue tie 756.0 Anomaly of skull/face bones **REIMBURSEMENT INFORMATION** Medicare ♦ Follow–up Days — 90 ♦ Assistant Surgeon — by report ♦ Supply Charges — not allowed ♦ Outpatient Limit — does not apply ♦ Major Surgery Rules Apply
41510	Suture of tongue to lip for micrognathia (Douglas type procedure)	524.0x Major anomaly of jaw size 756.0 Anomaly of skull/face bones **REIMBURSEMENT INFORMATION** Medicare ♦ Follow–up Days — 90 ♦ Assistant Surgeon — by report ♦ Supply Charges — not allowed ♦ Outpatient Limit — does not apply ♦ Major Surgery Rules Apply
41520	Frenoplasty (surgical revision of frenum, eg, with Z-plasty) **CPT NOTES** ♦ For frenotomy, see 4806, 41010.	141.3 M-Neoplasm, Tongue ventral surface 141.8 M-Neoplasm, Tongue NEC 524.5 Dentofacial functional abnormality 744.9 Congenital face/neck anomaly NOS 750.0 Tongue tie V13.6 Hx of congenital malformation **REIMBURSEMENT INFORMATION** Medicare ♦ Follow–up Days — 90 ♦ Assistant Surgeon — by report ♦ Supply Charges — not allowed ♦ Outpatient Limit — does not apply ♦ Major Surgery Rules Apply

CPT CODE	SERVICE	ICD–9–CM
41599	Unlisted procedure, tongue, floor of mouth	141.0 M-Neoplasm, Tongue base 141.9 M-Neoplasm, Tongue NOS 750.0 Tongue tie **REIMBURSEMENT INFORMATION** Medicare ♦ Follow–up Days — determined by local carrier ♦ Assistant Surgeon — determined by local carrier ♦ Supply Charges — determined by local carrier ♦ Outpatient Limit — determined by local carrier
41800*	Drainage of abscess, cyst, hematoma from dentoalveolar structures	522.0 Pulpitis 522.5 Periapical abscess w/o sinus 522.7 Periapical abscess w/sinus 522.8 Radicular cyst 523.3 Acute periodontitis 526.0 Developmental odontogenic cysts 526.1 Fissural cysts of jaw 526.2 Jaw cysts NEC 526.4 Inflammation of jaw 527.3 Salivary gland abscess 527.6 Salivary gland mucocele 528.3 Cellulitis/abscess of mouth 528.4 Oral soft tissue cyst 528.5 Diseases of lips **REIMBURSEMENT INFORMATION** General ♦ Starred procedure. Medicare ♦ Follow–up Days — 10 ♦ Assistant Surgeon — not paid ♦ Supply Charges — not allowed ♦ Outpatient Limit — does not apply ♦ Minor Surgery Rules Apply

CPT CODE	SERVICE	ICD–9–CM
41805	Removal of embedded foreign body from dentoalveolar structures; soft tissues	935.0 Foreign body in mouth
41806	Removal of embedded foreign body from dentoalveolar structures; bone	

REIMBURSEMENT INFORMATION

Medicare

- Follow–up Days — 10
- Assistant Surgeon — not paid
- Supply Charges — not allowed
- Outpatient Limit — does not apply
- Minor Surgery Rules Apply

CPT CODE	SERVICE	ICD–9–CM
41820	Gingivectomy, excision gingiva, each quadrant	523.0 Acute gingivitis 523.1 Chronic gingivitis 523.8 Periodontal disease NEC 523.9 Gingival/periodontal disease NOS

REIMBURSEMENT INFORMATION

Medicare

- Follow–up Days — global concept does not apply
- Assistant Surgeon — by report
- Supply Charges — not allowed
- Outpatient Limit — does not apply

CPT CODE	SERVICE	ICD–9–CM
41821	Operculectomy, excision pericoronal tissues	523.1 Chronic gingivitis 523.3 Acute periodontitis 523.4 Chronic periodontitis 523.5 Periodontosis 523.8 Periodontal disease NEC 528.6 Leukoplakia of oral mucosa/tongue 528.9 Oral soft tissue disease NEC

REIMBURSEMENT INFORMATION

Medicare

- Follow–up Days — global concept does not apply
- Assistant Surgeon — by report
- Supply Charges — not allowed
- Outpatient Limit — does not apply

CPT CODE	SERVICE	ICD-9-CM
41822	Excision of fibrous tuberosities, dentoalveolar structures	210.4 B-Neoplasm, Mouth NEC/NOS 523.9 Gingival/periodontal disease NOS 525.2 Atrophy, edentulous alveolar ridge 525.8 Dental disorder NEC 525.9 Dental disorder NOS 526.89 Jaw disease NEC 528.7 Oral epithelium disturbance NEC 528.8 Oral submucosal fibrosis, tongue 528.9 Oral soft tissue disease NEC **REIMBURSEMENT INFORMATION** Medicare ♦ Follow–up Days — 10 ♦ Assistant Surgeon — by report ♦ Supply Charges — not allowed ♦ Outpatient Limit — does not apply ♦ Minor Surgery Rules Apply
41823	Excision of osseous tuberosities, dentoalveolar structures	523.3 Acute periodontitis 523.4 Chronic periodontitis 523.5 Periodontosis 523.9 Gingival/periodontal disease NOS 525.8 Dental disorder NEC 525.9 Dental disorder NOS 526.81 Exostosis of jaw **REIMBURSEMENT INFORMATION** Medicare ♦ Follow–up Days — 90 ♦ Assistant Surgeon — by report ♦ Supply Charges — not allowed ♦ Outpatient Limit — does not apply ♦ Major Surgery Rules Apply

CPT CODE	SERVICE
41825	Excision of lesion or tumor (except listed above), dentoalveolar structures; without repair

CPT NOTES

- For nonexcisional destruction, see 41850.

ICD–9–CM

143.0	M-Neoplasm, Upper gum
143.1	M-Neoplasm, Lower gum
143.8	M-Neoplasm, Gum NEC
143.9	M-Neoplasm, Gum NOS
145.6	M-Neoplasm, Retromolar area
145.8	M-Neoplasm, Mouth NEC
145.9	M-Neoplasm, Mouth NOS
210.4	B-Neoplasm, Mouth NEC/NOS
230.0	CA in situ, Oral cavity/pharynx
235.1	UB-Neoplasm, Oral cavity/pharynx
522.5	Periapical abscess w/o sinus
522.6	Chronic apical periodontitis
522.7	Periapical abscess w/sinus
522.8	Radicular cyst
522.9	Pulp/periapical disease NEC
523.1	Chronic gingivitis
523.8	Periodontal disease NEC
526.0	Developmental odontogenic cysts
526.1	Fissural cysts of jaw
526.2	Jaw cysts NEC
526.3	Jaw, central giant cell granuloma
527.6	Salivary gland mucocele
528.0	Stomatitis
528.4	Oral soft tissue cyst
528.6	Leukoplakia of oral mucosa/tongue
528.7	Oral epithelium disturbance NEC
528.8	Oral submucosal fibrosis, tongue
528.9	Oral soft tissue disease NEC
697.0	Lichen planus

REIMBURSEMENT INFORMATION

Medicare

- Follow–up Days — 10
- Assistant Surgeon — not paid
- Supply Charges — not allowed
- Outpatient Limit — applies
- Minor Surgery Rules Apply

CPT CODE	SERVICE
41826	Excision of lesion or tumor (except listed above), dentoalveolar structures; with simple repair

CPT NOTES

- For nonexcisional destruction, see 41850.

ICD–9–CM

143.0	M-Neoplasm, Upper gum
143.1	M-Neoplasm, Lower gum
143.8	M-Neoplasm, Gum NEC
143.9	M-Neoplasm, Gum NOS
145.6	M-Neoplasm, Retromolar area
145.8	M-Neoplasm, Mouth NEC
145.9	M-Neoplasm, Mouth NOS
210.4	B-Neoplasm, Mouth NEC/NOS
230.0	CA in situ, Oral cavity/pharynx
235.1	UB-Neoplasm, Oral cavity/pharynx
239.0	Digestive neoplasm NOS
522.5	Periapical abscess w/o sinus
522.6	Chronic apical periodontitis
522.7	Periapical abscess w/sinus
522.8	Radicular cyst
522.9	Pulp/periapical disease NEC
523.5	Periodontosis
523.8	Periodontal disease NEC
523.9	Gingival/periodontal disease NOS
524.3	Tooth position anomaly
526.0	Developmental odontogenic cysts
526.1	Fissural cysts of jaw
526.2	Jaw cysts NEC
526.3	Jaw, central giant cell granuloma
527.6	Salivary gland mucocele
528.4	Oral soft tissue cyst
528.6	Leukoplakia of oral mucosa/tongue
528.7	Oral epithelium disturbance NEC
528.8	Oral submucosal fibrosis, tongue
528.9	Oral soft tissue disease NEC
701.1	Keratoderma, acquired

REIMBURSEMENT INFORMATION

Medicare

- Follow–up Days — 10
- Assistant Surgeon — not paid
- Supply Charges — not allowed
- Outpatient Limit — applies
- Minor Surgery Rules Apply

CPT CODE	SERVICE
41827	Excision of lesion or tumor (except listed above), dentoalveolar structures; with complex repair

CPT NOTES

- For nonexcisional destruction, see 41850.

ICD–9–CM

143.0	M-Neoplasm, Upper gum
143.1	M-Neoplasm, Lower gum
143.8	M-Neoplasm, Gum NEC
143.9	M-Neoplasm, Gum NOS
145.6	M-Neoplasm, Retromolar area
145.8	M-Neoplasm, Mouth NEC
145.9	M-Neoplasm, Mouth NOS
210.4	B-Neoplasm, Mouth NEC/NOS
214.1	Lipoma, Skin NEC
230.0	CA in situ, Oral cavity/pharynx
235.1	UB-Neoplasm, Oral cavity/pharynx
522.5	Periapical abscess w/o sinus
522.6	Chronic apical periodontitis
522.7	Periapical abscess w/sinus
522.8	Radicular cyst
523.8	Periodontal disease NEC
526.0	Developmental odontogenic cysts
526.1	Fissural cysts of jaw
526.2	Jaw cysts NEC
526.3	Jaw, central giant cell granuloma
527.6	Salivary gland mucocele
528.4	Oral soft tissue cyst
528.6	Leukoplakia of oral mucosa/tongue
528.7	Oral epithelium disturbance NEC
528.8	Oral submucosal fibrosis, tongue
528.9	Oral soft tissue disease NEC
701.1	Keratoderma, acquired

REIMBURSEMENT INFORMATION

Medicare

- Follow–up Days — 90
- Assistant Surgeon — not paid
- Supply Charges — not allowed
- Outpatient Limit — does not apply
- Major Surgery Rules Apply

CPT CODE	SERVICE	ICD–9–CM
▲ **41828**	Excision of hyperplastic alveolar mucosa, each quadrant (specify)	210.4 B-Neoplasm, Mouth NEC/NOS 213.1 B-Neoplasm, Lower jaw bone 523.8 Periodontal disease NEC 524.0x Major anomaly of jaw size 525.8 Dental disorder NEC 526.81 Exostosis of jaw 528.6 Leukoplakia of oral mucosa/tongue 528.9 Oral soft tissue disease NEC **REIMBURSEMENT INFORMATION** General ◆ Description changed in 1995 CPT. Medicare ◆ Follow–up Days — 10 ◆ Assistant Surgeon — not paid ◆ Supply Charges — not allowed ◆ Outpatient Limit — does not apply ◆ Minor Surgery Rules Apply
41830	Alveolectomy, including curettage of osteitis or sequestrectomy	523.8 Periodontal disease NEC 525.8 Dental disorder NEC 525.9 Dental disorder NOS 526.4 Inflammation of jaw 526.5 Alveolitis of jaw 526.81 Exostosis of jaw 909.2 Late effect of radiation V10.01 Hx of tongue malignancy V10.02 Hx of oral/pharynx malignancy NEC **REIMBURSEMENT INFORMATION** Medicare ◆ Follow–up Days — 10 ◆ Assistant Surgeon — by report ◆ Supply Charges — not allowed ◆ Outpatient Limit — does not apply ◆ Minor Surgery Rules Apply

CPT CODE	SERVICE	ICD-9-CM
41850	Destruction of lesion (except excision), dentoalveolar structures	210.3 B-Neoplasm, Floor of mouth 210.4 B-Neoplasm, Mouth NEC/NOS 228.00 Hemangioma NOS 230.0 CA in situ, Oral cavity/pharynx 235.1 UB-Neoplasm, Oral cavity/pharynx **REIMBURSEMENT INFORMATION** Medicare ◆ Follow-up Days — global concept does not apply ◆ Assistant Surgeon — by report ◆ Supply Charges — not allowed ◆ Outpatient Limit — does not apply
41870	Periodontal mucosal grafting	523.1 Chronic gingivitis 523.2 Gingival recession 523.3 Acute periodontitis 523.4 Chronic periodontitis 523.5 Periodontosis 523.8 Periodontal disease NEC 528.6 Leukoplakia of oral mucosa/tongue 528.9 Oral soft tissue disease NEC **REIMBURSEMENT INFORMATION** Medicare ◆ Follow-up Days — global concept does not apply ◆ Assistant Surgeon — by report ◆ Supply Charges — not allowed ◆ Outpatient Limit — does not apply
▲ 41872	Gingivoplasty, each quadrant (specify)	522.9 Pulp/periapical disease NEC 523.0 Acute gingivitis 523.1 Chronic gingivitis 523.3 Acute periodontitis 523.4 Chronic periodontitis 523.5 Periodontosis 523.8 Periodontal disease NEC 523.9 Gingival/periodontal disease NOS **REIMBURSEMENT INFORMATION** General ◆ Description changed in 1995 CPT. Medicare ◆ Follow-up Days — 90 ◆ Assistant Surgeon — by report ◆ Supply Charges — not allowed ◆ Outpatient Limit — does not apply ◆ Major Surgery Rules Apply

CPT CODE **SERVICE**

▲ **41874** Alveoplasty, each quadrant (specify)

CPT NOTES

- For closure of lacerations, see 40830, 40831.
- For segmental osteotomy, see 21206.
- For reduction of fractures, see 21421-21490.

ICD–9–CM

141.0	M-Neoplasm, Tongue base
141.3	M-Neoplasm, Tongue ventral surface
144.8	M-Neoplasm, Floor of mouth NEC
145.9	M-Neoplasm, Mouth NOS
146.9	M-Neoplasm, Oropharynx NOS
213.0	B-Neoplasm, Skull/Face bone
213.1	B-Neoplasm, Lower jaw bone
516.3	Idiopathic fibrosing alveolitis
523.3	Acute periodontitis
523.4	Chronic periodontitis
523.5	Periodontosis
523.9	Gingival/periodontal disease NOS
524.0x	Major anomaly of jaw size
524.1x	Jaw/cranial base relation anomaly
524.2	Dental arch relationship anomaly
524.3	Tooth position anomaly
525.0	Tooth exfoliation, systemic cause
525.2	Atrophy, edentulous alveolar ridge
525.8	Dental disorder NEC
526.4	Inflammation of jaw
526.81	Exostosis of jaw
526.89	Jaw disease NEC

REIMBURSEMENT INFORMATION

General

- Description changed in 1995 CPT.

Medicare

- Follow–up Days — 90
- Assistant Surgeon — by report
- Supply Charges — not allowed
- Outpatient Limit — does not apply
- Major Surgery Rules Apply

CPT CODE	SERVICE
41899	Unlisted procedure, dentoalveolar structures

ICD-9-CM

141.0	M-Neoplasm, Tongue base
144.8	M-Neoplasm, Floor of mouth NEC
145.2	M-Neoplasm, Hard palate
145.9	M-Neoplasm, Mouth NOS
146.9	M-Neoplasm, Oropharynx NOS
195.0	M-Neoplasm, Head/face/neck
213.1	B-Neoplasm, Lower jaw bone
473.0	Chronic maxillary sinusitis
520.1	Supernumerary teeth
520.2	Abnormal tooth size/form
520.3	Mottled teeth
520.4	Tooth formation disturbances
520.5	Hereditary tooth struct disturb NEC
520.6	Tooth eruption disturbances
520.7	Teething syndrome
520.8	Tooth devel/eruption disorder NEC
520.9	Tooth devel/eruption disorder NOS
521.8	Hard tissue disease teeth NEC
521.9	Hard tissue disease teeth NOS
524.3	Tooth position anomaly
524.6	Temporomandibular joint disorder
524.60	TMJ disorders NOS
524.61	TMJ adhesions/ankylosis
524.62	TMJ arthralgia
524.63	TMJ articular disc disorder
524.69	TMJ disorders NEC
524.9	Dentofacial anomaly NOS
525.0	Tooth exfoliation, systemic cause
525.1	Tooth loss, acquired
525.2	Atrophy, edentulous alveolar ridge
525.3	Retained dental root
525.9	Dental disorder NOS
526.2	Jaw cysts NEC
526.4	Inflammation of jaw
526.8	Jaw disease
526.81	Exostosis of jaw
528.6	Leukoplakia of oral mucosa/tongue
528.9	Oral soft tissue disease NEC
749.2x	Cleft palate w/cleft lip
802.35	Fx angle of jaw, open
873.60	Open wound of mouth NOS
873.61	Open wound of buccal mucosa
873.62	Open wound of gum
873.63	Broken tooth

REIMBURSEMENT INFORMATION

Medicare

- Follow–up Days — determined by local carrier
- Assistant Surgeon — determined by local carrier
- Supply Charges — determined by local carrier
- Outpatient Limit — determined by local carrier

CPT CODE	SERVICE	ICD–9–CM
42000*	Drainage of abscess of palate, uvula	526.4 Inflammation of jaw 528.3 Cellulitis/abscess of mouth

REIMBURSEMENT INFORMATION

General

- ♦ Starred procedure.

Medicare

- ♦ Follow–up Days — 10
- ♦ Assistant Surgeon — not paid
- ♦ Supply Charges — not allowed
- ♦ Outpatient Limit — does not apply
- ♦ Minor Surgery Rules Apply

42100 Biopsy of palate, uvula

145.2	M-Neoplasm, Hard palate
145.3	M-Neoplasm, Soft palate
145.4	M-Neoplasm, Uvula
145.5	M-Neoplasm, Palate NOS
145.8	M-Neoplasm, Mouth NEC
210.4	B-Neoplasm, Mouth NEC/NOS
230.0	CA in situ, Oral cavity/pharynx
235.1	UB-Neoplasm, Oral cavity/pharynx
522.6	Chronic apical periodontitis
522.7	Periapical abscess w/sinus
523.9	Gingival/periodontal disease NOS
527.2	Sialoadenitis
528.0	Stomatitis
528.4	Oral soft tissue cyst
528.6	Leukoplakia of oral mucosa/tongue
528.7	Oral epithelium disturbance NEC
528.8	Oral submucosal fibrosis, tongue
528.9	Oral soft tissue disease NEC
701.1	Keratoderma, acquired

REIMBURSEMENT INFORMATION

Medicare

- ♦ Follow–up Days — 10
- ♦ Assistant Surgeon — not paid
- ♦ Supply Charges — not allowed
- ♦ Outpatient Limit — applies
- ♦ Minor Surgery Rules Apply

CPT CODE SERVICE	ICD-9-CM
42104 Excision, lesion of palate, uvula; without closure	145.2 M-Neoplasm, Hard palate 145.3 M-Neoplasm, Soft palate 145.4 M-Neoplasm, Uvula 145.5 M-Neoplasm, Palate NOS 145.8 M-Neoplasm, Mouth NEC 210.4 B-Neoplasm, Mouth NEC/NOS 230.0 CA in situ, Oral cavity/pharynx 235.1 UB-Neoplasm, Oral cavity/pharynx 528.6 Leukoplakia of oral mucosa/tongue 528.7 Oral epithelium disturbance NEC 528.8 Oral submucosal fibrosis, tongue 528.9 Oral soft tissue disease NEC 701.1 Keratoderma, acquired

CPT NOTES

- For skin graft, see 14040-14300.
- For mucosal graft, see 40818.

REIMBURSEMENT INFORMATION

Medicare

- Follow–up Days — 10
- Assistant Surgeon — not paid
- Supply Charges — not allowed
- Outpatient Limit — does not apply
- Minor Surgery Rules Apply

CPT CODE SERVICE	ICD-9-CM
42106 Excision, lesion of palate, uvula; with simple primary closure	145.2 M-Neoplasm, Hard palate 145.3 M-Neoplasm, Soft palate 145.4 M-Neoplasm, Uvula 145.5 M-Neoplasm, Palate NOS 145.8 M-Neoplasm, Mouth NEC 210.4 B-Neoplasm, Mouth NEC/NOS 230.0 CA in situ, Oral cavity/pharynx 235.1 UB-Neoplasm, Oral cavity/pharynx 527.2 Sialoadenitis 527.7 Salivary secretion disturbance 528.6 Leukoplakia of oral mucosa/tongue 528.7 Oral epithelium disturbance NEC 528.8 Oral submucosal fibrosis, tongue 528.9 Oral soft tissue disease NEC

CPT NOTES

- For skin graft, see 14040-14300.
- For mucosal graft, see 40818.

REIMBURSEMENT INFORMATION

Medicare

- Follow–up Days — 10
- Assistant Surgeon — not paid
- Supply Charges — not allowed
- Outpatient Limit — does not apply
- Minor Surgery Rules Apply

CPT CODE	SERVICE	ICD-9-CM	
42107	Excision, lesion of palate, uvula; with local flap closure	145.2	M-Neoplasm, Hard palate
		145.3	M-Neoplasm, Soft palate
		145.4	M-Neoplasm, Uvula
		145.5	M-Neoplasm, Palate NOS
		145.8	M-Neoplasm, Mouth NEC
		210.4	B-Neoplasm, Mouth NEC/NOS
		214.1	Lipoma, Skin NEC
		230.0	CA in situ, Oral cavity/pharynx
		235.1	UB-Neoplasm, Oral cavity/pharynx
		528.7	Oral epithelium disturbance NEC
		528.8	Oral submucosal fibrosis, tongue
		528.9	Oral soft tissue disease NEC

CPT NOTES

- ♦ For skin graft, see 14040-14300.
- ♦ For mucosal graft, see 40818.

REIMBURSEMENT INFORMATION

Medicare

- ♦ Follow-up Days — 90
- ♦ Assistant Surgeon — not paid
- ♦ Supply Charges — not allowed
- ♦ Outpatient Limit — does not apply
- ♦ Major Surgery Rules Apply

CPT CODE	SERVICE	ICD-9-CM	
42120	Resection of palate or extensive resection of lesion	145.2	M-Neoplasm, Hard palate
		145.3	M-Neoplasm, Soft palate
		145.4	M-Neoplasm, Uvula
		145.5	M-Neoplasm, Palate NOS
		145.8	M-Neoplasm, Mouth NEC
		210.4	B-Neoplasm, Mouth NEC/NOS
		230.0	CA in situ, Oral cavity/pharynx
		235.1	UB-Neoplasm, Oral cavity/pharynx
		528.7	Oral epithelium disturbance NEC
		528.8	Oral submucosal fibrosis, tongue
		528.9	Oral soft tissue disease NEC

CPT NOTES

- ♦ For reconstruction of palate with extraoral tissue, see 14040-14300, 15050, 15120, 15240, 15576.

REIMBURSEMENT INFORMATION

Medicare

- ♦ Follow-up Days — 90
- ♦ Assistant Surgeon — paid
- ♦ Supply Charges — not allowed
- ♦ Outpatient Limit — does not apply
- ♦ Major Surgery Rules Apply

CPT CODE	SERVICE	ICD-9-CM
42140	Uvulectomy, excision of uvula	145.4 M-Neoplasm, Uvula 210.4 B-Neoplasm, Mouth NEC/NOS 230.0 CA in situ, Oral cavity/pharynx 239.0 Digestive neoplasm NOS 528.7 Oral epithelium disturbance NEC 528.8 Oral submucosal fibrosis, tongue 528.9 Oral soft tissue disease NEC **REIMBURSEMENT INFORMATION** Medicare ♦ Follow-up Days — 90 ♦ Assistant Surgeon — not paid ♦ Supply Charges — not allowed ♦ Outpatient Limit — does not apply ♦ Major Surgery Rules Apply
42145	Palatopharyngoplasty (eg, uvulopalatopharyngoplasty, uvulopharyngoplasty)	145.2 M-Neoplasm, Hard palate 145.3 M-Neoplasm, Soft palate 145.4 M-Neoplasm, Uvula 145.5 M-Neoplasm, Palate NOS 749.00 Cleft palate NOS 749.02 Unilateral cleft palate, incomplete **REIMBURSEMENT INFORMATION** Medicare ♦ Follow-up Days — 90 ♦ Assistant Surgeon — not paid ♦ Supply Charges — not allowed ♦ Outpatient Limit — does not apply ♦ Major Surgery Rules Apply
42160	Destruction of lesion, palate or uvula (thermal, cryo or chemical)	210.4 B-Neoplasm, Mouth NEC/NOS 228.00 Hemangioma NOS 230.0 CA in situ, Oral cavity/pharynx 235.1 UB-Neoplasm, Oral cavity/pharynx 239.2 Bone/Skin neoplasm NOS 527.2 Sialoadenitis 528.9 Oral soft tissue disease NEC **REIMBURSEMENT INFORMATION** Medicare ♦ Follow-up Days — 10 ♦ Assistant Surgeon — not paid ♦ Supply Charges — not allowed ♦ Outpatient Limit — does not apply ♦ Minor Surgery Rules Apply

CPT CODE	SERVICE	ICD-9-CM
42180	Repair, laceration of palate; up to 2 cm	873.65 Open wound of palate 873.75 Open wound of palate, complicated 998.3 Postop wound disruption V13.6 Hx of congenital malformation **REIMBURSEMENT INFORMATION** Medicare ◆ Follow-up Days — 10 ◆ Assistant Surgeon — by report ◆ Supply Charges — not allowed ◆ Outpatient Limit — does not apply ◆ Minor Surgery Rules Apply
42182	Repair, laceration of palate; over 2 cm or complex	
42200	Palatoplasty for cleft palate, soft and/or hard palate only	749.0x Cleft palate 749.20 Cleft palate w/cleft lip NOS 749.21 Unilat cleft palate/lip, complete 749.22 Unilat cleft palate/lip, incomplete 749.23 Bilat cleft palate/lip, complete 749.24 Bilat cleft palate/lip, incomplete V13.6 Hx of congenital malformation **REIMBURSEMENT INFORMATION** Medicare ◆ Follow-up Days — 90 ◆ Assistant Surgeon — paid ◆ Supply Charges — not allowed ◆ Outpatient Limit — does not apply ◆ Major Surgery Rules Apply
42205	Palatoplasty for cleft palate, with closure of alveolar ridge; soft tissue only	749.0x Cleft palate 749.20 Cleft palate w/cleft lip NOS 749.21 Unilat cleft palate/lip, complete 749.22 Unilat cleft palate/lip, incomplete 749.23 Bilat cleft palate/lip, complete 749.24 Bilat cleft palate/lip, incomplete V13.6 Hx of congenital malformation **REIMBURSEMENT INFORMATION** Medicare ◆ Follow-up Days — 90 ◆ Assistant Surgeon — paid ◆ Supply Charges — not allowed ◆ Outpatient Limit — does not apply ◆ Major Surgery Rules Apply
42210	Palatoplasty for cleft palate, with closure of alveolar ridge; with bone graft to alveolar ridge (includes obtaining graft)	

CPT CODE	SERVICE	ICD–9–CM
42215	Palatoplasty for cleft palate; major revision	749.0x Cleft palate 749.20 Cleft palate w/cleft lip NOS 749.21 Unilat cleft palate/lip, complete 749.22 Unilat cleft palate/lip, incomplete 749.23 Bilat cleft palate/lip, complete 749.24 Bilat cleft palate/lip, incomplete V13.6 Hx of congenital malformation
42220	Palatoplasty for cleft palate; secondary lengthening procedure	
42225	Palatoplasty for cleft palate; attachment pharyngeal flap	

REIMBURSEMENT INFORMATION

Medicare

- ◆ Follow–up Days — 90
- ◆ Assistant Surgeon — paid
- ◆ Supply Charges — not allowed
- ◆ Outpatient Limit — does not apply
- ◆ Major Surgery Rules Apply

CPT CODE	SERVICE	ICD–9–CM
42226	Lengthening of palate, and pharyngeal flap	749.00 Cleft palate NOS V13.6 Hx of congenital malformation

REIMBURSEMENT INFORMATION

Medicare

- ◆ Follow–up Days — 90
- ◆ Assistant Surgeon — paid
- ◆ Supply Charges — not allowed
- ◆ Outpatient Limit — does not apply
- ◆ Major Surgery Rules Apply

CPT CODE	SERVICE	ICD–9–CM
42227	Lengthening of palate, with island flap	749.0x Cleft palate 749.20 Cleft palate w/cleft lip NOS 749.21 Unilat cleft palate/lip, complete 749.22 Unilat cleft palate/lip, incomplete 749.23 Bilat cleft palate/lip, complete 749.24 Bilat cleft palate/lip, incomplete V13.6 Hx of congenital malformation

REIMBURSEMENT INFORMATION

Medicare

- ◆ Follow–up Days — 90
- ◆ Assistant Surgeon — paid
- ◆ Supply Charges — not allowed
- ◆ Outpatient Limit — does not apply
- ◆ Major Surgery Rules Apply

CPT CODE	SERVICE	ICD–9–CM
42235	Repair of anterior palate, including vomer flap	749.0x Cleft palate 749.20 Cleft palate w/cleft lip NOS 749.21 Unilat cleft palate/lip, complete 749.22 Unilat cleft palate/lip, incomplete 749.23 Bilat cleft palate/lip, complete 749.24 Bilat cleft palate/lip, incomplete 873.65 Open wound of palate 873.75 Open wound of palate, complicated **REIMBURSEMENT INFORMATION** Medicare ♦ Follow–up Days — 90 ♦ Assistant Surgeon — paid ♦ Supply Charges — not allowed ♦ Outpatient Limit — does not apply ♦ Major Surgery Rules Apply
42260	Repair of nasolabial fistula **CPT NOTES** ♦ For repair of cleft lip, see 40700 et seq.	528.5 Diseases of lips 749.00 Cleft palate NOS 750.25 Congenital fistula, lip **REIMBURSEMENT INFORMATION** Medicare ♦ Follow–up Days — 90 ♦ Assistant Surgeon — paid ♦ Supply Charges — not allowed ♦ Outpatient Limit — does not apply ♦ Major Surgery Rules Apply

CPT CODE	SERVICE	ICD-9-CM
42280	Maxillary impression for palatal prosthesis	524.0x Major anomaly of jaw size 524.1x Jaw/cranial base relation anomaly 524.2 Dental arch relationship anomaly 524.3 Tooth position anomaly 524.4 Malocclusion NOS 524.5 Dentofacial functional abnormality 749.0x Cleft palate 749.2x Cleft palate w/cleft lip 784.49 Voice disturbance NEC 802.20 Mandible Fx NOS, closed 802.30 Mandible Fx NOS, open 802.4 Fx malar/maxillary, closed 802.5 Fx malar/maxillary, open 905.0 Late effect, skull/face fracture 906.0 Late effect, open wound head/trunk **REIMBURSEMENT INFORMATION** Medicare ◆ Follow–up Days — 90 ◆ Assistant Surgeon — by report ◆ Supply Charges — not allowed ◆ Outpatient Limit — does not apply ◆ Major Surgery Rules Apply
42281	Insertion of pin-retained palatal prosthesis	524.0x Major anomaly of jaw size 524.1x Jaw/cranial base relation anomaly 524.2 Dental arch relationship anomaly 524.3 Tooth position anomaly 524.4 Malocclusion NOS 524.5 Dentofacial functional abnormality 749.0x Cleft palate 749.2x Cleft palate w/cleft lip 802.20 Mandible Fx NOS, closed 802.30 Mandible Fx NOS, open 802.4 Fx malar/maxillary, closed 802.5 Fx malar/maxillary, open **REIMBURSEMENT INFORMATION** Medicare ◆ Follow–up Days — 10 ◆ Assistant Surgeon — by report ◆ Supply Charges — not allowed ◆ Outpatient Limit — does not apply ◆ Minor Surgery Rules Apply

CPT CODE	SERVICE	ICD–9–CM
42300*	Drainage of abscess; parotid, simple	527.3 Salivary gland abscess 528.3 Cellulitis/abscess of mouth
42305	Drainage of abscess; parotid, complicated	**REIMBURSEMENT INFORMATION** General ♦ Starred procedure. (42300) Medicare ♦ Follow–up Days 42300 — 10 42305 — 90 ♦ Assistant Surgeon — not paid ♦ Supply Charges — not allowed ♦ Outpatient Limit — does not apply ♦ Minor Surgery Rules Apply (42300) Major Surgery Rules Apply (42305)
42310*	Drainage of abscess; submaxillary or sublingual, intraoral	527.3 Salivary gland abscess 528.3 Cellulitis/abscess of mouth 528.9 Oral soft tissue disease NEC 682.0 Cellulitis of face **REIMBURSEMENT INFORMATION** General ♦ Starred procedure. Medicare ♦ Follow–up Days — 10 ♦ Assistant Surgeon — not paid ♦ Supply Charges — not allowed ♦ Outpatient Limit — does not apply ♦ Minor Surgery Rules Apply
42320*	Drainage of abscess; submaxillary, external	527.3 Salivary gland abscess 682.0 Cellulitis of face **REIMBURSEMENT INFORMATION** General ♦ Starred procedure. Medicare ♦ Follow–up Days — 10 ♦ Assistant Surgeon — by report ♦ Supply Charges — not allowed ♦ Outpatient Limit — does not apply ♦ Minor Surgery Rules Apply

CPT CODE	SERVICE	ICD-9-CM
42325	Fistulization of sublingual salivary cyst (ranula)	527.6 Salivary gland mucocele 750.24 Congenital fistula, salivary gland **REIMBURSEMENT INFORMATION** Medicare ◆ Follow-up Days — 90 ◆ Assistant Surgeon — paid ◆ Supply Charges — not allowed ◆ Outpatient Limit — does not apply ◆ Major Surgery Rules Apply
42326	Fistulization of sublingual salivary cyst (ranula); with prothesis	
42330	Sialolithotomy; submandibular (submaxillary), sublingual or parotid, uncomplicated, intraoral	527.2 Sialoadenitis 527.4 Salivary gland fistula 527.5 Sialolithiasis 527.6 Salivary gland mucocele 527.8 Salivary gland disease NEC 527.9 Salivary gland disease NOS **REIMBURSEMENT INFORMATION** Medicare ◆ Follow-up Days — 10 ◆ Assistant Surgeon — not paid ◆ Supply Charges — not allowed ◆ Outpatient Limit — applies ◆ Minor Surgery Rules Apply
42335	Sialolithotomy; submandibular (submaxillary), complicated, intraoral	527.2 Sialoadenitis 527.4 Salivary gland fistula 527.5 Sialolithiasis 527.6 Salivary gland mucocele 527.8 Salivary gland disease NEC **REIMBURSEMENT INFORMATION** Medicare ◆ Follow-up Days — 90 ◆ Assistant Surgeon — not paid ◆ Supply Charges — not allowed ◆ Outpatient Limit — does not apply ◆ Major Surgery Rules Apply

CPT CODE	SERVICE	ICD-9-CM
42340	Sialolithotomy; parotid, extraoral or complicated intraoral	527.2 Sialoadenitis 527.4 Salivary gland fistula 527.5 Sialolithiasis 527.6 Salivary gland mucocele 527.8 Salivary gland disease NEC **REIMBURSEMENT INFORMATION** Medicare ◆ Follow–up Days — 90 ◆ Assistant Surgeon — not paid ◆ Supply Charges — not allowed ◆ Outpatient Limit — does not apply ◆ Major Surgery Rules Apply
42400*	Biopsy of salivary gland; needle	135. Sarcoidosis 142.0 M-Neoplasm, Parotid gland 142.1 M-Neoplasm, Submandibular gland 142.2 M-Neoplasm, Sublingual gland 142.8 M-Neoplasm, Major salivary glnd NEC 142.9 M-Neoplasm, Salivary gland NOS 145.1 M-Neoplasm, Mouth vestibule 198.89 M2-Neoplasm NEC 210.2 B-Neoplasm, Major salivary glands 230.0 CA in situ, Oral cavity/pharynx 235.0 UB-Neoplasm, Major salivary glands 239.0 Digestive neoplasm NOS 527.1 Salivary gland hypertrophy 527.6 Salivary gland mucocele 527.8 Salivary gland disease NEC 527.9 Salivary gland disease NOS **REIMBURSEMENT INFORMATION** General ◆ Starred procedure. Medicare ◆ Follow–up Days — 0 ◆ Assistant Surgeon — not paid ◆ Supply Charges — not allowed ◆ Outpatient Limit — applies ◆ Minor Surgery Rules Apply

CPT CODE	SERVICE	ICD-9-CM
42405	Biopsy of salivary gland; incisional	135. Sarcoidosis 142.0 M-Neoplasm, Parotid gland 142.1 M-Neoplasm, Submandibular gland 142.2 M-Neoplasm, Sublingual gland 142.8 M-Neoplasm, Major salivary glnd NEC 142.9 M-Neoplasm, Salivary gland NOS 198.89 M2-Neoplasm NEC 210.2 B-Neoplasm, Major salivary glands 230.0 CA in situ, Oral cavity/pharynx 235.0 UB-Neoplasm, Major salivary glands 239.0 Digestive neoplasm NOS 527.1 Salivary gland hypertrophy 527.5 Sialolithiasis 527.6 Salivary gland mucocele 527.8 Salivary gland disease NEC 527.9 Salivary gland disease NOS **REIMBURSEMENT INFORMATION** Medicare ◆ Follow–up Days — 10 ◆ Assistant Surgeon — not paid ◆ Supply Charges — not allowed ◆ Outpatient Limit — does not apply ◆ Minor Surgery Rules Apply
42408	Excision of sublingual salivary cyst (ranula)	527.6 Salivary gland mucocele 750.24 Congenital fistula, salivary gland **REIMBURSEMENT INFORMATION** Medicare ◆ Follow–up Days — 90 ◆ Assistant Surgeon — not paid ◆ Supply Charges — not allowed ◆ Outpatient Limit — does not apply ◆ Major Surgery Rules Apply
42409	Marsupialization of sublingual salivary cyst (ranula) **CPT NOTES** ◆ For fistulization of sublingual salivary cyst, see 42325.	527.4 Salivary gland fistula 527.6 Salivary gland mucocele 750.24 Congenital fistula, salivary gland **REIMBURSEMENT INFORMATION** Medicare ◆ Follow–up Days — 90 ◆ Assistant Surgeon — paid ◆ Supply Charges — not allowed ◆ Outpatient Limit — does not apply ◆ Major Surgery Rules Apply

CPT CODE	SERVICE	ICD–9–CM
42410	Excision of parotid tumor or parotid gland; lateral lobe, without nerve dissection	142.0 M-Neoplasm, Parotid gland
		198.89 M2-Neoplasm NEC
42415	Excision of parotid tumor or parotid gland; lateral lobe, with dissection and preservation of facial nerve	210.2 B-Neoplasm, Major salivary glands
		230.0 CA in situ, Oral cavity/pharynx
		235.0 UB-Neoplasm, Major salivary glands
		527.0 Salivary gland atrophy
		527.1 Salivary gland hypertrophy
		527.6 Salivary gland mucocele
		527.8 Salivary gland disease NEC
		527.9 Salivary gland disease NOS

CPT NOTES

- For suture or grafting of facial nerve, see 64864, 64865, 69740, 69745.

REIMBURSEMENT INFORMATION

Medicare

- Follow–up Days — 90
- Assistant Surgeon — paid
- Supply Charges — not allowed
- Outpatient Limit — does not apply
- Major Surgery Rules Apply

CPT CODE	SERVICE	ICD–9–CM
42420	Excision of parotid tumor or parotid gland; total, with dissection and preservation of facial nerve	142.0 M-Neoplasm, Parotid gland
		198.89 M2-Neoplasm NEC
42425	Excision of parotid tumor or parotid gland; total, en bloc removal with sacrifice of facial nerve	210.2 B-Neoplasm, Major salivary glands
		230.0 CA in situ, Oral cavity/pharynx
		234.8 CA in situ NEC
		235.0 UB-Neoplasm, Major salivary glands
		527.0 Salivary gland atrophy
		527.1 Salivary gland hypertrophy
		527.8 Salivary gland disease NEC
		527.9 Salivary gland disease NOS

CPT NOTES

- For suture or grafting of facial nerve, see 64864, 64865, 69740, 69745.

REIMBURSEMENT INFORMATION

Medicare

- Follow–up Days — 90
- Assistant Surgeon — paid
- Supply Charges — not allowed
- Outpatient Limit — does not apply
- Major Surgery Rules Apply

CPT CODE	SERVICE	ICD–9–CM
42426	Excision of parotid tumor or parotid gland; total, with unilateral radical neck dissection **CPT NOTES** ♦ For suture or grafting of facial nerve, see 64864, 64865, 69740, 69745.	142.0 M-Neoplasm, Parotid gland 198.89 M2-Neoplasm NEC 210.2 B-Neoplasm, Major salivary glands 234.8 CA in situ NEC 527.9 Salivary gland disease NOS **REIMBURSEMENT INFORMATION** Medicare ♦ Follow–up Days — 90 ♦ Assistant Surgeon — paid ♦ Supply Charges — not allowed ♦ Outpatient Limit — does not apply ♦ Major Surgery Rules Apply
42440	Excision of submandibular (submaxillary) gland	142.1 M-Neoplasm, Submandibular gland 210.2 B-Neoplasm, Major salivary glands 230.0 CA in situ, Oral cavity/pharynx 235.0 UB-Neoplasm, Major salivary glands 239.0 Digestive neoplasm NOS 527.2 Sialoadenitis 527.5 Sialolithiasis 527.9 Salivary gland disease NOS **REIMBURSEMENT INFORMATION** Medicare ♦ Follow–up Days — 90 ♦ Assistant Surgeon — paid ♦ Supply Charges — not allowed ♦ Outpatient Limit — does not apply ♦ Major Surgery Rules Apply
42450	Excision of sublingual gland	142.1 M-Neoplasm, Submandibular gland 142.2 M-Neoplasm, Sublingual gland 210.2 B-Neoplasm, Major salivary glands 210.3 B-Neoplasm, Floor of mouth 230.0 CA in situ, Oral cavity/pharynx 235.0 UB-Neoplasm, Major salivary glands 239.0 Digestive neoplasm NOS 527.6 Salivary gland mucocele 527.9 Salivary gland disease NOS 784.2 Swelling in head/neck **REIMBURSEMENT INFORMATION** Medicare ♦ Follow–up Days — 90 ♦ Assistant Surgeon — not paid ♦ Supply Charges — not allowed ♦ Outpatient Limit — does not apply ♦ Major Surgery Rules Apply

CPT CODE	SERVICE	ICD–9–CM
42500	Plastic repair of salivary duct, sialodochoplasty; primary or simple	135. Sarcoidosis 142.0 M-Neoplasm, Parotid gland 142.1 M-Neoplasm, Submandibular gland 142.2 M-Neoplasm, Sublingual gland 142.8 M-Neoplasm, Major salivary glnd NEC 142.9 M-Neoplasm, Salivary gland NOS 198.89 M2-Neoplasm NEC 210.2 B-Neoplasm, Major salivary glands 235.0 UB-Neoplasm, Major salivary glands 527.1 Salivary gland hypertrophy 527.5 Sialolithiasis 527.8 Salivary gland disease NEC 527.9 Salivary gland disease NOS 873.51 Open wound of cheek, complicated 906.0 Late effect, open wound head/trunk **REIMBURSEMENT INFORMATION** Medicare ◆ Follow–up Days — 90 ◆ Assistant Surgeon 42500 — not paid 42505 — paid ◆ Supply Charges — not allowed ◆ Outpatient Limit — does not apply ◆ Major Surgery Rules Apply
42505	Plastic repair of salivary duct, sialodochoplasty; secondary or complicated	
42507	Parotid duct diversion, bilateral (Wilke type procedure)	135. Sarcoidosis 142.0 M-Neoplasm, Parotid gland 142.1 M-Neoplasm, Submandibular gland 142.2 M-Neoplasm, Sublingual gland 142.8 M-Neoplasm, Major salivary glnd NEC 142.9 M-Neoplasm, Salivary gland NOS 198.89 M2-Neoplasm NEC 210.2 B-Neoplasm, Major salivary glands 235.0 UB-Neoplasm, Major salivary glands 527.1 Salivary gland hypertrophy **REIMBURSEMENT INFORMATION** Medicare ◆ Follow–up Days — 90 ◆ Assistant Surgeon 42507–42508, 42510 — paid 42509 — by report ◆ Supply Charges — not allowed ◆ Outpatient Limit — does not apply ◆ Major Surgery Rules Apply
42508	Parotid duct diversion, bilateral (Wilke type procedure); with excision of one submandibular gland	
42509	Parotid duct diversion, bilateral (Wilke type procedure); with excision of both submandibular glands	
42510	Parotid duct diversion, bilateral (Wilke type procedure); with ligation of both submandibular (Wharton's) ducts	

CPT CODE	SERVICE	ICD-9-CM

42550 Injection procedure for sialography

CPT NOTES

- For radiological supervision and interpretation, see 70390.

ICD-9-CM	
142.0	M-Neoplasm, Parotid gland
142.1	M-Neoplasm, Submandibular gland
142.2	M-Neoplasm, Sublingual gland
142.8	M-Neoplasm, Major salivary glnd NEC
142.9	M-Neoplasm, Salivary gland NOS
210.2	B-Neoplasm, Major salivary glands
230.0	CA in situ, Oral cavity/pharynx
235.0	UB-Neoplasm, Major salivary glands
527.0	Salivary gland atrophy
527.1	Salivary gland hypertrophy
527.2	Sialoadenitis
527.3	Salivary gland abscess
527.4	Salivary gland fistula
527.5	Sialolithiasis
527.6	Salivary gland mucocele
527.7	Salivary secretion disturbance
527.8	Salivary gland disease NEC
527.9	Salivary gland disease NOS

REIMBURSEMENT INFORMATION

Medicare

- Follow-up Days — 0
- Assistant Surgeon — not paid
- Supply Charges — not allowed
- Outpatient Limit — does not apply
- Minor Surgery Rules Apply

42600 Closure salivary fistula

ICD-9-CM	
527.4	Salivary gland fistula
527.6	Salivary gland mucocele
527.9	Salivary gland disease NOS
906.0	Late effect, open wound head/trunk

REIMBURSEMENT INFORMATION

Medicare

- Follow-up Days — 90
- Assistant Surgeon — by report
- Supply Charges — not allowed
- Outpatient Limit — does not apply
- Major Surgery Rules Apply

CPT CODE / SERVICE	ICD–9–CM
42650* Dilation salivary duct	527.2 Sialoadenitis 527.3 Salivary gland abscess 527.4 Salivary gland fistula 527.5 Sialolithiasis 527.6 Salivary gland mucocele 527.8 Salivary gland disease NEC 527.9 Salivary gland disease NOS 906.0 Late effect, open wound head/trunk **REIMBURSEMENT INFORMATION** <u>General</u> ◆ Starred procedure. <u>Medicare</u> ◆ Follow–up Days — 0 ◆ Assistant Surgeon — not paid ◆ Supply Charges — not allowed ◆ Outpatient Limit — applies ◆ Minor Surgery Rules Apply
42660* Dilation and catheterization of salivary duct, with or without injection	210.2 B-Neoplasm, Major salivary glands 527.5 Sialolithiasis 527.8 Salivary gland disease NEC 527.9 Salivary gland disease NOS 906.0 Late effect, open wound head/trunk **REIMBURSEMENT INFORMATION** <u>General</u> ◆ Starred procedure. <u>Medicare</u> ◆ Follow–up Days — 0 ◆ Assistant Surgeon — by report ◆ Supply Charges — not allowed ◆ Outpatient Limit — applies ◆ Minor Surgery Rules Apply
42665 Ligation salivary duct, intraoral	527.7 Salivary secretion disturbance **REIMBURSEMENT INFORMATION** <u>Medicare</u> ◆ Follow–up Days — 90 ◆ Assistant Surgeon — by report ◆ Supply Charges — not allowed ◆ Outpatient Limit — does not apply ◆ Major Surgery Rules Apply

CPT CODE	SERVICE	ICD–9–CM
42699	Unlisted procedure, salivary glands or ducts	210.2 B-Neoplasm, Major salivary glands 527.5 Sialolithiasis 527.6 Salivary gland mucocele **REIMBURSEMENT INFORMATION** Medicare ♦ Follow–up Days — determined by local carrier ♦ Assistant Surgeon — determined by local carrier ♦ Supply Charges — determined by local carrier ♦ Outpatient Limit — determined by local carrier
42700*	Incision and drainage abscess; peritonsillar	475. Peritonsillar abscess **REIMBURSEMENT INFORMATION** General ♦ Starred procedure. Medicare ♦ Follow–up Days — 10 ♦ Assistant Surgeon — not paid ♦ Supply Charges — not allowed ♦ Outpatient Limit — does not apply ♦ Minor Surgery Rules Apply
42720 **42725**	Incision and drainage abscess; retropharyngeal or parapharyngeal, intraoral approach Incision and drainage abscess; retropharyngeal or parapharyngeal, external approach	478.22 Parapharyngeal abscess 478.24 Retropharyngeal abscess **REIMBURSEMENT INFORMATION** Medicare ♦ Follow–up Days 42720 — 10 42725 — 90 ♦ Assistant Surgeon 42720 — not paid 42725 — paid ♦ Supply Charges — not allowed ♦ Outpatient Limit — does not apply ♦ Minor Surgery Rules Apply (42720) Major Surgery Rules Apply (42725)

CPT CODE	SERVICE	ICD–9–CM	
42800	Biopsy; oropharynx	141.4	M-Neoplasm, Tongue anterior 2/3 NOS
		141.6	M-Neoplasm, Lingual tonsil
		141.9	M-Neoplasm, Tongue NOS
		146.x	Malignant neoplasm, Oropharynx
		149.0	M-Neoplasm, Pharynx NOS
		149.8	M-Neoplasm, Oral cavity/pharynx NEC
		210.1	B-Neoplasm, Tongue
		210.4	B-Neoplasm, Mouth NEC/NOS
		210.5	B-Neoplasm, Tonsil
		210.6	B-Neoplasm, Oropharynx NEC
		210.9	B-Neoplasm, Pharynx NOS
		230.0	CA in situ, Oral cavity/pharynx
		235.1	UB-Neoplasm, Oral cavity/pharynx
		239.0	Digestive neoplasm NOS
		474.8	Chronic tonsil/adenoid disease NEC
		478.29	Disease of pharynx NEC

CPT NOTES

- For laryngoscopic biopsy, see 31510, 31535, 31536.

REIMBURSEMENT INFORMATION

Medicare

- Follow–up Days — 10
- Assistant Surgeon — not paid
- Supply Charges — not allowed
- Outpatient Limit — applies
- Minor Surgery Rules Apply

CPT CODE	SERVICE	ICD–9–CM	
42802	Biopsy; hypopharynx	148.0	M-Neoplasm, Postcricoid hypopharynx
		148.1	M-Neoplasm, Pyriform sinus
		148.2	M-Neoplasm, Aryepiglottic fold
		148.3	M-Neoplasm, Posterior hypopharynx
		148.8	M-Neoplasm, Hypopharynx NEC
		210.8	B-Neoplasm, Hypopharynx
		478.26	Cyst of pharynx/nasopharynx

CPT NOTES

- For laryngoscopic biopsy, see 31510, 31535, 31536.

REIMBURSEMENT INFORMATION

Medicare

- Follow–up Days — 10
- Assistant Surgeon — not paid
- Supply Charges — not allowed
- Outpatient Limit — does not apply
- Minor Surgery Rules Apply

CPT CODE	SERVICE	ICD-9-CM

42804 Biopsy; nasopharynx, visible lesion, simple

CPT NOTES

- For laryngoscopic biopsy, see 31510, 31535, 31536.

ICD-9-CM	
147.x	Malignant neoplasm, Nasopharynx
239.8	Neoplasm NOS, site NEC

REIMBURSEMENT INFORMATION

Medicare

- Follow-up Days — 10
- Assistant Surgeon — not paid
- Supply Charges — not allowed
- Outpatient Limit — does not apply
- Minor Surgery Rules Apply

42806 Biopsy; nasopharynx, survey for unknown primary lesion

CPT NOTES

- For laryngoscopic biopsy, see 31510, 31535, 31536.

ICD-9-CM	
147.x	Malignant neoplasm, Nasopharynx
787.2	Dysphagia

REIMBURSEMENT INFORMATION

Medicare

- Follow-up Days — 10
- Assistant Surgeon — not paid
- Supply Charges — not allowed
- Outpatient Limit — does not apply
- Minor Surgery Rules Apply

42808 Excision or destruction of lesion of pharynx, any method

ICD-9-CM	
146.9	M-Neoplasm, Oropharynx NOS
147.9	M-Neoplasm, Nasopharynx NOS
148.9	M-Neoplasm, Hypopharynx NOS
149.0	M-Neoplasm, Pharynx NOS
161.0	M-Neoplasm, Glottis
210.4	B-Neoplasm, Mouth NEC/NOS
210.5	B-Neoplasm, Tonsil
210.6	B-Neoplasm, Oropharynx NEC
210.7	B-Neoplasm, Nasopharynx
210.8	B-Neoplasm, Hypopharynx
230.0	CA in situ, Oral cavity/pharynx
235.1	UB-Neoplasm, Oral cavity/pharynx
239.0	Digestive neoplasm NOS
478.26	Cyst of pharynx/nasopharynx

REIMBURSEMENT INFORMATION

Medicare

- Follow-up Days — 10
- Assistant Surgeon — not paid
- Supply Charges — not allowed
- Outpatient Limit — does not apply
- Minor Surgery Rules Apply

CPT CODE	SERVICE	ICD-9-CM
42809	Removal of foreign body from pharynx	933.0 Foreign body in pharynx 938. Foreign body, digestive system NOS **REIMBURSEMENT INFORMATION** Medicare ◆ Follow-up Days — 10 ◆ Assistant Surgeon — not paid ◆ Supply Charges — not allowed ◆ Outpatient Limit — does not apply ◆ Minor Surgery Rules Apply
42810	Excision branchial cleft cyst or vestige, confined to skin and subcutaneous tissues	744.41 Branchial cleft sinus/fistula 744.42 Branchial cleft cyst 785.6 Enlargement of lymph nodes **REIMBURSEMENT INFORMATION** Medicare ◆ Follow-up Days — 90 ◆ Assistant Surgeon — paid ◆ Supply Charges — not allowed ◆ Outpatient Limit — does not apply ◆ Major Surgery Rules Apply
42815	Excision branchial cleft cyst, vestige, or fistula, extending beneath subcutaneous tissues and/or into pharynx	744.41 Branchial cleft sinus/fistula 744.42 Branchial cleft cyst **REIMBURSEMENT INFORMATION** Medicare ◆ Follow-up Days — 90 ◆ Assistant Surgeon — paid ◆ Supply Charges — not allowed ◆ Outpatient Limit — does not apply ◆ Major Surgery Rules Apply

CPT CODE	SERVICE	ICD–9–CM
42842	Radical resection of tonsil, tonsillar pillars, and/or retromolar trigone; without closure	141.6 M-Neoplasm, Lingual tonsil 145.6 M-Neoplasm, Retromolar area 146.0 M-Neoplasm, Tonsil 146.2 M-Neoplasm, Tonsillar pillars 210.5 B-Neoplasm, Tonsil 235.1 UB-Neoplasm, Oral cavity/pharynx 463. Acute tonsillitis 474.0 Chronic tonsillitis 474.10 Hypertrophy of tonsils/adenoids 474.11 Hypertrophy of tonsils 474.12 Hypertrophy of adenoids 475. Peritonsillar abscess 478.26 Cyst of pharynx/nasopharynx
42844	Radical resection of tonsil, tonsillar pillars, and/or retromolar trigone; closure with local flap (eg, tongue, buccal)	
42845	Radical resection of tonsil, tonsillar pillars, and/or retromolar trigone; closure with other flap	

CPT NOTES

- ♦ For closure with other flap(s), use appropriate number for flap(s).
- ♦ When combined with radical neck dissection, use also 38720.

REIMBURSEMENT INFORMATION

Medicare

- ♦ Follow–up Days — 90
- ♦ Assistant Surgeon
  42842 — not paid
  42844–42845 — paid
- ♦ Supply Charges — not allowed
- ♦ Outpatient Limit — does not apply
- ♦ Major Surgery Rules Apply

42860 Excision of tonsil tags

474.8 Chronic tonsil/adenoid disease NEC

REIMBURSEMENT INFORMATION

Medicare

- ♦ Follow–up Days — 90
- ♦ Assistant Surgeon — not paid
- ♦ Supply Charges — not allowed
- ♦ Outpatient Limit — does not apply
- ♦ Major Surgery Rules Apply

42870 Excision or destruction lingual tonsil, any method (separate procedure)

141.6 M-Neoplasm, Lingual tonsil
198.89 M2-Neoplasm NEC
210.1 B-Neoplasm, Tongue
235.1 UB-Neoplasm, Oral cavity/pharynx

REIMBURSEMENT INFORMATION

General

- ♦ Separate procedure rules apply.

Medicare

- ♦ Follow–up Days — 90
- ♦ Assistant Surgeon — not paid
- ♦ Supply Charges — not allowed
- ♦ Outpatient Limit — does not apply
- ♦ Major Surgery Rules Apply

CPT CODE / SERVICE	ICD-9-CM
42880 Excision nasopharyngeal lesion (eg, fibroma) **CPT NOTES** ♦ For excision and repair of hypopharyngeal diverticulum, cervical approach, see 43130.	147.x Malignant neoplasm, Nasopharynx 210.7 B-Neoplasm, Nasopharynx 230.0 CA in situ, Oral cavity/pharynx 235.1 UB-Neoplasm, Oral cavity/pharynx 239.0 Digestive neoplasm NOS **REIMBURSEMENT INFORMATION** Medicare ♦ Follow–up Days — 90 ♦ Assistant Surgeon — not paid ♦ Supply Charges — not allowed ♦ Outpatient Limit — does not apply ♦ Major Surgery Rules Apply
42890 Limited pharyngectomy	141.0 M-Neoplasm, Tongue base 149.0 M-Neoplasm, Pharynx NOS **REIMBURSEMENT INFORMATION** Medicare ♦ Follow–up Days — 90 ♦ Assistant Surgeon — paid ♦ Supply Charges — not allowed ♦ Outpatient Limit — does not apply ♦ Major Surgery Rules Apply
42892 Resection of lateral pharyngeal wall or pyriform sinus, direct closure by advancement of lateral and posterior pharyngeal walls **CPT NOTES** ♦ When combined with radical neck dissection, use also 38720.	141.0 M-Neoplasm, Tongue base 149.0 M-Neoplasm, Pharynx NOS **REIMBURSEMENT INFORMATION** Medicare ♦ Follow–up Days — 90 ♦ Assistant Surgeon — paid ♦ Supply Charges — not allowed ♦ Outpatient Limit — does not apply ♦ Major Surgery Rules Apply
42894 Resection of pharyngeal wall requiring closure with myocutaneous flap **CPT NOTES** ♦ When combined with radical neck dissection, use also 38720.	141.0 M-Neoplasm, Tongue base 149.0 M-Neoplasm, Pharynx NOS **REIMBURSEMENT INFORMATION** Medicare ♦ Follow–up Days — 90 ♦ Assistant Surgeon — paid ♦ Supply Charges — not allowed ♦ Outpatient Limit — does not apply ♦ Major Surgery Rules Apply

CPT CODE	SERVICE	ICD–9–CM
42900	Suture pharynx for wound or injury	874.4 Open wound of pharynx 874.5 Open wound of pharynx, complicated 998.3 Postop wound disruption **REIMBURSEMENT INFORMATION** Medicare ♦ Follow–up Days — 10 ♦ Assistant Surgeon — by report ♦ Supply Charges — not allowed ♦ Outpatient Limit — does not apply ♦ Minor Surgery Rules Apply
42950	Pharyngoplasty (plastic or reconstructive operation on pharynx) **CPT NOTES** ♦ For pharyngeal flap, see 42225.	149.0 M-Neoplasm, Pharynx NOS 874.4 Open wound of pharynx 874.5 Open wound of pharynx, complicated **REIMBURSEMENT INFORMATION** Medicare ♦ Follow–up Days — 90 ♦ Assistant Surgeon — paid ♦ Supply Charges — not allowed ♦ Outpatient Limit — does not apply ♦ Major Surgery Rules Apply
42953	Pharyngoesophageal repair **CPT NOTES** ♦ For closure with myocutaneous or other flap, use appropriate number in addition.	149.0 M-Neoplasm, Pharynx NOS 874.4 Open wound of pharynx 874.5 Open wound of pharynx, complicated **REIMBURSEMENT INFORMATION** Medicare ♦ Follow–up Days — 90 ♦ Assistant Surgeon — paid ♦ Supply Charges — not allowed ♦ Outpatient Limit — does not apply ♦ Major Surgery Rules Apply

CPT CODE	SERVICE	ICD-9-CM
42960	Control oropharyngeal hemorrhage (primary or secondary, eg, posttonsillectomy); simple	459.0 Hemorrhage NOS 474.8 Chronic tonsil/adenoid disease NEC 523.8 Periodontal disease NEC 528.9 Oral soft tissue disease NEC 784.8 Hemorrhage from throat 958.2 Secondary/recurrent hemorrhage 998.1 Hemorrhage complicating a procedure 998.2 Accidental op laceration/puncture
42961	Control oropharyngeal hemorrhage (primary or secondary, eg, posttonsillectomy); complicated, requiring hospitalization	
42962	Control oropharyngeal hemorrhage (primary or secondary, eg, posttonsillectomy); with secondary surgical intervention	

REIMBURSEMENT INFORMATION

Medicare

- Follow-up Days
  42960 — 10
  42961–42962 — 90
- Assistant Surgeon
  42960 — not paid
  42961–42962 — paid
- Supply Charges — not allowed
- Outpatient Limit — does not apply
- Minor Surgery Rules Apply (42960)
  Major Surgery Rules Apply (42961–42962)

CPT CODE	SERVICE	ICD-9-CM
42970	Control of nasopharyngeal hemorrhage (primary or secondary, eg, postadenoidectomy); simple, with posterior nasal packs, with or without anterior packs and/or cauterization	459.0 Hemorrhage NOS 474.8 Chronic tonsil/adenoid disease NEC 478.29 Disease of pharynx NEC 784.7 Epistaxis 784.8 Hemorrhage from throat 958.2 Secondary/recurrent hemorrhage 998.1 Hemorrhage complicating a procedure

REIMBURSEMENT INFORMATION

Medicare

- Follow-up Days — 90
- Assistant Surgeon — not paid
- Supply Charges — not allowed
- Outpatient Limit — does not apply
- Major Surgery Rules Apply

CPT CODE	SERVICE
42971	Control of nasopharyngeal hemorrhage (primary or secondary, eg, postadenoidectomy); complicated, requiring hospitalization
42972	Control of nasopharyngeal hemorrhage (primary or secondary, eg, postadenoidectomy); with secondary surgical intervention

ICD–9–CM

784.7	Epistaxis
784.8	Hemorrhage from throat
998.1	Hemorrhage complicating a procedure

REIMBURSEMENT INFORMATION

Medicare

- Follow–up Days — 90
- Assistant Surgeon — paid
- Supply Charges — not allowed
- Outpatient Limit — does not apply
- Major Surgery Rules Apply

CPT CODE	SERVICE	ICD–9–CM

61304 Craniectomy or craniotomy, exploratory; supratentorial

CPT NOTES

- For injection procedure for cerebral angiography, see 36100-36218.
- For injection procedure for ventriculography, see 61026, 61120, 61130.
- For injection procedure for pneumoencephalography, see 61055.

323.9	Encephalitis NOS
432.0	Nontraumatic extradural hemorrhage
854.00	Brain injury NEC
854.10	Brain injury NEC w/open wound
873.9	Open wound of head NEC, complicated

REIMBURSEMENT INFORMATION

Medicare

- Follow–up Days — 90
- Assistant Surgeon — paid
- Supply Charges — not allowed
- Outpatient Limit — does not apply
- Major Surgery Rules Apply

61330 Decompression of orbit only, transcranial approach

CPT NOTES

- For injection procedure for cerebral angiography, see 36100-36218.
- For injection procedure for ventriculography, see 61026, 61120, 61130.
- For injection procedure for pneumoencephalography, see 61055.

192.0	M-Neoplasm, Cranial nerves
376.21	Thyrotoxic exophthalmos
376.22	Exophthalmic ophthalmoplegia
376.31	Constant exophthalmos
376.36	Lateral globe displacement
376.42	Exostosis of orbit
376.43	Orbit deformity d/t bone disease
376.47	Orbit deformity d/t trauma/surgery

REIMBURSEMENT INFORMATION

Medicare

- Follow–up Days — 90
- Assistant Surgeon — paid
- Supply Charges — not allowed
- Outpatient Limit — does not apply
- Major Surgery Rules Apply

CPT CODE	SERVICE	ICD–9–CM

61332 Exploration of orbit (transcranial approach); with biopsy

CPT NOTES

- For injection procedure for cerebral angiography, see 36100-36218.
- For injection procedure for ventriculography, see 61026, 61120, 61130.
- For injection procedure for pneumoencephalography, see 61055.

ICD–9–CM	
170.0	M-Neoplasm, Skull/Face bone
190.1	M-Neoplasm, Orbit
190.8	M-Neoplasm, Eye NEC
198.4	M2-Neoplasm, Nervous system NEC
198.5	M2-Neoplasm, Bone and bone marrow
213.0	B-Neoplasm, Skull/Face bone
224.1	B-Neoplasm, Orbit
234.0	CA in situ, Eye
238.0	UB-Neoplasm, Bone
238.8	Uncertain behavior, neoplasm NEC
239.2	Bone/Skin neoplasm NOS
239.8	Neoplasm NOS, site NEC
376.11	Orbital granuloma
376.12	Orbital myositis
376.81	Orbital cysts

REIMBURSEMENT INFORMATION

Medicare

- Follow–up Days — 90
- Assistant Surgeon — paid
- Supply Charges — not allowed
- Outpatient Limit — does not apply
- Major Surgery Rules Apply

61333 Exploration of orbit (transcranial approach); with removal of lesion

CPT NOTES

- For injection procedure for cerebral angiography, see 36100-36218.
- For injection procedure for ventriculography, see 61026, 61120, 61130.
- For injection procedure for pneumoencephalography, see 61055.

ICD–9–CM	
170.0	M-Neoplasm, Skull/Face bone
190.1	M-Neoplasm, Orbit
190.8	M-Neoplasm, Eye NEC
198.4	M2-Neoplasm, Nervous system NEC
198.5	M2-Neoplasm, Bone and bone marrow
213.0	B-Neoplasm, Skull/Face bone
224.1	B-Neoplasm, Orbit
234.0	CA in situ, Eye
238.0	UB-Neoplasm, Bone
238.1	UB-Neoplasm, Soft tissue
238.8	Uncertain behavior, neoplasm NEC
239.2	Bone/Skin neoplasm NOS
239.8	Neoplasm NOS, site NEC
376.81	Orbital cysts

REIMBURSEMENT INFORMATION

Medicare

- Follow–up Days — 90
- Assistant Surgeon — paid
- Supply Charges — not allowed
- Outpatient Limit — does not apply
- Major Surgery Rules Apply

CPT CODE **SERVICE**

61334 Exploration of orbit (transcranial approach); with removal of foreign body

CPT NOTES

- For injection procedure for cerebral angiography, see 36100-36218.
- For injection procedure for ventriculography, see 61026, 61120, 61130.
- For injection procedure for pneumoencephalography, see 61055.

ICD–9–CM

376.6	Old foreign body, orbit
870.4	Penetrating orbit wound w/FB

REIMBURSEMENT INFORMATION

Medicare

- Follow–up Days — 90
- Assistant Surgeon — paid
- Supply Charges — not allowed
- Outpatient Limit — does not apply
- Major Surgery Rules Apply

CPT CODE	SERVICE
62000	Elevation of depressed skull fracture; simple, extradural
62005	Elevation of depressed skull fracture; compound or comminuted, extradural

CPT NOTES

- For injection procedure for cerebral angiography, see 36100-36218.
- For injection procedure for ventriculography, see 61026, 61120, 61130.
- For injection procedure for pneumoencephalography, see 61055.

ICD–9–CM

800.00	Closed skull vault Fx
800.01	Closed skull vault Fx w/o coma
800.02	Closed skull vault Fx, brief coma
800.03	Closed skull vlt Fx, moderate coma
800.04	Closed skull vlt Fx, prolonged coma
800.05	Closed skull vault Fx, deep coma
800.06	Closed skull vault Fx, coma NOS
800.10	Closed skull vlt Fx, cerebr lacer
800.11	Closed skull vault Fx w/o coma
800.12	Closed skull vault Fx, brief coma
800.13	Closed skull vlt Fx, moderate coma
800.14	Closed skull vlt Fx, prolonged coma
800.15	Closed skull vault Fx, deep coma
800.16	Closed skull vault Fx, coma NOS
800.20	Closed skull vault Fx, mening hem
800.21	Closed skull vault Fx w/o coma
800.22	Closed skull vault Fx, brief coma
800.23	Closed skull vlt Fx, moderate coma
800.24	Closed skull vlt Fx, prolonged coma
800.25	Closed skull vault Fx, deep coma
800.26	Closed skull vault Fx, coma NOS
800.30	Closed skull vlt Fx, hemorrhage NEC
800.31	Closed skull vault Fx w/o coma
800.32	Closed skull vault Fx, brief coma
800.33	Closed skull vlt Fx, moderate coma
800.34	Closed skull vlt Fx, prolonged coma
800.35	Closed skull vault Fx, deep coma
800.36	Closed skull vault Fx, coma NOS
800.40	Closed skull vlt Fx, brain inj NEC
800.41	Closed skull vault Fx w/o coma
800.42	Closed skull vault Fx, brief coma
800.43	Closed skull vlt Fx, moderate coma
800.44	Closed skull vlt Fx, prolonged coma
800.45	Closed skull vault Fx, deep coma
800.46	Closed skull vault Fx, coma NOS
801.00	Closed skull base fracture
801.01	Closed skull base Fx w/o coma
801.02	Closed skull base Fx, brief coma
801.03	Closed skull base Fx, moderate coma
801.04	Closed skull base Fx, prolong coma
801.05	Closed skull base Fx, deep coma
801.06	Closed skull base Fx, coma NOS
801.10	Closed skull base Fx, cerebr lacer
801.11	Closed skull base Fx w/o coma
801.12	Closed skull base Fx, brief coma
801.13	Closed skull base Fx, moderate coma
801.14	Closed skull base Fx, prolong coma
801.15	Closed skull base Fx, deep coma
801.16	Closed skull base Fx, coma NOS
801.20	Closed skull base Fx, mening hem
801.21	Closed skull base Fx w/o coma
801.22	Closed skull base Fx, brief coma
801.23	Closed skull base Fx, moderate coma
801.24	Closed skull base Fx, prolong coma
801.25	Closed skull base Fx, deep coma
801.26	Closed skull base Fx, coma NOS

CPT CODE	SERVICE	ICD–9–CM

62000, 62005 (Cont'd.)

801.30 Closed skull base Fx, hemorr NEC
801.31 Closed skull base Fx w/o coma
801.32 Closed skull base Fx, brief coma
801.33 Closed skull base Fx, moderate coma
801.34 Closed skull base Fx, prolong coma
801.35 Closed skull base Fx, deep coma
801.36 Closed skull base Fx, coma NOS
801.40 Closed skull base Fx, brain inj NEC
801.41 Closed skull base Fx w/o coma
801.42 Closed skull base Fx, brief coma
801.43 Closed skull base Fx, moderate coma
801.44 Closed skull base Fx, prolong coma
801.45 Closed skull base Fx, deep coma
801.46 Closed skull base Fx, coma NOS

REIMBURSEMENT INFORMATION

Medicare

- Follow–up Days — 90
- Assistant Surgeon — paid
- Supply Charges — not allowed
- Outpatient Limit — does not apply
- Major Surgery Rules Apply

62120 Repair of encephalocele, skull vault, including cranioplasty

CPT NOTES

- For injection procedure for cerebral angiography, see 36100-36218.
- For injection procedure for ventriculography, see 61026, 61120, 61130.
- For injection procedure for pneumoencephalography, see 61055.

742.0 Encephalocele

REIMBURSEMENT INFORMATION

Medicare

- Follow–up Days — 90
- Assistant Surgeon — paid
- Supply Charges — not allowed
- Outpatient Limit — does not apply
- Major Surgery Rules Apply

CPT CODE	SERVICE	ICD–9–CM
62121	Craniotomy with repair of encephalocele, skull base **CPT NOTES** ♦ For injection procedure for cerebral angiography, see 36100-36218. ♦ For injection procedure for ventriculography, see 61026, 61120, 61130. ♦ For injection procedure for pneumoencephalography, see 61055.	742.0 Encephalocele **REIMBURSEMENT INFORMATION** Medicare ♦ Follow–up Days — 90 ♦ Assistant Surgeon — paid ♦ Supply Charges — not allowed ♦ Outpatient Limit — does not apply ♦ Major Surgery Rules Apply
62140	Cranioplasty for skull defect; up to 5 cm diameter **CPT NOTES** ♦ For injection procedure for cerebral angiography, see 36100-36218. ♦ For injection procedure for ventriculography, see 61026, 61120, 61130. ♦ For injection procedure for pneumoencephalography, see 61055.	738.1 Acquired head deformity NEC 756.0 Anomaly of skull/face bones **REIMBURSEMENT INFORMATION** Medicare ♦ Follow–up Days — 90 ♦ Assistant Surgeon — paid ♦ Supply Charges — not allowed ♦ Outpatient Limit — does not apply ♦ Major Surgery Rules Apply
62141	Cranioplasty for skull defect; larger than 5 cm diameter **CPT NOTES** ♦ For injection procedure for cerebral angiography, see 36100-36218. ♦ For injection procedure for ventriculography, see 61026, 61120, 61130. ♦ For injection procedure for pneumoencephalography, see 61055.	738.1 Acquired head deformity NEC 756.0 Anomaly of skull/face bones 905.0 Late effect, skull/face fracture 906.0 Late effect, open wound head/trunk **REIMBURSEMENT INFORMATION** Medicare ♦ Follow–up Days — 90 ♦ Assistant Surgeon — paid ♦ Supply Charges — not allowed ♦ Outpatient Limit — does not apply ♦ Major Surgery Rules Apply
63700	Repair of meningocele; less than 5 cm diameter **CPT NOTES** ♦ For application of caliper tongs, see 20660. ♦ For treatment of fracture or dislocation of spine, see 22305-22327.	741.90 Spina bifida, region NOS 742.0 Encephalocele **REIMBURSEMENT INFORMATION** Medicare ♦ Follow–up Days — 90 ♦ Assistant Surgeon — paid ♦ Supply Charges — not allowed ♦ Outpatient Limit — does not apply ♦ Major Surgery Rules Apply

CPT CODE	SERVICE	ICD-9-CM

63702 Repair of meningocele; larger than 5 cm diameter

CPT NOTES

- ♦ For application of caliper tongs, see 20660.
- ♦ For treatment of fracture or dislocation of spine, see 22305-22327.

742.0 Encephalocele

REIMBURSEMENT INFORMATION

Medicare

- ♦ Follow–up Days — 90
- ♦ Assistant Surgeon — paid
- ♦ Supply Charges — not allowed
- ♦ Outpatient Limit — does not apply
- ♦ Major Surgery Rules Apply

63704 Repair of myelomeningocele; less than 5 cm diameter

63706 Repair of myelomeningocele; larger than 5 cm diameter

CPT NOTES

- ♦ For application of caliper tongs, see 20660.
- ♦ For treatment of fracture or dislocation of spine, see 22305-22327.
- ♦ For complex skin closure, see Integumentary System.

741.01 Spina bifida w/hydrocephalus cervix
741.02 Spina bifida w/hydrocephalus dorsal
741.03 Spina bifida w/hydrocephalus lumbar
741.90 Spina bifida, region NOS
741.91 Spina bifida, cervical
741.92 Spina bifida, dorsal
741.93 Spina bifida, lumbar

REIMBURSEMENT INFORMATION

Medicare

- ♦ Follow–up Days — 90
- ♦ Assistant Surgeon — paid
- ♦ Supply Charges — not allowed
- ♦ Outpatient Limit — does not apply
- ♦ Major Surgery Rules Apply

64400* Injection, anesthetic agent; trigeminal nerve, any division or branch

CPT NOTES

- ♦ For intracranial surgery on cranial nerves, see 61450, 61460, 61790.
- ♦ For phenol destruction, see 64600-64640.
- ♦ For subarachnoid or subdural injection, see 62274-62277.
- ♦ For epidural or caudal injection, see 62278, 62279.

239.8 Neoplasm NOS, site NEC
350.1 Trigeminal neuralgia
350.2 Atypical face pain
350.8 Trigeminal nerve disorder NEC

REIMBURSEMENT INFORMATION

General

- ♦ Starred procedure.

Medicare

- ♦ Follow–up Days — 0
- ♦ Assistant Surgeon — not paid
- ♦ Supply Charges — not allowed
- ♦ Outpatient Limit — applies
- ♦ Minor Surgery Rules Apply

CPT CODE **SERVICE** | **ICD–9–CM**

64402* Injection, anesthetic agent; facial nerve

CPT NOTES

- ♦ For intracranial surgery on cranial nerves, see 61450, 61460, 61790.
- ♦ For phenol destruction, see 64600-64640.
- ♦ For subarachnoid or subdural injection, see 62274-62277.
- ♦ For epidural or caudal injection, see 62278, 62279.

350.1	Trigeminal neuralgia
350.2	Atypical face pain
351.1	Geniculate ganglionitis
351.8	Facial nerve disorder NEC
374.30	Ptosis of eyelid NOS
375.15	Tear film insufficiency NOS
729.2	Neuralgia/neuritis NOS

REIMBURSEMENT INFORMATION

General

- ♦ Starred procedure.

Medicare

- ♦ Follow–up Days — 0
- ♦ Assistant Surgeon — not paid
- ♦ Supply Charges — not allowed
- ♦ Outpatient Limit — applies
- ♦ Minor Surgery Rules Apply

64413* Injection, anesthetic agent; cervical plexus

CPT NOTES

- ♦ For intracranial surgery on cranial nerves, see 61450, 61460, 61790.
- ♦ For phenol destruction, see 64600-64640.
- ♦ For subarachnoid or subdural injection, see 62274-62277.
- ♦ For epidural or caudal injection, see 62278, 62279.

353.2	Cervical root lesion NEC
715.9	Osteoarthrosis NOS
721.0	Cervical spondylosis
721.1	Cervical spondylosis w/myelopathy
722.0	Cervical disc displacement
722.4	Cervical disc degeneration
723.0	Cervical spinal stenosis
723.1	Cervicalgia
723.4	Brachial neuritis NOS
726.10	Rotator cuff syndrome NOS

REIMBURSEMENT INFORMATION

General

- ♦ Starred procedure.

Medicare

- ♦ Follow–up Days — 0
- ♦ Assistant Surgeon — not paid
- ♦ Supply Charges — not allowed
- ♦ Outpatient Limit — applies
- ♦ Minor Surgery Rules Apply

CPT CODE **SERVICE**

64415* Injection, anesthetic agent; brachial plexus

CPT NOTES

- For intracranial surgery on cranial nerves, see 61450, 61460, 61790.
- For phenol destruction, see 64600-64640.
- For subarachnoid or subdural injection, see 62274-62277.
- For epidural or caudal injection, see 62278, 62279.

ICD–9–CM

337.21	Reflex sympath dystrophy upper limb
353.0	Brachial plexus lesions
723.4	Brachial neuritis NOS
812.03	Fx greater tuberos humerus, closed
813.06	Fx radius neck, closed
813.41	Colles' fracture, closed
813.42	Fx distal radius NEC, closed

REIMBURSEMENT INFORMATION

General

- Starred procedure.

Medicare

- Follow–up Days — 0
- Assistant Surgeon — not paid
- Supply Charges — not allowed
- Outpatient Limit — applies
- Minor Surgery Rules Apply

CPT CODE **SERVICE**

64450* Injection, anesthetic agent; other peripheral nerve or branch

CPT NOTES

- ♦ For intracranial surgery on cranial nerves, see 61450, 61460, 61790.
- ♦ For phenol destruction, see 64600-64640.
- ♦ For subarachnoid or subdural injection, see 62274-62277.
- ♦ For epidural or caudal injection, see 62278, 62279.

ICD-9-CM

337.0	Idiopathic autonomic neuropathy
337.21	Reflex sympath dystrophy upper limb
337.22	Reflex sympath dystrophy lower limb
337.9	Autonomic nerve system disease NEC
354.0	Carpal tunnel syndrome
354.1	Lesion of median nerve NEC
354.2	Ulnar nerve lesion
354.3	Radial nerve lesion
354.4	Causalgia of upper limb
354.5	Mononeuritis multiplex
354.8	Mononeuritis of arm NEC
355.1	Meralgia paresthetica
355.2	Femoral nerve lesion NEC
355.3	Lateral popliteal nerve lesion
355.4	Medial popliteal nerve lesion
355.5	Tarsal tunnel syndrome
355.6	Plantar nerve lesion
355.7	Mononeuritis of leg NEC
356.0	Hereditary peripheral neuropathy
357.5	Alcoholic polyneuropathy
357.6	Polyneuropathy due to drugs
357.7	Polyneuropathy d/t toxic agents NEC
528.9	Oral soft tissue disease NEC
703.0	Ingrowing nail
729.2	Neuralgia/neuritis NOS
784.0	Headache
882.1	Open wound of hand, complicated
883.1	Open wound of finger, complicated
894.1	Open wound of leg NEC, complicated

REIMBURSEMENT INFORMATION

General

- ♦ Starred procedure.

Medicare

- ♦ Follow–up Days — 0
- ♦ Assistant Surgeon — not paid
- ♦ Supply Charges — not allowed
- ♦ Outpatient Limit — applies
- ♦ Minor Surgery Rules Apply

CPT CODE	SERVICE	ICD-9-CM
64600	Destruction by neurolytic agent, trigeminal nerve; supraorbital, infraorbital, mental, or inferior alveolar branch	171.0 M-Neoplasm, Soft tissue, head 225.1 B-Neoplasm, Cranial nerve 238.1 UB-Neoplasm, Soft tissue 350.1 Trigeminal neuralgia 350.2 Atypical face pain 350.8 Trigeminal nerve disorder NEC 350.9 Trigeminal nerve disorder NOS 351.8 Facial nerve disorder NEC 951.2 Injury to trigeminal nerve
64605	Destruction by neurolytic agent, trigeminal nerve; second and third division branches at foramen ovale	
64610	Destruction by neurolytic agent, trigeminal nerve; second and third division branches at foramen ovale under radiologic monitoring	

CPT NOTES

- ♦ For intracranial surgery on cranial nerves, see 61450, 61460, 61790.

REIMBURSEMENT INFORMATION

Medicare

- ♦ Follow-up Days — 10
- ♦ Assistant Surgeon — not paid
- ♦ Supply Charges — not allowed
- ♦ Outpatient Limit — does not apply
- ♦ Minor Surgery Rules Apply

64702 Neuroplasty; digital, one or both, same digit

CPT NOTES

- ♦ For intracranial surgery on cranial nerves, see 61450, 61460, 61790.
- ♦ Neuroplasty is the decompression or freeing of intact nerve from scar tissue, including external neurolysis and/or transposition.
- ♦ For internal neurolysis requiring use of operating microscope, use 64727.
- ♦ For facial nerve decompression, see 69720.

883.x	Open wound of finger(s)
893.x	Open wound of toe(s)
906.1	Late effect, open wound extremity
955.6	Injury digital nerve

REIMBURSEMENT INFORMATION

Medicare

- ♦ Follow-up Days — 90
- ♦ Assistant Surgeon — not paid
- ♦ Supply Charges — not allowed
- ♦ Outpatient Limit — does not apply
- ♦ Major Surgery Rules Apply

64704 Neuroplasty; nerve of hand or foot

CPT NOTES

- ♦ For intracranial surgery on cranial nerves, see 61450, 61460, 61790.
- ♦ Neuroplasty is the decompression or freeing of intact nerve from scar tissue, including external neurolysis and/or transposition.
- ♦ For internal neurolysis requiring use of operating microscope, use 64727.
- ♦ For facial nerve decompression, see 69720.

882.x	Open wound of hand
892.x	Open wound of foot
906.1	Late effect, open wound extremity
956.4	Injury cutaneous sensory nerve/leg

REIMBURSEMENT INFORMATION

Medicare

- ♦ Follow-up Days — 90
- ♦ Assistant Surgeon — paid
- ♦ Supply Charges — not allowed
- ♦ Outpatient Limit — does not apply
- ♦ Major Surgery Rules Apply

CPT CODE / SERVICE	ICD-9-CM
64708 Neuroplasty, major peripheral nerve, arm or leg; other than specified **CPT NOTES** ♦ For intracranial surgery on cranial nerves, see 61450, 61460, 61790. ♦ Neuroplasty is the decompression or freeing of intact nerve from scar tissue, including external neurolysis and/or transposition. ♦ For internal neurolysis requiring use of operating microscope, use 64727. ♦ For facial nerve decompression, see 69720.	955.1 Injury median nerve 955.2 Injury ulnar nerve 955.4 Injury musculocutaneous nerve 956.1 Injury femoral nerve 956.2 Injury posterior tibial nerve 956.3 Injury peroneal nerve 956.4 Injury cutaneous sensory nerve/leg **REIMBURSEMENT INFORMATION** Medicare ♦ Follow–up Days — 90 ♦ Assistant Surgeon — paid ♦ Supply Charges — not allowed ♦ Outpatient Limit — does not apply ♦ Major Surgery Rules Apply
64712 Neuroplasty, major peripheral nerve, arm or leg; sciatic nerve **CPT NOTES** ♦ For intracranial surgery on cranial nerves, see 61450, 61460, 61790. ♦ Neuroplasty is the decompression or freeing of intact nerve from scar tissue, including external neurolysis and/or transposition. ♦ For internal neurolysis requiring use of operating microscope, use 64727. ♦ For facial nerve decompression, see 69720.	956.0 Injury sciatic nerve **REIMBURSEMENT INFORMATION** Medicare ♦ Follow–up Days — 90 ♦ Assistant Surgeon — paid ♦ Supply Charges — not allowed ♦ Outpatient Limit — does not apply ♦ Major Surgery Rules Apply
64713 Neuroplasty, major peripheral nerve, arm or leg; brachial plexus **CPT NOTES** ♦ For intracranial surgery on cranial nerves, see 61450, 61460, 61790. ♦ Neuroplasty is the decompression or freeing of intact nerve from scar tissue, including external neurolysis and/or transposition. ♦ For internal neurolysis requiring use of operating microscope, use 64727. ♦ For facial nerve decompression, see 69720.	953.4 Brachial plexus injury **REIMBURSEMENT INFORMATION** Medicare ♦ Follow–up Days — 90 ♦ Assistant Surgeon — paid ♦ Supply Charges — not allowed ♦ Outpatient Limit — does not apply ♦ Major Surgery Rules Apply

CPT CODE	SERVICE	ICD-9-CM

64714 Neuroplasty, major peripheral nerve, arm or leg; lumbar plexus

CPT NOTES

- For intracranial surgery on cranial nerves, see 61450, 61460, 61790.
- Neuroplasty is the decompression or freeing of intact nerve from scar tissue, including external neurolysis and/or transposition.
- For internal neurolysis requiring use of operating microscope, use 64727.
- For facial nerve decompression, see 69720.

953.5 Lumbosacral plexus injury

REIMBURSEMENT INFORMATION

Medicare

- Follow-up Days — 90
- Assistant Surgeon — paid
- Supply Charges — not allowed
- Outpatient Limit — does not apply
- Major Surgery Rules Apply

64716 Neuroplasty and/or transposition; cranial nerve (specify)

CPT NOTES

- For intracranial surgery on cranial nerves, see 61450, 61460, 61790.
- Neuroplasty is the decompression or freeing of intact nerve from scar tissue, including external neurolysis and/or transposition.
- For internal neurolysis requiring use of operating microscope, use 64727.
- For facial nerve decompression, see 69720.
- For arthroscopic procedure, see 29848.

171.0	M-Neoplasm, Soft tissue, head
225.1	B-Neoplasm, Cranial nerve
951.0	Injury to oculomotor nerve
951.1	Injury to trochlear nerve
951.2	Injury to trigeminal nerve
951.3	Injury to abducens nerve
951.4	Injury to facial nerve
951.5	Injury to acoustic nerve
951.6	Injury to accessory nerve
951.7	Injury to hypoglossal nerve
951.8	Injury to cranial nerve NEC
951.9	Injury to cranial nerve NOS

REIMBURSEMENT INFORMATION

Medicare

- Follow-up Days — 90
- Assistant Surgeon — paid
- Supply Charges — not allowed
- Outpatient Limit — does not apply
- Major Surgery Rules Apply

CPT CODE	SERVICE	ICD-9-CM

64718 Neuroplasty and/or transposition; ulnar nerve at elbow

CPT NOTES

- For intracranial surgery on cranial nerves, see 61450, 61460, 61790.
- Neuroplasty is the decompression or freeing of intact nerve from scar tissue, including external neurolysis and/or transposition.
- For internal neurolysis requiring use of operating microscope, use 64727.
- For facial nerve decompression, see 69720.
- For arthroscopic procedure, see 29848.

354.2	Ulnar nerve lesion
812.40	Fx lower humerus NOS, closed
812.41	Supracondylar Fx humerus, closed
812.42	Fx humerus, lateral condyle, closed
812.43	Fx humerus, medial condyle, closed
812.44	Fx humerus, condyle NOS, closed
812.49	Fx lower humerus NEC, closed
812.50	Fx lower humerus NOS, open
812.51	Supracondylar Fx humerus, open
812.52	Fx humerus, lateral condyle, open
812.53	Fx humerus, medial condyle, open
812.54	Fx humerus, condyle NOS, open
812.59	Fx lower humerus NEC, open
955.2	Injury ulnar nerve

REIMBURSEMENT INFORMATION

Medicare

- Follow-up Days — 90
- Assistant Surgeon — paid
- Supply Charges — not allowed
- Outpatient Limit — does not apply
- Major Surgery Rules Apply

64719 Neuroplasty and/or transposition; ulnar nerve at wrist

CPT NOTES

- For intracranial surgery on cranial nerves, see 61450, 61460, 61790.
- Neuroplasty is the decompression or freeing of intact nerve from scar tissue, including external neurolysis and/or transposition.
- For internal neurolysis requiring use of operating microscope, use 64727.
- For facial nerve decompression, see 69720.
- For arthroscopic procedure, see 29848.

354.2	Ulnar nerve lesion
955.2	Injury ulnar nerve

REIMBURSEMENT INFORMATION

Medicare

- Follow-up Days — 90
- Assistant Surgeon — not paid
- Supply Charges — not allowed
- Outpatient Limit — does not apply
- Major Surgery Rules Apply

CPT CODE **SERVICE**

64721 Neuroplasty and/or transposition; median nerve at carpal tunnel

CPT NOTES

- For intracranial surgery on cranial nerves, see 61450, 61460, 61790.
- Neuroplasty is the decompression or freeing of intact nerve from scar tissue, including external neurolysis and/or transposition.
- For internal neurolysis requiring use of operating microscope, use 64727.
- For facial nerve decompression, see 69720.
- For arthroscopic procedure, see 29848.

ICD–9–CM

354.0	Carpal tunnel syndrome
354.2	Ulnar nerve lesion
682.4	Cellulitis of hand
727.03	Trigger finger
727.05	Tenosynovitis of hand/wrist NEC
727.41	Ganglion of joint
727.42	Ganglion of tendon sheath
813.4x	Fracture of radius/ulna, lower end
813.5x	Fracture of radius/ulna, lower end
814.00	Fx carpal bone NOS, closed
814.10	Fx carpal bone NOS, open
882.x	Open wound of hand
927.21	Crushing injury, wrist
955.1	Injury median nerve

REIMBURSEMENT INFORMATION

Medicare

- Follow–up Days — 90
- Assistant Surgeon — not paid
- Supply Charges — not allowed
- Outpatient Limit — does not apply
- Major Surgery Rules Apply
- Fragments — 20550, 29075, 29125

CPT CODE **SERVICE**

64722 Decompression; unspecified nerve(s) (specify)

CPT NOTES

- For intracranial surgery on cranial nerves, see 61450, 61460, 61790.
- Neuroplasty is the decompression or freeing of intact nerve from scar tissue, including external neurolysis and/or transposition.
- For internal neurolysis requiring use of operating microscope, use 64727.
- For facial nerve decompression, see 69720.

ICD–9–CM

171.0	M-Neoplasm, Soft tissue, head
225.1	B-Neoplasm, Cranial nerve
337.9	Autonomic nerve system disease NEC
344.6	Cauda equina syndrome
350.8	Trigeminal nerve disorder NEC
353.0	Brachial plexus lesions
353.1	Lumbosacral plexus lesions
353.2	Cervical root lesion NEC
353.4	Lumbosacral root lesion NEC
353.5	Neuralgic amyotrophy
353.8	Nerve root/plexus disorder NEC
354.0	Carpal tunnel syndrome
354.1	Lesion of median nerve NEC
354.2	Ulnar nerve lesion
354.3	Radial nerve lesion
354.5	Mononeuritis multiplex
354.8	Mononeuritis of arm NEC
354.9	Mononeuritis of arm NOS
355.0	Sciatic nerve lesion
355.1	Meralgia paresthetica
355.2	Femoral nerve lesion NEC
355.3	Lateral popliteal nerve lesion
355.4	Medial popliteal nerve lesion
355.5	Tarsal tunnel syndrome
355.8	Mononeuritis of leg NOS
356.x	Peripheral neuropathy
722.0	Cervical disc displacement
722.10	Lumbar disc displacement
722.11	Thoracic disc displacement
722.2	Disc displacement NOS
722.71	Cervical disc disorder w/myelopathy
722.72	Thoracic disc disorder w/myelopathy
722.73	Lumbar disc disorder w/myelopathy
722.81	Postlaminectomy syndrome, cervical
722.82	Postlaminectomy syndrome, thoracic
722.83	Postlaminectomy syndrome, lumbar
723.4	Brachial neuritis NOS
724.9	Back disorder NOS
951.2	Injury to trigeminal nerve
951.4	Injury to facial nerve

REIMBURSEMENT INFORMATION

Medicare

- Follow–up Days — 90
- Assistant Surgeon — paid
- Supply Charges — not allowed
- Outpatient Limit — does not apply
- Major Surgery Rules Apply

CPT CODE	SERVICE
64726	Decompression; plantar digital nerve

CPT NOTES

- For intracranial surgery on cranial nerves, see 61450, 61460, 61790.
- Neuroplasty is the decompression or freeing of intact nerve from scar tissue, including external neurolysis and/or transposition.
- For internal neurolysis requiring use of operating microscope, use 64727.
- For facial nerve decompression, see 69720.

ICD–9–CM

355.5	Tarsal tunnel syndrome
355.6	Plantar nerve lesion
892.x	Open wound of foot
893.x	Open wound of toe(s)
924.20	Contusion of foot
924.3	Contusion of toe
928.20	Crushing injury, foot
928.3	Crushing injury, toe
955.6	Injury digital nerve

REIMBURSEMENT INFORMATION

Medicare

- Follow–up Days — 90
- Assistant Surgeon — paid
- Supply Charges — not allowed
- Outpatient Limit — does not apply
- Major Surgery Rules Apply

CPT CODE	SERVICE
64727	Internal neurolysis, requiring use of operating microscope (list separately in addition to code for neuroplasty) (Neuroplasty includes external neurolysis)

CPT NOTES

- For intracranial surgery on cranial nerves, see 61450, 61460, 61790.
- Neuroplasty is the decompression or freeing of intact nerve from scar tissue, including external neurolysis and/or transposition.
- For internal neurolysis requiring use of operating microscope, use 64727.
- For facial nerve decompression, see 69720.

ICD–9–CM

171.0	M-Neoplasm, Soft tissue, head
225.1	B-Neoplasm, Cranial nerve
237.9	UB-Neoplasm, Nervous system NEC
238.1	UB-Neoplasm, Soft tissue
239.2	Bone/Skin neoplasm NOS
337.0	Idiopathic autonomic neuropathy
337.9	Autonomic nerve system disease NEC
350.1	Trigeminal neuralgia
350.2	Atypical face pain
350.8	Trigeminal nerve disorder NEC
350.9	Trigeminal nerve disorder NOS
354.0	Carpal tunnel syndrome
354.2	Ulnar nerve lesion
355.0	Sciatic nerve lesion
355.1	Meralgia paresthetica
355.3	Lateral popliteal nerve lesion
355.4	Medial popliteal nerve lesion
355.5	Tarsal tunnel syndrome
355.6	Plantar nerve lesion
356.0	Hereditary peripheral neuropathy
356.2	Hereditary sensory neuropathy
356.4	Idiopathic prog polyneuropathy
357.6	Polyneuropathy due to drugs
357.7	Polyneuropathy d/t toxic agents NEC
907.1	Late effect, cranial nerve injury
951.2	Injury to trigeminal nerve

REIMBURSEMENT INFORMATION

Medicare

- Follow–up Days — none; falls within global period of another procedure
- Assistant Surgeon — not paid
- Supply Charges — not allowed
- Outpatient Limit — does not apply

CPT CODE	SERVICE	ICD-9-CM	
64732	Transection or avulsion of; supraorbital nerve	171.0	M-Neoplasm, Soft tissue, head
64734	Transection or avulsion of; infraorbital nerve	225.1	B-Neoplasm, Cranial nerve
64736	Transection or avulsion of; mental nerve	237.9	UB-Neoplasm, Nervous system NEC
		238.1	UB-Neoplasm, Soft tissue
		239.2	Bone/Skin neoplasm NOS
		350.1	Trigeminal neuralgia
		350.2	Atypical face pain
		350.8	Trigeminal nerve disorder NEC
		350.9	Trigeminal nerve disorder NOS
		907.1	Late effect, cranial nerve injury
		951.2	Injury to trigeminal nerve

CPT NOTES

- For intracranial surgery on cranial nerves, see 61450, 61460, 61790.
- For stereotactic lesion of gasserian ganglion, see 61790.
- For section of recurrent laryngeal nerve, see 31595.

REIMBURSEMENT INFORMATION

Medicare

- Follow–up Days — 90
- Assistant Surgeon
  64732, 64736 — paid
  64734 — not paid
- Supply Charges — not allowed
- Outpatient Limit — does not apply
- Major Surgery Rules Apply

CPT CODE	SERVICE	ICD-9-CM	
64738	Transection or avulsion of; inferior alveolar nerve by osteotomy	171.0	M-Neoplasm, Soft tissue, head
		225.1	B-Neoplasm, Cranial nerve
		237.9	UB-Neoplasm, Nervous system NEC
		238.1	UB-Neoplasm, Soft tissue
		239.2	Bone/Skin neoplasm NOS
		350.1	Trigeminal neuralgia
		350.2	Atypical face pain
		350.8	Trigeminal nerve disorder NEC
		350.9	Trigeminal nerve disorder NOS
		351.8	Facial nerve disorder NEC
		907.1	Late effect, cranial nerve injury
		951.2	Injury to trigeminal nerve
		998.2	Accidental op laceration/puncture

CPT NOTES

- For intracranial surgery on cranial nerves, see 61450, 61460, 61790.
- For stereotactic lesion of gasserian ganglion, see 61790.
- For section of recurrent laryngeal nerve, see 31595.

REIMBURSEMENT INFORMATION

Medicare

- Follow–up Days — 90
- Assistant Surgeon — paid
- Supply Charges — not allowed
- Outpatient Limit — does not apply
- Major Surgery Rules Apply

CPT CODE	SERVICE	ICD–9–CM
64740	Transection or avulsion of; lingual nerve **CPT NOTES** ◆ For intracranial surgery on cranial nerves, see 61450, 61460, 61790. ◆ For stereotactic lesion of gasserian ganglion, see 61790. ◆ For section of recurrent laryngeal nerve, see 31595.	171.0 M-Neoplasm, Soft tissue, head 225.1 B-Neoplasm, Cranial nerve 237.9 UB-Neoplasm, Nervous system NEC 238.1 UB-Neoplasm, Soft tissue 239.2 Bone/Skin neoplasm NOS 350.1 Trigeminal neuralgia 350.2 Atypical face pain 350.8 Trigeminal nerve disorder NEC 350.9 Trigeminal nerve disorder NOS 907.1 Late effect, cranial nerve injury 951.2 Injury to trigeminal nerve 998.2 Accidental op laceration/puncture **REIMBURSEMENT INFORMATION** Medicare ◆ Follow–up Days — 90 ◆ Assistant Surgeon — paid ◆ Supply Charges — not allowed ◆ Outpatient Limit — does not apply ◆ Major Surgery Rules Apply
64742	Transection or avulsion of; facial nerve, differential or complete **CPT NOTES** ◆ For intracranial surgery on cranial nerves, see 61450, 61460, 61790. ◆ For stereotactic lesion of gasserian ganglion, see 61790. ◆ For section of recurrent laryngeal nerve, see 31595.	171.0 M-Neoplasm, Soft tissue, head 225.1 B-Neoplasm, Cranial nerve 237.9 UB-Neoplasm, Nervous system NEC 238.1 UB-Neoplasm, Soft tissue 239.2 Bone/Skin neoplasm NOS 351.0 Bell's palsy 351.1 Geniculate ganglionitis 351.8 Facial nerve disorder NEC 351.9 Facial nerve disorder NOS 907.1 Late effect, cranial nerve injury 998.2 Accidental op laceration/puncture **REIMBURSEMENT INFORMATION** Medicare ◆ Follow–up Days — 90 ◆ Assistant Surgeon — paid ◆ Supply Charges — not allowed ◆ Outpatient Limit — does not apply ◆ Major Surgery Rules Apply

CPT CODE	SERVICE	ICD-9-CM

64744 Transection or avulsion of; greater occipital nerve

CPT NOTES

- For intracranial surgery on cranial nerves, see 61450, 61460, 61790.
- For stereotactic lesion of gasserian ganglion, see 61790.
- For section of recurrent laryngeal nerve, see 31595.

238.1	UB-Neoplasm, Soft tissue
239.2	Bone/Skin neoplasm NOS
998.2	Accidental op laceration/puncture

REIMBURSEMENT INFORMATION

Medicare

- Follow–up Days — 90
- Assistant Surgeon — not paid
- Supply Charges — not allowed
- Outpatient Limit — does not apply
- Major Surgery Rules Apply

64772 Transection or avulsion of other spinal nerve, extradural

CPT NOTES

- For intracranial surgery on cranial nerves, see 61450, 61460, 61790.
- For stereotactic lesion of gasserian ganglion, see 61790.
- For excision of tender scar, skin and subcutaneous tissue, with or without tiny neuroma, see 11400-11446, 13100-13300.

343.x	Infantile cerebral palsy
998.2	Accidental op laceration/puncture

REIMBURSEMENT INFORMATION

Medicare

- Follow–up Days — 90
- Assistant Surgeon — paid
- Supply Charges — not allowed
- Outpatient Limit — does not apply
- Major Surgery Rules Apply

CPT CODE **SERVICE**

64774 Excision of neuroma; cutaneous nerve, surgically identifiable

CPT NOTES

- For intracranial surgery on cranial nerves, see 61450, 61460, 61790.
- For Morton neurectomy, see 28080.

ICD–9–CM

215.0	B-Neoplasm, Soft tissue, head
215.2	B-Neoplasm, Soft tissue, arm
215.3	B-Neoplasm, Soft tissue, leg
237.70	Neurofibromatosis NOS
337.9	Autonomic nerve system disease NEC
350.1	Trigeminal neuralgia
350.8	Trigeminal nerve disorder NEC
353.0	Brachial plexus lesions
353.1	Lumbosacral plexus lesions
353.2	Cervical root lesion NEC
354.8	Mononeuritis of arm NEC
354.9	Mononeuritis of arm NOS
355.1	Meralgia paresthetica
355.8	Mononeuritis of leg NOS
355.9	Mononeuritis NOS
356.9	Idiopathic periph neuropathy NOS
722.0	Cervical disc displacement
722.10	Lumbar disc displacement
722.11	Thoracic disc displacement
722.2	Disc displacement NOS
722.7x	Intervertebral disc disorder
722.8x	Postlaminectomy syndrome
722.9x	Intervertebral disc disorder NOS
723.4	Brachial neuritis NOS
724.9	Back disorder NOS
955.4	Injury musculocutaneous nerve
955.5	Injury cutaneous sensory nerve/arm
956.4	Injury cutaneous sensory nerve/leg
957.0	Injury superficial nerve head/neck
997.61	Neuroma of amputation stump

REIMBURSEMENT INFORMATION

Medicare

- Follow–up Days — 90
- Assistant Surgeon — not paid
- Supply Charges — not allowed
- Outpatient Limit — does not apply
- Major Surgery Rules Apply

CPT CODE	SERVICE
64776	Excision of neuroma; digital nerve, one or both, same digit

CPT NOTES

- For intracranial surgery on cranial nerves, see 61450, 61460, 61790.
- For Morton neurectomy, see 28080.

ICD–9–CM

215.2	B-Neoplasm, Soft tissue, arm
215.3	B-Neoplasm, Soft tissue, leg
237.70	Neurofibromatosis NOS
337.9	Autonomic nerve system disease NEC
344.6	Cauda equina syndrome
350.8	Trigeminal nerve disorder NEC
353.0	Brachial plexus lesions
353.1	Lumbosacral plexus lesions
353.2	Cervical root lesion NEC
354.8	Mononeuritis of arm NEC
354.9	Mononeuritis of arm NOS
355.1	Meralgia paresthetica
355.7	Mononeuritis of leg NEC
355.8	Mononeuritis of leg NOS
355.9	Mononeuritis NOS
356.9	Idiopathic periph neuropathy NOS
723.4	Brachial neuritis NOS
724.9	Back disorder NOS
955.6	Injury digital nerve
956.4	Injury cutaneous sensory nerve/leg

REIMBURSEMENT INFORMATION

Medicare

- Follow–up Days — 90
- Assistant Surgeon — not paid
- Supply Charges — not allowed
- Outpatient Limit — does not apply
- Major Surgery Rules Apply

CPT CODE **SERVICE**

64778 Excision of neuroma; digital nerve, each additional digit (list separately by this number)

CPT NOTES

- For intracranial surgery on cranial nerves, see 61450, 61460, 61790.
- For Morton neurectomy, see 28080.

ICD–9–CM

215.2	B-Neoplasm, Soft tissue, arm
215.3	B-Neoplasm, Soft tissue, leg
237.71	Neurofibromatosis, type 1
337.9	Autonomic nerve system disease NEC
344.6	Cauda equina syndrome
350.8	Trigeminal nerve disorder NEC
353.0	Brachial plexus lesions
353.1	Lumbosacral plexus lesions
353.2	Cervical root lesion NEC
354.8	Mononeuritis of arm NEC
354.9	Mononeuritis of arm NOS
355.1	Meralgia paresthetica
355.7	Mononeuritis of leg NEC
355.8	Mononeuritis of leg NOS
355.9	Mononeuritis NOS
356.9	Idiopathic periph neuropathy NOS
723.4	Brachial neuritis NOS
724.9	Back disorder NOS
955.6	Injury digital nerve
956.4	Injury cutaneous sensory nerve/leg
997.61	Neuroma of amputation stump

REIMBURSEMENT INFORMATION

Medicare

- Follow–up Days — none; falls within global period of another procedure
- Assistant Surgeon — paid
- Supply Charges — not allowed
- Outpatient Limit — does not apply
- Major Surgery Rules Apply

CPT CODE **SERVICE**

64782 Excision of neuroma; hand or foot, except digital nerve

CPT NOTES

- For intracranial surgery on cranial nerves, see 61450, 61460, 61790.
- For Morton neurectomy, see 28080.

ICD–9–CM

215.2	B-Neoplasm, Soft tissue, arm
215.3	B-Neoplasm, Soft tissue, leg
237.70	Neurofibromatosis NOS
337.9	Autonomic nerve system disease NEC
344.6	Cauda equina syndrome
350.8	Trigeminal nerve disorder NEC
353.0	Brachial plexus lesions
353.1	Lumbosacral plexus lesions
353.2	Cervical root lesion NEC
354.8	Mononeuritis of arm NEC
354.9	Mononeuritis of arm NOS
355.1	Meralgia paresthetica
355.5	Tarsal tunnel syndrome
355.6	Plantar nerve lesion
355.8	Mononeuritis of leg NOS
355.9	Mononeuritis NOS
356.8	Idiopathic periph neuropathy NEC
356.9	Idiopathic periph neuropathy NOS
723.4	Brachial neuritis NOS
724.9	Back disorder NOS
955.4	Injury musculocutaneous nerve
955.5	Injury cutaneous sensory nerve/arm
956.4	Injury cutaneous sensory nerve/leg
956.5	Injury nerve pelvis/leg NEC
997.61	Neuroma of amputation stump

REIMBURSEMENT INFORMATION

Medicare

- Follow–up Days — 90
- Assistant Surgeon — paid
- Supply Charges — not allowed
- Outpatient Limit — does not apply
- Major Surgery Rules Apply

CPT CODE	SERVICE
64783	Excision of neuroma; hand or foot, each additional nerve, except same digit (list separately by this number)

CPT NOTES

- For intracranial surgery on cranial nerves, see 61450, 61460, 61790.
- For Morton neurectomy, see 28080.

ICD–9–CM

215.2	B-Neoplasm, Soft tissue, arm
215.3	B-Neoplasm, Soft tissue, leg
237.70	Neurofibromatosis NOS
337.9	Autonomic nerve system disease NEC
344.6	Cauda equina syndrome
350.8	Trigeminal nerve disorder NEC
353.0	Brachial plexus lesions
353.1	Lumbosacral plexus lesions
353.2	Cervical root lesion NEC
354.8	Mononeuritis of arm NEC
354.9	Mononeuritis of arm NOS
355.1	Meralgia paresthetica
355.5	Tarsal tunnel syndrome
355.6	Plantar nerve lesion
355.8	Mononeuritis of leg NOS
355.9	Mononeuritis NOS
356.8	Idiopathic periph neuropathy NEC
356.9	Idiopathic periph neuropathy NOS
723.4	Brachial neuritis NOS
724.9	Back disorder NOS
955.4	Injury musculocutaneous nerve
955.5	Injury cutaneous sensory nerve/arm
956.4	Injury cutaneous sensory nerve/leg
956.5	Injury nerve pelvis/leg NEC
997.61	Neuroma of amputation stump

REIMBURSEMENT INFORMATION

Medicare

- Follow–up Days — none; falls within global period of another procedure
- Assistant Surgeon — paid
- Supply Charges — not allowed
- Outpatient Limit — does not apply
- Major Surgery Rules Apply

CPT CODE **SERVICE**

64784 Excision of neuroma; major peripheral nerve, except sciatic

CPT NOTES

- For intracranial surgery on cranial nerves, see 61450, 61460, 61790.
- For Morton neurectomy, see 28080.

ICD–9–CM

215.2	B-Neoplasm, Soft tissue, arm
215.3	B-Neoplasm, Soft tissue, leg
215.6	B-Neoplasm, Soft tissue, pelvis
237.70	Neurofibromatosis NOS
337.9	Autonomic nerve system disease NEC
344.6	Cauda equina syndrome
350.8	Trigeminal nerve disorder NEC
353.0	Brachial plexus lesions
353.1	Lumbosacral plexus lesions
353.2	Cervical root lesion NEC
354.x	Mononeuritis of upper limb
355.x	Mononeuritis of lower limb
356.x	Peripheral neuropathy
722.0	Cervical disc displacement
722.10	Lumbar disc displacement
722.11	Thoracic disc displacement
722.2	Disc displacement NOS
722.7x	Intervertebral disc disorder
722.8x	Postlaminectomy syndrome
723.4	Brachial neuritis NOS
724.9	Back disorder NOS
955.0	Injury axillary nerve
955.1	Injury median nerve
955.2	Injury ulnar nerve
955.3	Injury radial nerve
956.1	Injury femoral nerve
956.2	Injury posterior tibial nerve
956.3	Injury peroneal nerve
997.61	Neuroma of amputation stump

REIMBURSEMENT INFORMATION

Medicare

- Follow–up Days — 90
- Assistant Surgeon — paid
- Supply Charges — not allowed
- Outpatient Limit — does not apply
- Major Surgery Rules Apply

CPT CODE	SERVICE	ICD–9–CM	
64787	Implantation of nerve end into bone or muscle (list separately in addition to neuroma excision)	215.0	B-Neoplasm, Soft tissue, head
		215.2	B-Neoplasm, Soft tissue, arm
		215.3	B-Neoplasm, Soft tissue, leg
		215.4	B-Neoplasm, Soft tissue, thorax
		215.5	B-Neoplasm, Soft tissue, abdomen
		215.6	B-Neoplasm, Soft tissue, pelvis
		215.8	B-Neoplasm, Soft tissue NEC
		237.70	Neurofibromatosis NOS
		955.x	Injury to peripheral nerve(s)
		956.x	Pelvic/lower limb nerve injury
		957.0	Injury superficial nerve head/neck
		957.1	Injury to nerve NEC

CPT NOTES

- For intracranial surgery on cranial nerves, see 61450, 61460, 61790.
- For Morton neurectomy, see 28080.

REIMBURSEMENT INFORMATION

Medicare

- Follow–up Days — none; falls within global period of another procedure
- Assistant Surgeon — not paid
- Supply Charges — not allowed
- Outpatient Limit — does not apply
- Major Surgery Rules Apply

CPT CODE	SERVICE	ICD–9–CM	
64788	Excision of neurofibroma or neurolemmoma; cutaneous nerve	171.0	M-Neoplasm, Soft tissue, head
		215.0	B-Neoplasm, Soft tissue, head
		215.7	B-Neoplasm, Trunk NOS
		237.7	UB-Neoplasm, Neurofibromatosis
		237.70	Neurofibromatosis NOS
		238.1	UB-Neoplasm, Soft tissue
		239.2	Bone/Skin neoplasm NOS

CPT NOTES

- For intracranial surgery on cranial nerves, see 61450, 61460, 61790.
- For Morton neurectomy, see 28080.

REIMBURSEMENT INFORMATION

Medicare

- Follow–up Days — 90
- Assistant Surgeon — paid
- Supply Charges — not allowed
- Outpatient Limit — does not apply
- Major Surgery Rules Apply

CPT CODE	SERVICE	ICD–9–CM
64790	Excision of neurofibroma or neurolemmoma; major peripheral nerve	171.0 M-Neoplasm, Soft tissue, head 215.0 B-Neoplasm, Soft tissue, head 215.2 B-Neoplasm, Soft tissue, arm 215.3 B-Neoplasm, Soft tissue, leg 215.6 B-Neoplasm, Soft tissue, pelvis 237.7 UB-Neoplasm, Neurofibromatosis 237.70 Neurofibromatosis NOS 238.1 UB-Neoplasm, Soft tissue 239.2 Bone/Skin neoplasm NOS

CPT NOTES

- For intracranial surgery on cranial nerves, see 61450, 61460, 61790.
- For Morton neurectomy, see 28080.

REIMBURSEMENT INFORMATION

Medicare

- Follow–up Days — 90
- Assistant Surgeon — paid
- Supply Charges — not allowed
- Outpatient Limit — does not apply
- Major Surgery Rules Apply

CPT CODE	SERVICE	ICD–9–CM
64792	Excision of neurofibroma or neurolemmoma; extensive (including malignant type)	171.0 M-Neoplasm, Soft tissue, head 171.4 M-Neoplasm, Soft tissue, thorax 171.5 M-Neoplasm, Soft tissue, abdomen 171.7 M-Neoplasm, Trunk NOS 215.4 B-Neoplasm, Soft tissue, thorax 215.5 B-Neoplasm, Soft tissue, abdomen 237.70 Neurofibromatosis NOS 238.1 UB-Neoplasm, Soft tissue 239.0 Digestive neoplasm NOS 239.2 Bone/Skin neoplasm NOS

CPT NOTES

- For intracranial surgery on cranial nerves, see 61450, 61460, 61790.
- For Morton neurectomy, see 28080.

REIMBURSEMENT INFORMATION

Medicare

- Follow–up Days — 90
- Assistant Surgeon — paid
- Supply Charges — not allowed
- Outpatient Limit — does not apply
- Major Surgery Rules Apply

CPT CODE **SERVICE**

64795 Biopsy of nerve

CPT NOTES

- For intracranial surgery on cranial nerves, see 61450, 61460, 61790.
- For Morton neurectomy, see 28080.

ICD–9–CM

030.0	Lepromatous leprosy
171.0	M-Neoplasm, Soft tissue, head
171.2	M-Neoplasm, Soft tissue, arm
171.3	M-Neoplasm, Soft tissue, leg
171.4	M-Neoplasm, Soft tissue, thorax
171.5	M-Neoplasm, Soft tissue, abdomen
171.6	M-Neoplasm, Soft tissue, pelvis
171.7	M-Neoplasm, Trunk NOS
215.0	B-Neoplasm, Soft tissue, head
234.8	CA in situ NEC
237.7	UB-Neoplasm, Neurofibromatosis
237.9	UB-Neoplasm, Nervous system NEC
238.1	UB-Neoplasm, Soft tissue
239.2	Bone/Skin neoplasm NOS
336.8	Myelopathy NEC
337.9	Autonomic nerve system disease NEC
356.9	Idiopathic periph neuropathy NOS
357.9	Inflammatory/toxic neuropathy NOS
781.1	Smell/taste sensation disturbance
781.2	Abnormality of gait
781.4	Transient limb paralysis
781.9	Nervous/musculoskeletal symptom NEC

REIMBURSEMENT INFORMATION

Medicare

- Follow–up Days — 0
- Assistant Surgeon — not paid
- Supply Charges — not allowed
- Outpatient Limit — does not apply
- Minor Surgery Rules Apply

CPT CODE	SERVICE
64830	Microdissection and/or microrepair of nerve (list separately in addition to code for nerve repair)

CPT NOTES

- For intracranial surgery on cranial nerves, see 61450, 61460, 61790.

ICD–9–CM

171.0	M-Neoplasm, Soft tissue, head
171.2	M-Neoplasm, Soft tissue, arm
171.3	M-Neoplasm, Soft tissue, leg
171.4	M-Neoplasm, Soft tissue, thorax
171.5	M-Neoplasm, Soft tissue, abdomen
171.6	M-Neoplasm, Soft tissue, pelvis
171.7	M-Neoplasm, Trunk NOS
171.8	M-Neoplasm, Soft tissue NEC
215.0	B-Neoplasm, Soft tissue, head
215.2	B-Neoplasm, Soft tissue, arm
215.3	B-Neoplasm, Soft tissue, leg
215.4	B-Neoplasm, Soft tissue, thorax
215.5	B-Neoplasm, Soft tissue, abdomen
215.6	B-Neoplasm, Soft tissue, pelvis
215.7	B-Neoplasm, Trunk NOS
215.8	B-Neoplasm, Soft tissue NEC
238.1	UB-Neoplasm, Soft tissue
239.2	Bone/Skin neoplasm NOS
842.1x	Hand sprain/strain
881.22	Open wound of wrist w/tendon
882.2	Open wound of hand, w/tendon
884.2	Open wound of arm NOS w/tendon
907.1	Late effect, cranial nerve injury
951.2	Injury to trigeminal nerve
954.0	Injury cervical sympathetic nerve
954.1	Injury sympathetic nerve NEC
954.8	Injury trunk nerve NEC
955.x	Injury to peripheral nerve(s)
956.x	Pelvic/lower limb nerve injury
957.0	Injury superficial nerve head/neck
957.1	Injury to nerve NEC
957.8	Injury to multiple nerves

REIMBURSEMENT INFORMATION

Medicare

- Follow–up Days — none; falls within global period of another procedure
- Assistant Surgeon — not paid
- Supply Charges — not allowed
- Outpatient Limit — does not apply

CPT CODE	SERVICE	ICD–9–CM

64831 Suture of digital nerve, hand or foot; one nerve

CPT NOTES

- For intracranial surgery on cranial nerves, see 61450, 61460, 61790.

443.0	Raynaud's syndrome
882.x	Open wound of hand
883.x	Open wound of finger(s)
886.x	Traumatic finger amputation
892.x	Open wound of foot
893.0	Open wound of toe
893.1	Open wound of toe, complicated
906.1	Late effect, open wound extremity
927.3	Crushing injury, finger
955.6	Injury digital nerve
956.4	Injury cutaneous sensory nerve/leg

REIMBURSEMENT INFORMATION

Medicare

- Follow–up Days — 90
- Assistant Surgeon — not paid
- Supply Charges — not allowed
- Outpatient Limit — does not apply
- Major Surgery Rules Apply

64832 Suture of digital nerve, hand or foot; each additional digital nerve

CPT NOTES

- For intracranial surgery on cranial nerves, see 61450, 61460, 61790.

443.0	Raynaud's syndrome
883.x	Open wound of finger(s)
886.x	Traumatic finger amputation
892.x	Open wound of foot
893.0	Open wound of toe
893.1	Open wound of toe, complicated
906.1	Late effect, open wound extremity
927.3	Crushing injury, finger
955.6	Injury digital nerve
956.4	Injury cutaneous sensory nerve/leg

REIMBURSEMENT INFORMATION

Medicare

- Follow–up Days — none; falls within global period of another procedure
- Assistant Surgeon — not paid
- Supply Charges — not allowed
- Outpatient Limit — does not apply

CPT CODE	SERVICE	ICD-9-CM
64834	Suture of one nerve, hand or foot; common sensory nerve **CPT NOTES** ♦ For intracranial surgery on cranial nerves, see 61450, 61460, 61790.	906.1 Late effect, open wound extremity 955.1 Injury median nerve 955.2 Injury ulnar nerve 955.3 Injury radial nerve 955.5 Injury cutaneous sensory nerve/arm 956.4 Injury cutaneous sensory nerve/leg **REIMBURSEMENT INFORMATION** Medicare ♦ Follow-up Days — 90 ♦ Assistant Surgeon — not paid ♦ Supply Charges — not allowed ♦ Outpatient Limit — does not apply ♦ Major Surgery Rules Apply
64835	Suture of one nerve, hand or foot; median motor thenar **CPT NOTES** ♦ For intracranial surgery on cranial nerves, see 61450, 61460, 61790.	906.1 Late effect, open wound extremity 955.1 Injury median nerve **REIMBURSEMENT INFORMATION** Medicare ♦ Follow-up Days — 90 ♦ Assistant Surgeon — paid ♦ Supply Charges — not allowed ♦ Outpatient Limit — does not apply ♦ Major Surgery Rules Apply
64836	Suture of one nerve, hand or foot; ulnar motor **CPT NOTES** ♦ For intracranial surgery on cranial nerves, see 61450, 61460, 61790.	906.1 Late effect, open wound extremity 955.2 Injury ulnar nerve **REIMBURSEMENT INFORMATION** Medicare ♦ Follow-up Days — 90 ♦ Assistant Surgeon — paid ♦ Supply Charges — not allowed ♦ Outpatient Limit — does not apply ♦ Major Surgery Rules Apply

CPT CODE SERVICE	ICD–9–CM
64837 Suture of each additional nerve, hand or foot **CPT NOTES** ◆ For intracranial surgery on cranial nerves, see 61450, 61460, 61790.	906.1 Late effect, open wound extremity 955.1 Injury median nerve 955.2 Injury ulnar nerve 955.6 Injury digital nerve 956.2 Injury posterior tibial nerve 956.4 Injury cutaneous sensory nerve/leg **REIMBURSEMENT INFORMATION** Medicare ◆ Follow–up Days — none; falls within global period of another procedure ◆ Assistant Surgeon — paid ◆ Supply Charges — not allowed ◆ Outpatient Limit — does not apply
64840 Suture of posterior tibial nerve **CPT NOTES** ◆ For intracranial surgery on cranial nerves, see 61450, 61460, 61790.	906.1 Late effect, open wound extremity 956.2 Injury posterior tibial nerve **REIMBURSEMENT INFORMATION** Medicare ◆ Follow–up Days — 90 ◆ Assistant Surgeon — paid ◆ Supply Charges — not allowed ◆ Outpatient Limit — does not apply ◆ Major Surgery Rules Apply
64856 Suture of major peripheral nerve, arm or leg, except sciatic; including transposition **64857** Suture of major peripheral nerve, arm or leg, except sciatic; without transposition **CPT NOTES** ◆ For intracranial surgery on cranial nerves, see 61450, 61460, 61790.	906.1 Late effect, open wound extremity 955.0 Injury axillary nerve 955.1 Injury median nerve 955.2 Injury ulnar nerve 955.3 Injury radial nerve 955.4 Injury musculocutaneous nerve 956.1 Injury femoral nerve 956.2 Injury posterior tibial nerve 956.3 Injury peroneal nerve 956.4 Injury cutaneous sensory nerve/leg **REIMBURSEMENT INFORMATION** Medicare ◆ Follow–up Days — 90 ◆ Assistant Surgeon — paid ◆ Supply Charges — not allowed ◆ Outpatient Limit — does not apply ◆ Major Surgery Rules Apply

CPT CODE / SERVICE	ICD-9-CM
64861 Suture of; brachial plexus **CPT NOTES** ♦ For intracranial surgery on cranial nerves, see 61450, 61460, 61790.	906.0 Late effect, open wound head/trunk 953.4 Brachial plexus injury **REIMBURSEMENT INFORMATION** Medicare ♦ Follow-up Days — 90 ♦ Assistant Surgeon — paid ♦ Supply Charges — not allowed ♦ Outpatient Limit — does not apply ♦ Major Surgery Rules Apply
64864 Suture of facial nerve; extracranial **CPT NOTES** ♦ For intracranial surgery on cranial nerves, see 61450, 61460, 61790.	171.0 M-Neoplasm, Soft tissue, head 225.1 B-Neoplasm, Cranial nerve 906.0 Late effect, open wound head/trunk 907.1 Late effect, cranial nerve injury 951.4 Injury to facial nerve 951.8 Injury to cranial nerve NEC **REIMBURSEMENT INFORMATION** Medicare ♦ Follow-up Days — 90 ♦ Assistant Surgeon — paid ♦ Supply Charges — not allowed ♦ Outpatient Limit — does not apply ♦ Major Surgery Rules Apply
64865 Suture of facial nerve; infratemporal, with or without grafting **CPT NOTES** ♦ For intracranial surgery on cranial nerves, see 61450, 61460, 61790.	951.4 Injury to facial nerve **REIMBURSEMENT INFORMATION** Medicare ♦ Follow-up Days — 90 ♦ Assistant Surgeon — paid ♦ Supply Charges — not allowed ♦ Outpatient Limit — does not apply ♦ Major Surgery Rules Apply

CPT CODE	SERVICE	ICD–9–CM
64868	Anastomosis; facial-hypoglossal	351.0 Bell's palsy 951.4 Injury to facial nerve

CPT NOTES

- For intracranial surgery on cranial nerves, see 61450, 61460, 61790.

REIMBURSEMENT INFORMATION

Medicare

- Follow–up Days — 90
- Assistant Surgeon — paid
- Supply Charges — not allowed
- Outpatient Limit — does not apply
- Major Surgery Rules Apply

64872 Suture of nerve; requiring secondary or delayed suture (list separately in addition to code for primary neurorrhaphy)

CPT NOTES

- For intracranial surgery on cranial nerves, see 61450, 61460, 61790.

ICD–9–CM	
171.0	M-Neoplasm, Soft tissue, head
225.1	B-Neoplasm, Cranial nerve
905.2	Late effect, arm fracture
905.4	Late effect, leg fracture
907.4	Late effect, nerve injury shld/arm
907.5	Late effect, nerve inj pelvis/leg
951.4	Injury to facial nerve
953.0	Cervical root injury
953.1	Dorsal root injury
953.2	Lumbar root injury
953.3	Sacral root injury
953.4	Brachial plexus injury
953.5	Lumbosacral plexus injury
955.0	Injury axillary nerve
955.1	Injury median nerve
955.2	Injury ulnar nerve
955.3	Injury radial nerve
955.4	Injury musculocutaneous nerve
955.5	Injury cutaneous sensory nerve/arm
955.6	Injury digital nerve
956.0	Injury sciatic nerve
956.1	Injury femoral nerve
956.2	Injury posterior tibial nerve
956.3	Injury peroneal nerve
956.4	Injury cutaneous sensory nerve/leg
998.2	Accidental op laceration/puncture

REIMBURSEMENT INFORMATION

Medicare

- Follow–up Days — none; falls within global period of another procedure
- Assistant Surgeon — paid
- Supply Charges — not allowed
- Outpatient Limit — does not apply

CPT CODE	SERVICE	ICD-9-CM
64874	Suture of nerve; requiring extensive mobilization, or transposition of nerve (list separately in addition to code for nerve suture) **CPT NOTES** ♦ For intracranial surgery on cranial nerves, see 61450, 61460, 61790.	171.0 M-Neoplasm, Soft tissue, head 225.1 B-Neoplasm, Cranial nerve 951.2 Injury to trigeminal nerve 951.4 Injury to facial nerve 955.0 Injury axillary nerve 955.1 Injury median nerve 955.2 Injury ulnar nerve 955.4 Injury musculocutaneous nerve **REIMBURSEMENT INFORMATION** Medicare ♦ Follow-up Days — none; falls within global period of another procedure ♦ Assistant Surgeon — paid ♦ Supply Charges — not allowed ♦ Outpatient Limit — does not apply
64885	Nerve graft (includes obtaining graft), head or neck; up to 4 cm in length **CPT NOTES** ♦ For intracranial surgery on cranial nerves, see 61450, 61460, 61790.	951.4 Injury to facial nerve 951.6 Injury to accessory nerve 957.0 Injury superficial nerve head/neck **REIMBURSEMENT INFORMATION** Medicare ♦ Follow-up Days — 90 ♦ Assistant Surgeon — paid ♦ Supply Charges — not allowed ♦ Outpatient Limit — does not apply ♦ Major Surgery Rules Apply
64886	Nerve graft (includes obtaining graft), head or neck; more than 4 cm in length **CPT NOTES** ♦ For intracranial surgery on cranial nerves, see 61450, 61460, 61790.	907.1 Late effect, cranial nerve injury 951.4 Injury to facial nerve 951.6 Injury to accessory nerve 957.0 Injury superficial nerve head/neck **REIMBURSEMENT INFORMATION** Medicare ♦ Follow-up Days — 90 ♦ Assistant Surgeon — paid ♦ Supply Charges — not allowed ♦ Outpatient Limit — does not apply ♦ Major Surgery Rules Apply

CPT CODE	SERVICE	ICD-9-CM

64890 Nerve graft (includes obtaining graft), single strand, hand or foot; up to 4 cm length

CPT NOTES

- For intracranial surgery on cranial nerves, see 61450, 61460, 61790.

905.2	Late effect, arm fracture
905.4	Late effect, leg fracture
907.1	Late effect, cranial nerve injury
907.4	Late effect, nerve injury shld/arm
907.5	Late effect, nerve inj pelvis/leg
955.1	Injury median nerve
955.2	Injury ulnar nerve
955.3	Injury radial nerve
955.6	Injury digital nerve
956.1	Injury femoral nerve
956.2	Injury posterior tibial nerve
956.3	Injury peroneal nerve
956.4	Injury cutaneous sensory nerve/leg

REIMBURSEMENT INFORMATION

Medicare

- Follow-up Days — 90
- Assistant Surgeon — paid
- Supply Charges — not allowed
- Outpatient Limit — does not apply
- Major Surgery Rules Apply

64891 Nerve graft (includes obtaining graft), single strand, hand or foot; more than 4 cm length

CPT NOTES

- For intracranial surgery on cranial nerves, see 61450, 61460, 61790.

905.2	Late effect, arm fracture
905.4	Late effect, leg fracture
907.4	Late effect, nerve injury shld/arm
907.5	Late effect, nerve inj pelvis/leg
955.1	Injury median nerve
955.2	Injury ulnar nerve
955.3	Injury radial nerve
955.6	Injury digital nerve
956.1	Injury femoral nerve
956.2	Injury posterior tibial nerve
956.3	Injury peroneal nerve
956.4	Injury cutaneous sensory nerve/leg

REIMBURSEMENT INFORMATION

Medicare

- Follow-up Days — 90
- Assistant Surgeon — paid
- Supply Charges — not allowed
- Outpatient Limit — does not apply
- Major Surgery Rules Apply

CPT CODE	SERVICE	ICD-9-CM

64892 Nerve graft (includes obtaining graft), single strand, arm or leg; up to 4 cm length

64893 Nerve graft (includes obtaining graft), single strand, arm or leg; more than 4 cm length

CPT NOTES

- For intracranial surgery on cranial nerves, see 61450, 61460, 61790.

ICD-9-CM

905.2 Late effect, arm fracture
905.4 Late effect, leg fracture
907.4 Late effect, nerve injury shld/arm
907.5 Late effect, nerve inj pelvis/leg
953.4 Brachial plexus injury
953.5 Lumbosacral plexus injury
955.0 Injury axillary nerve
955.1 Injury median nerve
955.2 Injury ulnar nerve
955.3 Injury radial nerve
955.4 Injury musculocutaneous nerve
955.5 Injury cutaneous sensory nerve/arm
956.1 Injury femoral nerve
956.2 Injury posterior tibial nerve
956.3 Injury peroneal nerve
956.4 Injury cutaneous sensory nerve/leg

REIMBURSEMENT INFORMATION

Medicare

- Follow-up Days — 90
- Assistant Surgeon — paid
- Supply Charges — not allowed
- Outpatient Limit — does not apply
- Major Surgery Rules Apply

64895 Nerve graft (includes obtaining graft), multiple strands (cable), hand or foot; up to 4 cm length

64896 Nerve graft (includes obtaining graft), multiple strands (cable), hand or foot; more than 4 cm length

CPT NOTES

- For intracranial surgery on cranial nerves, see 61450, 61460, 61790.

905.2 Late effect, arm fracture
905.4 Late effect, leg fracture
907.4 Late effect, nerve injury shld/arm
907.5 Late effect, nerve inj pelvis/leg
955.1 Injury median nerve
955.2 Injury ulnar nerve
955.3 Injury radial nerve
955.4 Injury musculocutaneous nerve
955.6 Injury digital nerve
956.1 Injury femoral nerve
956.2 Injury posterior tibial nerve
956.3 Injury peroneal nerve
956.4 Injury cutaneous sensory nerve/leg

REIMBURSEMENT INFORMATION

Medicare

- Follow-up Days — 90
- Assistant Surgeon — paid
- Supply Charges — not allowed
- Outpatient Limit — does not apply
- Major Surgery Rules Apply

CPT CODE	SERVICE	ICD-9-CM

64897 Nerve graft (includes obtaining graft), multiple strands (cable), arm or leg; up to 4 cm length

64898 Nerve graft (includes obtaining graft), multiple strands (cable), arm or leg; more than 4 cm length

CPT NOTES

- For intracranial surgery on cranial nerves, see 61450, 61460, 61790.

905.2	Late effect, arm fracture
905.4	Late effect, leg fracture
907.4	Late effect, nerve injury shld/arm
907.5	Late effect, nerve inj pelvis/leg
955.0	Injury axillary nerve
955.1	Injury median nerve
955.2	Injury ulnar nerve
955.3	Injury radial nerve
955.4	Injury musculocutaneous nerve
955.5	Injury cutaneous sensory nerve/arm
956.1	Injury femoral nerve
956.2	Injury posterior tibial nerve
956.3	Injury peroneal nerve
956.4	Injury cutaneous sensory nerve/leg

REIMBURSEMENT INFORMATION

Medicare

- Follow-up Days — 90
- Assistant Surgeon — paid
- Supply Charges — not allowed
- Outpatient Limit — does not apply
- Major Surgery Rules Apply

64901 Nerve graft, each additional nerve; single strand

CPT NOTES

- For intracranial surgery on cranial nerves, see 61450, 61460, 61790.

905.2	Late effect, arm fracture
905.4	Late effect, leg fracture
907.4	Late effect, nerve injury shld/arm
907.5	Late effect, nerve inj pelvis/leg
955.0	Injury axillary nerve
955.1	Injury median nerve
955.2	Injury ulnar nerve
955.3	Injury radial nerve
955.4	Injury musculocutaneous nerve
955.5	Injury cutaneous sensory nerve/arm
955.6	Injury digital nerve
955.7	Injury nerve shoulder/arm NEC
956.0	Injury sciatic nerve
956.1	Injury femoral nerve
956.2	Injury posterior tibial nerve
956.3	Injury peroneal nerve
956.4	Injury cutaneous sensory nerve/leg
956.5	Injury nerve pelvis/leg NEC

REIMBURSEMENT INFORMATION

Medicare

- Follow-up Days — none; falls within global period of another procedure
- Assistant Surgeon — paid
- Supply Charges — not allowed
- Outpatient Limit — does not apply

CPT CODE	SERVICE	ICD–9–CM

64902 Nerve graft, each additional nerve; multiple strands (cable)

CPT NOTES

- For intracranial surgery on cranial nerves, see 61450, 61460, 61790.

905.2	Late effect, arm fracture
905.4	Late effect, leg fracture
907.4	Late effect, nerve injury shld/arm
907.5	Late effect, nerve inj pelvis/leg
955.0	Injury axillary nerve
955.1	Injury median nerve
955.2	Injury ulnar nerve
955.3	Injury radial nerve
955.4	Injury musculocutaneous nerve
955.5	Injury cutaneous sensory nerve/arm
955.6	Injury digital nerve
955.7	Injury nerve shoulder/arm NEC
955.8	Injury multiple nerves shoulder/arm
956.0	Injury sciatic nerve
956.1	Injury femoral nerve
956.2	Injury posterior tibial nerve
956.3	Injury peroneal nerve
956.4	Injury cutaneous sensory nerve/leg
956.5	Injury nerve pelvis/leg NEC
956.8	Injury multiple nerves pelvis/leg

REIMBURSEMENT INFORMATION

Medicare

- Follow–up Days — none; falls within global period of another procedure
- Assistant Surgeon — paid
- Supply Charges — not allowed
- Outpatient Limit — does not apply

67350 Biopsy of extraocular muscle

CPT NOTES

- For diagnostic and treatment ophthalmological services, see Medicine, Ophthalmology, and 92002 et seq.
- For repair of wound, extraocular muscle, tendon or Tenon's capsule, see 65290.

190.1	M-Neoplasm, Orbit
190.8	M-Neoplasm, Eye NEC
198.4	M2-Neoplasm, Nervous system NEC
198.89	M2-Neoplasm NEC
199.0	M-Neoplasm, Disseminated
224.1	B-Neoplasm, Orbit
234.0	CA in situ, Eye
238.1	UB-Neoplasm, Soft tissue
238.8	Uncertain behavior, neoplasm NEC

REIMBURSEMENT INFORMATION

Medicare

- Follow–up Days — 0
- Assistant Surgeon — by report
- Supply Charges — not allowed
- Outpatient Limit — does not apply
- Minor Surgery Rules Apply

CPT CODE	SERVICE	ICD–9–CM

▲ 67400 Orbitotomy without bone flap (frontal or transconjunctival approach); for exploration, with or without biopsy

CPT NOTES

- ♦ For diagnostic and treatment ophthalmological services, see Medicine, Ophthalmology, and 92002 et seq.

173.1	M-Neoplasm, Skin of eyelid/canthus
190.1	M-Neoplasm, Orbit
190.8	M-Neoplasm, Eye NEC
198.4	M2-Neoplasm, Nervous system NEC
198.89	M2-Neoplasm NEC
199.0	M-Neoplasm, Disseminated
224.1	B-Neoplasm, Orbit
234.0	CA in situ, Eye
238.1	UB-Neoplasm, Soft tissue
238.8	Uncertain behavior, neoplasm NEC
376.01	Orbital cellulitis
376.11	Orbital granuloma
376.30	Exophthalmos NOS
376.42	Exostosis of orbit
376.6	Old foreign body, orbit
376.81	Orbital cysts
905.0	Late effect, skull/face fracture

REIMBURSEMENT INFORMATION

General

- ♦ Description changed in 1995 CPT.

Medicare

- ♦ Follow–up Days — 90
- ♦ Assistant Surgeon — paid
- ♦ Supply Charges — not allowed
- ♦ Outpatient Limit — does not apply
- ♦ Major Surgery Rules Apply

67405 Orbitotomy without bone flap (frontal or transconjunctival approach); with drainage only

CPT NOTES

- ♦ For diagnostic and treatment ophthalmological services, see Medicine, Ophthalmology, and 92002 et seq.

376.01	Orbital cellulitis
376.11	Orbital granuloma
376.30	Exophthalmos NOS
376.32	Orbital hemorrhage
376.33	Orbital edema
376.81	Orbital cysts
905.0	Late effect, skull/face fracture
921.2	Contusion of orbital tissue

REIMBURSEMENT INFORMATION

Medicare

- ♦ Follow–up Days — 90
- ♦ Assistant Surgeon — paid
- ♦ Supply Charges — not allowed
- ♦ Outpatient Limit — does not apply
- ♦ Major Surgery Rules Apply

CPT CODE	SERVICE	ICD-9-CM
67412	Orbitotomy without bone flap (frontal or transconjunctival approach); with removal of lesion	190.1 M-Neoplasm, Orbit 190.8 M-Neoplasm, Eye NEC 198.4 M2-Neoplasm, Nervous system NEC 198.89 M2-Neoplasm NEC 199.0 M-Neoplasm, Disseminated 224.1 B-Neoplasm, Orbit 234.0 CA in situ, Eye 238.1 UB-Neoplasm, Soft tissue 238.8 Uncertain behavior, neoplasm NEC 239.2 Bone/Skin neoplasm NOS 376.30 Exophthalmos NOS 376.32 Orbital hemorrhage 376.6 Old foreign body, orbit 376.81 Orbital cysts

CPT NOTES

- For diagnostic and treatment ophthalmological services, see Medicine, Ophthalmology, and 92002 et seq.

REIMBURSEMENT INFORMATION

Medicare

- Follow-up Days — 90
- Assistant Surgeon — paid
- Supply Charges — not allowed
- Outpatient Limit — does not apply
- Major Surgery Rules Apply

CPT CODE	SERVICE	ICD-9-CM
67413	Orbitotomy without bone flap (frontal or transconjunctival approach); with removal of foreign body	376.6 Old foreign body, orbit 870.4 Penetrating orbit wound w/FB

CPT NOTES

- For diagnostic and treatment ophthalmological services, see Medicine, Ophthalmology, and 92002 et seq.

REIMBURSEMENT INFORMATION

Medicare

- Follow-up Days — 90
- Assistant Surgeon — paid
- Supply Charges — not allowed
- Outpatient Limit — does not apply
- Major Surgery Rules Apply

CPT CODE	SERVICE
67415	Fine needle aspiration of orbital contents

CPT NOTES

- For diagnostic and treatment ophthalmological services, see Medicine, Ophthalmology, and 92002 et seq.
- For exenteration, enucleation, and repair, see 65101 et. seq; for optic nerve decompression, see 67570.

ICD–9–CM

190.1	M-Neoplasm, Orbit
190.8	M-Neoplasm, Eye NEC
198.4	M2-Neoplasm, Nervous system NEC
198.89	M2-Neoplasm NEC
199.0	M-Neoplasm, Disseminated
224.1	B-Neoplasm, Orbit
234.0	CA in situ, Eye
238.1	UB-Neoplasm, Soft tissue
238.8	Uncertain behavior, neoplasm NEC
376.01	Orbital cellulitis
376.11	Orbital granuloma
376.33	Orbital edema
376.81	Orbital cysts
377.32	Retrobulbar neuritis

REIMBURSEMENT INFORMATION

Medicare

- Follow–up Days — 0
- Assistant Surgeon — not paid
- Supply Charges — not allowed
- Outpatient Limit — does not apply
- Minor Surgery Rules Apply

CPT CODE **SERVICE**

67420 Orbitotomy with bone flap or window, lateral approach (eg, Kroenlein); with removal of lesion

CPT NOTES

- For diagnostic and treatment ophthalmological services, see Medicine, Ophthalmology, and 92002 et seq.
- For optic nerve sheath decompression, see 67570.
- For orbitotomy, transcranial approach, see 61330-62334.
- For orbital implant, see 67550, 67560.
- For removal of eyeball or for repair after removal, see 65091-65175.

ICD–9–CM

190.1	M-Neoplasm, Orbit
190.8	M-Neoplasm, Eye NEC
198.4	M2-Neoplasm, Nervous system NEC
198.89	M2-Neoplasm NEC
224.1	B-Neoplasm, Orbit
234.0	CA in situ, Eye
238.1	UB-Neoplasm, Soft tissue
238.8	Uncertain behavior, neoplasm NEC
376.11	Orbital granuloma
376.21	Thyrotoxic exophthalmos
376.22	Exophthalmic ophthalmoplegia
376.31	Constant exophthalmos
376.32	Orbital hemorrhage
376.33	Orbital edema
376.34	Intermittent exophthalmos
376.35	Pulsating exophthalmos
376.36	Lateral globe displacement
376.41	Hypertelorism of orbit
376.42	Exostosis of orbit
376.43	Orbit deformity d/t bone disease
376.44	Craniofacial orbit deformity
376.45	Atrophy of orbit
376.46	Enlargement of orbit
376.47	Orbit deformity d/t trauma/surgery
376.6	Old foreign body, orbit
376.81	Orbital cysts

REIMBURSEMENT INFORMATION

Medicare

- Follow–up Days — 90
- Assistant Surgeon — paid
- Supply Charges — not allowed
- Outpatient Limit — does not apply
- Major Surgery Rules Apply

CPT CODE	SERVICE	ICD-9-CM

67550 Orbital implant (implant outside muscle cone); insertion

CPT NOTES

- For diagnostic and treatment ophthalmological services, see Medicine, Ophthalmology, and 92002 et seq.
- For ocular implant (implant inside muscle cone), see 65093-65015, 65130-65175.
- For treatment of fractures of malar area, orbit, see 21355 et seq.

190.0	M-Neoplasm, Eyeball
190.1	M-Neoplasm, Orbit
190.4	M-Neoplasm, Cornea
224.1	B-Neoplasm, Orbit
360.11	Sympathetic uveitis
360.81	Luxation of globe
376.00	Acute inflammation NOS of orbit
376.01	Orbital cellulitis
376.02	Orbital periostitis
376.03	Orbital osteomyelitis
376.04	Orbital tenonitis
376.40	Deformity of orbit NOS
376.41	Hypertelorism of orbit
376.43	Orbit deformity d/t bone disease
376.44	Craniofacial orbit deformity
376.45	Atrophy of orbit
376.46	Enlargement of orbit
376.47	Orbit deformity d/t trauma/surgery
376.51	Enophthalmos d/t orbit atrophy
376.52	Enophthalmos d/t trauma/surgery
743.66	Specified congenital orbit anomaly
871.2	Rupture of eye w/tissue loss
871.3	Avulsion of eye
905.0	Late effect, skull/face fracture
951.0	Injury to oculomotor nerve

REIMBURSEMENT INFORMATION

Medicare

- Follow–up Days — 90
- Assistant Surgeon — paid
- Supply Charges — not allowed
- Outpatient Limit — does not apply
- Major Surgery Rules Apply

67560 Orbital implant (implant outside muscle cone); removal or revision

CPT NOTES

- For diagnostic and treatment ophthalmological services, see Medicine, Ophthalmology, and 92002 et seq.
- For ocular implant (implant inside muscle cone), see 65093-65015, 65130-65175.
- For treatment of fractures of malar area, orbit, see 21355 et seq.

376.47	Orbit deformity d/t trauma/surgery
905.0	Late effect, skull/face fracture
996.59	Malfunction other device/graft
996.69	Reaction, intern prosth device NEC
998.3	Postop wound disruption
998.5	Postoperative infection
998.89	Surgical complications NEC

REIMBURSEMENT INFORMATION

Medicare

- Follow–up Days — 90
- Assistant Surgeon — not paid
- Supply Charges — not allowed
- Outpatient Limit — does not apply
- Major Surgery Rules Apply

CPT CODE / SERVICE	ICD-9-CM
67700* Blepharotomy, drainage of abscess, eyelid	

67700* Blepharotomy, drainage of abscess, eyelid

CPT NOTES

- For diagnostic and treatment ophthalmological services, see Medicine, Ophthalmology, and 92002 et seq.

ICD-9-CM

373.11 Hordeolum externum
373.12 Hordeolum internum
373.2 Chalazion
374.84 Cysts of eyelids

REIMBURSEMENT INFORMATION

General

- Starred procedure.

Medicare

- Follow-up Days — 10
- Assistant Surgeon — not paid
- Supply Charges — not allowed
- Outpatient Limit — applies
- Minor Surgery Rules Apply

67710* Severing of tarsorrhaphy

CPT NOTES

- For diagnostic and treatment ophthalmological services, see Medicine, Ophthalmology, and 92002 et seq.

351.0 Bell's palsy
370.34 Exposure keratoconjunctivitis
374.10 Ectropion NOS
374.30 Ptosis of eyelid NOS
710.2 Sicca syndrome
940.0 Chemical burn, eyelid/periocular
940.1 Burn, eyelid/periocular area NEC
940.2 Alkaline burn, cornea/conjunctiva
940.3 Acid burn, cornea/conjunctiva
940.4 Burn, cornea/conjunctiva NEC
951.4 Injury to facial nerve

REIMBURSEMENT INFORMATION

General

- Starred procedure.

Medicare

- Follow-up Days — 10
- Assistant Surgeon — not paid
- Supply Charges — not allowed
- Outpatient Limit — applies
- Minor Surgery Rules Apply

CPT CODE	SERVICE	ICD–9–CM

67715* Canthotomy (separate procedure)

CPT NOTES

- For diagnostic and treatment ophthalmological services, see Medicine, Ophthalmology, and 92002 et seq.
- For canthoplasty, see 67950.
- For division of symblepharon, see 68340.

372.73 Conjunctival edema
374.46 Blepharophimosis
376.32 Orbital hemorrhage
376.33 Orbital edema

REIMBURSEMENT INFORMATION

General

- Starred procedure.
- Separate procedure rules apply.

Medicare

- Follow–up Days — 10
- Assistant Surgeon — not paid
- Supply Charges — not allowed
- Outpatient Limit — does not apply

67800 Excision of chalazion; single

67801 Excision of chalazion; multiple, same lid

67805 Excision of chalazion; multiple, different lids

67808 Excision of chalazion; under general anesthesia and/or requiring hospitalization, single or multiple

CPT NOTES

- For diagnostic and treatment ophthalmological services, see Medicine, Ophthalmology, and 92002 et seq.
- Codes for removal of lesion include more than skin (i.e., involving lid margin, tarsus, and/or palpebral conjunctiva).
- For removal of lesion, involving mainly skin of eyelid, see 11440-11446; 11640-11646; 17000-17010.
- For repair of wounds, blepharoplasty, grafts, reconstruction surgery, see 67930-67975.

373.2 Chalazion

REIMBURSEMENT INFORMATION

Medicare

- Follow–up Days
  67800–67805 — 10
  67808 — 90
- Assistant Surgeon — not paid
- Supply Charges — not allowed
- Outpatient Limit
  67800–67805 — applies
  67808 — does not apply
- Minor Surgery Rules Apply (67800–67805)
  Major Surgery Rules Apply (67808)

CPT CODE **SERVICE**

67810* Biopsy of eyelid

CPT NOTES

- For diagnostic and treatment ophthalmological services, see Medicine, Ophthalmology, and 92002 et seq.
- Codes for removal of lesion include more than skin (i.e., involving lid margin, tarsus, and/or palpebral conjunctiva).
- For removal of lesion, involving mainly skin of eyelid, see 11440-11446; 11640-11646; 17000-17010.
- For repair of wounds, blepharoplasty, grafts, reconstruction surgery, see 67930-67975.

ICD-9-CM

078.10	Viral warts NOS
171.0	M-Neoplasm, Soft tissue, head
172.1	Malignant melanoma, eyelid/canthus
173.1	M-Neoplasm, Skin of eyelid/canthus
215.0	B-Neoplasm, Soft tissue, head
216.1	B-Neoplasm, Skin of eyelid/canthus
232.1	CA in situ, Eyelid/canthus
238.2	UB-Neoplasm, Skin
374.84	Cysts of eyelids

REIMBURSEMENT INFORMATION

General

- Starred procedure.

Medicare

- Follow–up Days — 0
- Assistant Surgeon — not paid
- Supply Charges — not allowed
- Outpatient Limit — applies
- Minor Surgery Rules Apply

67820* Correction of trichiasis; epilation, by forceps only

CPT NOTES

- For diagnostic and treatment ophthalmological services, see Medicine, Ophthalmology, and 92002 et seq.
- Codes for removal of lesion include more than skin (i.e., involving lid margin, tarsus, and/or palpebral conjunctiva).
- For removal of lesion, involving mainly skin of eyelid, see 11440-11446; 11640-11646; 17000-17010.
- For repair of wounds, blepharoplasty, grafts, reconstruction surgery, see 67930-67975.

374.01	Senile entropion
374.04	Cicatricial entropion
374.05	Trichiasis w/o entropion
374.54	Hypertrichosis of eyelid
375.15	Tear film insufficiency NOS

REIMBURSEMENT INFORMATION

General

- Starred procedure.

Medicare

- Follow–up Days — 0
- Assistant Surgeon — not paid
- Supply Charges — not allowed
- Outpatient Limit — applies
- Minor Surgery Rules Apply

CPT CODE	SERVICE	ICD-9-CM

67825* Correction of trichiasis; epilation, (eg, by electrosurgery or cryotherapy)

67830 Correction of trichiasis; incision of lid margin

67835 Correction of trichiasis; incision of lid margin, with free mucous membrane graft

CPT NOTES

- For diagnostic and treatment ophthalmological services, see Medicine, Ophthalmology, and 92002 et seq.
- Codes for removal of lesion include more than skin (i.e., involving lid margin, tarsus, and/or palpebral conjunctiva).
- For removal of lesion, involving mainly skin of eyelid, see 11440-11446; 11640-11646; 17000-17010.
- For repair of wounds, blepharoplasty, grafts, reconstruction surgery, see 67930-67975.

374.05 Trichiasis w/o entropion
374.54 Hypertrichosis of eyelid

REIMBURSEMENT INFORMATION

General

- Starred procedure. (67825)

Medicare

- Follow-up Days
  67825–67830 — 10
  67835 — 90
- Assistant Surgeon — not paid
- Supply Charges — not allowed
- Outpatient Limit
  67825 — applies
  67830–67835 — does not apply
- Minor Surgery Rules Apply (67825–67830)
  Major Surgery Rules Apply (67835)

67840* Excision of lesion of eyelid (except chalazion) without closure or with simple direct closure

CPT NOTES

- For diagnostic and treatment ophthalmological services, see Medicine, Ophthalmology, and 92002 et seq.
- Codes for removal of lesion include more than skin (i.e., involving lid margin, tarsus, and/or palpebral conjunctiva).
- For removal of lesion, involving mainly skin of eyelid, see 11440-11446; 11640-11646; 17000-17010.
- For repair of wounds, blepharoplasty, grafts, reconstruction surgery, see 67930-67975.
- For excision and repair of eyelid by reconstructive surgery, see 67961, 67966.

078.10 Viral warts NOS
171.0 M-Neoplasm, Soft tissue, head
173.1 M-Neoplasm, Skin of eyelid/canthus
215.0 B-Neoplasm, Soft tissue, head
216.1 B-Neoplasm, Skin of eyelid/canthus
238.2 UB-Neoplasm, Skin
239.2 Bone/Skin neoplasm NOS
373.11 Hordeolum externum
373.12 Hordeolum internum
373.13 Abscess of eyelid
374.51 Xanthelasma
374.84 Cysts of eyelids

REIMBURSEMENT INFORMATION

General

- Starred procedure.

Medicare

- Follow-up Days — 10
- Assistant Surgeon — not paid
- Supply Charges — not allowed
- Outpatient Limit — applies
- Minor Surgery Rules Apply

CPT CODE / SERVICE	ICD-9-CM
67850* Destruction of lesion of lid margin (up to 1 cm)	171.0 M-Neoplasm, Soft tissue, head 173.1 M-Neoplasm, Skin of eyelid/canthus 215.0 B-Neoplasm, Soft tissue, head 216.1 B-Neoplasm, Skin of eyelid/canthus 373.11 Hordeolum externum 373.12 Hordeolum internum 373.13 Abscess of eyelid 374.51 Xanthelasma 374.84 Cysts of eyelids

CPT NOTES

- For diagnostic and treatment ophthalmological services, see Medicine, Ophthalmology, and 92002 et seq.
- Codes for removal of lesion include more than skin (i.e., involving lid margin, tarsus, and/or palpebral conjunctiva).
- For removal of lesion, involving mainly skin of eyelid, see 11440-11446; 11640-11646; 17000-17010.
- For repair of wounds, blepharoplasty, grafts, reconstruction surgery, see 67930-67975.
- For Mohs' micrographic surgery, see 17304-17310.
- For initiation or follow-up care of topical chemotherapy (e.g., 5-FU or similar agents), see appropriate office visits.

REIMBURSEMENT INFORMATION

General

- Starred procedure.

Medicare

- Follow–up Days — 10
- Assistant Surgeon — not paid
- Supply Charges — not allowed
- Outpatient Limit — applies
- Minor Surgery Rules Apply

CPT CODE / SERVICE	ICD-9-CM
67880 Construction of intermarginal adhesions, median tarsorrhaphy, or canthorrhaphy **67882** Construction of intermarginal adhesions, median tarsorrhaphy, or canthorrhaphy; with transposition of tarsal plate	351.0 Bell's palsy 370.34 Exposure keratoconjunctivitis 374.10 Ectropion NOS 374.21 Paralytic lagophthalmos 870.0 Laceration eyelid skin/periocular 870.1 Full-thickness laceration eyelid 870.2 Eyelid laceration inv lacrimal pas 940.2 Alkaline burn, cornea/conjunctiva 940.3 Acid burn, cornea/conjunctiva 940.4 Burn, cornea/conjunctiva NEC 951.4 Injury to facial nerve

CPT NOTES

- For diagnostic and treatment ophthalmological services, see Medicine, Ophthalmology, and 92002 et seq.
- For severing of tarsorrhaphy, see 67710.
- For canthoplasty, reconstruction canthus, see 67950.
- For canthotomy, see 67715.

REIMBURSEMENT INFORMATION

Medicare

- Follow–up Days — 90
- Assistant Surgeon — not paid
- Supply Charges — not allowed
- Outpatient Limit — does not apply
- Major Surgery Rules Apply

CPT CODE	SERVICE	ICD-9-CM	
67901	Repair of blepharoptosis; frontalis muscle technique with suture or other material	374.04	Cicatricial entropion
		374.30	Ptosis of eyelid NOS
		374.31	Paralytic ptosis
		374.32	Myogenic ptosis
		374.33	Mechanical ptosis
		374.34	Blepharochalasis
		374.43	Abnormal innervation syndrome
		374.44	Sensory disorder, eyelid
		374.46	Blepharophimosis
		742.8	Nervous system anomaly NEC
		743.61	Congenital ptosis
		743.62	Congenital eyelid deformity

CPT NOTES

- For diagnostic and treatment ophthalmological services, see Medicine, Ophthalmology, and 92002 et seq.

REIMBURSEMENT INFORMATION

Medicare

- Follow-up Days — 90
- Assistant Surgeon — not paid
- Supply Charges — not allowed
- Outpatient Limit — does not apply
- Major Surgery Rules Apply

67902	Repair of blepharoptosis; frontalis muscle technique with fascial sling (includes obtaining fascia)	374.10	Ectropion NOS
		374.30	Ptosis of eyelid NOS
		374.31	Paralytic ptosis
		374.32	Myogenic ptosis
		374.33	Mechanical ptosis
		374.34	Blepharochalasis
		374.43	Abnormal innervation syndrome
		374.44	Sensory disorder, eyelid
		374.46	Blepharophimosis
		742.8	Nervous system anomaly NEC
		743.61	Congenital ptosis
		743.62	Congenital eyelid deformity

CPT NOTES

- For diagnostic and treatment ophthalmological services, see Medicine, Ophthalmology, and 92002 et seq.

REIMBURSEMENT INFORMATION

Medicare

- Follow-up Days — 90
- Assistant Surgeon — paid
- Supply Charges — not allowed
- Outpatient Limit — does not apply
- Major Surgery Rules Apply

CPT CODE	SERVICE	ICD-9-CM

67903 Repair of blepharoptosis; (tarso)levator resection or advancement, internal approach

CPT NOTES

- For diagnostic and treatment ophthalmological services, see Medicine, Ophthalmology, and 92002 et seq.

374.30	Ptosis of eyelid NOS
374.31	Paralytic ptosis
374.32	Myogenic ptosis
374.33	Mechanical ptosis
374.34	Blepharochalasis
374.43	Abnormal innervation syndrome
374.44	Sensory disorder, eyelid
374.46	Blepharophimosis
742.8	Nervous system anomaly NEC
743.61	Congenital ptosis
743.62	Congenital eyelid deformity

REIMBURSEMENT INFORMATION

Medicare

- Follow–up Days — 90
- Assistant Surgeon — paid
- Supply Charges — not allowed
- Outpatient Limit — does not apply
- Major Surgery Rules Apply

67904 Repair of blepharoptosis; (tarso)levator resection or advancement, external approach

CPT NOTES

- For diagnostic and treatment ophthalmological services, see Medicine, Ophthalmology, and 92002 et seq.

374.10	Ectropion NOS
374.30	Ptosis of eyelid NOS
374.31	Paralytic ptosis
374.32	Myogenic ptosis
374.33	Mechanical ptosis
374.34	Blepharochalasis
374.43	Abnormal innervation syndrome
374.44	Sensory disorder, eyelid
374.46	Blepharophimosis
742.8	Nervous system anomaly NEC
743.61	Congenital ptosis
743.62	Congenital eyelid deformity

REIMBURSEMENT INFORMATION

Medicare

- Follow–up Days — 90
- Assistant Surgeon — paid
- Supply Charges — not allowed
- Outpatient Limit — does not apply
- Major Surgery Rules Apply
- Fragments — 15822, 15823

CPT CODE	SERVICE	ICD–9–CM

67906 Repair of blepharoptosis; superior rectus technique with fascial sling (includes obtaining fascia)

CPT NOTES

- ♦ For diagnostic and treatment ophthalmological services, see Medicine, Ophthalmology, and 92002 et seq.

374.30	Ptosis of eyelid NOS
374.31	Paralytic ptosis
374.32	Myogenic ptosis
374.33	Mechanical ptosis
374.34	Blepharochalasis
374.43	Abnormal innervation syndrome
374.44	Sensory disorder, eyelid
374.46	Blepharophimosis
742.8	Nervous system anomaly NEC
743.61	Congenital ptosis
743.62	Congenital eyelid deformity

REIMBURSEMENT INFORMATION

Medicare

- ♦ Follow–up Days — 90
- ♦ Assistant Surgeon — paid
- ♦ Supply Charges — not allowed
- ♦ Outpatient Limit — does not apply
- ♦ Major Surgery Rules Apply

67908 Repair of blepharoptosis; conjunctivo-tarso-Muller's muscle- levator resection (eg, Fasanella-Servat type)

CPT NOTES

- ♦ For diagnostic and treatment ophthalmological services, see Medicine, Ophthalmology, and 92002 et seq.

374.30	Ptosis of eyelid NOS
374.31	Paralytic ptosis
374.32	Myogenic ptosis
374.33	Mechanical ptosis
374.34	Blepharochalasis
374.43	Abnormal innervation syndrome
374.44	Sensory disorder, eyelid
374.46	Blepharophimosis
742.8	Nervous system anomaly NEC
743.61	Congenital ptosis
743.62	Congenital eyelid deformity

REIMBURSEMENT INFORMATION

Medicare

- ♦ Follow–up Days — 90
- ♦ Assistant Surgeon — not paid
- ♦ Supply Charges — not allowed
- ♦ Outpatient Limit — does not apply
- ♦ Major Surgery Rules Apply

CPT CODE SERVICE	ICD-9-CM
67909 Reduction of overcorrection of ptosis **CPT NOTES** ♦ For diagnostic and treatment ophthalmological services, see Medicine, Ophthalmology, and 92002 et seq.	374.23 Cicatricial lagophthalmos 374.30 Ptosis of eyelid NOS 374.33 Mechanical ptosis 374.34 Blepharochalasis 374.41 Eyelid retraction or lag 998.89 Surgical complications NEC **REIMBURSEMENT INFORMATION** Medicare ♦ Follow-up Days — 90 ♦ Assistant Surgeon — not paid ♦ Supply Charges — not allowed ♦ Outpatient Limit — does not apply ♦ Major Surgery Rules Apply
67911 Correction of lid retraction **CPT NOTES** ♦ For diagnostic and treatment ophthalmological services, see Medicine, Ophthalmology, and 92002 et seq. ♦ For obtaining autogenous graft materials, see 20920, 20922 or 20926. ♦ For correction of trichiasis by mucous membrane graft, see 67835.	242.00 Toxic diffuse goiter, no crisis 351.0 Bell's palsy 374.10 Ectropion NOS 374.41 Eyelid retraction or lag 376.21 Thyrotoxic exophthalmos 376.22 Exophthalmic ophthalmoplegia 743.62 Congenital eyelid deformity 951.4 Injury to facial nerve **REIMBURSEMENT INFORMATION** Medicare ♦ Follow-up Days — 90 ♦ Assistant Surgeon — not paid ♦ Supply Charges — not allowed ♦ Outpatient Limit — does not apply ♦ Major Surgery Rules Apply
67914 Repair of ectropion; suture **CPT NOTES** ♦ For diagnostic and treatment ophthalmological services, see Medicine, Ophthalmology, and 92002 et seq. ♦ For correction of everted punctum, see 68705.	374.10 Ectropion NOS 374.11 Senile ectropion 374.12 Mechanical ectropion 374.13 Spastic ectropion 374.14 Cicatricial ectropion 375.20 Epiphora NOS 743.62 Congenital eyelid deformity 906.0 Late effect, open wound head/trunk 906.5 Late effect of head/neck burn **REIMBURSEMENT INFORMATION** Medicare ♦ Follow-up Days — 90 ♦ Assistant Surgeon — not paid ♦ Supply Charges — not allowed ♦ Outpatient Limit — does not apply ♦ Major Surgery Rules Apply

CPT CODE	SERVICE	ICD-9-CM

67915 Repair of ectropion; thermocauterization

CPT NOTES

- For diagnostic and treatment ophthalmological services, see Medicine, Ophthalmology, and 92002 et seq.
- For correction of everted punctum, see 68705.

374.10	Ectropion NOS
374.11	Senile ectropion
374.12	Mechanical ectropion
374.13	Spastic ectropion
374.14	Cicatricial ectropion
743.62	Congenital eyelid deformity
906.0	Late effect, open wound head/trunk
906.5	Late effect of head/neck burn

REIMBURSEMENT INFORMATION

Medicare

- Follow–up Days — 90
- Assistant Surgeon — not paid
- Supply Charges — not allowed
- Outpatient Limit — applies
- Major Surgery Rules Apply

67916 Repair of ectropion; blepharoplasty, excision tarsal wedge

CPT NOTES

- For diagnostic and treatment ophthalmological services, see Medicine, Ophthalmology, and 92002 et seq.
- For correction of everted punctum, see 68705.

171.0	M-Neoplasm, Soft tissue, head
173.1	M-Neoplasm, Skin of eyelid/canthus
374.10	Ectropion NOS
374.11	Senile ectropion
374.12	Mechanical ectropion
374.13	Spastic ectropion
374.14	Cicatricial ectropion
374.34	Blepharochalasis
375.51	Lacrimal punctum eversion

REIMBURSEMENT INFORMATION

Medicare

- Follow–up Days — 90
- Assistant Surgeon — not paid
- Supply Charges — not allowed
- Outpatient Limit — does not apply
- Major Surgery Rules Apply

CPT CODE	SERVICE	ICD–9–CM
67917	Repair of ectropion; blepharoplasty, extensive (eg, Kuhnt- Szymanowski or tarsal strip operations) **CPT NOTES** ♦ For diagnostic and treatment ophthalmological services, see Medicine, Ophthalmology, and 92002 et seq. ♦ For correction of everted punctum, see 68705.	351.0 Bell's palsy 374.10 Ectropion NOS 374.11 Senile ectropion 374.12 Mechanical ectropion 374.13 Spastic ectropion 374.14 Cicatricial ectropion 374.34 Blepharochalasis 375.22 Epiphora d/t insufficient drainage 743.62 Congenital eyelid deformity 906.0 Late effect, open wound head/trunk 906.5 Late effect of head/neck burn **REIMBURSEMENT INFORMATION** Medicare ♦ Follow-up Days — 90 ♦ Assistant Surgeon — not paid ♦ Supply Charges — not allowed ♦ Outpatient Limit — does not apply ♦ Major Surgery Rules Apply ♦ Fragments — 67500, 67914, 67916, 67950
67921	Repair of entropion; suture **CPT NOTES** ♦ For diagnostic and treatment ophthalmological services, see Medicine, Ophthalmology, and 92002 et seq. ♦ For repair of cicatricial ectropion or entropian requiring scar excision or skin grafts, see also 67961 et seq.	374.01 Senile entropion 374.02 Mechanical entropion 374.03 Spastic entropion 374.04 Cicatricial entropion 374.34 Blepharochalasis 743.62 Congenital eyelid deformity **REIMBURSEMENT INFORMATION** Medicare ♦ Follow-up Days — 90 ♦ Assistant Surgeon — not paid ♦ Supply Charges — not allowed ♦ Outpatient Limit — does not apply ♦ Major Surgery Rules Apply
67922	Repair of entropion; thermocauterization **CPT NOTES** ♦ For diagnostic and treatment ophthalmological services, see Medicine, Ophthalmology, and 92002 et seq. ♦ For repair of cicatricial ectropion or entropian requiring scar excision or skin grafts, see also 67961 et seq.	374.01 Senile entropion 374.02 Mechanical entropion 374.03 Spastic entropion 374.04 Cicatricial entropion 743.62 Congenital eyelid deformity **REIMBURSEMENT INFORMATION** Medicare ♦ Follow-up Days — 90 ♦ Assistant Surgeon — not paid ♦ Supply Charges — not allowed ♦ Outpatient Limit — applies ♦ Major Surgery Rules Apply

CPT CODE	SERVICE	ICD-9-CM
67923	Repair of entropion; blepharoplasty, excision tarsal wedge **CPT NOTES** ◆ For diagnostic and treatment ophthalmological services, see Medicine, Ophthalmology, and 92002 et seq. ◆ For repair of cicatricial ectropion or entropian requiring scar excision or skin grafts, see also 67961 et seq.	374.01 Senile entropion 374.02 Mechanical entropion 374.03 Spastic entropion 374.04 Cicatricial entropion 374.05 Trichiasis w/o entropion 374.34 Blepharochalasis 743.62 Congenital eyelid deformity **REIMBURSEMENT INFORMATION** Medicare ◆ Follow-up Days — 90 ◆ Assistant Surgeon — not paid ◆ Supply Charges — not allowed ◆ Outpatient Limit — does not apply ◆ Major Surgery Rules Apply
67924	Repair of entropion; blepharoplasty, extensive (eg, Wheeler operation) **CPT NOTES** ◆ For diagnostic and treatment ophthalmological services, see Medicine, Ophthalmology, and 92002 et seq. ◆ For repair of cicatricial ectropion or entropian requiring scar excision or skin grafts, see also 67961 et seq.	374.00 Entropion NOS 374.01 Senile entropion 374.02 Mechanical entropion 374.03 Spastic entropion 374.04 Cicatricial entropion 374.05 Trichiasis w/o entropion 374.34 Blepharochalasis 743.62 Congenital eyelid deformity **REIMBURSEMENT INFORMATION** Medicare ◆ Follow-up Days — 90 ◆ Assistant Surgeon — not paid ◆ Supply Charges — not allowed ◆ Outpatient Limit — does not apply ◆ Major Surgery Rules Apply ◆ Fragments — 67500, 67921, 67923, 67950
67930 **67935**	Suture of recent wound, eyelid, involving lid margin, tarsus, and/or palpebral conjunctiva) direct closure; partial thickness Suture of recent wound, eyelid, involving lid margin, tarsus, and/or palpebral conjunctiva) direct closure; full thickness **CPT NOTES** ◆ For diagnostic and treatment ophthalmological services, see Medicine, Ophthalmology, and 92002 et seq. ◆ Codes for blepharoplasty involve more than skin (i.e., involving lid margin, tarsus, and/or palpebral conjunctiva).	870.0 Laceration eyelid skin/periocular 870.1 Full-thickness laceration eyelid 870.2 Eyelid laceration inv lacrimal pas **REIMBURSEMENT INFORMATION** Medicare ◆ Follow-up Days — 10 ◆ Assistant Surgeon — not paid ◆ Supply Charges — not allowed ◆ Outpatient Limit — applies ◆ Major Surgery Rules Apply

CPT CODE	SERVICE
67950	Canthoplasty (reconstruction of canthus)

CPT NOTES

- For diagnostic and treatment ophthalmological services, see Medicine, Ophthalmology, and 92002 et seq.
- Codes for blepharoplasty involve more than skin (i.e., involving lid margin, tarsus, and/or palpebral conjunctiva).

ICD–9–CM

173.1	M-Neoplasm, Skin of eyelid/canthus
238.1	UB-Neoplasm, Soft tissue
351.0	Bell's palsy
374.01	Senile entropion
374.04	Cicatricial entropion
374.10	Ectropion NOS
374.11	Senile ectropion
374.14	Cicatricial ectropion
374.21	Paralytic lagophthalmos
374.30	Ptosis of eyelid NOS
374.41	Eyelid retraction or lag
374.46	Blepharophimosis
376.21	Thyrotoxic exophthalmos
743.62	Congenital eyelid deformity
905.0	Late effect, skull/face fracture
906.0	Late effect, open wound head/trunk
951.4	Injury to facial nerve

REIMBURSEMENT INFORMATION

Medicare

- Follow–up Days — 90
- Assistant Surgeon — paid
- Supply Charges — not allowed
- Outpatient Limit — does not apply
- Major Surgery Rules Apply

CPT CODE	SERVICE
67961	Excision and repair of eyelid, involving lid margin, tarsus, conjunctiva, canthus, or full thickness, may include preparation for skin graft or pedicle flap with adjacent tissue transfer or rearrangement; up to one-fourth of lid margin

CPT NOTES

- For diagnostic and treatment ophthalmological services, see Medicine, Ophthalmology, and 92002 et seq.
- Codes for blepharoplasty involve more than skin (i.e., involving lid margin, tarsus, and/or palpebral conjunctiva).
- For canthoplasty, see 67950.
- For free skin grafts, see 15120, 15121, 15260, 15261.
- For tubed pedicle flap preparation, see 15576; for delay, see 15630; for attachment, see 15630.

ICD–9–CM

173.1	M-Neoplasm, Skin of eyelid/canthus
214.0	Lipoma, Skin of face
215.0	B-Neoplasm, Soft tissue, head
216.1	B-Neoplasm, Skin of eyelid/canthus
216.3	B-Neoplasm, Skin of face NEC
232.1	CA in situ, Eyelid/canthus
238.1	UB-Neoplasm, Soft tissue
238.2	UB-Neoplasm, Skin
239.2	Bone/Skin neoplasm NOS
374.10	Ectropion NOS
374.11	Senile ectropion
374.14	Cicatricial ectropion
374.83	Elephantiasis of eyelid
374.84	Cysts of eyelids
374.85	Vascular anomaly, eyelid
374.86	Old foreign body, eyelid
870.0	Laceration eyelid skin/periocular
870.1	Full-thickness laceration eyelid
870.2	Eyelid laceration inv lacrimal pas

REIMBURSEMENT INFORMATION

Medicare

- Follow–up Days — 90
- Assistant Surgeon — paid
- Supply Charges — not allowed
- Outpatient Limit — does not apply
- Major Surgery Rules Apply

CPT CODE	SERVICE
67966	Excision and repair of eyelid, involving lid margin, tarsus, conjunctiva, canthus, or full thickness, may include preparation for skin graft or pedicle flap with adjacent tissue transfer or rearrangement; over one-fourth of lid margin

CPT NOTES

- For diagnostic and treatment ophthalmological services, see Medicine, Ophthalmology, and 92002 et seq.
- Codes for blepharoplasty involve more than skin (i.e., involving lid margin, tarsus, and/or palpebral conjunctiva).
- For canthoplasty, see 67950.
- For free skin grafts, see 15120, 15121, 15260, 15261.
- For tubed pedicle flap preparation, see 15576; for delay, see 15630; for attachment, see 15630.

ICD–9–CM

171.0	M-Neoplasm, Soft tissue, head
172.1	Malignant melanoma, eyelid/canthus
173.1	M-Neoplasm, Skin of eyelid/canthus
214.0	Lipoma, Skin of face
215.0	B-Neoplasm, Soft tissue, head
216.1	B-Neoplasm, Skin of eyelid/canthus
216.3	B-Neoplasm, Skin of face NEC
232.1	CA in situ, Eyelid/canthus
238.1	UB-Neoplasm, Soft tissue
238.2	UB-Neoplasm, Skin
239.2	Bone/Skin neoplasm NOS
374.04	Cicatricial entropion
374.10	Ectropion NOS
374.14	Cicatricial ectropion
374.34	Blepharochalasis
374.83	Elephantiasis of eyelid
374.85	Vascular anomaly, eyelid
374.86	Old foreign body, eyelid
686.1	Pyogenic granuloma
706.2	Sebaceous cyst
870.0	Laceration eyelid skin/periocular
870.1	Full-thickness laceration eyelid
870.2	Eyelid laceration inv lacrimal pas

REIMBURSEMENT INFORMATION

Medicare

- Follow–up Days — 90
- Assistant Surgeon — not paid
- Supply Charges — not allowed
- Outpatient Limit — does not apply
- Major Surgery Rules Apply

CPT CODE	SERVICE	ICD-9-CM	

67971 Reconstruction of eyelid, full thickness by transfer of tarsoconjunctival flap from opposing eyelid; up to two-thirds of eyelid, one stage or first stage

CPT NOTES

- For diagnostic and treatment ophthalmological services, see Medicine, Ophthalmology, and 92002 et seq.
- Codes for blepharoplasty involve more than skin (i.e., involving lid margin, tarsus, and/or palpebral conjunctiva).

ICD-9-CM	
172.1	Malignant melanoma, eyelid/canthus
173.1	M-Neoplasm, Skin of eyelid/canthus
216.1	B-Neoplasm, Skin of eyelid/canthus
232.1	CA in situ, Eyelid/canthus
238.2	UB-Neoplasm, Skin
743.62	Congenital eyelid deformity
870.0	Laceration eyelid skin/periocular
870.1	Full-thickness laceration eyelid
870.2	Eyelid laceration inv lacrimal pas
906.0	Late effect, open wound head/trunk
906.5	Late effect of head/neck burn
V10.82	Hx of malignant skin melanoma
V10.83	Hx of skin malignancy NEC

REIMBURSEMENT INFORMATION

Medicare

- Follow–up Days — 90
- Assistant Surgeon — paid
- Supply Charges — not allowed
- Outpatient Limit — does not apply
- Major Surgery Rules Apply

67973 Reconstruction of eyelid, full thickness by transfer of tarsoconjunctival flap from opposing eyelid; total eyelid, lower, one stage or first stage

CPT NOTES

- For diagnostic and treatment ophthalmological services, see Medicine, Ophthalmology, and 92002 et seq.
- Codes for blepharoplasty involve more than skin (i.e., involving lid margin, tarsus, and/or palpebral conjunctiva).

ICD-9-CM	
172.1	Malignant melanoma, eyelid/canthus
173.1	M-Neoplasm, Skin of eyelid/canthus
216.1	B-Neoplasm, Skin of eyelid/canthus
232.1	CA in situ, Eyelid/canthus
239.2	Bone/Skin neoplasm NOS
374.04	Cicatricial entropion
374.05	Trichiasis w/o entropion
374.23	Cicatricial lagophthalmos
374.34	Blepharochalasis
743.62	Congenital eyelid deformity
870.0	Laceration eyelid skin/periocular
870.1	Full-thickness laceration eyelid
870.2	Eyelid laceration inv lacrimal pas
906.0	Late effect, open wound head/trunk
906.5	Late effect of head/neck burn
V10.82	Hx of malignant skin melanoma
V10.83	Hx of skin malignancy NEC

REIMBURSEMENT INFORMATION

Medicare

- Follow–up Days — 90
- Assistant Surgeon — paid
- Supply Charges — not allowed
- Outpatient Limit — does not apply
- Major Surgery Rules Apply

CPT CODE	SERVICE	ICD–9–CM

67974 Reconstruction of eyelid, full thickness by transfer of tarsoconjunctival flap from opposing eyelid; total eyelid, upper, one stage or first stage

CPT NOTES

- For diagnostic and treatment ophthalmological services, see Medicine, Ophthalmology, and 92002 et seq.
- Codes for blepharoplasty involve more than skin (i.e., involving lid margin, tarsus, and/or palpebral conjunctiva).

172.1	Malignant melanoma, eyelid/canthus
173.1	M-Neoplasm, Skin of eyelid/canthus
216.1	B-Neoplasm, Skin of eyelid/canthus
232.1	CA in situ, Eyelid/canthus
374.23	Cicatricial lagophthalmos
374.41	Eyelid retraction or lag
743.62	Congenital eyelid deformity
870.0	Laceration eyelid skin/periocular
870.1	Full-thickness laceration eyelid
870.2	Eyelid laceration inv lacrimal pas
906.0	Late effect, open wound head/trunk
906.5	Late effect of head/neck burn
V10.82	Hx of malignant skin melanoma
V10.83	Hx of skin malignancy NEC

REIMBURSEMENT INFORMATION

Medicare

- Follow–up Days — 90
- Assistant Surgeon — paid
- Supply Charges — not allowed
- Outpatient Limit — does not apply
- Major Surgery Rules Apply

67975 Reconstruction of eyelid, full thickness by transfer of tarsoconjunctival flap from opposing eyelid; second stage

CPT NOTES

- For diagnostic and treatment ophthalmological services, see Medicine, Ophthalmology, and 92002 et seq.
- Codes for blepharoplasty involve more than skin (i.e., involving lid margin, tarsus, and/or palpebral conjunctiva).

171.0	M-Neoplasm, Soft tissue, head
173.1	M-Neoplasm, Skin of eyelid/canthus
216.1	B-Neoplasm, Skin of eyelid/canthus
232.1	CA in situ, Eyelid/canthus
374.01	Senile entropion
374.23	Cicatricial lagophthalmos
374.41	Eyelid retraction or lag
743.62	Congenital eyelid deformity
870.0	Laceration eyelid skin/periocular
870.1	Full-thickness laceration eyelid
870.2	Eyelid laceration inv lacrimal pas
906.0	Late effect, open wound head/trunk
906.5	Late effect of head/neck burn
V10.82	Hx of malignant skin melanoma
V10.83	Hx of skin malignancy NEC

REIMBURSEMENT INFORMATION

Medicare

- Follow–up Days — 90
- Assistant Surgeon — not paid
- Supply Charges — not allowed
- Outpatient Limit — does not apply
- Major Surgery Rules Apply

CPT CODE	SERVICE	ICD–9–CM

67999 Unlisted procedure, eyelids

CPT NOTES

- ♦ For diagnostic and treatment ophthalmological services, see Medicine, Ophthalmology, and 92002 et seq.

351.0	Bell's palsy
374.31	Paralytic ptosis
374.32	Myogenic ptosis
374.33	Mechanical ptosis
374.34	Blepharochalasis
374.43	Abnormal innervation syndrome
374.46	Blepharophimosis
742.8	Nervous system anomaly NEC
743.61	Congenital ptosis
743.62	Congenital eyelid deformity

REIMBURSEMENT INFORMATION

Medicare

- ♦ Follow–up Days — determined by local carrier
- ♦ Assistant Surgeon — determined by local carrier
- ♦ Supply Charges — determined by local carrier
- ♦ Outpatient Limit — determined by local carrier

68400 Incision, drainage of lacrimal gland

CPT NOTES

- ♦ For diagnostic and treatment ophthalmological services, see Medicine, Ophthalmology, and 92002 et seq.
- ♦ For removal of foreign body, see 65205, et seq.

375.01	Acute dacryoadenitis
375.02	Chronic dacryoadenitis
375.03	Chronic enlargement lacrimal gland
375.11	Dacryops
375.12	Lacrimal gland cyst NEC
375.13	Primary lacrimal atrophy
375.14	Secondary lacrimal atrophy

REIMBURSEMENT INFORMATION

Medicare

- ♦ Follow–up Days — 10
- ♦ Assistant Surgeon — not paid
- ♦ Supply Charges — not allowed
- ♦ Outpatient Limit — applies
- ♦ Minor Surgery Rules Apply

CPT CODE	SERVICE	ICD-9-CM

68420 Incision, drainage of lacrimal sac (dacryocystotomy or dacryocystostomy)

CPT NOTES

- For diagnostic and treatment ophthalmological services, see Medicine, Ophthalmology, and 92002 et seq.
- For removal of foreign body, see 65205, et seq.

375.21 Epiphora d/t excess lacrimation
375.30 Dacryocystitis NOS
375.31 Acute canaliculitis
375.32 Acute dacryocystitis
375.33 Phlegmonous dacryocystitis
375.42 Chronic dacryocystitis
375.56 Acquired nasolacrimal duct stenosis

REIMBURSEMENT INFORMATION

Medicare

- Follow-up Days — 10
- Assistant Surgeon — not paid
- Supply Charges — not allowed
- Outpatient Limit — applies
- Minor Surgery Rules Apply

68440* Snip incision of lacrimal punctum

CPT NOTES

- For diagnostic and treatment ophthalmological services, see Medicine, Ophthalmology, and 92002 et seq.
- For removal of foreign body, see 65205, et seq.

374.11 Senile ectropion
374.12 Mechanical ectropion
374.13 Spastic ectropion
374.14 Cicatricial ectropion
375.22 Epiphora d/t insufficient drainage
375.30 Dacryocystitis NOS
375.32 Acute dacryocystitis
375.51 Lacrimal punctum eversion
375.52 Lacrimal punctum stenosis

REIMBURSEMENT INFORMATION

General

- Starred procedure

Medicare

- Follow-up Days — 10
- Assistant Surgeon — not paid
- Supply Charges — not allowed
- Outpatient Limit — applies
- Minor Surgery Rules Apply

CPT CODE	SERVICE	ICD–9–CM

68500 Excision of lacrimal gland (dacryoadenectomy), except for tumor; total

CPT NOTES

- For diagnostic and treatment ophthalmological services, see Medicine, Ophthalmology, and 92002 et seq.
- For removal of foreign body, see 65205, et seq.

375.01 Acute dacryoadenitis
375.02 Chronic dacryoadenitis
375.03 Chronic enlargement lacrimal gland
375.11 Dacryops
375.16 Lacrimal gland dislocation
375.21 Epiphora d/t excess lacrimation
375.22 Epiphora d/t insufficient drainage

REIMBURSEMENT INFORMATION

Medicare

- Follow–up Days — 90
- Assistant Surgeon — paid
- Supply Charges — not allowed
- Outpatient Limit — does not apply
- Major Surgery Rules Apply

68505 Excision of lacrimal gland (dacryoadenectomy), except for tumor; partial

CPT NOTES

- For diagnostic and treatment ophthalmological services, see Medicine, Ophthalmology, and 92002 et seq.
- For removal of foreign body, see 65205, et seq.

375.01 Acute dacryoadenitis
375.02 Chronic dacryoadenitis
375.03 Chronic enlargement lacrimal gland
375.11 Dacryops
375.16 Lacrimal gland dislocation
375.21 Epiphora d/t excess lacrimation
375.22 Epiphora d/t insufficient drainage

REIMBURSEMENT INFORMATION

Medicare

- Follow–up Days — 90
- Assistant Surgeon — paid
- Supply Charges — not allowed
- Outpatient Limit — does not apply
- Major Surgery Rules Apply

68520 Excision of lacrimal sac (dacryocystectomy)

CPT NOTES

- For diagnostic and treatment ophthalmological services, see Medicine, Ophthalmology, and 92002 et seq.
- For removal of foreign body, see 65205, et seq.

190.7 M-Neoplasm, Lacrimal duct
224.7 B-Neoplasm, Lacrimal duct
375.32 Acute dacryocystitis

REIMBURSEMENT INFORMATION

Medicare

- Follow–up Days — 90
- Assistant Surgeon — not paid
- Supply Charges — not allowed
- Outpatient Limit — does not apply
- Major Surgery Rules Apply

CPT CODE / SERVICE	ICD-9-CM
68525 Biopsy of lacrimal sac **CPT NOTES** ◆ For diagnostic and treatment ophthalmological services, see Medicine, Ophthalmology, and 92002 et seq. ◆ For removal of foreign body, see 65205, et seq.	190.7 M-Neoplasm, Lacrimal duct 224.1 B-Neoplasm, Orbit 224.7 B-Neoplasm, Lacrimal duct 238.8 Uncertain behavior, neoplasm NEC 375.30 Dacryocystitis NOS 375.56 Acquired nasolacrimal duct stenosis 375.81 Lacrimal passage granuloma **REIMBURSEMENT INFORMATION** Medicare ◆ Follow–up Days — 0 ◆ Assistant Surgeon — paid ◆ Supply Charges — not allowed ◆ Outpatient Limit — does not apply ◆ Minor Surgery Rules Apply
68530 Removal of foreign body or dacryolith, lacrimal passages **CPT NOTES** ◆ For diagnostic and treatment ophthalmological services, see Medicine, Ophthalmology, and 92002 et seq. ◆ For removal of foreign body, see 65205, et seq.	375.57 Dacryolith 930.2 Foreign body in lacrimal punctum **REIMBURSEMENT INFORMATION** Medicare ◆ Follow–up Days — 10 ◆ Assistant Surgeon — not paid ◆ Supply Charges — not allowed ◆ Outpatient Limit — applies ◆ Minor Surgery Rules Apply
68540 Excision of lacrimal gland tumor; frontal approach **68550** Excision of lacrimal gland tumor; involving osteotomy **CPT NOTES** ◆ For diagnostic and treatment ophthalmological services, see Medicine, Ophthalmology, and 92002 et seq. ◆ For removal of foreign body, see 65205, et seq.	190.2 M-Neoplasm, Lacrimal gland 224.2 B-Neoplasm, Lacrimal gland **REIMBURSEMENT INFORMATION** Medicare ◆ Follow–up Days — 90 ◆ Assistant Surgeon — paid ◆ Supply Charges — not allowed ◆ Outpatient Limit — does not apply ◆ Major Surgery Rules Apply

CPT CODE / SERVICE	ICD-9-CM
68700 Plastic repair of canaliculi **CPT NOTES** ◆ For diagnostic and treatment ophthalmological services, see Medicine, Ophthalmology, and 92002 et seq. ◆ For removal of foreign body, see 65205, et seq.	173.1 M-Neoplasm, Skin of eyelid/canthus 375.22 Epiphora d/t insufficient drainage 375.53 Lacrimal canaliculi stenosis 375.56 Acquired nasolacrimal duct stenosis 870.2 Eyelid laceration inv lacrimal pas **REIMBURSEMENT INFORMATION** Medicare ◆ Follow-up Days — 90 ◆ Assistant Surgeon — not paid ◆ Supply Charges — not allowed ◆ Outpatient Limit — does not apply ◆ Major Surgery Rules Apply
68705 Correction of everted punctum, cautery **CPT NOTES** ◆ For diagnostic and treatment ophthalmological services, see Medicine, Ophthalmology, and 92002 et seq. ◆ For removal of foreign body, see 65205, et seq.	374.10 Ectropion NOS 374.11 Senile ectropion 374.12 Mechanical ectropion 374.13 Spastic ectropion 374.14 Cicatricial ectropion 375.20 Epiphora NOS 375.22 Epiphora d/t insufficient drainage 375.51 Lacrimal punctum eversion 375.52 Lacrimal punctum stenosis **REIMBURSEMENT INFORMATION** Medicare ◆ Follow-up Days — 10 ◆ Assistant Surgeon — not paid ◆ Supply Charges — not allowed ◆ Outpatient Limit — applies ◆ Minor Surgery Rules Apply
68720 Dacryocystorhinostomy (fistulization of lacrimal sac to nasal cavity) **CPT NOTES** ◆ For diagnostic and treatment ophthalmological services, see Medicine, Ophthalmology, and 92002 et seq. ◆ For removal of foreign body, see 65205, et seq.	375.20 Epiphora NOS 375.21 Epiphora d/t excess lacrimation 375.22 Epiphora d/t insufficient drainage 375.30 Dacryocystitis NOS 375.32 Acute dacryocystitis 375.42 Chronic dacryocystitis 375.43 Lacrimal mucocele 375.55 Neonatal nasolacrimal obstruction **REIMBURSEMENT INFORMATION** Medicare ◆ Follow-up Days — 90 ◆ Assistant Surgeon — paid ◆ Supply Charges — not allowed ◆ Outpatient Limit — does not apply ◆ Major Surgery Rules Apply

CPT CODE	SERVICE	ICD–9–CM

68745 Conjunctivorhinostomy (fistulization of conjunctiva to nasal cavity); without tube

CPT NOTES

- ♦ For diagnostic and treatment ophthalmological services, see Medicine, Ophthalmology, and 92002 et seq.
- ♦ For removal of foreign body, see 65205, et seq.

375.21	Epiphora d/t excess lacrimation
375.22	Epiphora d/t insufficient drainage
375.41	Chronic canaliculitis
375.42	Chronic dacryocystitis
375.43	Lacrimal mucocele
375.51	Lacrimal punctum eversion
375.52	Lacrimal punctum stenosis
375.53	Lacrimal canaliculi stenosis
375.54	Lacrimal sac stenosis
375.55	Neonatal nasolacrimal obstruction
375.56	Acquired nasolacrimal duct stenosis
375.57	Dacryolith
743.65	Spec congen lacrimal passage anom
905.0	Late effect, skull/face fracture

REIMBURSEMENT INFORMATION

Medicare

- ♦ Follow–up Days — 90
- ♦ Assistant Surgeon — paid
- ♦ Supply Charges — not allowed
- ♦ Outpatient Limit — does not apply
- ♦ Major Surgery Rules Apply

68750 Conjunctivorhinostomy (fistulization of conjunctiva to nasal cavity); with insertion of tube or stent

CPT NOTES

- ♦ For diagnostic and treatment ophthalmological services, see Medicine, Ophthalmology, and 92002 et seq.
- ♦ For removal of foreign body, see 65205, et seq.

375.20	Epiphora NOS
375.21	Epiphora d/t excess lacrimation
375.22	Epiphora d/t insufficient drainage
375.41	Chronic canaliculitis
375.42	Chronic dacryocystitis
375.43	Lacrimal mucocele
375.51	Lacrimal punctum eversion
375.52	Lacrimal punctum stenosis
375.53	Lacrimal canaliculi stenosis
375.54	Lacrimal sac stenosis
375.55	Neonatal nasolacrimal obstruction
375.56	Acquired nasolacrimal duct stenosis
375.57	Dacryolith
743.65	Spec congen lacrimal passage anom
905.0	Late effect, skull/face fracture

REIMBURSEMENT INFORMATION

Medicare

- ♦ Follow–up Days — 90
- ♦ Assistant Surgeon — paid
- ♦ Supply Charges — not allowed
- ♦ Outpatient Limit — does not apply
- ♦ Major Surgery Rules Apply

CPT CODE	SERVICE	ICD-9-CM

68760 Closure of lacrimal punctum; by thermocauterization, ligation, or laser surgery

CPT NOTES

- For diagnostic and treatment ophthalmological services, see Medicine, Ophthalmology, and 92002 et seq.
- For removal of foreign body, see 65205, et seq.

370.34	Exposure keratoconjunctivitis
375.13	Primary lacrimal atrophy
375.14	Secondary lacrimal atrophy
375.15	Tear film insufficiency NOS
375.56	Acquired nasolacrimal duct stenosis
710.2	Sicca syndrome

REIMBURSEMENT INFORMATION

Medicare

- Follow-up Days — 10
- Assistant Surgeon — not paid
- Supply Charges — not allowed
- Outpatient Limit — applies
- Minor Surgery Rules Apply

68770 Closure of lacrimal fistula (separate procedure)

CPT NOTES

- For diagnostic and treatment ophthalmological services, see Medicine, Ophthalmology, and 92002 et seq.
- For removal of foreign body, see 65205, et seq.

375.22	Epiphora d/t insufficient drainage
375.55	Neonatal nasolacrimal obstruction
375.61	Lacrimal fistula

REIMBURSEMENT INFORMATION

General

- Separate procedure rules apply.

Medicare

- Follow-up Days — 90
- Assistant Surgeon — not paid
- Supply Charges — not allowed
- Outpatient Limit — applies
- Major Surgery Rules Apply

CPT CODE	SERVICE	ICD-9-CM

68800* Dilation of lacrimal punctum, with or without irrigation, unilateral or bilateral

CPT NOTES

- ♦ For diagnostic and treatment ophthalmological services, see Medicine, Ophthalmology, and 92002 et seq.
- ♦ For removal of foreign body, see 65205, et seq.

ICD-9-CM

375.20 Epiphora NOS
375.21 Epiphora d/t excess lacrimation
375.22 Epiphora d/t insufficient drainage
375.30 Dacryocystitis NOS
375.32 Acute dacryocystitis
375.52 Lacrimal punctum stenosis
375.53 Lacrimal canaliculi stenosis
375.55 Neonatal nasolacrimal obstruction
375.56 Acquired nasolacrimal duct stenosis

REIMBURSEMENT INFORMATION

General

- ♦ Starred procedure.

Medicare

- ♦ Follow-up Days — 10
- ♦ Assistant Surgeon — not paid
- ♦ Supply Charges — not allowed
- ♦ Outpatient Limit — applies
- ♦ Minor Surgery Rules Apply

68820* Probing of nasolacrimal duct, with or without irrigation, unilateral or bilateral

CPT NOTES

- ♦ For diagnostic and treatment ophthalmological services, see Medicine, Ophthalmology, and 92002 et seq.
- ♦ For removal of foreign body, see 65205, et seq.

ICD-9-CM

375.20 Epiphora NOS
375.30 Dacryocystitis NOS
375.51 Lacrimal punctum eversion
375.52 Lacrimal punctum stenosis
375.53 Lacrimal canaliculi stenosis
375.54 Lacrimal sac stenosis
375.55 Neonatal nasolacrimal obstruction
375.56 Acquired nasolacrimal duct stenosis
375.57 Dacryolith
771.6 Neonatal conjunctivitis

REIMBURSEMENT INFORMATION

General

- ♦ Starred procedure.

Medicare

- ♦ Follow-up Days — 10
- ♦ Assistant Surgeon — not paid
- ♦ Supply Charges — not allowed
- ♦ Outpatient Limit — applies
- ♦ Minor Surgery Rules Apply

CPT CODE	SERVICE	ICD–9–CM

68825 Probing of nasolacrimal duct, with or without irrigation, unilateral or bilateral; requiring general anesthesia

CPT NOTES

- For diagnostic and treatment ophthalmological services, see Medicine, Ophthalmology, and 92002 et seq.
- For removal of foreign body, see 65205, et seq.
- See also 92018.

ICD–9–CM

375.20	Epiphora NOS
375.30	Dacryocystitis NOS
375.32	Acute dacryocystitis
375.51	Lacrimal punctum eversion
375.52	Lacrimal punctum stenosis
375.53	Lacrimal canaliculi stenosis
375.54	Lacrimal sac stenosis
375.55	Neonatal nasolacrimal obstruction
375.56	Acquired nasolacrimal duct stenosis
375.57	Dacryolith
771.6	Neonatal conjunctivitis

REIMBURSEMENT INFORMATION

Medicare

- Follow–up Days — 10
- Assistant Surgeon — not paid
- Supply Charges — not allowed
- Outpatient Limit — does not apply
- Minor Surgery Rules Apply

68830 Probing of nasolacrimal duct, with or without irrigation, unilateral or bilateral; with insertion of tube or stent

CPT NOTES

- For diagnostic and treatment ophthalmological services, see Medicine, Ophthalmology, and 92002 et seq.
- For removal of foreign body, see 65205, et seq.

ICD–9–CM

375.20	Epiphora NOS
375.51	Lacrimal punctum eversion
375.52	Lacrimal punctum stenosis
375.53	Lacrimal canaliculi stenosis
375.54	Lacrimal sac stenosis
375.55	Neonatal nasolacrimal obstruction
375.56	Acquired nasolacrimal duct stenosis
375.57	Dacryolith
771.6	Neonatal conjunctivitis

REIMBURSEMENT INFORMATION

Medicare

- Follow–up Days — 10
- Assistant Surgeon — not paid
- Supply Charges — not allowed
- Outpatient Limit — applies
- Minor Surgery Rules Apply
- Fragments — 68820

CPT CODE **SERVICE**

68840* Probing of lacrimal canaliculi, with or without irrigation

CPT NOTES

- For diagnostic and treatment ophthalmological services, see Medicine, Ophthalmology, and 92002 et seq.
- For removal of foreign body, see 65205, et seq.

ICD–9–CM

375.13	Primary lacrimal atrophy
375.14	Secondary lacrimal atrophy
375.20	Epiphora NOS
375.22	Epiphora d/t insufficient drainage
375.30	Dacryocystitis NOS
375.31	Acute canaliculitis
375.41	Chronic canaliculitis
375.43	Lacrimal mucocele
375.52	Lacrimal punctum stenosis
375.53	Lacrimal canaliculi stenosis
375.54	Lacrimal sac stenosis
375.55	Neonatal nasolacrimal obstruction
375.56	Acquired nasolacrimal duct stenosis
375.57	Dacryolith
905.0	Late effect, skull/face fracture

REIMBURSEMENT INFORMATION

General

- Starred procedure.

Medicare

- Follow–up Days — 10
- Assistant Surgeon — not paid
- Supply Charges — not allowed
- Outpatient Limit — applies
- Minor Surgery Rules Apply

CPT CODE	SERVICE
68850*	Injection of contrast medium for dacryocystography

CPT NOTES

- ♦ For diagnostic and treatment ophthalmological services, see Medicine, Ophthalmology, and 92002 et seq.
- ♦ For removal of foreign body, see 65205, et seq.
- ♦ For radiological supervision and interpretation, see 70170.

ICD–9–CM

190.7	M-Neoplasm, Lacrimal duct
224.7	B-Neoplasm, Lacrimal duct
375.00	Dacryoadenitis NOS
375.01	Acute dacryoadenitis
375.02	Chronic dacryoadenitis
375.03	Chronic enlargement lacrimal gland
375.11	Dacryops
375.15	Tear film insufficiency NOS
375.20	Epiphora NOS
375.30	Dacryocystitis NOS
375.32	Acute dacryocystitis
375.33	Phlegmonous dacryocystitis
375.42	Chronic dacryocystitis
375.54	Lacrimal sac stenosis
375.56	Acquired nasolacrimal duct stenosis
375.57	Dacryolith
905.0	Late effect, skull/face fracture

REIMBURSEMENT INFORMATION

General

- ♦ Starred procedure.

Medicare

- ♦ Follow–up Days — 0
- ♦ Assistant Surgeon — not paid
- ♦ Supply Charges — not allowed
- ♦ Outpatient Limit — does not apply
- ♦ Minor Surgery Rules Apply

CPT CODE	SERVICE	ICD–9–CM

68899 Unlisted procedure, lacrimal system

CPT NOTES

- ♦ For diagnostic and treatment ophthalmological services, see Medicine, Ophthalmology, and 92002 et seq.
- ♦ For removal of foreign body, see 65205, et seq.

190.7	M-Neoplasm, Lacrimal duct
224.7	B-Neoplasm, Lacrimal duct
375.13	Primary lacrimal atrophy
375.14	Secondary lacrimal atrophy
375.22	Epiphora d/t insufficient drainage
375.30	Dacryocystitis NOS
375.32	Acute dacryocystitis
375.52	Lacrimal punctum stenosis
375.53	Lacrimal canaliculi stenosis
375.54	Lacrimal sac stenosis
375.56	Acquired nasolacrimal duct stenosis
375.61	Lacrimal fistula
375.81	Lacrimal passage granuloma
771.6	Neonatal conjunctivitis
905.0	Late effect, skull/face fracture

REIMBURSEMENT INFORMATION

Medicare

- ♦ Follow–up Days — determined by local carrier
- ♦ Assistant Surgeon — determined by local carrier
- ♦ Supply Charges — determined by local carrier
- ♦ Outpatient Limit — determined by local carrier

69000* Drainage external ear, abscess or hematoma; simple

69005 Drainage external ear, abscess or hematoma; complicated

CPT NOTES

- ♦ For diagnostic services (e.g., audiometry, vestibular tests), see 92502 et seq.

380.31	Hematoma of auricle/pinna
706.2	Sebaceous cyst
738.7	Cauliflower ear

REIMBURSEMENT INFORMATION

General

- ♦ Starred procedure. (69000)

Medicare

- ♦ Follow–up Days — 10
- ♦ Assistant Surgeon — not paid
- ♦ Supply Charges — not allowed
- ♦ Outpatient Limit — applies
- ♦ Minor Surgery Rules Apply

CPT CODE	SERVICE	ICD–9–CM

69020* Drainage external auditory canal, abscess

CPT NOTES

- For diagnostic services (e.g., audiometry, vestibular tests), see 92502 et seq.

380.31 Hematoma of auricle/pinna
706.2 Sebaceous cyst

REIMBURSEMENT INFORMATION

General

- Starred procedure.

Medicare

- Follow–up Days — 10
- Assistant Surgeon — not paid
- Supply Charges — not allowed
- Outpatient Limit — applies
- Minor Surgery Rules Apply

69090 Ear piercing

CPT NOTES

- For diagnostic services (e.g., audiometry, vestibular tests), see 92502 et seq.

V50.3 Ear piercing

REIMBURSEMENT INFORMATION

Medicare

- Follow–up Days — global concept does not apply
- Assistant Surgeon — not paid
- Supply Charges — not allowed
- Outpatient Limit — does not apply

69100 Biopsy external ear

CPT NOTES

- For diagnostic services (e.g., audiometry, vestibular tests), see 92502 et seq.

173.2 M-Neoplasm, Skin of ear
198.2 M2-Neoplasm, Skin
216.2 B-Neoplasm, Skin of ear
232.2 CA in situ, Skin of ear
238.2 UB-Neoplasm, Skin
380.89 External ear disorder NEC

REIMBURSEMENT INFORMATION

Medicare

- Follow–up Days — 0
- Assistant Surgeon — not paid
- Supply Charges — not allowed
- Outpatient Limit — applies
- Minor Surgery Rules Apply

CPT CODE	SERVICE	ICD-9-CM

69105 Biopsy external auditory canal

CPT NOTES

- ♦ For diagnostic services (e.g., audiometry, vestibular tests), see 92502 et seq.

173.2	M-Neoplasm, Skin of ear
198.2	M2-Neoplasm, Skin
216.2	B-Neoplasm, Skin of ear
380.23	Chronic otitis externa NEC
380.89	External ear disorder NEC

REIMBURSEMENT INFORMATION

Medicare

- ♦ Follow-up Days — 0
- ♦ Assistant Surgeon — not paid
- ♦ Supply Charges — not allowed
- ♦ Outpatient Limit — applies
- ♦ Minor Surgery Rules Apply

69110 Excision external ear; partial, simple repair

CPT NOTES

- ♦ For diagnostic services (e.g., audiometry, vestibular tests), see 92502 et seq.
- ♦ For reconstruction of ear, see 15120 et seq.

173.2	M-Neoplasm, Skin of ear
216.2	B-Neoplasm, Skin of ear
232.2	CA in situ, Skin of ear
706.2	Sebaceous cyst
709.2	Scar/fibrosis of skin
709.4	Foreign body granuloma, skin

REIMBURSEMENT INFORMATION

Medicare

- ♦ Follow-up Days — 90
- ♦ Assistant Surgeon — not paid
- ♦ Supply Charges — not allowed
- ♦ Outpatient Limit — does not apply
- ♦ Major Surgery Rules Apply

69120 Excision external ear; complete amputation

CPT NOTES

- ♦ For diagnostic services (e.g., audiometry, vestibular tests), see 92502 et seq.
- ♦ For reconstruction of ear, see 15120 et seq.

173.2	M-Neoplasm, Skin of ear
216.2	B-Neoplasm, Skin of ear
232.2	CA in situ, Skin of ear
706.2	Sebaceous cyst

REIMBURSEMENT INFORMATION

Medicare

- ♦ Follow-up Days — 90
- ♦ Assistant Surgeon — not paid
- ♦ Supply Charges — not allowed
- ♦ Outpatient Limit — does not apply
- ♦ Major Surgery Rules Apply

CPT CODE / SERVICE	ICD-9-CM
69140 Excision exostosis(es), external auditory canal **CPT NOTES** ◆ For diagnostic services (e.g., audiometry, vestibular tests), see 92502 et seq.	380.81 Exostosis of external ear canal **REIMBURSEMENT INFORMATION** Medicare ◆ Follow–up Days — 90 ◆ Assistant Surgeon — not paid ◆ Supply Charges — not allowed ◆ Outpatient Limit — does not apply ◆ Major Surgery Rules Apply
69145 Excision soft tissue lesion, external auditory canal **CPT NOTES** ◆ For diagnostic services (e.g., audiometry, vestibular tests), see 92502 et seq.	380.89 External ear disorder NEC **REIMBURSEMENT INFORMATION** Medicare ◆ Follow–up Days — 90 ◆ Assistant Surgeon — not paid ◆ Supply Charges — not allowed ◆ Outpatient Limit — does not apply ◆ Major Surgery Rules Apply
69150 Radical excision external auditory canal lesion; without neck dissection **CPT NOTES** ◆ For diagnostic services (e.g., audiometry, vestibular tests), see 92502 et seq. ◆ For resection of temporal bone, see 69535. ◆ For skin grafting, see 15000-15261.	173.2 M-Neoplasm, Skin of ear 198.2 M2-Neoplasm, Skin 216.2 B-Neoplasm, Skin of ear 380.89 External ear disorder NEC **REIMBURSEMENT INFORMATION** Medicare ◆ Follow–up Days — 90 ◆ Assistant Surgeon — paid ◆ Supply Charges — not allowed ◆ Outpatient Limit — does not apply ◆ Major Surgery Rules Apply
69155 Radical excision external auditory canal lesion; with neck dissection **CPT NOTES** ◆ For diagnostic services (e.g., audiometry, vestibular tests), see 92502 et seq. ◆ For resection of temporal bone, see 69535. ◆ For skin grafting, see 15000-15261.	173.2 M-Neoplasm, Skin of ear 198.2 M2-Neoplasm, Skin 216.2 B-Neoplasm, Skin of ear **REIMBURSEMENT INFORMATION** Medicare ◆ Follow–up Days — 90 ◆ Assistant Surgeon — paid ◆ Supply Charges — not allowed ◆ Outpatient Limit — does not apply ◆ Major Surgery Rules Apply

CPT CODE	SERVICE	ICD-9-CM

69200 Removal foreign body from external auditory canal; without general anesthesia

69205 Removal foreign body from external auditory canal; with general anesthesia

CPT NOTES

- For diagnostic services (e.g., audiometry, vestibular tests), see 92502 et seq.

931. Foreign body in ear

REIMBURSEMENT INFORMATION

Medicare

- Follow-up Days
  69200 — 0
- 69205 — 10
- Assistant Surgeon — not paid
- Supply Charges — not allowed
- Outpatient Limit
  69200 — applies
  69205 — does not apply
- Minor Surgery Rules Apply

69300 Otoplasty, protruding ear, with or without size reduction

CPT NOTES

- For diagnostic services (e.g., audiometry, vestibular tests), see 92502 et seq.
- For suture of wound or injury of external ear, see 12011-14300.

380.32 Acquired deformity auricle/pinna
744.22 Macrotia
744.29 Ear anomalies NEC
744.3 Ear anomaly NOS

REIMBURSEMENT INFORMATION

Medicare

- Follow-up Days — determined by local carrier
- Assistant Surgeon — by report
- Supply Charges — not allowed
- Outpatient Limit — does not apply

69310 Reconstruction of external auditory canal (meatoplasty) (eg, for stenosis due to trauma, infection), (separate procedure)

CPT NOTES

- For diagnostic services (e.g., audiometry, vestibular tests), see 92502 et seq.
- For suture of wound or injury of external ear, see 12011-14300.

380.32 Acquired deformity auricle/pinna
380.51 Stenosis ext ear canal d/t trauma
385.30 Cholesteatoma NOS
385.32 Cholesteatoma of middle ear
744.02 Ext ear anomaly NEC, hearing impair

REIMBURSEMENT INFORMATION

General

- Separate procedure rules apply.

Medicare

- Follow-up Days — 90
- Assistant Surgeon — not paid
- Supply Charges — not allowed
- Outpatient Limit — does not apply
- Major Surgery Rules Apply

CPT CODE	SERVICE	ICD-9-CM

69320 Reconstruction external auditory canal for congenital atresia, single stage

CPT NOTES

- For diagnostic services (e.g., audiometry, vestibular tests), see 92502 et seq.
- For suture of wound or injury of external ear, see 12011-14300.
- For combination with middle ear reconstruction, see 69631, 69641.
- For other reconstructive procedures with grafts (e.g., skin, cartilage, bone), see 13150-15760, 21230-21235.

744.02 Ext ear anomaly NEC, hearing impair
744.24 Eustachian tube anomaly NEC

REIMBURSEMENT INFORMATION

Medicare

- Follow–up Days — 90
- Assistant Surgeon — paid
- Supply Charges — not allowed
- Outpatient Limit — does not apply
- Major Surgery Rules Apply

69550 Excision aural glomus tumor; transcanal

69552 Excision aural glomus tumor; transmastoid

69554 Excision aural glomus tumor; extended (extratemporal)

CPT NOTES

- For diagnostic services (e.g., audiometry, vestibular tests), see 92502 et seq.

192.0 M-Neoplasm, Cranial nerves
198.4 M2-Neoplasm, Nervous system NEC
225.1 B-Neoplasm, Cranial nerve
237.9 UB-Neoplasm, Nervous system NEC

REIMBURSEMENT INFORMATION

Medicare

- Follow–up Days — 90
- Assistant Surgeon — paid
- Supply Charges — not allowed
- Outpatient Limit — does not apply
- Major Surgery Rules Apply

69700 Closure postauricular fistula, mastoid (separate procedure)

CPT NOTES

- For diagnostic services (e.g., audiometry, vestibular tests), see 92502 et seq.

383.81 Postauricular fistula

REIMBURSEMENT INFORMATION

General

- Separate procedure rules apply.

Medicare

- Follow–up Days — 90
- Assistant Surgeon — paid
- Supply Charges — not allowed
- Outpatient Limit — does not apply
- Major Surgery Rules Apply

CPT CODE / SERVICE	ICD-9-CM
69720 Decompression facial nerve, intratemporal; lateral to geniculate ganglion **CPT NOTES** ♦ For diagnostic services (e.g., audiometry, vestibular tests), see 92502 et seq.	389.10 Sensorineural hearing loss NOS 389.11 Sensory hearing loss 389.12 Neural hearing loss 389.14 Central hearing loss 389.18 Sensorineural hear loss comb type 951.4 Injury to facial nerve **REIMBURSEMENT INFORMATION** Medicare ♦ Follow–up Days — 90 ♦ Assistant Surgeon — paid ♦ Supply Charges — not allowed ♦ Outpatient Limit — does not apply ♦ Major Surgery Rules Apply
69725 Decompression facial nerve, intratemporal; including medial to geniculate ganglion **CPT NOTES** ♦ For diagnostic services (e.g., audiometry, vestibular tests), see 92502 et seq.	389.10 Sensorineural hearing loss NOS 389.11 Sensory hearing loss 389.12 Neural hearing loss 389.14 Central hearing loss 389.18 Sensorineural hear loss comb type 907.1 Late effect, cranial nerve injury 951.4 Injury to facial nerve **REIMBURSEMENT INFORMATION** Medicare ♦ Follow–up Days — 90 ♦ Assistant Surgeon — paid ♦ Supply Charges — not allowed ♦ Outpatient Limit — does not apply ♦ Major Surgery Rules Apply
69740 Suture facial nerve, intratemporal, with or without graft or decompression; lateral to geniculate ganglion **CPT NOTES** ♦ For diagnostic services (e.g., audiometry, vestibular tests), see 92502 et seq. ♦ For extracranial suture of facial nerve, see 64864.	389.10 Sensorineural hearing loss NOS 389.11 Sensory hearing loss 389.12 Neural hearing loss 389.14 Central hearing loss 389.18 Sensorineural hear loss comb type 951.4 Injury to facial nerve **REIMBURSEMENT INFORMATION** Medicare ♦ Follow–up Days — 90 ♦ Assistant Surgeon — paid ♦ Supply Charges — not allowed ♦ Outpatient Limit — does not apply ♦ Major Surgery Rules Apply

CPT CODE	SERVICE
69955	Total facial nerve decompression and/or repair (may include graft)

CPT NOTES

- For diagnostic services (e.g., audiometry, vestibular tests), see 92502 et seq.
- For external approach, see 69535.

ICD–9–CM

389.10	Sensorineural hearing loss NOS
389.11	Sensory hearing loss
389.12	Neural hearing loss
389.14	Central hearing loss
389.18	Sensorineural hear loss comb type
907.1	Late effect, cranial nerve injury
951.4	Injury to facial nerve

REIMBURSEMENT INFORMATION

Medicare

- Follow–up Days — 90
- Assistant Surgeon — paid
- Supply Charges — not allowed
- Outpatient Limit — does not apply
- Major Surgery Rules Apply

RADIOLOGY

CPT CODE	SERVICE	ICD-9-CM
70100	Radiologic examination, mandible; partial, less than four views	524.0x Major anomaly of jaw size 524.6x Temporomandibular joint disorder 526.81 Exostosis of jaw 526.89 Jaw disease NEC 802.2x Fracture, Mandible, closed 802.3x Fracture, Mandible, open 802.8 Fx facial bone NEC, closed V54.0 Removal of internal fixation device
70110	Radiologic examination, mandible; complete, minimum of four views	170.1 M-Neoplasm, Mandible 213.1 B-Neoplasm, Lower jaw bone 524.0x Major anomaly of jaw size 524.1x Jaw/cranial base relation anomaly 524.6x Temporomandibular joint disorder 526.0 Developmental odontogenic cysts 526.81 Exostosis of jaw 526.89 Jaw disease NEC 802.2x Fracture, Mandible, closed V54.0 Removal of internal fixation device **REIMBURSEMENT INFORMATION** Medicare ◆ Fragments — 70100
70140	Radiologic examination, facial bones; less than three views	682.0 Cellulitis of face 715.09 General osteoarthrosis, mult sites 733.19 Pathologic fracture, site NEC 754.0 Congen skull/face/jaw deformity 802.x Fracture of face bones 873.2x Nose, open wound 873.3x Nose, complex open wound 873.4x Face, open wound 873.5x Face, complicated open wound 959.0 Face and neck injury NOS 959.8 Injury, multiple sites, site NEC

CPT CODE	SERVICE	ICD-9-CM	
70150	Radiologic examination, facial bones; complete, minimum of three views	682.0	Cellulitis of face
		715.09	General osteoarthrosis, mult sites
		733.19	Pathologic fracture, site NEC
		754.0	Congen skull/face/jaw deformity
		802.x	Fracture of face bones
		873.2x	Nose, open wound
		873.3x	Nose, complex open wound
		873.4x	Face, open wound
		873.5x	Face, complicated open wound
		959.0	Face and neck injury NOS
		959.8	Injury, multiple sites, site NEC

REIMBURSEMENT INFORMATION

Medicare

- ♦ Fragments — 70140

CPT CODE	SERVICE	ICD-9-CM	
70160	Radiologic examination, nasal bones, complete, minimum of three views	738.0	Acquired nose deformity
		748.1	Congenital nose anomaly NEC
		749.0x	Cleft palate
		784.7	Epistaxis
		802.0	Nasal bone Fx, closed
		802.1	Nasal bone Fx, open
		848.0	Sprain of nasal septum
		873.2x	Nose, open wound
		932.	Foreign body in nose
		951.4	Injury to facial nerve
		959.0	Face and neck injury NOS
70200	Radiologic examination; orbits, complete, minimum of four views	160.2	M-Neoplasm, Maxillary sinus
		195.0	M-Neoplasm, Head/face/neck
		756.0	Anomaly of skull/face bones
		802.6	Fx orbital floor, closed
		802.7	Fx orbital floor, open
		870.0	Laceration eyelid skin/periocular
		870.3	Penetrating orbit wound w/o FB
		870.8	Open wound of ocular adnexa NEC
		920.	Contusion face/scalp/neck
		921.2	Contusion of orbital tissue
		921.9	Contusion of eye NOS
		959.0	Face and neck injury NOS
		959.8	Injury, multiple sites, site NEC

CPT CODE	SERVICE	ICD-9-CM	
70210	Radiologic examination, sinuses, paranasal, less than three views	212.0	B-Neoplasm, Nasal cavity/sinus
		289.1	Chronic lymphadenitis
		461.2	Acute ethmoidal sinusitis
		473.2	Chronic ethmoidal sinusitis
		715.18	Loc prim osteoarthritis NEC
		748.1	Congenital nose anomaly NEC
		748.8	Respiratory system anomaly NEC
		754.0	Congen skull/face/jaw deformity
		781.1	Smell/taste sensation disturbance
		802.6	Fx orbital floor, closed
		802.8	Fx facial bone NEC, closed
		802.9	Fx facial bone NEC, open
		872.6x	Open wound of ear
		873.9	Open wound of head NEC, complicated
		959.0	Face and neck injury NOS
70220	Radiologic examination, sinuses, paranasal, complete, minimum of three views	212.0	B-Neoplasm, Nasal cavity/sinus
		289.1	Chronic lymphadenitis
		461.2	Acute ethmoidal sinusitis
		473.2	Chronic ethmoidal sinusitis
		715.18	Loc prim osteoarthritis NEC
		754.0	Congen skull/face/jaw deformity
		781.1	Smell/taste sensation disturbance
		784.7	Epistaxis
		802.6	Fx orbital floor, closed
		802.8	Fx facial bone NEC, closed
		802.9	Fx facial bone NEC, open
		872.6x	Open wound of ear
		873.9	Open wound of head NEC, complicated
		959.0	Face and neck injury NOS
		REIMBURSEMENT INFORMATION	
		Medicare	
		♦ Fragments — 70210	
70250	Radiologic examination, skull; less than four views, with or without stereo	170.0	M-Neoplasm, Skull/Face bone
		800.00	Closed skull vault Fx
		V67.0	Surgery follow-up
		V67.4	Fracture follow-up

CPT CODE	SERVICE	ICD–9–CM
70260	Radiologic examination, skull; complete, minimum of four views, with or without stereo	170.0 M-Neoplasm, Skull/Face bone 733.29 Bone cyst NEC 800.00 Closed skull vault Fx V67.0 Surgery follow-up V67.4 Fracture follow-up **REIMBURSEMENT INFORMATION** Medicare ♦ Fragments — 70250
70350	Cephalogram, orthodontic	524.0x Major anomaly of jaw size 524.2 Dental arch relationship anomaly 756.0 Anomaly of skull/face bones 802.2x Fracture, Mandible, closed 802.3x Fracture, Mandible, open V67.0 Surgery follow-up V67.4 Fracture follow-up
70355	Orthopantogram	524.0x Major anomaly of jaw size 524.1x Jaw/cranial base relation anomaly 524.6x Temporomandibular joint disorder 528.3 Cellulitis/abscess of mouth 528.9 Oral soft tissue disease NEC 802.2x Fracture, Mandible, closed 802.4x Fx malar/maxillary, closed V67.0 Surgery follow-up
70450	Computerized axial tomography, head or brain; without contrast material **CPT NOTES** ♦ For coronal, sagittal, and/or oblique sections, see 76375.	733.3 Hyperostosis of skull 802.9 Fx facial bone NEC, open 803.x Skull fracture 870.4 Penetrating orbit wound w/FB 873.9 Open wound of head NEC, complicated V67.0 Surgery follow-up
70460	Computerized axial tomography, head or brain; with contrast material(s) **CPT NOTES** ♦ For coronal, sagittal, and/or oblique sections, see 76375.	733.3 Hyperostosis of skull 802.9 Fx facial bone NEC, open 803.x Skull fracture 870.4 Penetrating orbit wound w/FB 873.9 Open wound of head NEC, complicated V67.0 Surgery follow-up

CPT CODE	SERVICE	ICD–9–CM
70470	Computerized axial tomography, head or brain; without contrast material, followed by contrast material(s) and further sections **CPT NOTES** ♦ For coronal, sagittal, and/or oblique sections, see 76375.	733.3 Hyperostosis of skull 802.9 Fx facial bone NEC, open 803.x Skull fracture 870.4 Penetrating orbit wound w/FB 873.9 Open wound of head NEC, complicated V67.0 Surgery follow-up **REIMBURSEMENT INFORMATION** Medicare ♦ Fragments — 70450, 70460
70486	Computerized axial tomography, maxillofacial area; without contrast material **CPT NOTES** ♦ For coronal, sagittal, and/or oblique sections, see 76375.	524.6x Temporomandibular joint disorder 714.0 Rheumatoid arthritis 728.85 Spasm of muscle 756.0 Anomaly of skull/face bones 802.0 Nasal bone Fx, closed 802.2x Fracture, Mandible, closed 802.3x Fracture, Mandible, open 802.4 Fx malar/maxillary, closed 802.5 Fx malar/maxillary, open 802.8 Fx facial bone NEC, closed 830.0 Dislocation jaw, closed 830.1 Dislocation jaw, open 848.1 Sprain of jaw
70487	Computerized axial tomography, maxillofacial area; with contrast material(s) **CPT NOTES** ♦ For coronal, sagittal, and/or oblique sections, see 76375.	524.6x Temporomandibular joint disorder 714.0 Rheumatoid arthritis 728.85 Spasm of muscle 756.0 Anomaly of skull/face bones 784.0 Headache 802.0 Nasal bone Fx, closed 802.2x Fracture, Mandible, closed 802.3x Fracture, Mandible, open 802.4 Fx malar/maxillary, closed 802.5 Fx malar/maxillary, open 830.0 Dislocation jaw, closed 830.1 Dislocation jaw, open 848.1 Sprain of jaw

CPT CODE	SERVICE	ICD–9–CM
70488	Computerized axial tomography, maxillofacial area; without contrast material, followed by contrast material(s) and further sections **CPT NOTES** ◆ For coronal, sagittal, and/or oblique sections, see 76375.	524.6x Temporomandibular joint disorder 714.0 Rheumatoid arthritis 728.85 Spasm of muscle 756.0 Anomaly of skull/face bones 784.0 Headache 802.0 Nasal bone Fx, closed 802.2x Fracture, Mandible, closed 802.3x Fracture, Mandible, open 802.4 Fx malar/maxillary, closed 802.5 Fx malar/maxillary, open 830.0 Dislocation jaw, closed 830.1 Dislocation jaw, open 848.1 Sprain of jaw **REIMBURSEMENT INFORMATION** <u>Medicare</u> ◆ Fragments — 70486, 70487
71100	Radiologic examination, ribs, unilateral; two views	198.5 M2-Neoplasm, Bone and bone marrow 922.1 Contusion of chest wall 959.1 Trunk injury NOS 959.8 Injury, multiple sites, site NEC V10.3 Hx of breast malignancy
71101	Radiologic examination, ribs, unilateral; including posteroanterior chest, minimum of three views	198.5 M2-Neoplasm, Bone and bone marrow 922.1 Contusion of chest wall 959.1 Trunk injury NOS 959.8 Injury, multiple sites, site NEC V10.3 Hx of breast malignancy
73090	Radiologic examination; forearm, anteroposterior and lateral views	733.82 Nonunion of fracture 755.50 Upper limb anomaly NOS 756.51 Osteogenesis imperfecta 813.0x Fracture of radius/ulna, upper end 813.2x Fracture of radius and ulna shaft 813.8x Fracture of radius/ulna NOS 814.00 Fx carpal bone NOS, closed 881.00 Open wound of forearm 884.2 Open wound of arm NOS w/tendon 927.1x Crushing injury, elbow and forearm 927.2x Crushing injury, wrist and hand 927.3 Crushing injury, finger 927.9 Crushing injury arm NOS

CPT CODE	SERVICE	ICD–9–CM	
73100	Radiologic examination, wrist; anteroposterior and lateral views	714.0	Rheumatoid arthritis
		732.3	Juvenile osteochondrosis, arm
		732.8	Osteochondropathy NEC
		733.8	Malunion and nonunion of fracture
		736.0x	Acquired deformity of forearm
		755.50	Upper limb anomaly NOS
		813.4x	Fracture of radius/ulna, lower end
		813.5x	Fracture of radius/ulna, lower end
		814.0x	Carpal fracture, closed
		814.1x	Carpal fracture, open
		V67.0	Surgery follow-up
		V67.4	Fracture follow-up
73110	Radiologic examination, wrist; complete, minimum of three views	354.0	Carpal tunnel syndrome
		714.0	Rheumatoid arthritis
		729.5	Pain in limb
		733.82	Nonunion of fracture
		755.28	Longitudinal deficiency, hand
		755.50	Upper limb anomaly NOS
		813.51	Colles' fracture, open
		813.81	Fracture radius NOS, closed
		813.82	Fracture ulna NOS, closed
		814.01	Fx navicular, wrist, closed
		881.02	Open wound of wrist
		881.22	Open wound of wrist w/tendon
		V67.0	Surgery follow-up
		V67.4	Fracture follow-up

REIMBURSEMENT INFORMATION

Medicare

- ♦ Fragments — 73100

CPT CODE	SERVICE	ICD–9–CM	
73120	Radiologic examination, hand; two views	714.0	Rheumatoid arthritis
		714.30	Juvenile rheumatoid arthritis NOS
		726.4	Enthesopathy of wrist/carpus
		736.00	Forearm deformity NOS
		736.06	Claw hand
		736.20	Acquired finger deformity NOS
		736.29	Acquired finger deformity NEC
		755.00	Polydactyly NOS
		755.01	Polydactyly, fingers
		755.10	Syndactyly, multiple/NOS
		755.21	Transverse arm deficiency
		755.50	Upper limb anomaly NOS
		781.5	Clubbing of fingers
		813.41	Colles' fracture, closed
		813.42	Fx distal radius NEC, closed
		815.0x	Metacarpal fracture, closed
		816.01	Fx mid/prox phalanx, hand, closed
		882.0	Open wound of hand
		882.1	Open wound of hand, complicated
		882.2	Open wound of hand, w/tendon
		883.0	Open wound of finger
		883.1	Open wound of finger, complicated
		883.2	Open wound of finger w/tendon
		885.0	Traumatic thumb amputation
		885.1	Traumatic thumb amputation, compl
		886.0	Traumatic finger amputation
		886.1	Traumatic finger amputation, compl
73130	Radiologic examination, hand; minimum of three views	714.0	Rheumatoid arthritis
		714.30	Juvenile rheumatoid arthritis NOS
		755.50	Upper limb anomaly NOS
		813.41	Colles' fracture, closed
		813.42	Fx distal radius NEC, closed
		815.0x	Metacarpal fracture, closed
		816.01	Fx mid/prox phalanx, hand, closed
		882.0	Open wound of hand
		882.1	Open wound of hand, complicated
		882.2	Open wound of hand, w/tendon
		883.0	Open wound of finger
		883.1	Open wound of finger, complicated
		883.2	Open wound of finger w/tendon
		V67.0	Surgery follow-up

REIMBURSEMENT INFORMATION

Medicare

- ♦ Fragments — 73120

CPT CODE	SERVICE	ICD-9-CM
▲ 73140	Radiologic examination, finger(s), minimum of two views	681.00 Cellulitis, finger NOS 681.02 Onychia of finger 714.0 Rheumatoid arthritis 727.03 Trigger finger 736.1 Mallet finger 736.29 Acquired finger deformity NEC 755.11 Syndactyly of fingers, no fusion 755.50 Upper limb anomaly NOS 816.0x Phalanges fracture, closed 816.1x Phalanges fracture, open 883.0 Open wound of finger 883.1 Open wound of finger, complicated 883.2 Open wound of finger w/tendon 885.0 Traumatic thumb amputation 885.1 Traumatic thumb amputation, compl 886.0 Traumatic finger amputation 886.1 Traumatic finger amputation, compl **REIMBURSEMENT INFORMATION** Medicare ♦ Description changed in 1995 CPT.
73620	Radiologic examination, foot; anteroposterior and lateral views	714.0 Rheumatoid arthritis 727.1 Bunion 728.71 Plantar fascial fibromatosis 733.1x Pathologic fracture 735.x Acquired deformities of toe 736.7x Acquired deformity, ankle and foot 754.5x Varus deformities of feet 754.6x Valgus deformity of feet 754.7x Deformities of feet 755.02 Polydactyly, toes 755.13 Syndactyly of toes, no fusion 755.31 Transverse leg deficiency 755.35 Tibiofibular longitudinal defic 755.66 Anomalies of toes NEC 825.x Tarsal/metatarsal fracture 826.0 Fx phalanx, foot, closed 826.1 Fx phalanx, foot, open 892.x Open wound of foot 905.7 Late effect of sprain/strain 924.20 Contusion of foot 924.3 Contusion of toe 928.20 Crushing injury, foot 928.3 Crushing injury, toe

CPT CODE	SERVICE	ICD-9-CM	
73630	Radiologic examination, foot; complete, minimum of three views	714.0	Rheumatoid arthritis
		727.1	Bunion
		728.71	Plantar fascial fibromatosis
		733.1x	Pathologic fracture
		735.x	Acquired deformities of toe
		736.7x	Acquired deformity, ankle and foot
		754.5x	Varus deformities of feet
		754.6x	Valgus deformity of feet
		754.7x	Deformities of feet
		755.02	Polydactyly, toes
		755.13	Syndactyly of toes, no fusion
		755.31	Transverse leg deficiency
		755.35	Tibiofibular longitudinal defic
		755.66	Anomalies of toes NEC
		825.x	Tarsal/metatarsal fracture
		826.0	Fx phalanx, foot, closed
		826.1	Fx phalanx, foot, open
		892.x	Open wound of foot
		905.7	Late effect of sprain/strain
		924.20	Contusion of foot
		924.3	Contusion of toe
		928.20	Crushing injury, foot
		928.3	Crushing injury, toe

REIMBURSEMENT INFORMATION

Medicare

- ◆ Fragments — 73620

CPT CODE	SERVICE	ICD–9–CM	
▲ **73660**	Radiologic examination; toe(s), minimum of two views	681.10	Cellulitis, toe NOS
		681.11	Onychia of toe
		700.	Corns and callosities
		703.0	Ingrowing nail
		719.47	Pain in joint, ankle/foot
		726.91	Exostosis, site NOS
		727.1	Bunion
		735.x	Acquired deformities of toe
		755.02	Polydactyly, toes
		755.13	Syndactyly of toes, no fusion
		755.65	Macrodactylia of toes
		755.66	Anomalies of toes NEC
		785.4	Gangrene
		826.0	Fx phalanx, foot, closed
		826.1	Fx phalanx, foot, open
		893.0	Open wound of toe
		893.1	Open wound of toe, complicated
		895.0	Amputation of toe
		928.3	Crushing injury, toe
		V67.0	Surgery follow-up
		V67.4	Fracture follow-up

REIMBURSEMENT INFORMATION

Medicare

- Description changed in 1995 CPT.

76090 Mammography; unilateral

V10.3	Hx of breast malignancy
V16.3	Family Hx, breast malignancy
V76.1	Screening, malig neop, breast

CPT NOTES

- For injection procedure for venous system, see 36000-36015, 36400-36510.
- For injection procedure for lymphatic system, see 38790.
- For arthrography of shoulder, see 73040; elbow, see 73085; wrist, see 73115; hip, see 73525; knee, see 73580; ankle, see 73615.

76091 Mammography; bilateral

CPT NOTES

- For injection procedure for venous system, see 36000-36015, 36400-36510.
- For injection procedure for lymphatic system, see 38790.
- For arthrography of shoulder, see 73040; elbow, see 73085; wrist, see 73115; hip, see 73525; knee, see 73580; ankle, see 73615.

REIMBURSEMENT INFORMATION

Medicare

- Fragments — 76090

CPT CODE	SERVICE	ICD–9–CM	
76092	Screening mammography, bilateral (two view film study of each breast)	V10.3	Hx of breast malignancy
		V16.3	Family Hx, breast malignancy
		V76.1	Screening, malig neop, breast

CPT NOTES

- ♦ For injection procedure for venous system, see 36000-36015, 36400-36510.
- ♦ For injection procedure for lymphatic system, see 38790.
- ♦ For arthrography of shoulder, see 73040; elbow, see 73085; wrist, see 73115; hip, see 73525; knee, see 73580; ankle, see 73615.

CPT CODE	SERVICE	ICD–9–CM	
76140	Consultation on x-ray examination made elsewhere, written report	170.0	M-Neoplasm, Skull/Face bone
		213.0	B-Neoplasm, Skull/Face bone
		754.0	Congen skull/face/jaw deformity
		802.4	Fx malar/maxillary, closed
		802.6	Fx orbital floor, closed
		802.8	Fx facial bone NEC, closed

CPT NOTES

- ♦ For injection procedure for venous system, see 36000-36015, 36400-36510.
- ♦ For injection procedure for lymphatic system, see 38790.
- ♦ For arthrography of shoulder, see 73040; elbow, see 73085; wrist, see 73115; hip, see 73525; knee, see 73580; ankle, see 73615.

PATHOLOGY AND LABORATORY

CPT CODE	SERVICE	ICD–9–CM	
80003	Automated multichannel test; 3 clinical chemistry tests	V72.6	Laboratory examination
80004	Automated multichannel test; 4 clinical chemistry tests		
80006	Automated multichannel test; 6 clinical chemistry tests		
80007	Automated multichannel test; 7 clinical chemistry tests		
80008	Automated multichannel test; 8 clinical chemistry tests		
80016	Automated multichannel test; 13-16 clinical chemistry tests		
80019	Automated multichannel test; 19 or more clinical chemistry tests		

CPT NOTES

- The following list contains those tests that can be and are frequently done as groups and combinations ("profiles") on automated multichannel equipment. For any combination of tests among those listed immediately below, use the appropriate number 80002-80019. Groups of the tests listed here are distinguished from multiple tests performed individually for immediate or "stat" reporting. (For handling of specimen, see 99000 and 99001.)

  Alanine aminotransferase (ALT, SGPT)
  Albumin
  Aspartate aminotransferase (AST, SGOT)
  Bilirubin, direct
  Bilirubin, total
  Calcium
  Carbon dioxide content
  Chloride
  Cholesterol
  Creatinine
  Glucose
  Lactate dehydrogenase (LD)
  Phosphatase, alkaline
  Phosphorus (inorganic phosphate)
  Potassium
  Protein, total
  Sodium
  Urea Nitrogen (BUN)
  Uric acid

CPT CODE	SERVICE	ICD–9–CM	
80058	Hepatic function panel THIS PANEL MUST INCLUDE THE FOLLOWING: Albumin, serum (82040) Bilirubin, total or direct (82250) Phosphatase, alkaline (84075) Transferase, aspartate amino (AST) (SGOT) (84450) Transferase, alanine amino (ALT) (SGPT) (84460) **CPT NOTES** ♦ This panel was developed for coding purposes only and should not be interpreted as a clinical parameter. The tests listed identify the defined components of this panel only. This panel's components are not intended to limit the performance of other tests. If one performs tests in addition to those specifically indicated in this panel, those tests should be reported separately in addition to the panel code.	V10.82 V72.6	Hx of malignant skin melanoma Laboratory examination
81000	Urinalysis, by dip stick or tablet reagent for bilirubin, glucose, hemoglobin, ketones, leukocytes, nitrite, pH, protein, specific gravity, urobilinogen, any number of these constituents; with microscopy **CPT NOTES** ♦ For specific analyses, see appropriate section.	250.x 401.9 599.0 V72.6	Diabetes mellitus Essential hypertension NOS Urinary tract infection NOS Laboratory examination
81002	Urinalysis, by dip stick or tablet reagent for bilirubin, glucose, hemoglobin, ketones, leukocytes, nitrite, pH, protein, specific gravity, urobilinogen, any number of these constituents; without microscopy, non-automated **CPT NOTES** ♦ For specific analyses, see appropriate section.	V72.6	Laboratory examination

CPT CODE	SERVICE	ICD–9–CM
82565	Creatinine; blood	599.0 Urinary tract infection NOS V72.6 Laboratory examination V81.5 Screening, nephropathy
82947	Glucose; quantitative	250.x Diabetes mellitus V72.6 Laboratory examination

82565 Creatinine; blood

CPT NOTES

- ♦ The material for examination may be from any source. Examination is quantitative unless specified. (For list of automated, multichannel tests, see 80002-80019.)
- ♦ Clinical information derived from the results of laboratory data that is mathematically calculated (e.g., free thyroxine index (T7)) is considered part of the test procedure and therefore is not a separately reportable service.

82947 Glucose; quantitative

CPT NOTES

- ♦ The material for examination may be from any source. Examination is quantitative unless specified. (For list of automated, multichannel tests, see 80002-80019.)
- ♦ Clinical information derived from the results of laboratory data that is mathematically calculated (e.g., free thyroxine index (T7)) is considered part of the test procedure and therefore is not a separately reportable service.
- ♦ For insulin tolerance test, see 80434, 80435.
- ♦ For leucine tolerance test, see 80428.
- ♦ For semiquantitative urine glucose, see 81000, 81002, 81005, 81099.

CPT CODE	SERVICE	ICD-9-CM	
82948	Glucose; blood, reagent strip	250.x	Diabetes mellitus

CPT NOTES

- The material for examination may be from any source. Examination is quantitative unless specified. (For list of automated, multichannel tests, see 80002-80019.)
- Clinical information derived from the results of laboratory data that is mathematically calculated (e.g., free thyroxine index (T7)) is considered part of the test procedure and therefore is not a separately reportable service.
- For insulin tolerance test, see 80434, 80435.
- For leucine tolerance test, see 80428.
- For semiquantitative urine glucose, see 81000, 81002, 81005, 81099.

85002	Bleeding time	784.7	Epistaxis

CPT NOTES

- For blood banking procedures, see Transfusion Medicine.
- Agglutinins, see Immunology.
- Antiplasmin, see 85410.
- Antithrombin III, see 85300, 85301.

85007	Blood count; manual differential WBC count (includes RBC morphology and platelet estimation)	V72.6	Laboratory examination

CPT NOTES

- For blood banking procedures, see Transfusion Medicine.
- Agglutinins, see Immunology.
- Antiplasmin, see 85410.
- Antithrombin III, see 85300, 85301.
- See also 85585.
- For other fluids, (e.g., CSF), see 89050, 89051.

CPT CODE SERVICE	ICD-9-CM
85014 Blood count; other than spun hematocrit **CPT NOTES** ♦ For blood banking procedures, see Transfusion Medicine. ♦ Agglutinins, see Immunology. ♦ Antiplasmin, see 85410. ♦ Antithrombin III, see 85300, 85301. ♦ For other hemoglobin determination, see 83020-83069.	707.0 Decubitus ulcer V72.6 Laboratory examination
85022 Blood count; hemogram, automated, and manual differential WBC count (CBC) **CPT NOTES** ♦ For blood banking procedures, see Transfusion Medicine. ♦ Agglutinins, see Immunology. ♦ Antiplasmin, see 85410. ♦ Antithrombin III, see 85300, 85301.	682.3 Cellulitis of arm 682.4 Cellulitis of hand
85023 Blood count; hemogram and platelet count, automated, and manual differential WBC count (CBC) **CPT NOTES** ♦ For blood banking procedures, see Transfusion Medicine. ♦ Agglutinins, see Immunology. ♦ Antiplasmin, see 85410. ♦ Antithrombin III, see 85300, 85301.	465.9 Acute upper respiratory infect NOS 682.3 Cellulitis of arm 682.4 Cellulitis of hand
85024 Blood count; hemogram and platelet count, automated, and automated partial differential WBC count (CBC) **CPT NOTES** ♦ For blood banking procedures, see Transfusion Medicine. ♦ Agglutinins, see Immunology. ♦ Antiplasmin, see 85410. ♦ Antithrombin III, see 85300, 85301.	465.9 Acute upper respiratory infect NOS 490. Bronchitis NOS 782.2 Localized superficial swelling V72.6 Laboratory examination

CPT CODE	SERVICE	ICD-9-CM
85025	Blood count; hemogram and platelet count, automated, and automated complete differential WBC count (CBC) **CPT NOTES** ◆ For blood banking procedures, see Transfusion Medicine. ◆ Agglutinins, see Immunology. ◆ Antiplasmin, see 85410. ◆ Antithrombin III, see 85300, 85301.	799.9 Unk cause morbidity/mortality NEC V72.6 Laboratory examination
85651	Sedimentation rate, erythrocyte; non-automated **CPT NOTES** ◆ For blood banking procedures, see Transfusion Medicine. ◆ Agglutinins, see Immunology. ◆ Antiplasmin, see 85410. ◆ Antithrombin III, see 85300, 85301.	307.41 Transient insomnia 780.7 Malaise and fatigue V82.1 Screening, rheumatoid arthritis
86235	Extractable nuclear antigen, antibody to, any method (eg, nRNP, SS-A, SS-B, Sm, RNP, Sc170, J01), each antibody **CPT NOTES** ◆ Acteylcholine receptor antibody, see 86255, 86256. ◆ Actinomyces, antibodies to, use 86602. ◆ Adrenal cortex antibodies, see 86255, 86256.	V82.1 Screening, rheumatoid arthritis
86317	Immunoassay for infectious agent antibody, quantitative, not elsewhere specified **CPT NOTES** ◆ Acteylcholine receptor antibody, see 86255, 86256. ◆ Actinomyces, antibodies to, use 86602. ◆ Adrenal cortex antibodies, see 86255, 86256. ◆ For immunoassay techniques for antigens, see 83516, 83518, 83519, 83520, 86313, 86315. ◆ For particle agglutination procedures, see 86403.	V73.x Special screening for viral disease V75.x Screening for infectious diseases

CPT CODE	SERVICE	ICD-9-CM	
86430	Rheumatoid factor; qualitative **CPT NOTES** ◆ Acteylcholine receptor antibody, see 86255, 86256. ◆ Actinomyces, antibodies to, use 86602. ◆ Adrenal cortex antibodies, see 86255, 86256. ◆ Serologic test for syphilis, see 86592, 96593.	V82.1	Screening, rheumatoid arthritis
87060	Culture, bacterial, definitive; throat or nose **CPT NOTES** ◆ Includes bacteriology, mycology, parasitology, and virology. ◆ For urine, see 87086-87088.	462. 465.9 686.9	Acute pharyngitis Acute upper respiratory infect NOS Local skin infection NOS
87070	Culture, bacterial, definitive; any other source **CPT NOTES** ◆ Includes bacteriology, mycology, parasitology, and virology. ◆ For urine, see 87086-87088.	707.x 873.x 881.x 891.x 998.5 V67.0	Chronic ulcer of skin Open wound of head Elbow/forearm/wrist open wound Open wound of knee, leg, ankle Postoperative infection Surgery follow-up
87072	Culture or direct bacterial identification method, each organism, by commercial kit, any source except urine **CPT NOTES** ◆ Includes bacteriology, mycology, parasitology, and virology. ◆ For urine, see 87087.	707.x 873.x 881.x 891.x 998.5 V67.0	Chronic ulcer of skin Open wound of head Elbow/forearm/wrist open wound Open wound of knee, leg, ankle Postoperative infection Surgery follow-up
87075	Culture, bacterial, any source; anaerobic (isolation) **CPT NOTES** ◆ Includes bacteriology, mycology, parasitology, and virology. ◆ For anaerobe without GC, see 87072.	707.x 873.x 881.x 891.x 998.5 V67.0	Chronic ulcer of skin Open wound of head Elbow/forearm/wrist open wound Open wound of knee, leg, ankle Postoperative infection Surgery follow-up

CPT CODE	SERVICE	ICD-9-CM	
87083	Culture, presumptive, pathogenic organisms, screening only, by commercial kit (specify type); for multiple organisms **CPT NOTES** ♦ Includes bacteriology, mycology, parasitology, and virology. ♦ For urine colony count, see 87086.	465.9 873.x 881.x 891.x	Acute upper respiratory infect NOS Open wound of head Elbow/forearm/wrist open wound Open wound of knee, leg, ankle
87086	Culture, bacterial, urine; quantitative, colony count **CPT NOTES** ♦ Includes bacteriology, mycology, parasitology, and virology.	344.0x 344.1 599.0	Quadriplegia NOS Paraplegia NOS Urinary tract infection NOS
87101	Culture, fungi, isolation (with or without presumptive identification); skin **CPT NOTES** ♦ Includes bacteriology, mycology, parasitology, and virology.	110.4 V75.4	Dermatophytosis of foot Screening, mycotic infection
87163	Culture, any source, additional identification methods required (use in addition to primary culture code) **CPT NOTES** ♦ Includes bacteriology, mycology, parasitology, and virology.	682.0 707.x 873.x 881.x 891.x	Cellulitis of face Chronic ulcer of skin Open wound of head Elbow/forearm/wrist open wound Open wound of knee, leg, ankle
87184	Sensitivity studies, antibiotic; disk method, per plate (12 or less disks) **CPT NOTES** ♦ Includes bacteriology, mycology, parasitology, and virology.	707.x 998.5	Chronic ulcer of skin Postoperative infection

CPT CODE	SERVICE	ICD-9-CM
88104	Cytopathology, fluids, washings or brushings, except cervical or vaginal; smears with interpretation	611.72 Lump or mass in breast V76.42 Screening, malig neop, oral cavity V76.43 Screening, malig neop, skin
88106	Cytopathology, fluids, washings or brushings, except cervical or vaginal; filter method only with interpretation	202.80 Lymphoma NEC, site unspec 780.6 Pyrexia of unknown origin 786.6 Chest swelling/mass/lump V76.42 Screening, malig neop, oral cavity V76.43 Screening, malig neop, skin
88107	Cytopathology, fluids, washings or brushings, except cervical or vaginal; smears and filter preparation with interpretation	038.2 Pneumococcal septicemia 162.9 M-Neoplasm, Bronchus/Lung NOS 202.80 Lymphoma NEC, site unspec 611.72 Lump or mass in breast V76.1 Screening, malig neop, breast V76.42 Screening, malig neop, oral cavity V76.43 Screening, malig neop, skin
88108	Cytopathology, fluids, washings or brushings, except cervical or vaginal; concentration technique, smears and interpretation (eg, Saccomanno technique) **CPT NOTES** ♦ For cervical or vaginal smears, see 88150-88156. ♦ For gastric intubation with lavage, see 89130-89141, 91055. ♦ For x-ray localization, see 74340.	038.2 Pneumococcal septicemia V76.x Screening for malignant neoplasms
88170	Fine needle aspiration with or without preparation of smears; superficial tissue (eg, thyroid, breast, prostate) **CPT NOTES** ♦ For percutaneous needle biopsy, see 60100 for thyroid, 19100 for breast, 55700 for prostate.	193. M-Neoplasm, Thyroid gland 202.80 Lymphoma NEC, site unspec V76.1 Screening, malig neop, breast

CPT CODE	SERVICE	ICD–9–CM	
88172	Evaluation of fine needle aspirate with or without preparation of smears; immediate cytohistologic study to determine adequacy of specimen(s)	193.	M-Neoplasm, Thyroid gland
		202.80	Lymphoma NEC, site unspec
		V76.1	Screening, malig neop, breast
88173	Evaluation of fine needle aspirate with or without preparation of smears; interpretation and report	193.	M-Neoplasm, Thyroid gland
		202.80	Lymphoma NEC, site unspec
		611.72	Lump or mass in breast
		786.6	Chest swelling/mass/lump
		V76.1	Screening, malig neop, breast
88182	Flow cytometry; cell cycle or DNA analysis	174.8	M-Neoplasm, Female breast NEC
		V76.1	Screening, malig neop, breast
		V76.2	Screening, malig neop, cervix
		V76.3	Screening, malig neop, bladder

CPT NOTES

- For tumor morphometry and DNA and ploidy analysis by imaging techniques, use 88358.

SURGICAL PATHOLOGY
88300–88399

Services 88300 through 88309 include accession, examination, and reporting. They do not include the services designated in codes 88311 through 88365 and 88399, which are coded in addition when provided.

The unit of service for codes 88300 through 88309 is the specimen. A specimen is defined as tissue or tissues that is (are) submitted for individual and separate attention, requiring individual examination and pathologic diagnosis. Two or more such specimens from the same patient (e.g., separately identified endoscopic biopsies, skin lesions, etc.) are each appropriately assigned an individual code reflective of its proper level of service.

Service code 88300 is used for any specimen that in the opinion of the examining pathologist can be accurately diagnosed without microscopic examination. Service code 88302 is used when gross and microscopic examination is performed on a specimen to confirm identification and the absence of disease. Service codes 88304 through 88309 describe all other specimens requiring gross and microscopic examination, and represent additional ascending levels of physician work. Levels 88302 through 88309 are specifically defined by the assigned specimens.

Any unlisted specimen should be assigned to the code which most closely reflects the physician work involved when compared to other specimens assigned to that code.

See your CPT for the list of assigned specimens.

CPT CODE	SERVICE	ICD-9-CM
88300	LEVEL I - Surgical pathology, gross examination only	216.4 B-Neoplasm, Scalp/skin of neck 594.2 Urethral calculus 707.0 Decubitus ulcer **REIMBURSEMENT INFORMATION** <u>General</u> ♦ See notes on page 943.
88302	LEVEL II - Surgical pathology, gross and microscopic examination	172.2 Malignant melanoma, Ear 172.3 Malignant melanoma, Face NEC/NOS 173.2 M-Neoplasm, Skin of ear 173.3 M-Neoplasm, Skin of face NEC 238.2 UB-Neoplasm, Skin 702.x Other dermatosis **REIMBURSEMENT INFORMATION** <u>General</u> ♦ See notes on page 943.
88304	LEVEL III - Surgical pathology, gross and microscopic examination	173.x Malignant neoplasm, Skin 216.x Benign neoplasm, Skin 238.2 UB-Neoplasm, Skin 702.11 Inflamed seborrheic keratosis 706.2 Sebaceous cyst **REIMBURSEMENT INFORMATION** <u>General</u> ♦ See notes on page 943.
88305	LEVEL IV - Surgical pathology, gross and microscopic examination	173.x Malignant neoplasm, Skin 214.0 Lipoma, Skin of face 216.x Benign neoplasm, Skin 238.2 UB-Neoplasm, Skin 610.1 Diffuse cystic mastopathy 702.x Other dermatosis 795.4 Abnormal histological finding NEC **REIMBURSEMENT INFORMATION** <u>General</u> ♦ See notes on page 943.

CPT CODE	SERVICE	ICD–9–CM
88307	LEVEL V - Surgical pathology, gross and microscopic examination	173.x Malignant neoplasm, Skin 214.0 Lipoma, Skin of face 216.x Benign neoplasm, Skin 238.2 UB-Neoplasm, Skin 610.1 Diffuse cystic mastopathy 702.x Other dermatosis 795.4 Abnormal histological finding NEC **REIMBURSEMENT INFORMATION** General ♦ See notes on page 943.
88309	LEVEL VI - Surgical pathology, gross and microscopic examination	173.x Malignant neoplasm, Skin 214.0 Lipoma, Skin of face 216.x Benign neoplasm, Skin 238.2 UB-Neoplasm, Skin 610.1 Diffuse cystic mastopathy 702.x Other dermatosis 795.4 Abnormal histological finding NEC **REIMBURSEMENT INFORMATION** General ♦ See notes on page 943.
88311	Decalcification procedure (List separately in addition to code for surgical pathology examination)	170.0 M-Neoplasm, Skull/Face bone 170.1 M-Neoplasm, Mandible 198.5 M2-Neoplasm, Bone and bone marrow 733.90 Bone/Cartilage disorder NOS **REIMBURSEMENT INFORMATION** General ♦ See notes on page 943.
88329	Pathology consultation during surgery	140.x Malignant neoplasm of lip 173.x Malignant neoplasm, Skin 174.2 M-Neoplasm, Female breast, up/inner 174.4 M-Neoplasm, Female breast, up/outer 195.0 M-Neoplasm, Head/face/neck 216.x Benign neoplasm, Skin 232.3 CA in situ, Skin of face NEC **REIMBURSEMENT INFORMATION** General ♦ See notes on page 943.

CPT CODE	SERVICE	ICD–9–CM
88332	Pathology consultation during surgery; each additional tissue block with frozen section(s)	173.x Malignant neoplasm, Skin 174.2 M-Neoplasm, Female breast, up/inner 174.4 M-Neoplasm, Female breast, up/outer 702.x Other dermatosis **REIMBURSEMENT INFORMATION** General ♦ See notes on page 943.
88342	Immunocytochemistry (including tissue immunoperoxidase), each antibody	951.4 Injury to facial nerve 955.1 Injury median nerve 956.2 Injury posterior tibial nerve **REIMBURSEMENT INFORMATION** General ♦ See notes on page 943.

ISBN 0-07-600763-4
90000
9 780076 007639